Pediatric Psycho-oncology

Pediatric Psycho-oncology

Psychosocial Aspects and Clinical Interventions

Second Edition

Editors

Shulamith Kreitler, PhD

Professor, School of Psychological Sciences, Tel-Aviv University; Faculty of Social Welfare and Health Sciences, University of Haifa; Head, Psychooncology Research Center, Sheba Medical Center, Tel Hashomer, Israel

Myriam Weyl Ben-Arush, MD

Head, Department of Pediatric Hematology Oncology and Deputy Director, Meyer Children's Hospital, Rambam Health Care Campus, Technion Israel-Institute of Technology, the Bruce Rappaport Faculty of Medicine, Haifa, Israel

Andrés Martin, MPH

Riva Ariella Ritvo Professor of Pediatric Oncology Psychosocial Services, Child Study Center, Yale University School of Medicine; and Smilow Cancer Hospital at Yale-New Haven, New Haven, CT, USA

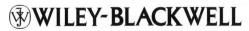

A John Wiley & Sons, Ltd., Publication

Library of Congress Cataloging-in-Publication Data

Pediatric psycho-oncology : psychosocial aspects and clinical interventions / editors, Shulamith Kreitler, Andrés Martin, Myriam Weyl Ben-Arush. – 2nd ed.
     p. cm.
  Includes bibliographical references and index.
  ISBN 978-1-119-99883-9 (cloth)
  1. Tumors in children–Psychological aspects. 2. Tumors in children–Social aspects. I. Kreitler,
Shulamith. II. Martin, Andrés. III. Weyl Ben-Arush, Myriam.
  RC281.C4P445 2012
  618.92'994–dc23
                                                                                        2012010170
A catalogue record for this book is available from the British Library.

Wiley also publishes its books in a variety of electronic formats. Some content that appears in print may not be available in electronic books.

Cover Image: © Sean Gladwell—fotolia.com

Set in 9/11pt Times New Roman by Thomson Digital, Noida, India.
Printed and bound in Singapore by Markono Print Media Pte Ltd.

First Impression 2012

The book is dedicated to all the children and families
we had the honor to take care of in the past
and who will benefit from it in the future.

Contents

List of Contributors

Annah N. Abrams, MD Child Psychiatrist, Department of Pediatric Hematology Oncology, Massachusetts General Hospital; Chief, Child Psychiatry Consultation Liaison Service, Massachusetts General Hospital; Assistant Professor of Psychiatry, Harvard Medical School, Boston, MA, USA

Melissa A. Alderfer, PhD Assistant Professor of Pediatrics, The Children's Hospital of Philadelphia and Perelman School of Medicine, The University of Pennsylvania, Philadelphia, PA, USA

Myriam Weyl Ben-Arush, MD Head, Department of Pediatric Hematology Oncology, Meyer Children's Hospital; Deputy Director, Meyer Children's Hospital, Rambam Health Care Campus, Technion Israel- Institute of Technology, the Bruce Rappaport Faculty of Medicine, Haifa, Israel

Matthew G. Biel, MD, MSc Chief, Section of Child and Adolescent Psychiatry; Assistant Professor, Departments of Psychiatry and Pediatrics, Georgetown University Hospital, Washington, DC, USA

Ryan W. Blum, AB Yale School of Medicine, Yale Child Study Center, Yale Pediatric Ethics Program, CT, USA

Laura Cousins, BA Pain and Palliative Care Program, Department of Pediatrics, David Geffen School of Medicine at University of California at Los Angeles, CA, USA

Ronit Elhasid, MD Head, Pediatric Hematology Oncology Department, Tel Aviv Sourasky Medical Center, Sackler Faculty of Medicine, Tel-Aviv University, Israel

Subhadra Evans, PhD Pain and Palliative Care Program, Department of Pediatrics, David Geffen School of Medicine at University of California at Los Angeles, CA, USA

Stefan J. Friedrichsdorf, MD Medical Director, Department of Pain Medicine, Palliative Care & Integrative Medicine. Children's Hospitals and Clinics of Minnesota. Minneapolis, MN, USA

Martha A. Grootenhuis, PhD, Professor of Pediatric Psychology, Emma Kinderziekenhuis, Academic Medical Centre, University of Amsterdam, Netherlands

Richard D. W. Hain, MBBS MSc MD MRCP(UK) FRCPCH Dip Pall Med FHEA PGCE Consultant and Lead Clinician, Wales Paediatric Palliative Medicine Managed Clinical Network, Children's Hospital for Wales, Cardiff, UK, Visiting Professor, University of Glamorgan, Wales, Honorary Senior Lecturer, Bangor University, Bangor, UK

Matthew C. Hocking, PhD Psychology Fellow, Division of Oncology, The Children's Hospital of Philadelphia, Philadelphia, PA, USA

Jimmie Holland, MD Wayne E. Chapman Chair in Psychiatric Oncology, Memorial Sloan-Kettering Cancer Center, New York, NY, USA

Shai Izraeli, MD Head, Functional Genomics and Childhood Cancer Research Section, Department of Pediatric Hemato-Oncology and the Cancer Research Center, Edmond and Lily Safra Children Hospital, Sheba Medical Center, Tel-Hashomer. Associate Professor, Sackler Faculty of Medicine, Tel-Aviv University, Israel

Meriel E.M. Jenney, MB ChB, MD, MRCP, FRCPCH Consultant Paediatric Oncologist, Children's Hospital for Wales, Cardiff, UK

Michal M. Kreitler, MA, School of Psychology, Tel-Aviv University, Israel; Psychooncology Research Center, and Pediatric Institute of

Hemato-Oncology, Sheba Medical Center, Tel-Hashomer, Israel

Shulamith Kreitler, PhD, Professor, School of Psychological Sciences, Tel-Aviv University; Faculty of Social Welfare and Health Sciences, University of Haifa; Head, Psychooncology Research Center, Sheba Medical Center, Tel Hashomer, Israel

Elena Krivoy, MSc Senior Clinical and Medical Psychologist. Department of Pediatric Hematology Oncology, Meyer Children's Hospital, Rambam Health Care Campus, Technion Israel- Institute of Technology, The Bruce Rappaport Faculty of Medicine, Haifa, Israel

Gary Kupfer, MD Professor of Pediatrics and Pathology, Chief, Section of Pediatric Hematology-Oncology, Yale School of Medicine, New Haven, CT, USA

Bob F. Last, PhD Emeritus Professor of Pediatric Psychology, VU University, Amsterdam and Emma Kinderziekenhuis, Academic Medical Centre, Amsterdam, Netherlands

Amita Mahajan, MD Department of Paediatric Oncology, Children's Hospital for Wales, Heath Park, Cardiff, UK

Andrés S. Martin, MPH Riva Ariella Ritvo Professor of Pediatric Oncology Psychosocial Services, Child Study Center, Yale University School of Medicine; and Smilow Cancer Hospital at Yale-New Haven, New Haven, CT, USA

Maria E. McGee, MD, MS, MPH Child and Adolescent Psychiatry Fellow, Georgetown University Hospital, Washington, DC, USA

Daniel Oppenheim, MD, PhD Psychoanalyst, Paris, France. Former senior psychiatrist, Gustave Roussy Cancer Institute, Villejuif, France

Maryland Pao, MD Clinical Director, National Institute of Mental Health, National Institutes of Health, Department of Health and Human Services, Bethesda, MD, USA

Monique Peretz Nahum, MD, Director Long Term Follow Up Outpatient Clinic, Department of Pediatric Hematology Oncology, Meyer

Children's Hospital, Rambam Health Care Campus, Haifa, Israel

Elizabeth G. Pinsky, MD Child and Adolescent Psychiatry Resident, Massachusetts General/ McLean Hospital, MA, USA

Sergey Postovsky, MD Deputy Director, Department of Pediatric Oncology/Hematology, Meyer Children's Hospital, Rambam Health Care Campus. Assistant Professor in Pediatrics, Faculty of Medicine, Technion – Israel Institute of Technology, Haifa, Israel

Paula Rauch, MD Department of Psychiatry, Massachusetts General Hospital, Harvard Medical School, Boston, MA, USA

Gideon Rechavi, MD, PhD Director, Cancer Research Center, Sheba Medical Center, Tel-Hashomer. The Gregorio and Dora Shapiro professor for Hematology Malignancies, Sackler School of Medicine, Tel-Aviv University, Israel

Rivka Rosenkranz, MEd BA Educational Counselor, Department of Pediatric Hematology Oncology, Meyer Children's Hospital, Rambam Health Care Campus, Haifa, Israel

David J. Schonfeld, MD, FAAP Director of National Center for School Crisis and Bereavement and Director of the Division of Developmental and Behavioral Pediatrics, Cincinnati Children's Hospital Medical Center, Cincinnati, OH, USA

Elsa Segev-Shoham, MA Pediatric Oncology Unit, Haemek Medical Center, Afula, Israel; Former member of the board of the Israeli Society for Psycho-Oncology; Inspector of Special Education for the Israeli Ministry of Education, Israel

Aziza T. Shad, MD Chief, Division of Pediatric Hematology/Oncology, Blood, and Marrow Transplantation, Amey Distinguished Professor of Neuro-Oncology and Childhood Cancer, Lombardi Comprehensive Cancer Center and Georgetown University Hospital, Washington, DC, USA

Dafna Munitz-Shenkar, R.N, M.A Research Coordinator Nurse, Pediatric Hemato-Oncology, Edmond and Lily Safra Children's Hospital, Sheba Medical Center, Tel Hashomer, Israel

Michael Silbermann, MD, PhD Executive Director, Middle East Cancer Consortium, Halifa, Israel

Jane E. Skeen, BSc, MBChB Pediatric Oncologist, Starship Blood and Cancer Centre, Starship Children's Hospital, Auckland, New Zealand

Margaret L. Stuber, MD Vice Chair for Education in Psychiatry, Daniel X. Freedman Professor, Psychiatry and Biobehavioral Sciences, David Geffen School of Medicine at UCLA, CA, USA

Susan D. Swick, MD, MPH Director, Parenting At a Challenging Time (PACT, Program at the Vernon Cancer Center, Newton Wellesley Hospital; Medical Director, Mental Health Services, Vernon Cancer Center at Newton Wellesley Hospital; Attending Psychiatrist, Massachusetts General Hospital, Division of Child Psychiatry; Instructor in Psychiatry Harvard Medical School; MA, USA

Ciporah S. Tadmor, PhD Hospital-Based Medical Psychologist, Department of Pediatric Hematology Oncology Specialist in Medical Psychology, Consultant in Primary Prevention, Meyer Children's Hospital, Rambam Health Care Campus, Haifa, Israel

Amos Toren, MD, PhD Head Pediatric Hemato-oocology Edmond and Lily Safra Children's Hospital, The Sheba Medical Center-Tel Hashomer affiliated to The Sackler School of Medicine, Tel-Aviv University, Tel-Aviv, Israel

M. Louise Webster, MBChB, FRACP, FRANZCP Child and Adolescent Psychiatrist, Department Psychological Medicine, University of Auckland, Pediatric Consultation Liaison Psychiatry Team, Starship Children's Hospital, Auckland, New Zealand

Lori Wiener, PhD Co-Director, Behavioral Science Core; Head, Psychosocial Support and Research, NCI, POB, Bethesda, MD, USA

Lonnie Zeltzer, MD Pain and Palliative Care Program, Department of Pediatrics, David Geffen School of Medicine at University of California at Los Angeles, CA, USA

Foreword

It is an honor and pleasure to write the Foreword for the second edition of this important textbook of pediatric psycho-oncology. By identifying the international leaders in the field, the editors present a remarkable view of the state of the art in pediatric psycho-oncology, as we know it today, of the management of symptoms and psychosocial care. I commend them for it and also I commend this book to the reader.

Since the first edition was published, several important studies have been carried out and the importance of the care of the total child, not just the tumor, has become more widely recognized. An acknowledgement of this is the fact that in 2010 the International Pediatric Oncology Society (SIOP) endorsed the statement of the International Psycho-Oncology Society and the International Union Against Cancer (UICC) that a new standard of quality cancer care has been established: quality cancer care today must integrate the psychosocial domain into routine cancer care. The SIOP Board, at its meeting in Boston, MA, in September, 2010, endorsed this statement as it applies to the care of children with cancer. These are landmark statements which will encourage the field to move forward more rapidly with this policy support from the major oncology international societies.

I dedicated the first edition to my grandson, Gabriel, who had just died of hepatoblastoma, aged 3. I continue to honor his memory, like other professionals in the field, who have shared a similar loss, to carry the work forward as a memorial to him and to the children whom many pediatric oncologists remember with equal love, sadness and yet joy for their short lives and the pleasure they brought us. The struggle goes on to reduce the numbers of children who do not survive, and also to continue making our own contribution to improve the quality of life of those children during their illness to be the best possible. This dedication of purpose is the least that we can do to remember those whom we have loved and lost. I am grateful to be a part of this important effort to make the most up-to-date research results available to pediatric oncology teams around the world.

Jimmie Holland, MD
Wayne E. Chapman Chair in Psychiatric Oncology
Memorial Sloan-Kettering Cancer Center
New York, NY
November 2011

Introduction: Embedding Psychosocial Care in Medicine: Pediatric Psycho-oncology as a Model

The history of pediatric oncology is a transcendent one. Until 1948, a patient with leukemia simply was provided with supportive care, itself most meager, and family and medical caregivers awaited the patient's death. Through the vision of many, including in no small part the pioneering Sidney Farber, clinical remissions were first achieved, and the modern age of chemotherapeutics in oncology began.

Concomitant with the provision of chemotherapeutics was the emergence of the modern age of supportive care. Blood-banking, so crucial to counteract the deleterious effects of chemotherapy, became more scientific in screening for antibodies and infection. Penicillin and the elaboration of multiple categories of antibiotics allowed aggressive infection-fighting efforts to combat rampant fever and neutropenia. A greater realization of the importance of treating pain allowed rational use of narcotics to combat the inevitable mucositis that accompanied dose intensification efforts that clearly resulted in improvements in overall survival.

In essence, knowledge culminating in the rise of rational cancer therapeutics was accompanied by the advancement of medical knowledge in the areas of hematological support and infectious diseases. The consistent rise in survival rates, as exemplified by steadily improving Kaplan-Meier curves in repeated acute lypmphoblastic leukemia clinical trials, could never have occurred without the remarkable progress in each of these areas.

The past 60 years also saw growing social awareness of mental health disorders and the (gradual) removal of the stigma of such disorders. Increasing acceptance of the importance of addressing mental health has led to present-day efforts to openly lead patients to mental health resources and to legally encode in practical terms access to such services.

Coincidentally, these efforts have strongly paralleled the diminishing negative connotations associated with those afflicted with cancer. Not so much time has elapsed since the diagnosis of cancer was sometimes hidden from the patient and certainly hidden from those around the patient, such as co-workers, for fear of ostracism or unemployment. The Western media today abounds with bold depictions of currently treated patients and survivors and with pink-shrouded football players raising cancer awareness.

The confluence of these factors makes it even starker that psychosocial challenges still abound for patients with cancer. First, there is a greater incidence of diagnosis of mental health disorders in cancer patients, whereby underlying or latent issues are enhanced or exposed by the anxieties of diagnosis, therapy, and disruption of activities of everyday living. Second, the stress of caring for and enduring the treatment of a child with cancer confers similarly increased risk of psychosocial disturbances upon both parents and siblings. Third, side effects of the therapy itself (chemotherapy, surgery, and radiation), especially in the developing child, can result in loss of cognition and coping skills, which imposes increased risk of disordered behavior. Of course, the challenges to our patients do not end with the final dose of chemotherapy, the pronouncement of cure, or a contrived 5-year window, but rather follow them through a lifetime as they grow, mature, go to school, and become job holders, spouses, and parents themselves.

In spite of the vast advantages of resources available in the developed countries, the provision of resources necessary for psychosocial care of patients and their families remains uneven. While more and more insurance plans cover some modicum of psychosocial services, reimbursements are often inadequate for the task. Even insurance that may be available does not guarantee that a given provider will accept that particular insurance, and examples abound of the most august institutions insisting that patients self-pay. In addition, when such services are obtained in the community and out of contiguity with the clinic experience, a disconnect occurs for both caregiver and patient.

We and others have found that the model of embedded psychosocial care, on an equal footing and integrated with chemotherapy, antibiotics, and blood products, has proved to be an especially effective manner of intervention. The typical pediatric oncology clinic has some combination of exam rooms and infusion space, often with therapy administered "in the round" with common areas for play for patient and siblings alike. A sense of community is created, as patients typically have recurring and regular days of the week for their visits, whereby patients and their families interact in an ongoing way with their caregivers: nurses, nursing assistants, nurse practitioners, and oncologists. It is within that community that the psychosocial team is able to introduce itself, becoming a seamless part of the caregiving team that encounters that particular patient and family during each visit.

The concept of the psychosocial team is one that can vary from program to program, depending on local custom and state regulatory agencies. A collaborative psychosocial team such as that we have constructed at Yale consists of such people as psychiatrists, psychologists, social workers, special education teachers, child life specialists, and volunteers. While very often overlapping in certain skill sets and abilities, each of these specialists brings a unique perspective that rounds out the entire team.

Ultimately, the greatest challenge in the embedded model is one of provision of resources. Hospitals and medical schools are under financial pressure due to decreasing reimbursements, increasing unfunded care, and increased regulatory environment. Psychosocial care, even in this age of enlightenment, in many circles is still viewed as a superfluous or unnecessary frill. The acquisition of resources to fund a full staff in order to run such a team requires the infusion of philanthropy and grant support in most centers. The challenge of funding is magnified by the fact that provision of services is never-ending; personnel are a constant cost center on the ledger sheet.

Fortunately, pediatric oncology is a specialty that attracts attention: bald-headed children on chemotherapy are head-turners on billboards, television, print media, and, of course, social media. Pediatric oncology also benefits from infrastructure in general pediatrics, in which focus on growth and development, school, and behavior figures prominently. Yet chronic disease or disease that requires long-term care abounds in pediatrics. Thus, the relationship between pediatrics and pediatric oncology has the chance to become symbiotic: pediatric oncology can gather resources and test the embedded model. Departments of Pediatrics, and as a result other subspecialties within it, can benefit from the ingathering of talent that is nucleated by such a paradigm.

The greatest barriers toward establishment of psychosocial services remain recognition and commitment at every level of a particular program from caregiver to hospital administrator. Pediatric oncology programs that understand that the concept of mental health care is as important as the chemotherapy and the antibiotics are well on their way to successful implementation and sustenance of a truly well-rounded program.

Gary M. Kupfer, MD
Professor of Pediatrics and Pathology
Yale School of Medicine
Section Chief, Pediatric Hematology-Oncology
Yale New Haven Children's Hospital and Smilow
Cancer Hospital New Haven, Connecticut

Preface

It has been eight years since the initial publication of *Psychosocial Aspects of Pediatric Oncology*. This second edition provides more than an update to the original volume: it reflects the expansion in the field of pediatric psycho-oncology and the growing incorporation of best practices in psychosocial care for children diagnosed with cancer. Pediatric oncology research and clinical practice have made remarkable strides toward improving recovery and survival of children with cancer. Psycho-oncology has enhanced awareness of the importance of considering the whole person in the course of the medical treatments designed to safeguard life and maximize the lifelong potential of the children. Enhancing the quality of life of the children and their families in all stages of diagnosis and treatment has become part of the goal of pediatric oncology at large. This book reflects an important step in the integration of psycho-oncology within the framework of pediatric oncology, by which we can strive to attain a complete cure.

This edition includes 22 chapters divided into four sections: Active Treatment, Survivorship, Death and Bereavement, and Additional Considerations. Sixteen chapters of the original edition have been thoroughly updated, and six new chapters address areas not previously covered, including psychopharmacology, bereavement, ethics, international collaborations, and addressing the emotional needs of children whose parents have cancer. In addition, a new appendix provides a comprehensive overview and description of research tools in pediatric psycho-oncology that we hope will help expand the field of evidence-based pediatric psycho-oncology.

As in the original edition, the volume's contributors are internationally recognized leaders in the field.

We are indebted to all contributors for their shared commitment to this work. We are especially thankful to Jimmie Holland for her heartfelt Foreword, and for her support of the volume from its original inception. We are grateful to Joan Marsh and Fiona Woods at Wiley-Blackwell for their guidance and high editorial standards.

It is our hope that these pages will contribute to improving the lives of children and families facing one of the hardest of conceivable challenges. Their strength and example inspire and energize us anew each day.

Shulamith Kreitler,
Myriam Weyl Ben-Arush and
Andrés Martin

Part A
Active Treatment

1

Cancer in Children: an Overview

Shai Izraeli, Gideon Rechavi

Introduction

Approximately one in every 350 children will develop cancer by adulthood, and despite the remarkable cure rate, cancer is still the leading cause of non-accidental death in children in affluent countries after the neonatal period. In this Introduction we shall highlight some unique medical aspects of childhood cancer that are especially pertinent to pediatric psycho-oncology. For more details about specific diseases, the reader is referred to the available textbooks in pediatric oncology.

The characteristic cancers of children are different from those encountered in adults. Typically they arise in tissues and organs that develop most rapidly during embryogenesis and the postnatal period. Indeed, it is likely that most cancers in children result from unfortunate developmental "accidents," often occurring *in utero*. In contrast, the typical "adult" malignancies arise in epithelial cells covering the surface of ducts and body cavities that are exposed for prolonged periods of time to a large variety of environmental carcinogens. Colon cancer, for example, is the end stage of a slow multistep transition from normal tissue through benign polyps to malignant invasive carcinomas. Colon cancer may be prevented by either modifying diet or by treatment with drugs such as aspirin, which affects the tumorogenic response of the colonic mucosa to carcinogens, or by removal of benign polyps. Unlike cancers in adults, most cancers in children cannot be prevented, are not preceded by obvious pre-malignant lesions and are not amenable to early diagnosis. Indeed, several international trials of massive screening for pre-malignant lesions or early stages of neuroblastoma, a childhood cancer of the sympathetic nervous system, have proved futile. These issues are relevant when dealing with the parents of a child with cancer, who are, naturally, overwhelmed by guilt and self-blame. It is important to explain to parents that to the best of our knowledge cancers in children are not caused by any wrongdoing of the child or his/her parents, nor could they have been diagnosed earlier (except, of course, in cases of clear medical neglect).

Most of the tumors arise spontaneously, although there are rare familial hereditary cancer syndromes. For example, retinoblastoma, a malignant tumor of the retina, is often hereditary. A child with hereditary retinoblastoma is likely to develop tumors in the other eye and later may also be diagnosed with osteosarcoma, a malignant bone tumor. Most of these children are cured and their chances of passing the hereditary trait are 50%. Families with hereditary cancer syndromes require therefore special lifelong attention and present the health care community with new challenges. One of these challenges is caused by modern genetic diagnostic techniques that enable identification of individuals carrying a cancer-predisposing mutation while they are still healthy. This medically helpful knowledge may also add a significant psychosocial burden to the patients and their families.

Another high-risk group is identical twins. An identical twin of a child with leukemia has a 25% risk of developing the same leukemia before the age of 10. This high risk of a non-genetic disease among identical twins has been puzzling. The mystery has been solved recently. As leukemia is commonly an "accident" during embryonic development, pre-leukemic cells can circulate from one embryonic twin to the other through their common vascular channels. Other than these examples, in most instances there is no substantial basis for the fear that other young members of the family will develop cancer as well. Moreover, the rate of cancer in offsprings of childhood cancer survivors is not significantly higher than in the normal population. Thus, in the majority of instances we can safely reassure the families that the cancer will not spread in the family.

The most common malignancy in children involves the lymphoid system, especially acute lymphoblastic

Pediatric Psycho-oncology: Psychosocial Aspects and Clinical Interventions, Second Edition.
Edited by Shulamith Kreitler, Myriam Weyl Ben-Arush and Andrés Martin.
© 2012 John Wiley & Sons, Ltd. Published 2012 by John Wiley & Sons, Ltd.

leukemia (ALL). During embryonic development and early childhood the normal lymphoid system has to develop rapidly and acquire the capabilities to mount specific immune responses against an enormous variety of foreign antigens. For efficient diversification of the various immune receptors, lymphoid cells possess an unusual type of genetic instability that predisposes them to rare genetic accidents leading to acute leukemia. ALL is most common in young children but occurs throughout childhood.

The nervous system is another rapidly developing organ that also involves substantial fine-tuned diversification and differentiation during embryogenesis and early childhood. The frequency of tumors of the nervous system is almost equal to ALL and together these malignancies are responsible for more than half of the cancers in children. Many of these tumors are relatively slow-growing gliomas, often implying living through childhood with slowly progressing brain tumors. A large fraction of childhood brain tumors have an embryonic and more aggressive phenotype. These include medulloblastoma, a cancer of the cerebellum, retinoblastoma, and neuroblastoma, a malignant tumor of the peripheral sympathetic nervous system. Embryonic tumors outside the nervous system such as Wilm's tumor of the kidney, hepatoblastoma and various tumors of the gonads are also typical of children.

The third most common type of malignancy of children is a diverse group of tumors of the musculoskeletal and the soft tissues. These sarcomas can arise at any age and have specific molecular, pathological and clinical characteristics. Many of those occur more frequently during adolescence, a period of robust musculoskeletal development.

Pediatric oncology is one of the greatest medical success stories of the past four decades. The cure rate of childhood cancer has increased from about 25% in the 1960s to more than 75% in the 1990s. This remarkable progress has occurred in almost all types of childhood malignancies and is due to the exquisite sensitivity of these malignancies to chemotherapy and to the series of carefully conducted collaborative empirical clinical trials in Europe and the USA.

The paradigm to this success is childhood ALL, a uniformly fatal disease in the 1960s that has become curable in almost 80% of children today. The treatment "protocol" of childhood ALL consists of 2–3 years of therapy utilizing up to ten chemotherapeutic drugs given in various combinations. Intensive remission induction and consolidation therapies, lasting up to half a year, are followed by prolonged and less intensive maintenance therapy. During the first half year,

the child requires frequent hospitalizations for administration of drugs or for combating infectious complications of chemotherapy. The child can attend kindergarten or school and function almost normally during the rest of the therapy.

A specific problem associated with ALL and relevant to the topic of this textbook is the need for prevention therapy to the central nervous system (CNS). Early trials with chemotherapy have failed because of the recurrence of the leukemia in the CNS. Apparently due to the poor penetration of most chemotherapeutic drugs into the CNS it serves as a "sanctuary" haven for leukemic cells. Cure of ALL became a reality only when routine irradiation of the brain was added to systemic chemotherapy. This success has proven to be a mixed blessing as the exposure of the brain of young children to a hefty dose of radiation resulted in severe long-term intellectual, behavioral and other neurological impairments. In most modern treatment protocols of ALL, cranial irradiation has been replaced by a combination of systemic high dose methotrexate and intrathecal chemotherapy. While this approach has been proven to be less toxic than irradiation, its long-term neurological implications still need to be studied.

The treatment of solid tumors combines usually at least two modalities. Local control is achieved through surgery or radiotherapy. Because of the severe long-term toxicities of radiating growing tissues, surgery is preferred when possible. Modern pediatric surgical oncology has become much less mutilating. Thus, in most instances, bone and soft tissue sarcomas can be removed by limb-sparing surgery. Still, in many instances, such as brain tumors, Hodgkin's disease and inoperable sarcomas, radiation is unavoidable. It is critically important that radiation will be delivered in centers specializing in treatment of children because of many specific considerations unique to these patients that are required to minimize the long-term side effects and encourage conservation of symmetric growth and development.

The most significant progress in the treatment of childhood solid tumors occurred when the concept of "adjuvant chemotherapy" was introduced, initially for treatment of Wilm's tumor and osteosarcoma. In the case of osteosarcoma, even when the tumor was localized to the limb, and the limb was amputated, the long-term survival was no more than 20%. Since all deaths were caused by distant metastases, the unavoidable conclusion was that micro-metastases were present in most of the patients with localized tumors at the time of diagnosis. The administration of "adjuvant chemotherapy"—chemotherapy that is delivered with the intention to destroy those unseen micro-metastases, has led to the current 70% survival rates. Typically these patients today are treated first with chemotherapy, followed by surgical removal of the tumor with sparing of the limb, and another period of intensive chemotherapy. The concept of adjuvant chemotherapy has been also adopted by the adult oncologists for chemotherapy-sensitive tumors such as breast cancer.

The recent decade has witnessed remarkable development in molecular biology and diagnostics. Techniques allowing the visualization and quantifications of genes and gene products have enabled molecular classification of tumors and personalized adjustment of therapy to the biological tumor subtype. Again, pediatric oncology has shown the way. Thus, for example, the identification of the BCR-ABL fusion gene in a child with leukemia or the detection of multiple copies of the NMYC oncogene in a child with neuroblastoma led to their classification as high risk patients and to assignment to especially intensive treatments that included bone marrow transplantation. The molecular determination of minimal residual disease has allowed tailoring of therapy to the molecular response to therapy. The identification of specific molecular abnormalities has also raised hopes for development of cancer-specific, less toxic therapies. In the recent years since the first edition of this book, several novel targeted therapies have been finally introduced for children with cancer, and others are in clinical trials. For example, the addition of inhibitors of BCR-ABL to chemotherapy has caused such a dramatic improvement to survival that the presence of this abnormality no longer constitutes an automatic indicator of stem cell transplantation. These novel therapies are not "magic bullets" free of side effects. Indeed, many of these novel drugs target pathways important for childhood growth and development and hence have a multitude of newer side effects different from those caused by chemotherapy.

While childhood cancer is a relatively rare disease, its high cure rate is having a significant impact in developed societies. Currently, one in every 900 young (less than 45-year-old) Americans has been cured of childhood cancer. It is estimated that within 20 years this rate will increase to more than one in every 400. Unlike adult cancer, occurring mostly in the post-retirement age, children cured from cancer are expected to live many more productive years. Thus the quality of life of childhood cancer survivors and late effects of the cancer and its treatment have become a major focus of modern pediatric oncology and are particularly relevant for the field of psycho-oncology.

Although children tolerate the acute toxicities of chemotherapy better than adults, growing children are more vulnerable to the delayed effects of cancer therapy such as effects on growth, the endocrine system, fertility, the myocardium, neuropsychological function, and the occurrence of secondary cancers. Moreover, because children tolerate chemotherapy better than adults, they often receive far greater dose-intensity and are therefore more likely to develop late sequelae. Of the different therapeutic modalities, radiation is associated with the highest rates of late effects in children.

Most relevant for this textbook are the late neuropsychological sequelae of childhood cancer therapy. Long-term neurological impairments are associated with leukemia and brain tumors, the two most common malignancies of children. Learning difficulties have been most commonly attributed to cranial irradiation and are related to the dose and the age at the time of irradiation. For example, cranial irradiation with 3,600 cGy of children with brain tumors who are younger than 36m is universally associated with marked decreases in I.Q. Newer therapeutic protocols are attempting to delay radiation and lower the dose in young children.

Although radiation doses in children with ALL are significantly lower than those used for children with brain tumors, they are still likely to have long-term neuropsychological sequelae. These effects are mainly in attention capacities and other nonverbal cognitive processing skills and not in the global IQ. These deficits correlate with focal findings in magnetic resonance imaging (MRI) of the brain and neurophysiological studies. As with brain tumors, the extent and timing of the deficits are related to the radiation dose and the age at the time of radiation. Girls less than 5 years old are most vulnerable. At the extreme end of the spectrum of neurological toxicity is progressive necrotizing leukoencephalopathy, a rare and devastating complication, occurring mainly in patients who have received a combination of higher dose radiotherapy and intrathecal methotrexate. Although significantly less neurological impairment is seen in children with ALL treated with intrathecal therapy only, it is premature to conclude that no neuropsychological deficits are expected. Indeed, minor abnormalities in brain imaging are commonly detected and the long-term significance of these changes is presently unknown.

It is impossible to write an introduction to a book on psychology of children without relating to adolescence. Surviving normal adolescence is a challenge to children, their parents and educators and provides the livelihood of pediatric psychologists. Cancer in this life period is extraordinarily more challenging. Adolescents tend to delay bringing medical problems to attention and are less compliant with therapy. For example, it has been clearly shown that adolescents with ALL tend to be less adherent to the oral chemotherapy regimen during the maintenance period and that their prognosis directly correlates with their degree of compliance. There are also some unique medical issues such as preservation of fertility, and a large list of psychosocial issues. Because of these issues, the need of a specific discipline for adolescent and young adults oncology is being considered now in the USA and Europe.

The final issue relates to the topic we all try to avoid. Despite the enormous success, one in every five children with cancer will die from the disease. The grim outlook of a particular child is often known soon after diagnosis. Yet studies have repeatedly shown that the prospect of dying is usually, if at all, addressed only very shortly before death. Even in the most hopeless cases, treatment is usually characterized by intensive attempts to cure and by ignoring the option of palliative care. This is one area where we, who deal with childhood cancer, can learn from our colleagues in the adult oncology field. Hospice and palliative care are new and much needed concepts in pediatric oncology that, naturally, combine medical and psychosocial approaches. And after the death, there are bereaved parents, siblings, and friends. They often cling to the pediatric oncology department and look for comfort and help. The "end of life" issue is a chapter in pediatric oncology waiting to be defined and written.

Pediatric oncology meets childhood psychology at the time of the diagnosis of these devastating diseases, during the difficulties associated with the toxicities of intensive chemotherapy, the rehabilitation period, during the follow-up of the majority who are long-term survivors, and the bereavement of those who lost the most precious of all. Although the child is the one with the cancer, the pediatric oncology team interacts intensively with the siblings, parents, grandparents, friends, schoolteachers and more. It becomes a community affair in which the pediatric oncology team is at the center.

2

Comprehensive and Family-Centered Psychosocial Care in Pediatric Oncology: Integration of Clinical Practice and Research

Lori Wiener, Maryland Pao

Introduction

Pediatric oncology programs aspire to provide comprehensive clinical care to patients and their family members. Patient and family-centered care is an approach to health care that is grounded in mutually beneficial partnerships among health care providers, patients, and families, and where the vital role that families play in ensuring the health and well-being of infants, children, and adolescents is recognized [1]. Within a family-centered care environment, emotional, social, and developmental support is an integral component of health care. Attending to the child's and family's emotional distress and psychosocial needs due to a cancer diagnosis requires many experts, in addition to the oncologist, such as social workers, psychologists, child life workers, rehabilitation therapists, child psychiatrists and many others. To incorporate this practice of psychosocial care within a pediatric oncology setting means that the health care providers listen to and honor patient and family perspectives, choices, values, beliefs and cultural differences. Providers also shape policies, programs and facility design, and facilitate day-to-day staff interactions through ongoing discussions and feedback with patients and families. In addition to seeking patient's and family's points of view, conducting clinical research is another excellent mechanism to assure that the developed programs and provided interventions are based on what patients and families experience and need and in fact are improving outcomes.

Recent developments in dissemination of empirically supported interventions [2] and evidence-based assessments [3] suggest that pediatric oncology programs need to continue to integrate psychosocial practice with research in order to maximize successful psychosocial and physical outcomes for children with cancer. Critical areas of clinical practice and research under exploration include distress assessments [4, 5], screening of psychosocial risk factors after cancer diagnosis [6, 7] and survivorship, particularly studies of the late effects of those who are cured. These questions highlight the need for ongoing concomitant psychosocial practice and research within pediatric psycho-oncology settings. In this chapter, we describe the necessary components to be incorporated into an ideal (or model) comprehensive family-centered psychosocial support program and propose that the integration of clinical research can enhance clinical services while reducing the research–practice gap.

Psychosocial Care

Diagnosis

Excellent psychosocial care begins at the time of diagnosis, incorporates early assessment, continuing and consistent care, a range of therapeutic interventions, and utilizes interdisciplinary resources for all family members [8]. A diagnosis of childhood cancer is an acute, often traumatic event for a family. The way in which the diagnosis of cancer is presented significantly influences the family's initial reactions and sets the stage for collaboration with the medical team. The initial meeting with the family, which should be held as

Pediatric Psycho-oncology: Psychosocial Aspects and Clinical Interventions, Second Edition.
Edited by Shulamith Kreitler, Myriam Weyl Ben-Arush and Andrés Martin.
© 2012 John Wiley & Sons, Ltd. Published 2012 by John Wiley & Sons, Ltd.

quickly as possible once a cancer diagnosis is reached, is an opportunity to establish a trusting physician–patient–family relationship. The psycho-oncologist has a fundamental role in determining whether the medical information is clearly communicated and understood by the family. Assessing each family member's coping and learning styles is a key component of helping a family at this critical time. For example, some caregivers might search for and request detailed information on their child's cancer and treatments ("monitors"), while others may feel overwhelmed by all the new information and only want what they absolutely need to know ("blunters") [9, 10]. "Monitors" may be quite distressed by all that they read and require considerable support with what they learn, but it is equally important to make sure that "blunters," while wishing to avoid detailed medical information, have sufficient information to make informed decisions.

The days and weeks following a new cancer diagnosis are an important time to be available and to offer support and guidance to the child and family. Nearly all caregivers report significant psychological distress in the form of anxiety. With the demand for frequent medical tests and treatment, lives are disrupted, roles and responsibilities within the family need to be renegotiated to ensure that basic needs of the family continue to be met (e.g., working to retain medical insurance and pay bills, care of healthy siblings), and highly technical medical information has to be understood. Having a roadmap of treatment can help the family focus on what needs to be done and provide some sense of relief, optimism, and improved mood. Families also benefit from knowing what "normal" emotional responses are and how to answer questions from family and friends.

Initiation of Treatment

For the child, psychosocial care at diagnosis and initiation of treatment includes offering age-appropriate interventions such as positive incentives for cooperation with procedures, breathing exercises and developmentally appropriate distraction techniques during procedures. Storytelling, fantasy play and puzzles are often useful for the preschool child whereas the school-age child may benefit from engaging in medical play. For those undergoing surgery, short preparatory visits to the operating and recovery rooms can help children to become familiar with surroundings and reduce anxiety. Working with families and the medical team to allow and encourage adolescents to participate in medical decisions (i.e., signing consents; when appropriate, control with scheduling; viewing and explaining the results of laboratory tests; involving them in discussions of treatments) helps establish a strong working relationship with the medical team from the outset.

Ongoing Psychosocial Care

Psychological and developmental problems in the patient or any family member can add significantly to the caregiver burden of dealing with cancer and can exhaust a family's emotional resources (and staff time). The early assessment of the family's strengths and vulnerabilities, psychosocial resources, and preexisting problems can help the team anticipate the psychological adjustment of families to cancer and allow for quick and efficient provision of psychosocial care based on their needs [8, 11]. As treatment progresses and families establish a "new normal," the availability of group support, and individual and family counseling for caregivers can be useful in order to address feelings of anxiety, sibling adaptation, the marital (or significant) relationship (divergent coping styles, intimacy and communication patterns under chronic stress), concerns associated with the child's prognosis or late effects, or simply for reassurance that they are coping adequately. Good psychosocial care does not encourage dependence on the medical team, but rather encourages development of effective coping strategies, the child's integration back to school and with peers as soon as possible and supports the family for maximal functioning. The longer the child is away from his or her pre-cancer activities, the harder the adjustment can be to re-establish friendships and to feel comfortable back at school following the completion of therapy.

When indicated, age-appropriate psychiatric interventions for our pediatric patients are equally helpful. Somatic symptoms of depression, such as difficulty sleeping or fatigue, are common symptoms of both depression and cancer, and therefore can be difficult to differentiate. Careful psychiatric assessment of severe distress or prolonged symptoms is important [12]. Regardless of whether these symptoms are normal rather than pathological in nature, the symptoms should be documented and addressed. Assessment of mental health and coping based on the child's age, development, and personality may be obtained in many ways. Therapeutic interventions are designed to reduce distress and to help the child integrate the facets of his or her illness and life into expression [13]. A therapeutic game has been created for children aged 7–16 that assesses coping skills, family relationships, stressful issues, adjustment/adaptation, self-esteem, peer relationships, depression/sadness, and a view of prognosis [14]. For others, talk therapy can provide a vehicle for communication. Different forms of self-expression are equally powerful and effective, including behavioral and cognitive techniques, play, the use of workbooks [15], bibliotherapy, storytelling, writing, art, music, humor, and animal-assisted therapy [12]. Most often, however, a combination of approaches is most effective and will change based on the child's current emotional needs and medical circumstances.

Non-adherence can be a significant and often overlooked issue in pediatric oncology. Anticipating, assessing, monitoring, and, when necessary, emphasizing adherence to the treatment regimen are critical components of comprehensive psychosocial care [16]. Additionally, continuous assessment of physical as well as emotional pain is critical. An ideal program documents quality of life from the time of diagnosis throughout survivorship and provides each family access to pharmacologic and nonpharmacologic approaches, including complementary and alternative interventions. This includes energy therapies (e.g., therapeutic massage, energy healing, REIKI), manipulative and body-based methods (e.g., chiropractic, massage) and body-based mind–body interventions (e.g., mindfulness, meditation, prayer, guided imagery, and hypnosis) and thoughtful counsel pertaining to homeopathic approaches taking into account potential drug interactions [17]. Other interventions that aid healing include art therapy [18], music therapy [19, 20], aroma therapy [21] and animal-assisted therapy [22].

Siblings

Paying attention to the siblings in the family is a critical element of psychosocial care. It is only in recent years that the needs of siblings have been identified as being met inadequately compared to other members of the family. Comprehensive care considers the needs of siblings from the time of diagnosis and continues throughout the course of illness, including bereavement and survivorship. Siblings often feel that their needs pale in comparison to those of their sick brother or sister and yet they experience the same emotional reactions to the diagnosis of cancer (shock, disbelief, helplessness, sadness, guilt) plus jealousy without the luxury of doctors and staff who are worried about their emotional needs. Throughout treatment, the healthy sibling may feel a sense of isolation as the family travels out of town to a new treatment facility or as he or she spends time at home with extended family or at a friend's home. Disruptions in daily routine and prognostic uncertainty can lead to difficulties in school, acting out behaviors at home and school, anger or withdrawal. Siblings respond well to support and

consistency and many siblings thrive with the additional responsibility thrust upon them. While most cancer centers do not spend time evaluating the psychosocial needs of pediatric cancer patient's siblings, it is the authors' hope that this practice will change in the near future. Hospital programs that include siblings in their child and teen programming and those that have specific programs for siblings (such as a hospital-wide Sibling Day) are increasingly recognized for their importance. National organizations such as SuperSibs. are working hard to ensure that children whose brothers and sisters have cancer are "supported, honored and recognized to help them face the future with strength, courage and hope" (www.supersibs.org).

Creating an Optimal Healing Environment

Integrated cancer care incorporates the use of complementary and alternative medicine (CAM) techniques, as well as insights from research in medicine, nutrition, interior design, architecture, exercise, and psychooncology [23]. This includes creating a physical space using principles that have been shown to promote health, healing and quality of life and incorporating evidence-based health care environment research findings into hospital design. Healing principles take into consideration the use of color, light, shapes, noise, music, and natural elements. For example, the use of color in a children's hospital has been shown to create a more cheerful environment [24] whereas exposure to art reduces stress [25]. Bright light has been shown to reduce depression and those in sunny rooms have shorter periods of stay compared to those in dull rooms [26]. In a group of parents of children with severely developmentally disabled children, a correlation has been found between their satisfaction with the building environment and their satisfaction with health care services [27]. In another study that focused on the interior of a hematology-oncology unit, patients, their parents, and hospital staff participated in objective ratings of the physical environment along with other measures to elucidate the network of relationships between physical design elements in children's hospital rooms, environmental satisfaction, and outcome measures including psychosocial functioning, parental health care satisfaction, staff co-worker satisfaction, and staff fatigue. Pediatric hematology-oncology patients, their parents, and hospital staff were more satisfied in environments with better physical amenities. For parents, significant relationships between environmental satisfaction, health care satisfaction, and psychosocial functioning emerged. Likewise, environmental satisfaction was associated with co-worker satisfaction, psychosocial functioning, and fatigue among hospital staff [28, 29]. These studies support the core concepts of patient- and family-centered care as patient and family choices are incorporated into the design of the hospital space and decisions are made that reflect and honor their preferences, not the preferences of the staff alone.

The Roy and Patricia Disney Family Cancer Center provides a wonderful example of how a health care system can address healing of mind, body, and spirit. After extensive consultation with many disciplines and family members, specific spaces within the center were designed to promote comfort and tranquility, including indoor and outdoor areas for quiet contemplation, a Zen garden, a meditation labyrinth, an outdoor seating area surrounded by water features, a private meditation room with views onto the garden, and a yoga studio and physical therapy suite which opened onto the garden. The colors and materials were selected from the natural environment to enhance a sense of healing, growth, and life rather than the customary sterile clinical atmosphere. A state-of-the-art radio-frequency identification system allows patients to control lighting, music, temperature and even video in their exam and treatment rooms. When patients enter the lobby, the system automatically sends a text message alerting the reception desk and nursing staff via wireless phones so they can be greeted by name in a timely fashion [30]. While most centers will not have the resources to create such an extensive and sophisticated physical environment, it is clear that attention to creating spaces where the child can relax, teens can independently find comfort, and caregivers can obtain a sense of peace should be an essential component of all psychosocial oncology programs. This is especially important when extended periods of time are spent in the medical environment, such as in transplantation.

Transplant and Donor Issues

Stem cell or bone marrow transplant is becoming standard therapy for many high-risk malignancies [31]. Attentive pediatric oncology programs recognize that psychosocial interventions can begin at the time a family decides to undergo transplant through the search for a donor, and continues with long-term follow-up post-transplant to assess psychosocial, neurocognitive and psychoeducational sequelae. Through the acute phase of transplant hospitalization, the child and family are faced with extended medically required isolation, concern about engraftment, sleep and appetite disturbances, and disruption in family processes. Helpful psychosocial interventions during this time include advocating for developmentally appropriate distraction techniques during isolation, utilizing recreation therapy or child life services, ongoing support by psychosocial clinicians using individual and group modalities as well as the availability of art and music, and respite, in the form of some time out of the room to care for oneself, for family caregivers. The period following the acute phase of treatment is referred to as the transition phase [32]. The loss of daily medical staff support and the process of school and social reintegration are stressful for most families. Ideally, after discharge, a psychosocial team member makes calls between clinic visits to assess for social functioning, mood, sleep, appetite and symptoms of post-traumatic stress. During the follow-up period, families benefit from knowing that the oncology team will continue monitoring potential neurocognitive and psychosocial late effects and that counseling and other nursing interventions will continue to be available, if needed.

Donors

There are inherent stresses for all siblings of children with cancer, but unique concerns for those who are an HLA-match. Feelings of ambivalence and distress are common as those who are able to be a donor are proud to be immunologically compatible but anxious about the hospital procedures. Non-matched siblings may feel relief but also rejection because they are not a match [33]. Younger siblings can find the HLA blood typing frightening and painful and therefore wish not to donate [34]. Individuals of all ages may find the pre-donation evaluation as anxiety producing as previously unknown medical conditions might be discovered and sensitive and confidential questions are asked (e.g., sexual practices, drug use), the answers to which might preclude donation [35]. Deferral from donation would be expected to result in family member inquiry as to the reason for such. Finally, results of family HLA-typing might indicate false paternity. These issues can have significant emotional impact on a possible sibling donor. The development of comprehensive preparation and follow-up procedures post-stem cell collection and transplantation can reduce the negative effects for pediatric donors. A model that includes ongoing assessment and support of the psychological well-being of the sibling donor could identify those who are psychologically vulnerable and ensure the receipt of timely and appropriate clinical interventions [35].

Completion of Therapy

When treatment is completed, families face new challenges. Many people in the child's life anticipate that completion of therapy is a joyous occasion for families.

Yet, for many, this transition phase from the security of the medical center to preparing for the future is a time of anxiety, uncertainty, and perceived vulnerability. While most long-term survivors are psychologically resilient, having had pediatric cancer is a risk factor for somatic symptoms, cognitive impairment and deficits or delays of normative developmental tasks [36]. Psychosocial interventions in preparation for the end of treatment should be part of a comprehensive care cancer program. This work entails helping families balance a desire to deny or minimize the possibility of recurrence while maintaining optimism and a focus on making future life plans. The team works with the family: (1) to monitor for treatment associated late effects; (2) to understand the importance of adhering to medical follow-up; and (3) for those with central nervous system disease or treatments, to continue assessment of neurocognitive and consequences of cancer, as these may require educational testing, adaptations in school or work environments, or vocational testing and counseling. Importantly, helping caregivers to allow their child a sense of autonomy, assessing readiness and preparing for the transition to adult care is essential. The medical team should provide the child/family with a clinical summary that details the cancer treatment and recommendations for health screening and risk-reducing behaviors [36]. Providing an opportunity to find a sense of purpose and meaning in the cancer experience can be an essential component of end of treatment care.

Recurrence

For many families, cancer recurrence can feel more overwhelming than the initial diagnosis. Many find it more difficult to maintain optimism. The relationships that have been formed throughout the illness will help sustain the family during these challenging times. The role of the psychosocial team is to help the family develop a new sense of normalcy and expectations as they learn about new treatment options and adapt to additional demands on their family. It is important for the family to identify the coping mechanisms that helped them adapt after the initial diagnosis. Coping improves once families are reassured that they are actually better prepared to cope after a recurrence than they had been when they first learned their child had cancer, especially as they are more knowledgeable about the disease and medical system, insurance, treatments, terminology, and have established relationships with doctors and nurses. At this point, if they have not been introduced to stress-reducing interventions, including community- and hospital-based support

groups, mind–body techniques, and more traditional psychological support services, this is a good time for to do so. While the literature on psychological responses to cancer recurrence is limited, some degree of depression and anxiety is common in youth who are faced with their disease returning, especially if they have been cancer-free for a period of time. Unfortunately, some patients experience multiple recurrences. Responses such as depressive symptoms, along with a loss of hope for a cure, anxieties surrounding an uncertain future and fears of death are common. With each recurrence, most children and families appreciate additional psychological support as they consider alternative, research and/or complementary therapies.

If additional treatment is not successful, the transition from curative to end-of-life care requires more intense involvement and difficult conversations with the child and family. The psycho-oncologist's role at this point is: (1) to ascertain that maximizing comfort is a valued treatment goal for parents in their child's end-of-life care [37]; (2) to encourage ongoing communication between the child and caregivers; (3) to assess the child's understanding and capacity to plan for his or her end of life; (4) to address where the child and family would like to be as the end of life nears; (5) to understand whether the child and family prefer a natural death or resuscitation if the child stops breathing; and (6) to provide accurate, sensitive, age-appropriate communication until the child's last breath. The pediatric cancer experience often leads to long-term relationships with staff. Most families wish to maintain relationships with their child's oncology team after their child has died. This is difficult for some clinicians and not possible in many programs. Parents often hold onto written cards that are sent from the team that cared for the child for years. Some centers offer bereavement services. For those that do not have bereavement counseling resources within their facility, working with the family to obtain individual or group counseling or to have referral information for such services, is an essential component of compassionate and comprehensive care.

Integrating Clinical Care and Research

As psycho-oncology clinicians who work with children and their family members throughout the trajectory of the cancer experience, we are in a unique position to recognize meaningful patterns and organize information in ways that reflect a deep understanding of what we observe. Our assessment skills, diagnostic judgment, systematic case formulation and treatment planning as well as treatment implementation and monitoring of patient progress, interpersonal expertise, continual self-reflection and ability to work with the treatment teams are essential traits in a successful clinical researcher. These integrative skills allow the clinician to think about the kind of research questions that should be asked and to identify areas where effective interventions are needed. Furthermore, research allows a researcher's collected clinical wisdom to be tested and disseminated to help others. This information dissemination sometimes mitigates compassion fatigue (formerly called "burnout") by keeping one intellectually engaged and helping to focus and compartmentalize difficult-to-handle emotions. However, many challenges and obstacles can get in the way of being able to turn these patterns of observation into meaningful research questions.

The most commonly reported challenges to bridging clinical work with research are not lack of interest, but a lack of time, limited resources (e.g., research assistants, data analytic support), lack of expertise and training, a sense that the role of clinician and scientist may be incompatible, and limited fiscal incentives (e.g., lack of billable hours). Additional perceived challenges involve the culture of one's work. For programs that are clinical by design, incorporating research may be perceived as intrusive or unnecessary and therefore, not encouraged by program administrators.

Examples of Integrated Clinical Care and Research

There are many types of research that can potentially support clinical utility including clinical observation, qualitative research, systematic case studies, process-outcome studies, randomized controlled trials (RCT) and even meta-analysis when a patient population is not available. This is by no means an exhaustive list of all possible research opportunities or designs. Below we describe some practical steps needed when designing straightforward research projects within one's practice. Specific types of research that require few resources and can be feasibly incorporated into a clinician's job responsibilities are described below. Please note, due to space limitations, only a brief overview is provided and should not be considered to be all the information or training needed for the research described.

Where Do I Start? How Do I Start?

This is often the hardest obstacle for many clinicians. It requires patience to develop a good question that provides clinical utility and an ability to tolerate some false starts while pursuing the best path to answering the question.

(1) *Define a research question in an area of personal interest.* For example, one might have a desire to know whether guided imagery reduces procedural distress, or be interested in learning the prevalence of sleep problems during radiation therapy to the brain. One way to develop research ideas is to listen carefully to many patient stories for similar and dissimilar themes.

(2) *Do a literature review.* Once one develops a question, search the literature for any studies that might have already tested the theory or question. Write a summary of everything that has been done that is relevant to the research question and why the question is an important one to ask. Ask how it might contribute to better diagnosis, prognosis or treatment. For example, if one wants to know if guided imagery can reduce procedural distress, describe how and for what guided imagery has been used, other interventions used for procedural distress, and how this intervention can be applied effectively to reduce distress prior to a medical procedure. If there is a specific conceptual model to guide the research question, describe the theory and how the research question fits into the theoretical design. If ever in doubt as to the best way to proceed, always seek the help of an experienced researcher for guidance.

(3) *Describe specific aims.* With a research question established and a literature review and theory completed, it is time to describe one's specific aims. What would one like or expect to learn from the study? List between three and five central hypotheses/expectations about what one can expect to find. For example, one might hypothesize that children who present with a history of separation anxiety will have more pronounced anxiety reactions at the onset of radiation therapy, or that playing a specific game with a child prior to radiation therapy will result in a reduced need for anesthesia. It is important to write aims that are "actionable" so that at the completion of the study, an objective reader can assess how well the aims were met.

(4) *Make a study design.* Next, outline a study design that seems best suited to answer the research question(s). A study design includes identifying who the subjects or participants will be, whether there will be a comparison group, and what the key independent and dependent variables are. The *independent variable* is the variable that is controlled, changed, or manipulated by the research. The *dependent variable* is the variable that is measured or observed. For example, if one is studying whether adolescents who receive a cell text message

reminder- are more adherent to their medications post transplant than those who do not receive such reminders, one might consider the need to obtain adolescent, caregiver and provider reports of adherence. The cell phone and text messages would be the independent variable (what can be changed or manipulated) and better adherence based on the results of adherence measures and blood counts would be the dependent variable (what is observed, the outcome). The sampling strategy, research design, selection of variables and operationalization (defining) of the variables are very important elements of the research as these can affect the validity of results substantially. List the strengths and weaknesses of the design and review them with colleagues knowledgeable in research design.

(5) *Identify collaborators.* Securing buy-in from key team members is another very important step in order to conduct psychosocial research. If the medical team has a sense of ownership over the design and study outcomes, they will be more likely to encourage patient/subject participation. It is also important to explore what costs (both financial and time) will be associated with one's research and whether the patient/subjects one is interested in studying are available at one's setting. There are creative ways to get around monetary barriers. For example, some clinical researchers hire student interns from local colleges as healthy volunteers for academic credit, or provide food for focus group participants (instead of cash) or provide patients with gift cards for a local grocery store.

Types of Research Designs

Research within a pediatric oncology program will generally fall into two different areas. The first is evaluation research, which is designed to describe and assess the worth of a service or resource in order to facilitate decisions regarding the service. Evaluation research can also be used for quality improvement. The second is scientific research, which is designed to describe, predict, and understand phenomena and their interrelationships in order to contribute to a body of empirical knowledge.

Needs Assessments

Most pediatric oncology programs would be strengthened by accurate data on the psychosocial needs of the patients and families in their program in order to improve care and programming. A needs assessment involves using a systematic process to collect and examine information. Needs assessments, a form of evaluation research, can be carried out in outpatient or inpatient settings. Within a pediatric oncology setting, data on the perceived and expressed needs of the patient (child, adolescent, young adult) and caregiver(s) can be utilized to determine priority goals when developing a program service delivery plan and to determine how best to allocate funds and resources. By administering needs assessments before a new program is introduced and administering the same assessment after the program is established, the team can determine if the perceived/expressed needs of the patients and family members are being met. These data can also provide information on individuals who are either not aware of the new program or services and those for whom current services are not adequate. Investigating whether the programs offered are what patients and family members feel they need promotes a sense of partnership, accountability, and honors the core concepts of family-centered care. Greater patient and family satisfaction will come from family involvement at the intervention level as well as the program level. Steps in conducting a needs assessment are well described in both the educational and psychological literature [38]. A well-done needs assessment involves the collection, analysis, and interpretation of data within the context of current knowledge about a topic [39].

Other steps include: clarifying the purpose of the needs assessment and planning for what one will do with the information collected; identifying the population to be studied (e.g., patients, caregivers, siblings); developing a system for collecting and organizing the data; analyzing the data, summarizing and sharing the findings. This descriptive data should be presented to the pediatric oncology clinical team to inform them of perceived needs and to discuss ways to improve psychosocial services. The results can also be presented in writing, where the strengths of the program (services/ education being provided) are listed, so that areas where needs are not being met and future programming is needed are documented. Then the psychosocial team can use the results to develop a plan of short- and long-term goals. This is a very important part of conducting any research, particularly needs assessment. The plan may also consist of allocating, redistributing, or seeking new resources to meet patient and family psychosocial needs.

Similar procedures would be used in conducting program evaluations. This would include the collection, analysis, and interpretation of data (before and after a program was instituted) in order to describe the worth of the program and decisions regarding whether the program should continue [39]. Needs and program evaluations are only differentiated by their goals [40]. Program evaluations also acknowledge the need for

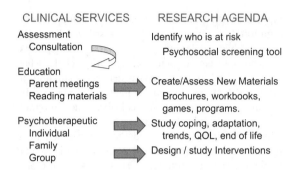

CLINICAL SERVICES

Assessment
  Consultation

Education
  Parent meetings
  Reading materials

Psychotherapeutic
  Individual
  Family
  Group

RESEARCH AGENDA

Identify who is at risk
  Psychosocial screening tool

Create/Assess New Materials
  Brochures, workbooks,
  games, programs.

Study coping, adaptation,
  trends, QOL, end of life

Design / study Interventions

Figure 2.1 Designing comprehensive and family-centered care programs in pediatric oncology.

patient and staff input regarding the problems that have been developed. Figure 2.1 shows the links between the comprehensive and family-centered care programs in pediatric oncology.

Single-Case Design

A single-case design falls into the category of *scientific* research and is the design of most interest to clinicians who are seeking to determine whether a specific intervention causes significant change for an individual or a group of individuals with whom they are working. Pediatric psychologists have successfully used single-case methodology in medical settings [41], including demonstrating the use of distraction for procedural pain [42] and tracheotomy weaning [43]. Due to the small sample size needed, a single-case design is well suited for busy clinicians. Importantly, the single-case study is recognized as a legitimate research methodology that can help establish empirically validated treatments and evidence-based practices. A single-case design has often been confused with a case report or case studies. In a single-case design, an experimental control is used, whereas in a case study, only a baseline and intervention are described [44]. There are many single-subject design options and those clinicians who are interested in this type of research are encouraged to consult references for when these designs might be useful [45–48]. For the purposes of this chapter, we will only describe one common design referred to as a reversal (withdrawal) design.

Within a single-case design, the experimental control is established by using the individual case as its own control. All conditions are kept the same, except for the independent variable, which is introduced and then withdrawn to see the effects on the participant's behavior. While a single-case design is the use of research design with one participant, and is a good

way to begin learning about research, the long-term goal is to identify multiple participants, systematically replicating the intervention effects with groups of children and allowing broader statements of generalizability to be made [44]. Changes in family life or health may lead some to drop out from the study and it is important to have additional eligible participants available to ensure completion of the study. Other challenges to single-case design include difficulty controlling for factors outside of the study that might cause changes in the child's behavior (family issues, progressive illness, treatment side effect).

A single-case design can be used to establish an empirically validated treatment. As a single-case design can be used to establish an empirically validated treatment, meticulous records of each research decision is required. When the results are written up, it is essential that the analyzed data supports the results/findings and discussion of the findings. It is essential to maintain meticulous records of each research decision. Finally, when writing up results, use the analyzed data to support all results/findings and to support the discussion of the findings. Once these results are published, larger and more complex study design (such as a randomized control trial) can determine whether the results can be generalizable to all children.

Further Integration of Psychosocial Research

While putting on one's research hat does not come naturally to most clinically trained psychosocial clinicians, the psychosocial clinician is already capturing important information about each child and family they work with. Learning to expand one's role, by systematically collecting and documenting this information is possible without the acquisition of considerable resources. A well-conceived psychosocial research program, however, can motivate and excite the oncology group and bring greater respect to the work already being provided. Involve other clinicians in your agency in identifying interesting and important research questions. Starting with relatively modest and short-term projects, such as a needs assessment or evaluation of a particular clinical program can instill a sense of collaboration and confidence in psychosocial research. Obtaining the commitment and endorsement of the medical director may be a critical ("top-down") step. By working together to incorporate psychosocial research into the organization's mission, one can ensure that one's research is both relevant and complements the mission of the pediatric oncology program [49]. Figure 2.2 presents one example of setting up a research program that includes social worker,

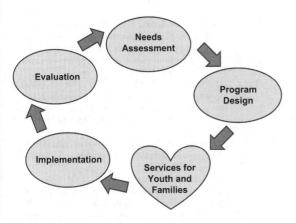

Figure 2.2 Psychosocial translational research in pediatric oncology.

psychologist, child psychiatrist and others (child life or recreation therapy), etc.

Over time, becoming a clinician-researcher becomes easier when one is able to synthesize research activities into one's clinical and programmatic responsibilities. If collaborations are not available within one's setting, explore collaborations with colleagues or professors at universities who share similar interests or connect with researchers at conferences. Universities often provide access to students, libraries, computer facilities, and technical assistance [49]. For those who are not interested in designing studies, psychosocial clinicians can participate or support the collection of important information in other ways. Of increasing importance is the need to assess more than treatment toxicity in clinical trials. Several reliable and valid health-related quality of life (HRQOL) measures are available that assess the physical, emotional, functional, and social impact on a child's life. Newer patient reported outcome measures are in development (PROMIS), these measures are especially useful in determining the effect of a new medication on a child's quality of life. The psychosocial clinician can recommend such measures be incorporated into clinical trials within their settings.

Caveats

As with most new tasks, caveats to the role of clinician-researcher exist. There may be confusion about one's role as a researcher or as a clinician and tensions exist between the goals of these activities. The primary goal of clinical care is caring for the patient but the primary goal of research is generalizable knowledge. If switching gears is not possible when working with certain families, training students and other colleagues to

assist with data collection data can be very useful. Most people appreciate learning new skills and being a part of an important project. Attend available lectures on clinical and research methodologies. The more familiar that research terms become, the more comfortable the clinician will become. Finally, remember that research can be fun, lead to greater insights and have impact. fun. It allows us an opportunity to increase the quality of care we provide while making our clinical work more meaningful.

Conclusion

Providing comprehensive multimodal clinical care in a family-centered care environment that attends to the emotional, social, cultural and developmental needs of patients and their family members is a worthy and rewarding pursuit, especially in the setting of heart-breaking cancer diagnoses. Patients and their families benefit from the expertise obtained from interdisciplinary psychosocial team members throughout the course of their cancers. They often learn that finding meaning and purpose from their medical experiences and the losses incurred throughout the cancer journey improves adjustment [50]. Clinicians too benefit from collaboration with interdisciplinary professionals, particularly when they can partner in producing new knowledge derived through psychosocial research. While most pediatric psychosocial oncology clinicians do not combine the roles of practitioner and researcher, the growing consensus is that psychological practice must be based on the best available evidence [51, 52], therefore we have a unique opportunity to revisit the integration of science and practice to improve patient and family function and outcomes.

References

1. Institute for Patient- and Family-Centered Care. Bethesda, MD: Institute for Patient- and Family-Centered Care; c1992–2011 [updated 2010 December 21; cited 2011 Apr 14]. Available from: http://www.ipfcc.org/about/index.html.
2. Spirito A, Kazak AE. *Effective and Emerging Treatments in Pediatric Psychology*. Oxford: Oxford University Press, 2006.
3. Cohen LL, Lemanek K, Blount RL, *et al.* (2008) Evidence-based assessment of pediatric pain. *Journal of Pediatric Psychology* 2008;**33**:939–955.
4. Patel SK, Mullins W, Turk A, *et al.* Distress screening, rater agreement, and services in pediatric oncology. *Psychooncology* 2010; Oct. 5 [E-pub ahead of print].
5. Zadeh S, Wiener L, Battles H, *et al.* Perceived benefit and burden for youth and for parents from participation in psychosocial research when undergoing treatment for cancer, NF-1, or HIV. Paper presented at International

Society of Paediatric Oncology SIOP XXXXII Congress, Boston, United States; Oct. 2010; 21–24. 2010 SIOP Abstracts. *Pediatric Blood & Cancer* 2010;**55** (in press). DOI: 10.1002/pbc.22779.

6. Kazak AE, Barakat LP, Hwang WT, *et al.* Association of psychosocial risk screening in pediatric cancer with psychosocial services provided. *Psychooncology* 2011; Apr 7 [E-pub ahead of print].

7. Kazak AE, Simms S, Alderfer MA, *et al.* Feasibility and preliminary outcomes from a pilot study of a brief psychological intervention for families and children with newly diagnosed cancer. *Journal of Pediatric Psychology* 2005;**30**:644–655.

8. Wiener L, Alderfer M. Psychosocial aspects of cancer for children and their families. In: Lanzkowsky P (ed.) *Manual of Pediatric Hematology and Oncology*. San Diego: Elsevier, 2011; pp. 952–968.

9. Miller SM, Mangan CE. Interesting effects of information and coping style in adapting to gynecological stress: should a doctor tell all? *Journal of Personality and Social Psychology* 1983;**45**:223–236.

10. van Zuuren FJ, Wolfs HM. Styles of information seeking under threat: personal and situational aspects of monitoring and blunting. *Personality and Individual Differences* 1991;**12**:141–149.

11. Wiener LS, Hersh SP, Alderfer MA. Psychosocial support for the child and family. In: Pizzo PA, Poplack DG (eds.) *Principles and Practices in Pediatric Oncology*, 6th edn. Philadelphia: Lippincott, Williams & Wilkins, 2010; pp. 1322–1346.

12. Pao M, Wiener L. Psychological symptoms. In: Wolfe J, Hinds PS, Sourkes BM (eds.) *Textbook of Interdisciplinary Pediatric Palliative Care*. Philadelphia: Elsevier, 2011; pp. 229–238.

13. Sourkes B, Frankel L, Brown M, *et al.* Food, toys, and love: pediatric palliative care. *Current Problems Pediatric Adolescent Health Care* 2005;**35**:350–386.

14. Wiener L, Battles H, Mamalian C, Zadeh S. ShopTalk: a pilot study of the feasibility and utility of a therapeutic board game for youth living with cancer. *Support Care Cancer* 2011; Mar 31 [E-pub ahead of print].

15. Wiener L. *This is My World*. An NCI, NIMH, NIH, DHHS publication available upon request from author, Washington, DC, 1998, reprinted 2011.

16. Drotar D, Witherspoon DO, Zebracki K, Peterson CC. *Psychological Interventions in Childhood Chronic Illness*. Washington, DC: American Psychological Association, 2006.

17. Brown RP, Gerbarg PG, Muskin PR. Alternative treatments in psychiatry. In: Tasman A, Kay J, Lieberman J (eds.) *Psychiatry*, 3rd edn. London: John Wiley & Sons, Ltd, 2003; pp. 2147–2183.

18. Nainis N, Paice, JA, Ratner J, *et al.* Relieving symptoms in cancer: innovative use of art therapy. *Journal of Pain and Symptom Management* 2006;**31**:162–169.

19. Barrera, ME, Rykov MH, Doyle SL. The effects of interactive music therapy on hospitalized children with cancer: a pilot study. *Psychooncology* 2002;**11**:379–388.

20. Stewart K. PATTERNS: A model for evaluating trauma in NICU Music Therapy: Part I –Theory and Design. *Music and Medicine* 2009;**1**:29–40.

21. Bonadies V. Guided imagery as a therapeutic recreation modality to reduce pain and anxiety. *Therapeutic Recreation Journal* 2009;**43**:43.

22. DeCourcey M, Russell AC, Keister KJ. Animal-assisted therapy: evaluation and implementation of a complementary therapy to improve the psychological and physiological health of critically ill patients. *Dimensions of Critical Care Nursing* 2010;**29**:211–214.

23. Block KI, Block P, Gyllenhall C. The role of optimal healing environments in patients undergoing cancer treatment: Clinical Research Protocol Guidelines. *The Journal of Alternative and Alternative Medicine* 2004;**10** (Suppl.1): S157–S170.

24. Park JG.Environmental color for pediatric patient room design. Doctoral dissertation, Texas A&M University, 2007.

25. Eisen SL, Ulrich RS, Shepley MM, *et al.* The stress-reducing effects of art in pediatric health care: art preferences of healthy children and hospitalized children. *Journal of Child Health Care: For Professionals Working with Children in the Hospital and Community* 2008;**12**:173.

26. Beauchemin KM, Hays P. Sunny hospital rooms expedite recovery from severe and refractory depressions. *Journal of Affective Disorders* 1996;**40**:49–51.

27. Varni JW, Burwinkle TM, Dickinson P, *et al.* Evaluation of the built environment at a children's convalescent hospital: development of the Pediatric Quality of Life Inventory parent and staff satisfaction measures for pediatric health care facilities. *Journal of Developmental and Behavioral Pediatrics* 2004;**25**:10–20.

28. Sherman S, Shepley MM, Varni JW. Children's environments and health-related quality of life: evidence informing pediatric healthcare environmental design. *Children, Youth and Environments* 2005;**15**:186–223.

29. Sherman-Bien S. An empirical approach to healthcare design: research on pediatric oncology units. *Psychooncology* 2011;**20** (Suppl. SI): 6.

30. Schwartz L, Sutton T. A cancer center dedicated to the healing of mind, body and spirit. *Psychooncology* 2011;**20** (Suppl. S1): 6.

31. Santos GW. Historical background to hematopoietic stem cell transplantation. In: Atkinson K (ed.) *Clinical Bone Marrow and Blood Stem Cell Transplantation*, 2nd edn. New York: Cambridge University Press, 2000; pp. 1–12.

32. Phipps S. Transplant and donor issues. In: Wiener LS, Pao M, Kazak AE, *et al.* (eds.) *Quick Reference for Pediatric Oncology Clinicians: The Psychiatric and Psychological Dimensions of Pediatric Cancer Symptom Management*. Charlottesville, VA: American Psychosocial Oncology Society, 2009.

33. Pot-Mees CC, Zeitlin H. Psychosocial consequences of bone marrow transplantation in children: a preliminary communication. *Journal Psychosocial Oncology* 1987;**5**: 73–81.

34. Kinrade, LC Preparation of sibling donor for bone marrow transplant harvest procedure. *Cancer Nursing* 1987;**10**:77–81.

35. Wiener LS, Steffen-Smith E, Fry T, Wayne AS. Hematopoietic stem cell donation in children: a review of the sibling donor experience. *Journal of Psychosocial Oncology* 2007;**25**:45–66.

36. Hobbie WL, Hudson MM, Rowland JH, Schwartz LA. Pediatric cancer survivors: moving beyond cure. In: Wiener LS, Pao M, Kazak AE, *et al.* (eds.) *Quick Reference for Pediatric Oncology Clinicians: The Psychiatric and Psychological Dimensions of Pediatric Cancer*

Symptom Management. Charlottesville, VA: American Psychosocial Oncology Society, 2009.

37. Breyer J. Talking to children and adolescents. In: Wiener LS, Pao M, Kazak AE, *et al.* (eds.) *Quick Reference for Pediatric Oncology Clinicians: The Psychiatric and Psychological Dimensions of Pediatric Cancer Symptom Management.* Charlottesville, VA: American Psychosocial Oncology Society, 2009; pp. 4–22.

38. North Dakota Department of Public Instruction [homepage on the Internet]. Bismarck, North Dakota: North Dakota Department of Public Instruction [cited 2011 April 14]. Available from: http://www.dpi.state.nd.us/grants/needs.pdf.

39. Popham WJ. *Educational Evaluation*, 3rd edn. London: Allyn & Bacon, 1993.

40. Peebles, J. The future of psychotherapy outcome research: science or political rhetoric. *The Journal of Psychology*, 2000;**134**:659–669.

41. Willis DJ. In memoriam: Logan Wright, Jr., Ph.D. (1933–1999). *Journal of Pediatric Psychology* 2000;**25**: 359–361.

42. Jay SM, Elliott CH, Ozolins M, *et al.* Behavioral management of children's distress during painful medical procedures. *Behavior Research and Therapy* 1985;**23**: 513–520.

43. Wright L, Nunnery A, Eichel B, Scott R. Application of conditioning principles to problems of tracheotomy addiction in children. *Journal of Consulting and Clinical Psychology* 1968;**32**:603–606.

44. Rapoff M, Stark L. Editorial: Journal of Pediatric Psychology Statement of Purpose: Section on Single-Subject Studies. *Journal of Pediatric Psychology* 2008; **33**:16–21.

45. Allen KD, Friman PC, Sanger WG. Small research designs in reproductive toxicology. *Reproductive Toxicology* 1992;**6**:115–121.

46. Horner RD, Baer DM. Multiple-probe technique: a variation of the multiple baseline. *Journal of Applied Behavior Analysis* 1978;**11**:189–196.

47. Barlow DH, Hersen M. Single case experimental designs. In: *Arthritis Care & Research*, 2nd edn. New York: Pergamon Press, 1984; pp. 132–135.

48. Kazdin AE. *Single-Case Research Designs: Methods for Clinical and Applied Setting.* New York: Oxford University Press, 1982.

49. Pfeiffer SI, Burd S, Wight A. Clinicians and research: recurring obstacles and some possible solutions. *Journal of Clinical Psychology* 1992;**48**:140–145.

50. Davis CG, Nolen-Hoeksema S. Loss and meaning: how do people make sense of loss? *American Behavioral Scientist. Special Issue: New Directions in Bereavement Research and Theory* 2001;**44**:726–741.

51. American Psychological Association Presidential Task Force on Evidence-Based, Practices. Evidence-based practice in psychology. *American Psychologist* 2006;**61**:271–285.

52. Norcross JC, Hogan TP, Koocher GP. *Clinician's Guide to Evidence-Based Practices: Mental Health and Addictions.* New York: Oxford University Press, 2008.

3

Quality of Life in Children with Cancer

Shulamith Kreitler, Michal M. Kreitler

Introduction

The initial signs of interest in the quality of life (QOL) of children with cancer started to appear at the end of the last century [1, 2]. The past decade has witnessed the further development of the interest in QOL in regard to pediatric cancer, spurred both by the availability of different assessment instruments of QOL [3] and the dramatic rise in survival of pediatric cancer patients from about 30% in the 1960s to over 80% long-term remissions in recent years [4]. The latter brought about a shift on the part of both professional and lay public from expectations of quality curative and palliative care to expectations of survival with good QOL [5]. The emphasis on QOL was further enhanced by awareness of both parents and patients of the price in terms of physical and psychological difficulties that the malignancy and the treatments bring about. Notably, two-thirds of the survivors suffer from at least one health problem, and 40% suffer from psychosocial or cognitive problems [6], which may affect adversely QOL.

Definition of QOL

QOL is defined as the individuals' perception of their functioning and well-being in different domains of life [7] or more specifically, the individuals' evaluation of their position in life, in the context of the culture and value systems in which they live, and in relation to their goals, expectations, standards and concerns [8]. These definitions emphasize the individuals' overall satisfaction or happiness in major domains of their life. Historically they were known as "life satisfaction" or "subjective well-being," and are now referred to as "global QOL" or "overall QOL." They refer to all domains that make up one's QOL or contribute to it, not just health. The above definition resembles in major features also the following definition that was specifically designed to represent pediatric cancer-related QOL: "an overall sense of well-being based on being able to participate in usual activities; to interact with others and feel cared about; to cope with uncomfortable physical, emotional, and cognitive reactions; and to find meaning in the illness experience" [9].

Related Constructs

QOL as defined above has to be distinguished from other related constructs. Major among these are the following:

(1) *Health status and perceived health status (or health perceptions)*: Health status is the person's relative status of health or illness, considering the presence of biological or physiological dysfunction, symptoms and functional impairment. Most definitions of health status refer to physical function, sensation, self-care and dexterity, cognition, pain and discomfort, and psychological well-being. The Health Utilities Index Mark 2 (HUI2) and the Health Utilities Index Mark 3 (HUI3) are common tools for assessing health status in pediatric oncology [10]. The Lansky play performance scale [11] is a health status measure in children with cancer which closely parallels the standard health status Karnovsky scale used with adult cancer patients. Perceived health status is the individual's subjective ratings of his or her health status. Though the two may coincide, they are not necessarily identical [12]. Symptoms and health perceptions are often included in health-related QOL.

(2) *Health-related quality of life (HRQL)*: This refers to the individual's satisfaction or happiness with domains of life insofar as they are affected by one's health (e.g., disease and its treatments). Most conceptualizations of HRQL refer to the effects of

Pediatric Psycho-oncology: Psychosocial Aspects and Clinical Interventions, Second Edition.
Edited by Shulamith Kreitler, Myriam Weyl Ben-Arush and Andrés Martin.
© 2012 John Wiley & Sons, Ltd. Published 2012 by John Wiley & Sons, Ltd.

disease in general (generic HRQL) or a particular disease or treatment (condition-specific HRQL) on physical, social, emotional and cognitive functioning [13]. The four listed domains are the basic ones defined by the European Organization for the Research and Treatment of Cancer (EORTC) [14].

(3) *Mood*: Emotional responses, usually negative ones, mainly depression, anxiety or anger that are often reported as part of QOL or the related constructs. The rationale is that emotions of this kind may result from or affect functional performance, health status and HRQL [12].

(4) *Symptoms*: Patients' reports of physical symptoms in general or those that are of particular interest in view of their disease or treatments they receive, such as fatigue or nausea in cancer.

(5) *Disease severity*: Scales of disease severity reflect the overall degree of severity of the patient's disease, which may be based on any or all of the following: objective symptoms, physicians' ratings and also on patients' reports.

(6) *Functional status*: Refers to the individual's ability to perform regular activities required to meet basic needs, fulfill one's roles and maintain well-being [15, 12]. It may include both functional capacity (based on actual assessment of capacity or on others' ratings) as well as functional performance (based on self-reports), which may or may not overlap.

In some cases, the boundaries between the constructs are difficult to draw and are blurred for theoretical or methodological reasons, such as between health status and HRQL or disease severity and functional status.

Major Characteristics of QOL

The standard approaches to QOL highlight the following characteristics of QOL [16]:

(1) QOL is a *subjective* construct, reflecting the individual's view of his or her well-being and functioning.

(2) QOL is a *phenomenological* construct, providing a surface image of the situation, without explaining how or why it arose.

(3) QOL is an *experiential or evaluative* construct, which presents judgments without any attempt to relate them to objectively verifiable facts.

(4) QOL is a *dynamic* construct, expected to be sensitive to significant changes in the individual's state.

(5) QOL is a *multidimensional* construct, based not merely on a single global measure but on evaluations in specific domains that have been identified as major constituents of QOL.

(6) QOL is a *quantifiable* construct, which may be assessed so that it provides scores comparable across different individuals or across different states or time points in the same individual.

The characterization of QOL would not be complete without specifying the negative defining features. Accordingly, QOL is not identical to (a) quantity of life (i.e., duration of life, survival); (b) health status; (c) functional status; and (d) disease severity.

Assessing QOL: General Issues

The Purpose of Assessing QOL

The assessment of QOL in pediatric cancer patients may have important implications in regard to the clinical care, research, policy development and psychosocial treatment of the affected children, in the course of treatment and afterwards. First, the assessment of QOL enables to identify the needs and difficulties of children undergoing oncological treatments or of the large numbers of survivors of pediatric cancer who may be impaired due to the highly toxic treatments they have undergone [17]. Hence, QOL assessments would enable us to address, anticipate and possibly remediate the difficulties of the disease and its treatments [18].

Further, QOL assessments complement the information we usually have about the effects of treatments. While most of this information reflects medically objective facts relevant for the cure, QOL focuses attention on additional effects that may reflect the costs of the cure in terms of impairments and suffering. Accordingly, QOL assessments provide a broader basis for evaluating treatments and for comparing them. This may be especially important in clinical situations when two considered treatments are expected to have similar outcomes in terms of survival but differing demands on the patients' life. Sometimes integrating the medical and QOL information sources enables an evaluation of the net effect of a treatment, which may be lower than the initially assumed one. Further, QOL information may help researchers set new goals for developing treatments reducing impairment of QOL without compromising clinical efficacy. In this context it is of interest to note that radiation to the brain was administered as a regular prophilactic therapy to patients with acute lymphoblastic leukemia but when QOL assessments identified serious sequelae of this therapy [19, 20], radiation-sparing treatments were developed as well as chemotherapy substituting for radiotherapy whenever possible [17].

Again, in cases of doubt about whether to apply a given treatment, QOL information may help physicians and parents reach a decision balancing probable cure effects against likely damage to QOL. When there is no possibility to choose among treatments, information about the likely QOL effects of the particular treatment may help in planning adequate interventions for moderating these likely effects or even preparing the children in advance with prophylactic measures [21].

It is customary to view QOL assessments as contributing also to screening, describing the beneficial effects of treatments, assisting in the management of individual patients, and contributing to decisions about clinical policy and resource allocation [22, 23].

Additionally, QOL assessments communicate to the child an important message—that regardless of how difficult the treatment that has to be applied is, the medical staff will not lose sight of the basic fact that the patient is first and foremost a human being.

Finally, it needs to be mentioned that assessment of QOL conforms to the requirement for patient-reported outcomes in clinical trials [24] at least for adults, although to date not for pediatric cancer patients [25].

Notably, the following two constructs that have been defined for QOL assessments facilitate the use of QOL assessments in clinical practice: (1) the determination of the "minimal clinically important difference" (i.e., the smallest difference in a score of some assessment that patients perceive to be beneficial and that could be used to change the treatment); and (2) the "cut-point for at-risk status scores" (i.e., about one standard deviation below the population mean for identifying at-risk status of QOL relative to population means) [26].

The Proxy Issue: QOL by Whom?

The question of whether the child or someone else should provide information about the child's QOL has turned into one of the most controversial issues in the assessment of QOL of pediatric patients. It is possible to present the involved issues in terms of three kinds of approach or three phases. The first and earliest one was characterized by arguments favoring the assessment of the child's QOL by a proxy, mostly a parent, rather than by the child. The distrust of children as a source of information was based primarily on the argument that children have a limited ability to report on their QOL, especially when the child is younger than 5 years old. But even in regard to children above 5, the tendency to overlook the child's view and rely instead on the parents' reports was based on arguments of the

following kind: children are limited or unable to understand, value and identify factors that "contribute or detract from HRQL" [27] or point out major functional domains for children (e.g., school, social relations) [28]; children may be too ill to respond [29]; children may continuously change their responses to a questionnaire which may impair psychometric standards [30]; children's responses are subjective and may contradict those of parents, so that a blurred view of the situation arises [27].

Several investigators openly stated that parents are a better source of information about the children's HRQL both from the points of view of reliability (presumably because they are adults), objectivity [31], and validity because parents "are usually the most knowledgeable about the child's behavior across time and situations" [28] and are "believed to be very familiar with their child's life" [32]. Further, it was claimed that it is no use bothering with the child's views since anyway "it is almost always the parents' view of their child's symptoms and behavior which is crucial in determining what is done about any health problem" at least up to the child's early adolescence. Another argument was that since it has always been the doctors' habit to ask the parents about the child's state of health [28], there is no special reason to change this age-honored procedure.

The second type of approach to dealing with the problem was characterized by studies comparing the responses of children and their parents. Most studies showed imperfect agreement between the responses of children and parents. Thus, on the subscales of the Behavioral, Affective and Somatic Experiences Scale, the correlations between the responses of the children (<6 to 12> years) and the parents were significant but low ($r = .29–.57$) and actually not very different from those between the responses of the parents and the nurse ($r = .19–.62$) [33]. On 10 of the 11 subscales of the Child Health Questionnaire (CHQ) the correlations between the responses of adolescents in treatment (aged 10–18-years-old) and their parents were significant but in the low to medium range except in regard to the Role/Social-Physical and Self-Esteem fields, in which the adolescents reported significantly higher scores than their parents. Hence, the parents reported a stronger impact of the illness on the adolescents' physical functioning, social and school activities and self-esteem than the adolescents themselves did [34]. Also in another study with the CHQ, greater discrepancies between the reports of parents and children were found in the cancer group (mean age 13.2, SD = 2.6 yrs) than in the healthy children's group [29]. The sick children reported significantly less bodily pain/distress, better general health perceptions, fewer limitations in performing activities requiring a lot or some energy, walking or climbing stairs, fewer limitations on the kind of school activities they could complete and the amount of time spent on that due to physical health (see also [35]). Similarly, on the PCQL-32 [36], children 6–12 years old reported higher scores on three scales (physical, psychological, disease-related) and lower on social functioning than their parents. The reports of children and parents were mostly not correlated.

In a study with children aged 6–16 years old, Challinor *et al.* [37] found on the Behavioral Assessment System for Children questionnaires that the scores of parents and children on the scale of somatization were unrelated at all, while the scores on the scales of anxiety and depression were correlated but those of parents were higher than those of children. Notably, also in another study the scores of parents and children for depression on the Child Behavior Checklist were not correlated and the parents reported higher levels of depression for the children than the children themselves [38]. A similar pattern emerged in a study with children aged 8–18 years old on the CHQ: on 50% of the items there were significant differences in the responses of the parents and the children, with the parents reporting typically higher levels of distress and restrictions for the children than the children themselves [29]. Similar findings were reported for a sample of children aged 5–12 undergoing bone marrow transplantation: the scores of parents on QOL and mental health were lower than those of the children [39].

A systematic review of the literature [40] examined the interrelations between parent and child reports of HRQL in the case of chronically sick children on the basis of 14 studies using 10 separate measures of HRQL. In regard to domains of HRQL, they found a tendency for somewhat greater agreement in regard to observable behaviors, such as physical functioning ($r > .50$) and less ($r < .30$) for non-observable ones, such as emotions and social functioning. Parents tended to report lower levels of functioning, more distress and in general a greater impact of the illness on the child's performance than the children did. Notably, another study found serious discrepancies between the importance assigned by pediatricians and sick children even to physical symptoms. For example, the pediatricians overestimated the importance of diarrhea and underestimated the importance of "worries about future health problems" [41]. The conclusion is that even the views of experts in a disease and in treating children cannot replace the views of the children themselves.

In sum, though there is some relation between the reports of parents and children on the children's QOL, the discrepancies are too large to justify substituting parents' reports for children's reports. It seems that agreement is higher when children are older and their health is better [42], for example, for children off treatment than on treatment [43], or for children during home stay than in the hospital [44]. The discrepancies tend to be particularly large in regard to content domains that are of greatest interest to the clinician and not accessible through direct observation (viz. emotional and social functioning) and in regard to the groups of children that are of greatest interest in this context (viz. sick children versus healthy children, and children in treatment versus children off treatment). Typically parents tend to report higher levels of distress and impairment than the children. This gap may be due, on the one hand, to the anxiety and stress of the parents evoked by the children's disease, and, on the other hand, to the tendency of children to cope by minimizing their reported distress and also to protect their parents.

The third phase, which largely dominates the present scene, is characterized by the commonly shared conclusion that the reports of parents cannot replace the children's reports, (common variance 15–25%) and should not replace them if we are to consider seriously the FDA Draft Guidance for Industry, that "some treatment effects are known only to the patient" [24]. Thus, it has become increasingly common practice to administer a QOL tool to the children and often to complement the information given there by getting in addition the responses of the parents to the QOL questionnaires. The latter are generally justified on the basis of the argument that it is desirable to rely on multiple sources of information, that the parents' views are crucial for clinical decisions [45] and that there may be situations when the children are actually unable to respond or unwilling to cooperate [46].

Assessment Tools of Pediatric QOL

There are a great many tools for the assessment of QOL in children and adolescents. They will not be reviewed here because there are many good and comprehensive descriptions and reviews of these tools [e.g., 25, 47–49] and because several of these tools are included in the Appendix A of this volume on pp. 271–297.

In general, the reviews show that most of the tools have been developed in line with standard and scientifically-based procedures, have good psychometric properties, including acceptable internal consistency, reliability, and tested validity, considering both construct validity and criterion validity [47]. Hence, we will not deal specifically with the psychometric properties of the individual tools.

This section will provide an overview, referring to major characteristics of the various existing tools, with the intent to highlight some of the issues and decisions involved in assessing QOL, especially those that may be of importance to the clinician or practitioners facing the need to choose an assessment tool for QOL.

Contents of the Assessment Tool

Almost all assessment tools include items that refer to several domains, in addition to a general question that refers to overall QOL. In the early phase of constructing tools for the assessment of QOL it apparently did not seem necessary to define the concept of pediatric QOL [50]. Thus, the pediatric QOL tools referred to the same domains that were covered in the tools for assessing QOL in adults. A survey of the domains found in most pediatric QOL tools shows that the ones that occur in most tools are the following: health status (including physical symptoms, pain, nausea, somatic distress), physical functioning, movement and balance, social functioning/friends (including social competence, intimate relations, playing with other children), family interactions or well-being, cognitive functioning, emotional functioning (including mood, procedural and treatment anxiety, worry), and body image. The following six domains occur in only one or two of the tools and are based on prior interviews with sick children: autonomy, outlook on life, the meaning of being ill, fun and enjoyment, hope, meaningfulness of life, creativity, the existence of something to live for. It is likely that focusing more on the perceptions and conceptions of the children would yield further domains that may be of interest for the clinician and practitioner, such as spiritual well-being, relations with one's siblings, fear of the recurrence of cancer, worries about fertility, and sexuality.

The following set of 18 themes based on a factor analysis of the 55 items in the Children's QOL questionnaire (CQOL) shows that the field of QOL in children may be differently structured than in adults and consists of a pattern of specific factors, each of which is focused on a definite theme and accounts for a small amount of variance: Negative feelings; School functioning; Pain; Motivation for living and coping; Fulfilling duties at home; Positive feelings; Mastery and control; Life at home (accommodation, playing, discussing problems); Cognitive functioning (solving problems, being oriented); Health and despair (health worries, feeling of health and low hopefulness); Jealousy in regard to health; Food and eating; Cognitive functioning (memory and thinking); Having close friends; Spending money on taking care of one's

appearance; Doing things that one likes; Being bothered and worried about something; and Having friends for keeping busy and active. A further factor analysis of these factors yielded the following three factors: Emotional distress (defined by negative feelings, confusion and stress); Coping with the disease (defined by positive feelings, body image, basic needs and motivation for living); and Worries (defined by pain, school and family).

Generic or Disease-Specific Tool

The meaning of the adjectives generic and disease-specific may vary in different contexts. Thus, generic may designate a tool that is adequate for assessing QOL of children with any kind of disease or none, in which case disease-specific would be a tool for assessing the QOL of a specific disease, say, cancer. Thus, the PedsQL™ 4.0 Generic Core Scales [51] and the Children's Inventory of Quality of Life (CQOL) [52] were designed for application in both healthy and patient populations, while the PedsQL™ modules for pediatric oncology were designed specifically for pediatric patients with cancer [53].

Or, again, generic may refer to some disease with all its variations, say, cancer including all its different kinds (e.g., [54–56]), whereas disease-specific would refer to the QOL of children diagnosed with a particular kind of cancer, for example, brain tumor [46, 57]. The advantages of a generic tool are that it enables comparisons across different pediatric populations and with healthy children, whereas the disease-specific measures provide information that refers specifically to a particular health condition. In recent years there has been a growing tendency to use both kinds of instruments so as to get a more comprehensive view of the patient's state [26].

General or Particular Tool

Also within the domain of the disease there are more general or more specific tools. Degrees of specificity may be defined in terms of symptoms, for example, some tools focus on a particular symptom, such as fatigue in children with cancer [53]. Alternately, specificity may be defined in terms of whether the tool was designed to measure QOL in pediatric patients undergoing any treatment [54, 58] or a specific treatment (stem cell transplantation [54] or bone marrow transplantation [59]). Some tools can be used to assess QOL in children on or off treatment [53, 60] and others are specific to pediatric cancer survivors [55, 61].

Further, specificity may be defined also in terms of the age of the child. Thus, some QOL tools are appropriate for use with children from 2 to 18 years [52] while others are targeted for children in specific age groups (e.g., the PedsQL 4.0 Generic Core Scales include parallel forms for ages 5–7, 8–12, 13–18 yrs) [53]. Furthermore, the versions differ not only in wording but also in the manner of administration (i.e., by an interviewer vs self-administered).

Finally, specificity may indicate also the period of time to which the QOL tool refers. In general, QOL tools measure functioning retrospectively for the past 7 days or the past 1 month. However, some tools allow for adapting instructions to the time period which is of interest (e.g., since the beginning or termination of a treatment) or do not specify any time period in the instructions but rather refer to "in general", or may even target the present time period (e.g., at-the-moment), which may prove useful especially for the measurement of constructs, such as pain, mood and fatigue [62].

It is evident that each type of specific or general tool will have its benefits or shortcomings. In general, the more specific a tool is, the more detailed and precise is the information obtained in regard to the particular aspect targeted. However, the highly specific tools narrow down the range of comparisons afforded with other values of the measured aspect, for example, the information provided by a tool targeted at measuring at-the-moment state can hardly be compared meaningfully with information about the last month.

Tools: For Whom and by Whom?

A review of this kind would not be complete without mentioning differences between tools in the persons for whom the tool is designed and in the administrators. It is important to note that some cancer QOL tools are meant to be filled in by caretakers and other adults about themselves, mostly parents or health professionals (e.g., SF-36 in [63]). These tools were used because of the assumptions that the disease of a child affects the QOL of all the family members, and that the sick child's QOL may in turn be affected by the QOL of its caretakers and family members. Notably, the Adult Quality of Life inventory (AQL) [64] refers to the adults or parents but the information may readily be compared with that of the parallel questionnaire for children (CQOL).

Tools that are designed to measure the child's QOL but are filled by a proxy, mostly a parent, represent a different situation (see tools in [58, 65]). As discussed above ("The Proxy Issue: QOL by Whom?"), the provided information does not tally completely with that provided by the child. Hence, some tools include two versions of measures: one for the child and one for the parent, which may be designed to correspond to each other, for example, PedsQL™ 4.0 Generic Core Scales [53] or not, for example, the Child Health Questionnaire (CHQ) [66].

Representative Findings on the QOL of Children with Cancer

This section is devoted to reviewing major findings concerning the QOL of children with cancer, focusing on the periods of diagnosis, active treatment and follow-up, but excluding studies of pediatric cancer survivors as well as children undergoing bone marrow transplantation which are dealt with in other chapters in the book (see Chapters 5 and 17).

On the Miami Pediatric QOL questionnaire [58] children with leukemias/lymphomas scored higher than children with brain tumors on the Total Index, social competence and self-competence (though not on emotional stability), but did not differ from those with solid tumors. Children who had received whole-brain radiation (mostly those diagnosed with ALL or high-grade brain tumors) scored significantly lower on the Total Index, social competence and self-competence than those who did not (but there was no difference on emotional stability). Physicians' global ratings of HRQL were not related to any of the four scores of QOL.

On the Pediatric Oncology QOL scale [65], there were high correlations among all three scale scores (physical restrictions, emotional distress and discomfort from medical treatment), which indicates that at least in this sample, QOL is a general global characteristic. The scores do not differ for the different ages (2.8 to 19.7) and the genders. Children out of treatment scored higher than those on intensive treatment on the scales of physical restrictions and discomfort from medical treatment, but not on emotional distress. Comparing only patients of leukemia and lymphoma differing in treatment status (off-treatment, on maintenance treatment and on intensive treatment) showed that those in intensive treatment scored higher on physical restrictions, but not higher on emotional distress, or on discomfort from medical treatment, and did not have an overall worse QOL. Comparing children with different diagnoses showed that those with leukemia or lymphoma had less emotional discomfort, less discomfort from treatment and overall better QOL than those with solid tumors (brain, solid, neuroblastoma). Time since diagnosis was correlated with physical restrictions, so that the longer the time, the fewer physical restrictions the child was reported to have.

On Watson *et al.*'s [28] *HRQL* (parental form), comparing the reports on children with a variety of cancer diagnoses on- and off treatment showed that in the course of treatment the children had more physical symptoms, but had *higher* scores on emotional status (perhaps due to a decline of the distress they have had earlier during diagnosis), and *better* cognitive functioning (perhaps "settling down to things" is easier for the children because they are busy with the physical effects of treatment). However, there were no differences on functional status, global health, social functioning, behavioral problems and global QOL.

A tool based on observing the children's play activities [67] showed that the ratings of the children's QOL were most influenced by the child's physical symptoms. There were significant differences between inpatients and outpatients, but not between outpatients receiving therapy and those patients who had completed therapy.

The PedsQL 4.0 Generic Core Scales were administered to a pediatric oncology sample that included 339 patients of both genders (mean age 8.72 yrs, range 2–18) with ALL, brain tumors, Hodgkin's and non-Hodgkin's lymphomas, Wilms' tumor and other cancers, with no co-morbidity, newly diagnosed and with recurrent disease, on- and off-treatment, with short or long remissions. Their scores on the Acute Version were compared with those of 157 healthy children (age range 2–18), and on the Standard Version with the scores of 730 healthy children [53]. In general, the oncology sample as a group scored lower on all four scale scores of physical, social, emotional and school functioning as well as on the total sum. However, there were many exceptions to this general description.

In the Generic scales, Child report, acute version, the oncology sample did not score lower than the healthy sample on the total score (children older than 12 off-treatment), on physical health (children younger or older than 12 off-treatment), on emotional functioning (children older than 12 off-treatment), on social functioning (children older than 12 off-treatment), and on school functioning (children younger or older than 12 off-treatment). In children younger than 12 there were no differences between the groups on-treatment and off-treatment in any of the scores, in contrast to children older than 12 where there were significant differences between the on- and off-treatment groups in the total score and in the scores of physical and emotional functioning.

On the Generic scales, Parent report, Acute Version, the on- and off-treatment groups scored in all cases less than the healthy controls (in children younger or older than 12). However, the on- and off-treatment groups did not differ from each other in all cases, for example,

they did not differ significantly in psychosocial health, social functioning and school functioning.

On the condition-specific module of *Multidimensional Fatigue* (child-report version), the findings are also not homogeneous. Thus, in the total score, the children on-treatment as well as the younger than 12 off-treatment scored lower than the healthy controls; in general fatigue and sleep/rest fatigue, those on treatment scored lower than those off-treatment older than 12 and also lower than the healthy controls; in cognitive fatigue only children on-treatment scored lower than the healthy controls but not those off-treatment regardless of age.

On the parent-report version of the Multidimensional Fatigue scale, all children with cancer, regardless of age and of treatment status, scored lower than the healthy controls on the total score and on all scales. However, only on two scales (i.e., general fatigue and sleep/rest fatigue) the on-treatment children scored lower than the off-treatment children, regardless of age. On total fatigue and cognitive fatigue, for example, there were no differences between the on- and off-treatment children younger than 12.

On the other condition-specific module of *Cancer*, the child form, there were no significant differences between children on- and off-treatment on 5 of the 8 scales, regardless of age; on the scales of worry, nausea and treatment anxiety, the on-treatment children scored lower than the off-treatment ones but only in the case of children older than 12.

On the parental form of the Cancer module, the on-treatment children scored lower than the off-treatment ones on five scales (pain, nausea, procedural anxiety, treatment anxiety and worry), but not always in regard to both age groups (in the case of pain, only older children; in the case of nausea, procedural anxiety and worry, both age groups; in the case of treatment anxiety, only the younger children).

Comparing 28 children with brain tumors with 28 children with other types of cancer, matched in demographic and medical characteristics showed that the former scored lower on the Pediatric Quality of Life Inventory in the domains of physical functioning, psychological functioning and social functioning and in the total score [68]. Comparing 125 on-treatment pediatric patients with 156 patients off-treatment (all diagnostic groups, age range 8–18 years) showed that they differed significantly only on the scale of physical functioning, but not on psychological and social functioning [56].

On the *Pediatric Cancer QOL Inventory* children 6–12 years old diagnosed with ALL in different stages of disease and treatment, had the highest scores in social functioning, followed in a descending order by psychological functioning, overall QOL, cognitive functioning, physical functioning, and disease and treatment problems. Parents rated the children lower than they themselves did [36].

On the Child Health Questionnaire (CHQ) [34] parents' reports showed that adolescents (mean age 13.6, SD = 2.2 yrs) with cancer were rated significantly lower than healthy controls on 7 of the 12 scales: Physical Functioning, Role/Social-Physical, General Health Perceptions, Family Activities, Role/Social-Emotional/Behavioral, Parental Impact –Emotional, and Self Esteem. There were no significant differences on Pain, Parental Impact-Time, Mental Health, Behavior and Family Cohesion. In the cancer group, the lowest scores were on the scales that rated the emotional impact that the adolescents' illness had on parents (the extent to which they were worried and concerned) and on the parents' perceptions of their adolescents' general health. However, on the bases of their own reports, adolescents with cancer scored significantly higher than healthy controls, on the scales of Mental Health and Role/Social Behavioral and lower on the scales of Self-Esteem and General Health Perceptions. The latter scale yielded the lowest scores they reported.

Further, the self-report form showed that adolescents in active treatment scored significantly lower than those off-treatment only on Physical Functioning and General Health Perceptions. However, the parent-report ratings indicated that adolescents in active treatment scored significantly lower than those off-treatment on 7 of the 12 scales: Physical Functioning, Role/Social-Physical, Bodily Pain, Family Activities, Role/Social-Emotional, Parental Impact-Time, and Parental Impact-Emotional.

The adolescents' self-reports yielded significant correlations between time since cancer diagnosis and the scales Physical Functioning, Role/Social-Physical, and General Health Perceptions. The parents' reports showed significant correlations between time since diagnosis and seven scales: Physical Functioning, Role/Social-Physical, Bodily Pain, Family Activities, Role/Social-Emotional/Behavioral, Parental Impact-Time, Parental Impact-Emotional. These findings suggest that parents assign a greater impact to the disease and the treatments than the adolescents tend to.

In a sample of adolescents of both genders, with different cancer diagnoses, those on-treatment scored lower than those off-treatment for one year in Global Health, Physical Functioning, Bodily Pain, Self-Esteem, General Health Perceptions, and Family Activities of the CHQ [69].

In a sample of children 6–14 years old, mostly with ALL, partly on- and partly off-treatment, parents reported for the children on the Behavioral Assessment System higher depression levels and higher anxiety than the teachers and the children themselves; the teachers and the parents reported for the children higher somatization levels than the children themselves. The reports of the parents and the children correlated moderately and significantly in regard to anxiety and depression but not in regard to somatization, and all three scales correlated significantly and positively in each respondent group [37].

In each of the scales a certain percentage of children scored in the "at risk" range (in regard to somatization 30.8–46.5%, in regard to anxiety 11.6–32.3%, in regard to depression 11.6–20.9%). In each case the highest numbers are those based on the parents' reports. Gender, treatment status, cranial irradiation and age (the latter except in regard to anxiety which was higher in adolescents) had no influence on who was identified as "at risk."

Comparing adolescents of both genders, with various cancer diagnoses, partly on- and partly off-treatment, with healthy controls showed that the cancer group scored significantly lower on 4 of the 8 scales of the Minneapolis-Manchester QOL Instrument: Physical functioning, Cognitive functioning, Psychological functioning, and Social functioning. There were no significant differences between the groups in Body image, Outlook on life, and Intimate relations, as well as in the total score. Patients on therapy scored lower than those off therapy in Physical functioning, Psychological functioning, and Outlook on life, and higher in Social functioning. Notably, the cancer patients off-treatment did not differ significantly from the healthy controls in half of the scales (Psychological functioning, Body image, Outlook on life, and Intimate relations) and in the total score [69].

Comparing children 8–18 years old, off-treatment showed that the QOL was lower in the leukemia/lymphoma patients than in those with solid tumors, especially in the scales of the Pediatric QOL Autonomy, Emotional Functioning, Cognition, Familial Interactions, Physical Functioning, and Body Image [70]. Lower scores on the Peds QL 4.0 Generic Core Scales, Acute Cancer Module, and Multidimensional Fatigue Scale, for children with leukemia/lymphoma than for those with brain tumors and solid tumors were reported also by others [71]. Leukemia patients have lower QOL also as compared with healthy controls [72, 73].

More detailed findings shedding light on the specific effects of medical and demographic variables on adn

CQOL will be presented [52]. Comparing children 9–14 years old with various cancer diagnoses (n = 35) and healthy controls (on a preliminary version of the CQOL (49 items) showed that the sick children scored significantly lower on the scales of school functioning, play, mastery and independence, cognitive functioning, satisfying basic needs, positive feelings, and negative feelings. Hence, the effect of disease on the children was negative and pervasive. Further, children in treatment scored lower on the scales of friends, cognitive functioning, negative feelings, and satisfying basic needs. Of particular interest is the finding that in regard to the children in treatment, the inpatients differed from the outpatients in higher scores on the scale of basic needs. In an interview after the study, the inpatients explained that during the treatment they felt more secure in the hospital where they could be sure that a doctor or nurse would be always available to offer professional help in any eventuality. Or, in the words of one child: "At home, if something happens and I feel sick, my parents don't know what to do and start arguing about whether to bring me to the hospital."

In a larger study the CQOL was administered to 217 children (6–18 years old) with cancer (different diagnoses, different disease stages, on-treatment and off-treatment). The five highest scores were in the domains of motivation, and positive feelings followed by body image, satisfying basic needs, and cognitive functioning. In contrast, the five lowest scores were in the domains of mastery and independence, pain, health worries, play and stress, which seem to be the domains hit the hardest in children with cancer.

Comparisons of CQOL scale scores in terms of demographic variables showed that children younger than 15 scored lower than the older ones on school, negative feelings, positive feelings, health, body image, play, stress, and the total QOL score; girls had more negative feelings than boys and scored lower on the total score; and children born in the country had lower negative feelings and stress and more mastery and independence than those who immigrated from other countries.

Comparisons of CQOL scale scores in terms of treatment variables showed that the scores of the children in remission reflect higher QOL than the scores of the children on-treatment in the scales of family, school, health, pain, mastery, basic needs, and the total, but lower scores in the motivation scale, probably because they do not have to deal any more with the difficult side-effects of the treatments. Further, comparisons in terms of current treatments showed that getting chemotherapy differed from getting other treatments only in lower scores on the scale of cognitive functioning. However, comparisons in terms of the chemotherapy load (heavy, medium or light) showed that those who got the heavy load had the lowest scores in overall QOL as well as in regard to pain, body image, and motivation. Comparisons of the effects of specific treatments showed that tamoxifen affected adversely more QOL aspects than other treatments, including pain, mobility, and play. Also pills adversely affected QOL but in other domains, including cognition, and negative emotions. Notably, the emotional effects were mostly limited to increasing negative emotions but not decreasing positive emotions. Findings of this kind may serve as guidelines for psychological interventions designed to help the child cope.

Comparisons focused on *disease-related variables* reveal the important effect on QOL of the kind of disease the child has. There is evidence that children with leukemia have the lowest levels of QOL in many domains (including school, cognition, health, body image, basic needs, and overall QOL), mostly lower than lymphoma patients. Further, sarcoma patients scored significantly lower than lymphoma patients on the scales of school, pain and play; children with head tumors scored lower than those with brain tumors, and in some domains lower than those with solid tumors.

Comparing children in different disease stages shows that children with a stage IV disease have the lowest QOL only in some of the variables (i.e., scales of health, negative feelings, and stress) whereas children with stage I disease score lowest on QOL in basic needs and cognitive functioning Thus, the major QOL concerns of stage IV disease are emotional, and of stage I disease functional. Finally, comparisons showed that longer disease duration (over 5 years as compared with less than 5 years) is related with lower QOL scores on negative feelings, stress and motivation.

Some Non-medical Factors Affecting Pediatric QOL

As shown in earlier sections of this chapter, there is ample evidence of the strong impact on the children's QOL exerted by medical factors, such as the kind of diagnosis, being on- or off-treatment, kind of treatment, stage of disease, number of symptoms, and duration of disease. There can be little doubt that the QOL of pediatric patients is affected also by further variables. An intriguing argument for assessing QOL has been put forward by Guyatt [74], who considers the assessment as an anchor for examining psychosocial and demographic correlates of good and poor QOL, so that children at risk for low QOL can be identified in time and adequate improvement interventions can be planned.

Actually, not much is known about the non-medical correlates of QOL. Thus, in regard to patients in therapy, in those with high-risk ALL, girls and older children had worse QOL, while in standard-risk ALL, those with lower household incomes and unmarried parents had worse QOL [72]. In children (6–12 years old) in different stages of disease and treatment, QOL was lower in older children and in children whose parents were depressed [36]. Further, parental overprotection, mediated by perceived child vulnerability, was found to be significantly related to the child's QOL [75]. Attitudes are correlates of a different order that affect QOL. Thus, in adolescents with cancer, optimism (assessed by the Life Orientation Test) was correlated with less reported pain and hurt, better communication with doctors, higher reported psychological functioning and higher overall QOL (assessed by the Pediatric QOL Inventory, Cancer Module, Acute Version and The Pediatric QOL Inventory, Generic Core Scale) [76]. Similarly, higher optimism was related to lower self-reports of pain and better motional/behavioral functioning, whereas pessimism was related to poorer mental health and general behavior, and greater impact on the family [77]. Attitudes affect QOL as a means of coping with the adversities of the disease and the treatments. It is well known that coping in general is a major factor affecting QOL [78]. The theme of coping lies, however, beyond the scope of the present chapter.

Some Conclusions

The purpose of this section is to deal briefly with the two following issues concerning QOL: "Where are we?" and "Where do we go from here?"

The presentation of tools and findings in the broad domain of QOL supports several general conclusions. The first is that QOL reflects an aspect of the child's functioning and state that is neither identical with nor fully predictable from the child's medical state. It is evident, for example, that diagnoses, disease stages and being on- or off-treatment affect QOL but the effects are not pervasive across the board and mostly not trivial. Thus, not all aspects of QOL are lower in the initial stage of the disease as compared with the advanced stage, or in "heavy" chemotherapy as compared with "light" chemotherapy (e.g., findings based on the CQL [79]); some aspects of QOL are not related with estimates of disease severity by the physicians (e.g., results with MPQOLQ [58]); QOL of children off-treatment is not always better than of children on-treatment (e.g., see results with the PPSC [67], or the generic PedsQL [53]); and the QOL of children with cancer is not lower in all respects than the QOL of healthy control children

(e.g., findings with the CHQ [69]) and may even be higher (e.g., findings with the CHQ [34]).

A second conclusion is that the domain of QOL in pediatric oncology samples is not a homogeneous field of functioning or experiencing. Factor analyses as well as findings comparing different subgroups suggest that it is multidimensional in its structure and contents, so that the variance of QOL is accounted for by a series of several factors or sets of items, each focused on a specific circumscribed theme (e.g., findings based on CQL [79], PedsQL [53]; yet, a more global structure found with the POQOLS [65]). This conclusion may seem to indicate the utility of broadening the scope of the domains and items represented in pediatric oncology QOL tools. Up to now, many though by no means all investigators seem to have followed the guidelines of the European Organization for Treatment of Cancer (EORTC) for constructing tools for assessing specific domains (i.e., school, social functioning, cognition, physical function, and emotional state). However, it may be advisable to reconsider these guidelines in view of the following arguments: (a) the represented domains do not seem to cover all important aspects of QOL, as shown by tools that were constructed on the basis of other assumptions (e.g., [80]; PPSC [67]); (b) in view of children's cognitive development and style, it is possible that children's tools may need to use more concrete and specific items than the normally used ones. This recommendation is of particular importance in view of the increasingly recognized need to rely primarily on children's reports of QOL rather than on those of proxy figures, including parents, nurses, siblings, physicians and friends, however trustworthy and easy to access they may seem (see "The Proxy Issue: QOL by Whom?" above).

A third conclusion is that the QOL of children with cancer is the product of a matrix including multiple factors. The major factors that have been identified in research up to now are diagnosis, disease stage, current treatment (its nature and difficulty), previous treatments (e.g., whole brain radiation), number of symptoms as well as the child's age and gender. Since all or most of these factors play a role in regard to the child's QOL, comparing groups defined by only one of the factors yields contradictory results in different studies. For the sake of illustration, let's take diagnosis. Thus, in a study with the Miami Pediatric QOL questionnaire, children with leukemia or lymphoma were found to have better QOL than children with brain tumors but equal to that of children with solid tumors [58]; similarly, in a study with the Pediatric Oncology QOL scale, children with leukemia or lymphoma had better QOL in terms of emotional distress and discomfort due to treatment than children with solid tumors [65]; but studies with the Pediatric QOL [70] or CQOL [79] showed that children with leukemia or lymphoma had lower QOL in most domains than children with brain tumors or solid tumors. Similar contradictions may be detected in the above-reported findings concerning the effects of treatment (being on- or off-treatment) (e.g., CHQ [34] vs. [79]), or age (e.g., Multidimensional Fatigue Scale [53] vs. CQL [79]). What these contradictions suggest is that it is probably not justified to compare groups by diagnosis without considering simultaneously at the very least whether the compared children are on- or off-treatment, and, if on-treatment, what kind of treatment they are getting, and how old they are.

Thus, for the time being, the reported findings seem to be context- or tool-bound and do not support sweeping generalizations about the effects of particular medical or therapeutic factors on the children's QOL. One reason for this may have to do with the way children experience themselves and situations. In contrast to adults who may be better able or for whom it may make more sense to focus on one or another major factor, children may tend to experience the situation as a whole. If that is the case, then we may expect larger fluctuations in the QOL of children when there is a change in some factor, such as the nature of treatment. Second, at the present stage of development of assessing QOL in pediatric oncology, still too little is known or understood about the factors operative in this domain. Hence, the findings may seem fragmentary or contradictory. The remedy for that would be to go on studying the field so as to unravel more of its components and dynamics. A third possibility is that in pediatric oncology the whole situation actually plays a larger role than in adults. If that is the case, we should beware of generalizations, not even pursue them and try instead to pose highly specific questions, exploring the QOL of groups defined precisely by a number of factors (e.g., "What are the effects on QOL of treatment X administered to boys younger than 12 with a particular diagnosis of leukemia, in the initial phase of disease?"). Finally, a fourth possibility is that the findings are largely tool-dependent.

Finally, a fourth conclusion concerns the tools of assessing QOL in children. It may be appropriate to consider whether the commonly used tools are appropriate for children and for the studied issue of QOL in terms of contents and form. Most importantly, in view of the definition of QOL in experiential and phenomenological terms, it may not be appropriate to use pediatric QOL instruments that require children to evaluate or judge the effects of factors, such as the treatment or

the disease on their QOL, as is common in Health-Related QOL instruments, or compare their present state with their state prior to the onset of the disease.

The four stated conclusions spell out at least two guidelines charting the way ahead in the research of QOL. One is to further explore the factors affecting the QOL of children with cancer, in an attempt to unravel the structure and dynamics of this important domain. The other is to refine and adapt the tools of assessment so that they are better adapted to the studied population and theme.

The third recommendation serves to extend the mentioned ones by suggesting that the study of QOL in children with cancer should move in the direction of identifying new factors that may affect the children's QOL. Two types of such factors appear significant. One type is factors that have to do with the child's personality and coping mechanisms. This type is important because it complements the set of studied factors (e.g., disease, treatments) which are external to the children themselves. A large body of data about QOL in adult cancer patients demonstrates the importance to QOL of coping mechanisms and other resources that the patient brings into the situation [78]. The other type of factors to be studied is those that may be expected to affect the sick child's QOL in a *positive* manner. Examples that come readily to mind would be the support of friends, family interactions, or art therapy. Extending the study of the effects of factors with positive contributions to QOL forms the bridge to the most important task of improving the sick children's QOL.

References

1. Bearison DJ, Mulhern RK. *Pediatric Psychooncology: Psychological Perspectives on Children with Cancer*. New York: Oxford University Press, 1994; pp. 220–221.
2. Bradlyn AS, Harris CV, Spieth LE. Quality of life assessment in pediatric oncology: a retrospective review of phase III reports. *Social Science and Medicine* 1995;**41**: 1463–1465.
3. Eiser C. *Children with Cancer: The Quality of Life*. Mahwah, NJ: Erlbaum, 2004.
4. Ries LAG, Melbert D, Krapcho M, *et al.* (eds.) *SEER Cancer Statistics Review*, Bethesda, MD: National Cancer Institute, 1975–2004. Available at: http://seer.cancer.gov/csr/1975_2004/, based on November 2006 SEER data submission (posted to the SEER website, 2007).
5. Oeffinger KC, Robinson LL. Childhood cancer survivors, late effects, and a new model for understanding survivorship. *JAMA* 2007;**297**:2762–2764.
6. Greenen MM, Cardous-Ubbink MC, Kremer LCM, *et al.* Medical assessment of adverse health outcomes in long-term survivors of childhood cancer. *JAMA* 2007; **297**:2705–2715.

7. Fayers PM, Machin D. *Quality of Life: Assessment, Analysis and Interpretation*. Chichester: John Wiley & Sons, Ltd., 2000.

8. WHOQOL Group, the World Health Organization Quality of Life assessment (WHOQOL). Position paper from the World Health Organization. *Social Science and Medicine* 1995;**41**:1403–1409.

9. Hinds PS, Gattuso JS, Fletcher A, *et al.* Quality of life as conveyed by pediatric patients with cancer. *Quality of Life Research* 2004;**13**:761–772.

10. Feeny D, Furlong W, Boyle M, *et al.* Multi-attribute health status classification systems: Health Utilities Index. *PharmacoEconomics* 1995;**7**:490–502.

11. Lansky SB, List MA, Lansky LL, *et al.* The measurement of performance in childhood cancer patients. *Cancer* 1987;**60**:1651–1656.

12. Wilson IB, Cleary PD. Linking clinical variables with health related quality of life. *JAMA* 1995;**1995**:59–65.

13. Ware JE. The status of health assessment. *Annual Review of Public Health* 1995;**16**:327–354.

14. Sprangers MAG, Cull A, Bjordal K, *et al.* The European Organization for Research and Treatment of Cancer Approach Quality of Life Assessment: guidelines for developing questionnaires modules. *Quality of Life Research* 1993;**2**:287–295.

15. Leidy NK. Functional status and the forward progress of merry-go-rounds: toward a coherent analytical framework. *Nursing Research* 1994;**43**:196–202.

16. Niv D, Kreitler S. Pain and quality of life. *Pain Practice* 2001;**1**:150–161.

17. Feeny D, Furlong W, Mulhern RK, *et al.* A framework for assessing health-related quality of life among children with cancer. *International Journal of Cancer* 1999;**83**: S12, 2–9.

18. Monaco GA. Commentary on assessing health-related quality of life in children with cancer. *International Journal of Cancer* 1999;**83**: S12, 10.

19. Green DM, Zevon MA, Hall B. Achievement of life goals by adult survivors of modern treatment of childhood cancer. *Cancer* 1991;**67**:206–213.

20. Mostow EN, Byrner J, Connelly RR, *et al.* Quality of life in long-term survivors of CNS tumors of childhood and adolescence. *Journal of Clinical Oncology* 1991;**9**: 592–599.

21. Lauria MM, Hockenberry-Eaton M, Pawletko TM, *et al.* Psychosocial protocol for childhood cancer: a conceptual model. *Cancer* 1996;**78**:1345–1356.

22. Osoba DL. Measuring the effects of cancer on health-related quality of life. *PharmacoEconomics* 1995;**7**: 308–319.

23. Parsons SK, Brown AP. Evaluation of quality of life of childhood cancer survivors: a methodological conundrum. *Medical and Pediatric Oncology* 1998; S1: 46–53.

24. FDA. *Guidance for Industry: Patient-Reported Outcome Measures: Use in Medical Product Development to Support Labeling Claims*. Rockville, MD: Center for Drug Evaluation and Research, Food and Drug Administration, 2006.

25. Clarke SA, Eiser C. The measurement of health-related quality of life in pediatric clinical trials: a systematic review. *Health and Quality of Life Outcomes* 2004;**2**:1–5.

26. Varni JW, Limbers C, Burwinkle TM. Literature review: health-related quality of life measurement in pediatric oncology: hearing the voices of the children. *Journal of Pediatric Psychology* 2007;**32**:1151–1163.

27. Mulhern RK, Horowitz ME, Ochs J, *et al.* Assessment of quality of life among pediatric patients with cancer. *Psychological Assessment* 1989;**1**:130–138.

28. Watson M, Edwards L, Von Essen L, *et al.* Development of the Royal Marsden Hospital pediatric oncology quality of life questionnaire. *International Journal of Cancer* 1999;**83**: S12, 65–70.

29. Levi RB, Drotar D. Health-related quality of life in childhood cancer: discrepancy in parent–child reports. *International Journal of Cancer* 1999;**83**: S12, 58–64.

30. Kamphuis RP. The concept of quality of life in pediatric oncology. In: Aronson NK, Beckmann J (eds.) *The Quality of Life in Cancer Patients*. New York: Raven Press, 1987; pp. 141–151.

31. Eiser C, Jenney MEM. Measuring symptomatic benefit and quality of life in paediatric oncology. *British Journal of Cancer* 1996;**73**:1313–1316.

32. Goodwin DAJ, Boggs SR, Graham-Pole J. Development and validation of the Pediatric Oncology Quality of Life Scale. *Psychological Assessment* 1994;**6**:321–328.

33. Phipps S, Dunavant M, Jayawardene D, *et al.* Assessment of health-related quality of life in acute in-patient settings: use of the BASES instrument in children undergoing bone marrow transplantation. *International Journal of Cancer* 1999;**83**: S12, 18–24.

34. Sawyer M, Antoniou G, Toogood I, *et al.* A comparison of parent and adolescent reports describing the health-related quality of life of adolescents treated for cancer. *International Journal of Cancer* 1999;**83**: S12, 39–45.

35. Canning EH, Canning RD, Boyce WT. Depressive symptoms and adaptive style in children with cancer. *Journal of the American Academy of Child and Adolescent Psychiatry* 1992;**31**:1120–1124.

36. Vance YH, Morse RC, Jenney ME, *et al.* Issues in measuring quality of life in childhood cancer: measures, proxies, and parental mental health. *Journal of Child Psychology & Psychiatry & Allied Disciplines* 2001;**42**: 661–667.

37. Challinor JM, Miaskowski CA, Franck LS, *et al.* Somatisation, anxiety and depression as measures of health-related quality of life in children/adolescents with cancer. *International Journal of Cancer* 1999;**83**: S12, 52–57.

38. Worchel FF, Nolan BF, Willson VL, *et al.* Assessment of depression in children with cancer. *Journal of Pediatric Psychology* 1988;**13**:101–112.

39. Parsons SK, Barlow SE, Levy SL, *et al.* Health-related quality of life in pediatric bone marrow transplant survivors: according to whom? *International Journal of Cancer* 1999;**83**: S12, 46–51.

40. Eiser C, Morse R. Can parents rate their child's health related quality of life? *Results of a systematic review. Quality of Life Research* 2001;**10**:347–357.

41. Loonen HJ, Drekx BHHF, Griffiths AM Pediatricians overestimate importance of physical symptoms upon children's health concerns. *Medical Care* 1991;**40**: 996–1001.

42. Cremeens J, Eiser C, Blades M. Factors influencing agreement between child self report and parent proxy-reports on the Pediatric Quality of Life Inventory™ 4.0 (PedsQLTM) Generic Core Scales. *Health and Quality of Life Outcomes* 2006;**4**:1–8.

43. Chang P, Yeh C. Agreement between child self-report and parent proxy-report to evaluate quality of life in children with cancer. *Psycho-Oncology* 2005;**14**:125–134.
44. Speyer E, Herbinet A, Vuillemin A, *et al.* Agreement between children with cancer and their parents in reporting the child's health-related quality of life during a stay at the hospital and at home. *Child: Care, Health and Development* 2009;**35**:489–495.
45. Campo JV, Comer D, Jansen-McWilliams L, *et al.* Recurrent pain, emotional distress, and health service use in childhood. *Journal of Pediatrics* 2002;**141**:76–83.
46. Palmer SN, Meeske KA, Katz ER, *et al.* The Peds-QL™ brain tumor module: initial reliability and validity. *Pediatric Blood & Cancer* 2007;**49**:287–293.
47. Klassen AF, Strohm SJ, Maurice-Stam H, *et al.* Quality of life questionnaires for children with cancer and childhood cancer survivors: a review of the development of available measures. *Support Care Cancer* 2010;**18**:1207–1217.
48. Creeman J, Eiser C, Blades M. Characteristics of health related self-report measures for children aged three to eight years: a review of the literature. *Quality of Life Research* 2006;**15**:739–754.
49. Spieth LE, Harris CV. Assessment of health related quality of life in children and adolescents: an integrative review. *Journal of Pediatric Psychology* 1996;**21**:175–193.
50. Hinds PS, Burghen EA, Haase JE, *et al.* Advances in defining, conceptualizing, and measuring quality of life in pediatric patients with cancer. *Oncology Nursing Forum* 2006;**33**:24–29.
51. Varni JW, Burwinkle TM, Seid M. The PedsQL™ 4. 0 as a school population health measure: feasibility, reliability, and validity. *Quality of Life Research* 2006;**15**:203–215.
52. Kreitler S, Kreitler MM. Quality of life in children with cancer: definition, assessment and results. In: Kreitler S, Weil Ben Arush M (eds.) *Psychosocial Aspects of Pediatric Oncology*. Chichester: John Wiley & Sons, Ltd., 2004; pp. 139–210.
53. Varni J, Burwinkle W, Katz TM, *et al.* The PedsQL™ in pediatric cancer: reliability and validity of the Pediatric Quality of Life Inventory™ Generic Core Scales, Multi-dimensional Fatigue Scale, and Cancer Module. *Cancer* 2002;**94**:2090–2106.
54. Parsons SK, Shih MC, Mayer DK, *et al.* Preliminary psychometric evaluation of the Child Health Ratings Inventory (CHRIs) and Disease-Specific Impairment Inventory-Hematopoietic Stem Cell Transplantation (DSII-HSCT) in parents and children. *Quality of Life Research* 2005;**14**:1613–1625.
55. Bhatia S, Jenney ME, Wu E, *et al.* The Minneapolis-Manchester quality of life instrument: reliability and validity of the youth form. *Journal of Pediatrics* 2004;**145**:39–46.
56. Varni JW, Seid M, Rode CA. The PedsQL™: measurement model for the Pediatric Quality of Life Inventory™ *Medical Care* 1999;**37**:126–139.
57. Lai J, Cella D, Tomita T, *et al.* Developing a health-related quality of life instrument for childhood brain tumor survivors. *Childs Nervous System* 2007;**23**:47–57.
58. Armstrong FD, Toledano SR, Miloslavich K, *et al.* The Miami Pediatric Quality of Life Questionnaire: parent scale. *International Journal of Cancer* 1999;**83**: S12, 11–17.
59. Phipps S, Dunavant M, Gray E, *et al.* Massage therapy in children undergoing hematopoietic stem cell transplant:

results of a pilot trial. *Journal of Cancer Integrated Medicine* 2005;**3**:62–70.
60. Ward-Smith P, McCaskie B, Rhoton S. Adolescent evaluated quality of life: a longitudinal study. *Journal of Pediatric Oncology Nursing* 2007;**24**:329–333.
61. Hutchings HA, Upton P, Cheung WY, *et al.* Development of a parent version of the Manchester-Minneapolis quality of life survey for use by parents and carers of UK children: MMQLUK (PF). *Health Quality Life Outcomes* 2008;**6**:19–26.
62. Feldman SI, Downey G, Schaffer-Neitz R. Pain, negative mood, and perceived support in chronic pain patients: a daily diary study of people with reflex sympathetic dystrophy syndrome. *Journal of Consulting and Clinical Psychology* 1999;**67**:776–785.
63. Yamazaki S, Sokejima S, Mizoue T, *et al.* Health-related quality of life of mothers of children with leukemia in Japan. *Quality of Life Research* 2005;**14**:1079–1085.
64. Kreitler S, Kreitler MM. *The Adult Quality of Life (ADL): Instrument and Manual.* Tel-Aviv, Israel: Psychooncology Unit, Tel-Aviv Medical Center, 2003.
65. Bijttebier P, Vercruysse T, Vertommen H, *et al.* New evidence on the reliability and validity of the Pediatric Oncology Quality of Life Scale. *Psychology and Health* 2001;**16**:461–469.
66. Landgraf JM, Abetz L, Ware JE. *The CHQ: The User's Manual,* 1st edn. Boston, MA: The Health Institute, New England Medical Center, 1996.
67. Mulhern RK, Fairclough DL, Friedman AG, *et al.* Play performance scale as an index of quality of life of children with cancer. *Psychological Assessment* 1990;**2**:149–155.
68. Stephenson RL. Health-related quality of life in pediatric patients with brain tumors. *Dissertation Abstracts International: Section B: The Sciences and Engineering* 2003; **62**:*(8-B)*, 3816.
69. Bhatia S, Jenney MEM, Bogue MK, *et al.* The Minneapolis-Manchester Quality of Life Instrument: reliability and validity of the adolescent form. *Journal of Clinical Oncology* 2002;**20**:4692–4698.
70. Calaminus G, Weinspach S, Teske C, *et al.* Quality of life in children and adolescents with cancer: first results of an evaluation of 49 patients with the PEDQOL questionnaire. *Klinische Pediatrie* 2000;**212**:211–215.
71. Tomlinson D, Hinds PS, Bartels U, *et al.* Parent reports of quality of life for pediatric patients with cancer with no realistic chance of cure. *Journal of Clinical Oncology* 2010;**29**:639–645.
72. Sung L, Yanofsky R, Klaassen RJ, *et al.* Quality of life during active treatment for pediatric acute lymphoblastic leukemia. *International Journal of Cancer* 2011;**128**: 1213–1220.
73. Waters EB, Wake MA, Hesketh KD, *et al.* Health-related quality of life of children with acute lymphoblastic leukemia: comparisons and correlations between parent and clinician reports. *International Journal of Cancer* 2003; **103**:514–518.
74. Guyatt GH. Measuring health-related quality of life in childhood cancer: lessons from the workshop (discussion). *International Journal of Cancer* 1999;**83**: S12, 143–146.
75. Hullmann SE, Wolfe-Christensen C, Meyer WH, *et al.* The relationship between parental overprotection and health-related quality of life in pediatric cancer: the mediating role of perceived child vulnerability. *International Journal of Quality of Life* 2010;**19**:1373–1380.

76. Mannix MM, Feldman JM, Moody K. Optimism and health-related quality of life in adolescents with cancer. *Child: Care, Health and Development* 2009;**35**:482–488.
77. Williams NA, Davis G, Hancock M, *et al.* Optimism and pessimism in children with cancer and healthy children: confirmatory factor analysis of the youth life orientation test and relations with health-related quality of life. *Journal of Pediatric Psychology* 2010;**35**:672–682.
78. Kreitler S. Coping and quality of life in the context of physical diseases. In: Lee AV (ed.) *Coping with Disease.* New York: Nova Biomedical Books, 2005; pp. 81–120.
79. Kreitler S, Kreitler MM. *The Children's Quality of Life (CQL): Instrument and Manual.* Tel-Aviv, Israel: Psychooncology Unit, Tel-Aviv Medical Center, 2003.
80. Eiser C, CotterI, Oades P, *et al.* Health-related quality of life measures for children. *International Journal of Cancer* 1999;**83**:S12, 87–90.

4

Pain in Pediatric Oncology

Richard D. W. Hain

Introduction

Ultimately the aim of all medical intervention is to improve the quality of life. The net value of any intervention must be considered by balancing its benefit against the burden it imposes on the patient. When there is the prospect of cure, it is often justifiable to impose measures that significantly impair the quality of life in the short term for the sake of long-term benefit. Chemotherapy is a good example.

If curative treatment is one way to improve a patient's quality of life, good symptom control is another. A curative and a palliative approach are not in any way mutually exclusive. Rather, the judgment of burden versus benefit is different depending on the stage of treatment. With this in mind, it is clear that there is no point in an illness at which good symptom control has no part to play.

As physicians, we often find it difficult to address problems that have no clear-cut solution. If cure of the disease is the only goal of our involvement with a patient, it is difficult to address issues of symptom control in which the possibility of cure, if any, is only incidental. On the other hand, for the child him- or herself, the immediacy of severe pain may eclipse any consideration of long-term survival.

The purpose of these guidelines is to demonstrate that good symptom control is an active adjunct to curative therapy. It demands the same rigorous and rational approach to assessment and treatment as all other medical interventions. This approach is familiar to doctors and should give them confidence dealing with children when there is little or no chance of cure and the goal of the doctor's involvement has become rather different.

Pain

Even today, pain is a common accompaniment to childhood cancer [1–4]. One rational and common-sense approach to pain in a child has been summarized in the letters "QUEST" [5]. That is: *Q*uestion the child, *U*se pain rating tools, *E*valuate behavior, *S*ensitize parents, and *T*ake action (or *T*reat). This is not very different from the approach we are taught at medical school for the rational diagnosis and management of other medical problems: history, examination, special tests, and treatment.

History

Points to note in the history of pain have been conveniently grouped under the headings "PQRST":

- *P*recipitating and relieving factors
- *Q*uality of pain
- *R*adiation of pain
- *S*everity
- *T*iming

- *Precipitating and relieving factors* can give an indication of cause of pain as well as for management. For example, pain that is experienced only during movement (incident pain) will need a specific management strategy and should lead one to consider the possibility of a pathological fracture.
- *Quality.* The quality of pain is perhaps the most important in making a differential diagnosis. It is usually possible to classify pain as one of the following:
  - *Bone pain.* Bone is characterized by a pain that is very intense and well circumscribed. Typically the patient points to the area with one finger. The pain may be described as "like toothache." Children can be very imaginative in their descriptions and will often use a far wider range of adjectives than their adult counterparts. It is important to consider the context in which the pain is occurring. For example, bony metastasis is common in osteosarcoma but very rare in brain tumors.

Pediatric Psycho-oncology: Psychosocial Aspects and Clinical Interventions, Second Edition.
Edited by Shulamith Kreitler, Myriam Weyl Ben-Arush and Andrés Martin.
© 2012 John Wiley & Sons, Ltd. Published 2012 by John Wiley & Sons, Ltd.

○ *Neuropathic pain*. This is characterized by altered sensation, that is, hyperesthesia (increased sensitivity, including to pain), paresthesia (pins and needles) and numbness. Patients will describe burning, pins and needles, electric shock or lightning pains. Patients will often use a whole hand in sweeping movement to illustrate that the pain is not localized but occurs in a distribution that is often recognizably dermatomal. The context is often tumors pressing on the spinal cord or those that cause bony metastasis in the spinal column itself. Neuropathic pain is also encountered in the soft tissue components of Ewing's and neuroblastoma (these being of neural origin).

- *Radiation*. Neuropathic pain is classically characterized by its radiation in a recognizable distribution. If the distribution is dermatomal, this may be easy to recognize but neuropathic pain may be in a less familiar distribution. For example, tumors that impinge on the coeliac plexus, such as advanced Wilms' or neuroblastoma, can cause a "boring" type pain which radiates from the epigastrium to the back or vice versa. Neuropathic pain may also follow the distribution of the sympathetic nerves, that is to say in a vascular rather than obviously nerve distribution. Bone pain is typically characterized by its very well-circumscribed nature with little or no radiation. However, it is common for many bony pains to occur simultaneously in different locations and this may masquerade as radiation. Children are adept at distinguishing between the same pain occurring in two places, and two different pains. Colicky pain is typically localized to the abdomen, but painful muscle spasms can occur elsewhere and are particularly common in non-malignant pain.

- *Severity*. It is important to make some assessment of the severity of pain in order to judge the effectiveness of an intervention. This is not always easy as children may lack the necessary abstract and verbal skills to rate pain effectively. There are a large number of scales available for children, many of which are modifications of a visual analogue scale (VAS) using faces [6]. Such scales simply ask the patient to select the severity of pain between two extremes, usually 0–10 or 0–100. In order for there to be some kind of fixed anchor point at either end, it is essential to explain beforehand that "0 means no pain at all and 10 represents the worst pain you can imagine."

Children who are too young to express pain may demonstrate it by behavior changes [7]. The child may, for example, adopt a posture that minimizes pain or over time appear to become resigned to it. This syndrome, termed "psychomotor atonia," has been likened to adult depression [8], and measuring it is the basis of an observational pain scale developed in France that is well suited to the management of a child's cancer pain [9, 10].

It is always important to ask those who are with the child all the time—usually the parents—for their opinion. This should only allow a revision of estimates of pain severity upwards. It is not usually appropriate to conclude that a child is overstating the severity of pain, only that he or she is understating it. Ideally, pain scales should be in routine use for all children receiving analgesia of any kind. Realistically, such scales are not yet always practical.

- *Timing*. The timing of pain can give valuable clues as to the cause. For example, abdominal pain that is relieved by defecation is likely to be due to constipation while pain that is at its most severe immediately before attending hospital is likely to have a large psychological component. This in no way argues, of course, that the pain is any less "real"—only that the strategy used to treat it needs to be considered accordingly.

Examination

As always, the examination should be guided by the history. At the end of the history, it should be possible to make a reasonable clinical diagnosis of the nature of the pain and to have a differential diagnosis of the causes. The aims of the examination are:

- to distinguish between the differential diagnoses;
- to exclude related pain problems (for example, other painful metastases that have not been reported);
- to identify factors that might complicate treatment.

The examination itself is no different from other Pediatric examinations. It should start with a global assessment of the child. The site of pain may be immediately obvious if the child adopts an antalgic posture or is simply able to indicate the area of pain. However, the signs may be more subtle. It has been said that a normal child is always sleeping, eating or playing. If the child is doing none of these things, pain may be the explanation. It is rarely possible to distinguish definitively between signs of anxiety and pain. Where pain is likely (either because the child has reported it or simply because knowledge of the clinical context leads one to expect it), it is usually better to assume it than to diagnose anxiety alone. Pain and anxiety are only definitively distinguished by a response to pure analgesics such as opioids. If it later becomes clear that prescribing adequate doses of analgesia has made no difference to the child's clinical state, it is reasonable to assume that pain was not the cause and to review the need for analgesia.

The rest of the examination is guided by the history. If neuropathic pain is considered, it is important to delineate the distribution. This will not only help establish the underlying cause of the pain but may also be important in managing it, for example, if a local nerve block is to be considered. Where the history suggests bone pain, it is particularly important to exclude the possibility of pathological fracture as these require a different therapeutic approach from other causes of bone pain. Colicky pain should prompt careful examination to exclude intestinal obstruction. This is not because surgical intervention will necessarily be appropriate, but because the management of other symptoms, particularly nausea and vomiting, is quite different if it is present. Soft tissue pain should prompt careful examination of the area. Soft tissue pain is common around the site of the tumor itself but may also occur at sites of metastasis, particularly the liver. Again, this is important as the management of pain due to stretching of the capsule around the liver or a tumor is different from other forms of pain.

Lastly, the examination should identify factors that might complicate the management of symptoms. For example, demonstrating severe epigastric pain would suggest that caution will be necessary in prescribing non-steroidal anti-inflammatory drugs.

Investigations

Investigations are often considered inappropriate when there is no longer any prospect of cure. Certainly it is true that the benefit of an investigation (how it will help improve the patient's symptoms) has to be weighed very carefully against the need for the child to come to the hospital and perhaps to undergo venepuncture. However, this is only a special case of something that is always true of medical interventions; that is, that they should only be undertaken when the benefit outweighs the burden. This balance should be carefully considered before undertaking any investigations, but the balance will sometimes mean that they are justified even where palliation is the only aim.

Plain X-Ray

Plain X-rays are usually painless but require the child to attend hospital. During the period of treatment when a cure is still possible, this may be very appropriate but at other times children may choose to avoid all contact with the hospital. In practice, the potential value of a plain X-ray is usually relatively small. Metastases that are symptomatic do not need to be demonstrated; those that cause no symptoms do not need to be treated. The main clinical situation in which a plain X-ray can be very helpful is in distinguishing the pain of a metastasis from that of a pathological fracture; this will have an impact on management and is therefore a real benefit.

Bone Scan

The bone scan is of considerable diagnostic value in demonstrating for the first time that there has been disease progression or metastasis. Once this has been established, however, there is usually little benefit in repeating the procedure. It is uncomfortable and demands a hospital visit. It is not usually necessary to demonstrate the presence of a metastasis if there are clinical signs and symptoms to suggest one. Once again, bony lesions that are symptomatic do not need to be demonstrated radiologically and those that are not require no treatment. Palliative radiation of bone metastases does not usually require them to be demonstrated radiologically.

MRI or CT Scan

These tests are often surprisingly frightening and uncomfortable for children and should be avoided unless there is a good reason. Such good reasons include excluding imminent cord compression or to localize a tumor prior to neurolytic procedure such as coeliac access block. Missing a cord compression can mean a child's being paraplegic for the last weeks or even months of his or her life so that despite being uncomfortable, these scans can be very valuable investigations. MRI and CT can also be required in preparation for palliative radiotherapy.

Blood Tests

Generally speaking, blood tests should be avoided even in patients who have indwelling central lines. For the child, accessing these lines can often be an unpleasant reminder of uncomfortable treatment that has ultimately failed. At the very least, it runs the risk of further medicalizing the child. However, once again there are circumstances under which blood tests can be of value. For example, anemia that is symptomatic may benefit from palliative transfusion and sudden onset of opioid toxicity can be caused by an acute deterioration in renal function which should be demonstrated.

Other Investigations

The exact judgement as to when an investigation becomes justifiable will depend not only on the

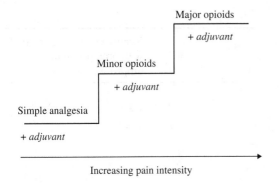

Figure 4.1 The WHO Pain Ladder.

individual situation but on the individual patient. Many continue to see the hospital as a lifeline and welcome evidence that palliative care is an active plan of management. Others prefer to forget they were ever ill and to cut themselves off from the hospital. The important thing is not whether investigations are ordered more or less often for the purposes of symptom control, but that they continue to be ordered appropriately after considering the balance of burden and benefit.

Pain Management

Before the 1980s, management of pain tended to be chaotic and ill-thought through. The World Health Organisation sought to improve the delivery of analgesia by clarifying and simplifying it [11–13]. They did this by means of the concept of the 'Pain Ladder' (Figure 4.1).

While this was developed and validated in adults, the principles on which it was based can be applied to children [14]. They are:

- As pain increases in severity, more powerful analgesia should be offered.
- There is no advantage in exchanging one analgesia for another of similar type and potency. If a previously useful analgesic becomes inadequate, either the dose should be reviewed or a more powerful drug substituted.
- The simplest medication and the oral route should be selected wherever possible.
- Adjuvant therapy (that is, medications that are not usually considered to be analgesics but which become analgesic in certain situations) should be used as soon as a specific diagnosis of pain is made. This means, for example, that NSAID therapy should be instituted as soon as a diagnosis of bone pain is made, rather than waiting until other measures have failed.

- Opioid medication should be given regularly and never only "as needed."
- Breakthrough medication should remain a fixed proportion of the regular medication and always be prescribed simultaneously.

The WHO Pain Ladder

Step 1 (Simple Analgesia)

In pediatrics, the only simple analgesia widely available is paracetamol. In palliative situations, it may sometimes be appropriate to consider using aspirin which is a powerful anti-inflammatory, antipyretic and analgesic.

Step 2 (Minor Opioid)

Minor opioids include codeine, dihydrocodeine and dextropropoxyphene. These are often conveniently combined with paracetamol. This may improve compliance but imposes a ceiling dose as there is a maximum safe daily dose of paracetamol.

In practice, the middle step (minor opioid) is probably unnecessary in children. There is no difference in effect between a large dose of a minor opioid and a small dose of a major opioid. Even in adults there is considerable overlap; in children who are resistant to the effects of opioids and who clear them very quickly, it is often justifiable to go straight from simple analgesia (step 1) to a small dose of a major opioid (step 3).

Step 3 (Major Opioid)

It is the third step in which there is most variety. Morphine is the archetype major opioid and is both effective and relatively non-toxic. Unlike many opioids, the pharmacology of morphine has been studied in children with cancer [15–17]. There have been numerous commercial attempts to develop superior major opioids to morphine, most of which have yet to show a definite advantage over the parent drug. However, a small number of synthetic or semi-synthetic opioids do potentially offer genuine benefits over morphine and some of these are listed in Table 4.1. As a rule of thumb, the best approach is to use morphine orally unless there is a good reason not to.

Patient- (or Nurse-)Controlled Analgesia

Patient-controlled or nurse-controlled analgesia (P(N) CA) is used in palliative care in children, particularly in Oceania and North America. Rather than being seen as contradictory to the WHO approach [18], P(N) CA should properly be seen simply as another route

Table 4.1 Conversion of common major opioids in children.

Opioid	Advantage over morphine	Relative potency compared with oral morphine (approx)
Morphine		
Diamorphine (po)	More soluble	1.5
Fentanyl (patch)	Patch formulation	100
	Less constipation	
	Less itch (?)	
	Less retention (?)	
	Suitable for opioid rotation	
Buprenorphine (patch)	Patch formulation (available at low dose)	40–60
	Less constipation	
Methadone (po)	Possible anti-neuropathic activity	Variable – seek specialist advice
	Suitable for opioid rotation	
Hydromorphone (po)	Greater potency	5–7.5
	Suitable for opioid rotation	
Pethidine	None	0.125
Tramadol (non-opioid)	None, but often preferred by patients anxious about taking major opioids	0.25 (but additional non-opioid analgesic mechanisms)
Oxycodone	Probably none (though anti-neuropathic activity has been suggested), but more easily available than morphine in some countries.	1
	Suitable for opioid rotation.	

that can be used to deliver the WHO approach. It offers advantages of convenience and immediacy that, for most children, largely offset the need for additional needles and equipment. If P(N)CA is used, it is critically important that background and breakthrough doses are adequate, and in line with correct use of opioids in palliative care. Otherwise, there is a risk that children will need to experience pain before they can access analgesia, in contravention of the WHO guidelines.

Practical Application

There are essentially three phases in managing a child's pain:

(1) Choosing a starting dose.
(2) Finding the right dose (titration).
(3) Maintenance of analgesia.

Choosing a Starting Dose

The starting point on the WHO pain ladder must depend on a clinical assessment, as outlined above. In selecting a starting dose for a major opioid, one of two approaches can be taken. Either an empiric starting point can be selected (usually the equivalent of 0.5–1mg/kg/day of oral morphine) or a conversion can be made from existing opioid requirements using conversions in Table 4.2. The most appropriate approach is usually the one that will result in the higher dose of opioid.

A prescription of both *regular* and *breakthrough* dose must be made.

Regular Medication

Having established the dose, the starting opioid should usually be immediate release morphine 4-hourly by mouth. Rarely, it may be preferable to commence

Table 4.2 Principles of symptom management in children.

1   All pain is multidimensional, having physical, psychosocial and existential (spiritual) aspects.

2   Pain is subjective: "It is what the child says it is."

3   Management of pain should be rational, based on an understanding of the pathophysiology of pain and of the underlying condition after systematic history, examination and investigation. However, it should also be empirical; if something works, use it and if it doesn't, reconsider.

4   Like all medical interventions, palliative maneuvers should be undertaken only when the benefit outweighs the burden in the individual child. Appropriate weight needs to be given to non-physical aspects, both of burden and benefit, in making this judgment, particularly in the palliative phase.

immediately on parenteral opioids (usually subcutaneous diamorphine or transdermal fentanyl, see Table 4.1).

Breakthrough Medication

The dose of breakthrough medication is calculated simply by prescribing the regular 4-hourly dose of immediate release morphine and prescribing the same dose PRN. Children appear to clear morphine more quickly than adults and it is a common practice to prescribe half the 4-hourly dose but increase the frequency to 2-hourly PRN. Usually medication for breakthrough pain should be the same as that for regular pain. However, there is sometimes an advantage in using two different formulations. For example, children having a fentanyl patch for regular analgesia will prefer to have oral morphine for breakthrough than fentanyl, which is currently only available as an injection.

Finding the Right Dose (Titration)

The primary purpose of breakthrough medication is to ensure adequate analgesia during the period of assessment of the correct dose of opioids. A secondary purpose, however, is to provide an indirect measure of the child's experience of pain. It is therefore very important to encourage the child and/or parents to administer breakthrough medication as soon as there is any sign of pain. Unless this is clearly articulated to the child's family, his or her requirements for analgesia will almost always be underestimated.

The requirements for breakthrough pain should ideally be reviewed after 48 hours. If there have been two or more requirements for breakthrough pain in each 24-hour period, the regular dose should be increased by the amount of breakthrough that has been required. To do these calculations, all doses should be converted to milligram equivalents of oral morphine (Table 4.1).

It is sometimes necessary to titrate more quickly. Where possible, this should be avoided as it typically takes 48 hours for the full effect of any modification of the regular dose to become apparent. Too rapid an escalation of opioid dose can cause intolerable adverse effects which can jeopardize future symptom management by causing the patient to lose confidence in the medications.

Adverse Effects

Morphine is a well-tried and trusted medication. The adverse effects are few and well recognized. Fortunately, the body develops tolerance to many of these effects well before the analgesic effectiveness of morphine is lost. The following are side effects of morphine:

(1) *Drowsiness.* During the first 48 hours of opioid therapy, or following an increase in opioid dose, drowsiness is universal. This will resolve spontaneously with no modification of the dose and it is important to warn the patient and family that it will occur. It is caused partly by the direct central effect of morphine but also by the relief of pain which can sometimes allow sleep for the first time in many weeks.

(2) *Constipation.* Constipation is one of the adverse effects for which no tolerance develops. A stimulant laxative should always be prescribed. Lactulose is not appropriate for this purpose as it is mainly osmotic. A combination of senna and magnesium hydroxide, or codanthrusate in the palliative phase should be considered. Oral opioid antagonists have been used [19]. Alternatively, constipation may be an indication to change to an alternative opioid (see Table 4.3).

(3) *Urinary hesitancy.* Urinary retention and hesitancy appear anecdotally to be more common in children than in adults. It is still relatively unusual, but if it occurs is an indication to consider an alternative

Table 4.3 Adjuvant therapies in management of pain in children.

Physical pain	Characteristic	Suggested adjuvants
Neuropathic pain	Altered sensation (numbness, dysaesthesia, hyperaesthesia, paraesthesia), weakness, characteristic distribution	Tricyclic antidepressants
		Anticonvulsants
		Steroids in first 48 hours
		Radiotherapy
		Neurolytic procedures
Bone pain	Severe, well-circumscribed "like toothache,", in context of metastatic cancer	Radiotherapy (local)
		Non-steroidal anti-inflammatory drugs
Colicky pain	Constipation	Anticholinergics
	Malignant obstruction	
Incident pain	Worse on movement	Reduce movement (eg immobilize pathological fracture).
		Parenteral opioids 20 mins before procedure
		Entonox

Note: most pains are at least partially opioid responsive. Adjuvants should accompany rather than replace appropriate opioid therapy.

opioid, particularly fentanyl which is a synthetic opioid and appears much less likely to cause the problem.

(4) *Pruritus.* Again, skin itching as a result of histamine release from mast cells that have been directly activated by the morphine molecule, is much more common in children than in adults. It is still rare. Antihistamines and topical preparations such as calamine can be very helpful but once again this is probably an indication to select an alternative from a different class, such as fentanyl.

(5) *Nausea and vomiting.* Nausea and vomiting due to opioids in children are distinctly unusual. There is usually no need to prescribe prophylactic antiemetics. If they do occur, the most effective antiemetics are ondansetron or other $5HT_3$ or dopamine D_2 antagonists.

(6) *Dysphoria.* Dysphoria is relatively uncommon in children but may simply be under-reported. It is often transient and self-limiting but, again, fentanyl may be a suitable alternative if it is difficult to treat.

Maintaining Analgesia

The result of titration should be a clear idea of what the patient's immediate analgesia needs are. Clearly, as the disease progresses, it may be necessary to increase the dose of opioids. However, this is not universal and the complex and multidimensional nature of pain means that despite disease progression opioid requirements sometimes even decrease [1]. The process of reviewing 48-hourly requirements for breakthrough should therefore continue. This relies on good record keeping so that the health care professional (usually doctor or nurse) advising on prescription can see exactly how much has been required. It is unlikely that regular medication will be able to provide complete pain relief and it is acceptable for a patient to require breakthrough medication once every day, or even occasionally twice. Again, it is often helpful to make the child and family aware of this before embarking on therapy.

Once the dose of opioid has become clear, the next stage is to simplify its prescription. Morphine is conveniently available as slow release (MST). In adults, the dosage interval is 12-hourly and the starting dose interval in children should be the same. However, a large proportion of children require a smaller interval than this [20], and it is often necessary to change the dosing interval to 8-hourly. Once daily preparations of slow release morphine are also available, though not licensed in children.

Fentanyl patches offer numerous potential advantages over morphine for some children (see Table 4.1).

The patches are designed to last for 72 hours but, again, the more rapid clearance of opioids in children means that this not uncommonly needs to be reduced to 48 hourly. The conversion from morphine dose to fentanyl patch is given in the product insert. Calculating the conversion without this is complex. The "size" of the patch that is usually quoted refers not to the total amount of drug in the patch but to the hourly rate of fentanyl delivered by it. Other fentanyl formulations are also available [21, 22], though research is on adults.

Non-Opioid and Adjuvant Therapy

It has already been seen that a rational and analytical approach to the history and examination of a child in pain should mean that some attempt can be made to categorize it. An alternative and very practical way to categorize pain is into opioid-sensitive, opioid-partially sensitive, and opioid-resistant. These three categories obviously represent points on a spectrum. The clinician should consider pain under these headings at the same time as considering the diagnostic category of the pain. The two systems are linked but are not the same. For example, neuropathic pain is typically relatively resistant to treatment with opioids but the individual child with neuropathic pain may nevertheless experience great relief from opioid therapy.

The WHO Guidelines suggest that once a diagnosis of pain is made, an appropriate adjuvant therapy should be used [11–13]. The use of such adjuvants does not replace the rest of the pain ladder—simple analgesia, minor opioid, major opioid—but proceeds in parallel with it. For example, as soon as a diagnosis of bone pain is made, non-steroidals should be considered even if the severity of the pain warrants only simple analgesia. In other words, the selection of an adjuvant is on the basis of the nature of the pain rather than just the severity of it. It is worth emphasizing that even in pain that is only partially sensitive to opioids, few adjuvants can offer the chance of good analgesia provided by morphine.

Adjuvants

A drug that is not usually considered to be an analgesic, but can provide pain relief in certain situations, is termed an "adjuvant" medication. Some drugs in this category have, in fact, been shown to have analgesic properties in their own right, for example, non-steroidal anti-inflammatory drugs (NSAID).

Bone Pain

The classical adjuvant for bone pain are the non-steroidal anti-inflammatory drugs (NSAIDs), though evidence for their use in children with cancer is unclear [14]. The side effect profile in children, even of stronger NSAID such as diclofenac [23] appears to be very good. Most children experience no adverse effects. Others experience mild gastrointestinal upset, which resolves spontaneously, without a need for a change in dose. Where adverse effects are more persistent and mean that the child is unable to tolerate them, enteric-coated preparations are available. It is probably prudent to prescribe proton blockers such as omeprazole if non-steroidals are co-prescribed with steroids for more than a few days. All non-steroidal anti-inflammatory drugs inhibit platelet aggregation through their effect on the cyclo-oxygenase system and should be used with caution in children with a low platelet count or defective coagulation. H_2 blockers such as ranitidine may be useful in managing established gastrointestinal irritation but appear to be of little or no help in prophylaxis.

All children with bone pain due to proven or probable metastatic disease should be assessed for radiotherapy. A small, localized dose of radiation as a single fraction can often provide lasting relief of symptoms with little or no side effects. It is therefore worth considering even in relatively radio-resistant tumors such as osteosarcoma.

Neuropathic Pain

Neuropathic pain is usually at least partially opioid responsive. The pain is typically caused by compression or outright damage of a peripheral nerve, for example, by tumor at the spinal cord. Within the first 48 hours of the onset of neuropathic pain, compression can be relieved with the use of steroids (dexamethasone is the most widely used in palliative care, see section 'Liver Capsular Pain' below). This may be enough to convert an opioid-resistant to an opioid-sensitive pain. For pain of longer duration, it is likely that actual nerve damage has occurred and that steroids will be ineffective. Anti-depressants are effective in management of neuropathic pain [24], but anticonvulsants such as gabapentin and pregabalin are often the first line in palliative medicine [25].

Drugs that interfere with the n-methyl D-aspartate system are also effective in relieving neuropathic pain. They have a particular role in managing phantom limb pain and the "wind up phenomenon" in which chronic exposure to repeated painful procedures leads to ever increasing sensation of pain on each occasion. Of these, ketamine is the one most often used in children. Methadone is unusual among opioids in possessing additional NMDA blocking activity [26] which might make it ideal for neuropathic pain. Despite its idiosyncratic pharmacology [27–29], methadone has been extensively used in pediatric palliative medicine [30] without incident. Nevertheless, good practice is that it should be treated with caution.

Episodic Pain

The difficulty in managing episodic pain is that a dose of analgesic that is adequate for pain at its worst is likely to be too toxic for pain at its least. Breakthrough morphine is often ineffective for severe episodic pain, since the time taken for it to reach its effective serum levels means that the pain has subsided before the medication can work.

Pain may be episodic for three reasons. The dose of regular medication may be too small, resulting in intermittent breakthrough pain for which the solution is to review the regular medication. The cause of the pain may be episodic, for example, pain from a pathological fracture of from some bone metastases can be provoked by movement ("incident pain"). Management of the underlying lesion (for example, using radiotherapy), and identifying and avoiding the provoking factors (for example, by immobilization of a fracture) may be practical. Anticipating the need for breakthrough medications before painful procedures can be helpful if it is impossible to avoid them. Rapid-acting analgesics such as Entonox, or buccal, sublingual or parenteral opioids [31, 32] moderate but rarely abolish procedure-related pain [33].

Finally, the pain may simply be of an episodic nature, for example, intestinal colic or muscle spasm. The pain from intestinal colic can be excruciating but is typically short-lived. Where possible, the frequency of colic spasms should be reduced. Pain caused by muscle spasm is relatively unusual in the context of cancer, though it is a common problem among other life-limiting diseases such as cerebral palsy. It may respond to benzodiazepines or anti-spasmodics such as baclofen.

P(N)CA can be particularly useful in episodic pain; arranging for the child or parent to be able to administer the analgesia, rather than having to wait for a health care professional to do so, allows a sense of control as well as minimizing the lag period between experiencing pain and experiencing relief.

Psychological Components to Pain

Properly speaking, the syndrome of "total pain" describes all pain. It embodies the concept that the physical, nociceptive aspect is only one factor among many in determining the degree of discomfort caused by the pain. Thus, the pain of an ankle injury acquired during a game of football is very different from the pain of the same intensity when relapsed osteosarcoma is the proven or even the suspected cause.

However, total pain is often used to describe those pains in which the psychological, emotional and existential elements of the pain are such that analgesics alone are unlikely to provide adequate analgesia. Ideally, these aspects should be dealt with by discussion, exploration and where necessary support from pastoral or psychology services. In practice, it is often necessary to supplement these with medications that have some influence on the psyche. Depression is typically underdiagnosed in childhood, but anxiety is more common. This can be moderated with careful use antidepressants or anxiolytics alongside psychological intervention. Further details about these and other drugs useful in the management of depression and anxiety are provided in Chapter 11 (Pinsky and Abrams).

Liver Capsular Pain

Liver capsular pain is characterized by severe pain in the right upper quadrant of the abdomen. It occurs in the context of metastatic disease, particularly neuroblastoma, Wilm's or osteosarcoma where spread to the liver is relatively common, and is often accompanied by nausea and vomiting.

Like most pains, it is usually at least partially sensitive to opioids but adjuvant therapy using steroids is often helpful (dexamethasone orally). Anecdotally, it is best given in two divided doses, one at 6.00 and one at 12.00 md to minimize mood and sleep disturbance. The adverse effects of long-term steroids mean that for most indications their use in children should be restricted to five-day courses. The course can if necessary be repeated if symptoms recur.

Neurolytic Procedures

Some forms of neuropathic pain can respond well to carefully performed infusion of local anesthetic or even permanent blockade using phenol. This requires great expertise and the services of a specialized pediatric anesthesiologist. Since the procedure involves both needles and general anesthetic, it is less often used in treating pain in children than in adults. Epidurals are much more readily available in children and can be very helpful in the management of pain in the lower limbs unresponsive to other modalities, particularly where mobility is not an issue.

Conclusion

The clinical evidence is accumulating that major opioids can be used safely and effectively in children with moderate to severe pain. They should be used as part of a rational approach to the diagnosis, assessment and management of pain. The WHO pain ladder gives a straightforward structure to such an approach and is recommended to all those who wish to approach the management of a child with pain.

The evolution of clinical expertise and experience has been paralleled and supported by an expansion of the research evidence base. This seems to show that, where children differ from adults in their handling of morphine, the result is that they are more resilient rather than more sensitive to its effects.

Good symptom control should be seen as an active intervention which at different stages in the progress of a disease will complement or replace potentially curative interventions. Like them, interventions for symptom control should be a judicious mix of the empirical and the evidence-based but should always be rigorously rational.

References

1. Goldman, A, Hewitt M, Collins GS, et al. Symptoms in children/young people with progressive malignant disease: United Kingdom Children's Cancer Study Group/ Pediatric Oncology Nurses Forum survey. Pediatrics 2006;117:e1179–e1186.
2. Hendricks-Ferguson V.Physical symptoms of children receiving pediatric hospice care at home during the last week of life.Oncology Nursing Forum2008;35:e108–e115.
3. Jalmsell L, Kreicbergs U, Onelov E, et al. Symptoms affecting children with malignancies during the last month of life: a nationwide follow-up. Pediatrics 2006;117:1314–1320.
4. Pritchard M, Burghen E, Srivastava DK, et al. Cancer-related symptoms most concerning to parents during the last week and last day of their child's life. Pediatrics 2008;121:e1301–e1309.
5. Baker CM, Wong DL. QUEST: a process of pain assessment in children. Orthopaedic Nursing 1987;6:11–21.
6. Tomlinson D, von Baeyer CL, Stinson JN, Sung L. A systematic review of faces scales for the self-report of pain intensity in children. Pediatrics 2008;126:e1168–e1198.
7. von Baeyer CL, Spagrud LJ. Systematic review of observational (behavioral) measures of pain for children and adolescents aged 3 to 18 years. Pain 2007;127:140–150.
8. Gauvain-Piquard A, Rodary C, Lemerle J. L'atonie psychomotrice: signe majeur de douleur chez l'enfant de moins de 6 ans. Journées parisiennes de pédiatrie 1988;5:249–252.
9. Gauvain-Piquard A, Rodary C, Rezvani A, Serbouti S. The development of the DEGR(R): a scale to assess pain in young children with cancer. European Journal of Pain 1999;3:165–176.
10. Gauvain-Piquard A, Rodary C, François, RA, et al. Validity assessment of DEGR scale for observational rating of 2–6 year old child pain. Journal of Pain Symptom Management 1991;6:171.
11. Ventafridda V, Tamburini M, Caraceni A, et al. A validation study of the WHO method for cancer pain relief. Cancer 1989; 856.
12. World Health, Organisation. Cancer as a Global Problem. Geneva: WHO, 1984.
13. World Health, Organisation. Guidelines for analgesic drug therapy. In: Cancer Pain Relief and Palliative Care in Children. Geneva: WHO/IASP, 1998; pp. 24–28.
14. Zernikow B, Smale H, Michel E, et al. Pediatric cancer pain management using the WHO analgesic ladder: results of a prospective analysis from 2265 treatment days during a quality improvement study. European Journal of Pain 2006;10:587–595.
15. Hain RD, Hardcastle A, Pinkerton CR, Aherne GW. Morphine and morphine-6-glucuronide in the plasma and cerebrospinal fluid of children. British Journal of Clinical Pharmacology 1999;48:37–42.
16. Mashayekhi SO, Ghandforoush-Sattari M, Routledge PA, Hain RD. Pharmacokinetic and pharmacodynamic study of morphine and morphine 6-glucuronide after oral and intravenous administration of morphine in children with cancer. Biopharmaceutics and Drug Disposition 2009;30:99–106.
17. Mashayekhi SO, Hain RD, Buss DC, Routledge PA. Morphine in children with cancer: impact of age, chemotherapy and other factors on protein binding. Journal of Pain and Palliative Care Pharmacotherapy 2007;21:5–12.
18. Vargas-Schaffer G. Is the WHO analgesic ladder still valid? Twenty-four years of experience. Canadian Family Physician 2010;56:514–517, e202–e205.
19. Healy R. Effectiveness of two opioid antagonists in treating opioid-induced constipation. British Journal of Nursing 2009;18:998–1002.
20. Hunt TL, Kaiko RF. Comparison of the pharmacokinetic profiles of two oral controlled- release morphine formulations in healthy young adults. Clinical Therapeutics 1991;13 (4): 482–488.
21. Droney J, Riley J. Recent advances in the use of opioids for cancer pain. Journal of Pain Research 2009;2: 135–155.
22. Zeppetella G. Sublingual fentanyl citrate for cancer-related breakthrough pain: a pilot study. Palliative Medicine 2001;15:323–328.
23. Standing JF, Savage I, Pritchard D, Waddington M. Diclofenac for acute pain in children. Cochrane Database of Systematic Reviews 2009;4:CD005538.
24. Saarto T, Wiffen PJ. Antidepressants for neuropathic pain. Cochrane Database of Systematic Reviews 2007;4: CD005454.
25. Mishra S, Bhatnagar S, Gupta D, Nirwani Goyal G, Jain R, Chauhan H. Management of neuropathic cancer pain following WHO analgesic ladder: a prospective study. American Journal of Hospital Palliaive Care 2008;25: 447–451.
26. Stringer M, Makin MK, Miles J, Morley JS. D-morphine, but not l-morphine, has low micromolar affinity for the non-competitive N-methyl-D-aspartate site in rat forebrain: possible clinical implications for the management of neuropathic pain. Neuroscience Letters 2000;295: 21–24.
27. Lugo RA, Satterfield KL, Kern SE. Pharmacokinetics of methadone. Journal of Pain and Palliative Care Pharmacotherapy 2005;19:13–24.

28. Nicholson A. Methadone for cancer pain. *Cochrane Database of Systematic Reviews* 2006;**4**. DOI: 10.1002/14651858. CD003971.pub3.

29. Shaiova L, Berger A, Blinderman CD, *et al.* Consensus guideline on parenteral methadone use in pain and palliative care. *Palliative Support Care* 2008;**6**:165–176.

30. Davies D, DeVlaming D, Haines C. Methadone analgesia for children with advanced cancer. *Pediatric Blood & Cancer* 2008;**51**:393–397.

31. Mercadante S, Radbruch L, Caraceni A, *et al.* Episodic (breakthrough) pain: consensus conference of an expert working group of the European Association for Palliative Care. *Cancer* 2002;**94**:832–839.

32. Mercadante S, Villari P, Ferrera P, *et al.* Safety and effectiveness of intravenous morphine for episodic breakthrough pain in patients receiving transdermal buprenorphine. *Journal of Pain and Symptom Management* 2006;**32**:175–179.

33. Martin JP, Sexton BF, Saunders BP, Atkin WS. Inhaled patient-administered nitrous oxide/oxygen mixture does not impair driving ability when used as analgesia during screening flexible sigmoidoscopy. *Gastrointestinal Endoscience* 2000;**51**:701–703.

5

Psychiatric Impact of Childhood Cancer

Margaret L. Stuber

Introduction

In the United States, childhood cancer is almost always treated in large pediatric oncology centers. The American Academy of Pediatrics (AAP) has had specific guidelines regarding treatment facilities for childhood cancer since 1986. These were updated in 1997 and in 2004, with a reaffirmation of the 2004 guidelines in 2009. These most recent guidelines include the direction that pediatric cancer should be managed using the types of "facilities available only at a tertiary center" [1]. The list of personnel who should be a part of a pediatric oncology treatment center includes

Board-certified pediatric subspecialists available to participate actively in all areas of the care of the child with cancer, including anesthesiology, intensive care, infectious diseases, cardiology, neurology, endocrinology and metabolism, genetics, gastroenterology, *child and adolescent psychiatry*, nephrology, and pulmonology.

(emphasis added; [1], p. 1833)

The AAP guideline also states that the "pediatric hematologist/oncologist must be assisted by skilled nurses, social workers, pharmacists, nutritionists, and psychologists who specialize in pediatric oncology" ([1], p. 1834). Thus it is expected that children with cancer and their parents should have access to clinical social workers, psychologists, and child and adolescent psychiatrists.

Along with these more stringent guidelines has come a greatly improved prognosis for pediatric cancer [2]. Long-term survival of over 80% for most childhood cancers has changed the primary focus of psychiatric concern from dying and bereavement to issues of coping and survivorship. However, some life threat remains, and the intensity of this more successful treatment (and subsequent toxicity) is significant. This chapter will examine the psychiatric impact of cancer on children and their families. The chapter will start, as does the child or adolescent, with diagnosis and treatment, and then consider the long-term psychiatric sequelae of childhood cancer and its treatment. The chapter ends with a consideration of the types of intervention which have been found useful and future directions for research.

Diagnosis and Treatment

The diagnosis of a malignancy is difficult for any child, adolescent, or parent. Despite medical progress, the word cancer conjures up mental images of bald heads, emaciated bodies, vomiting, suffering, and death. Over time and with experience and education, most families learn to differentiate between what they have seen in the movies and what they are facing. The majority of families are impressively resilient [3]. In this section we will consider some of the types of psychiatric issues that are commonly encountered in the acute phase of the cancer experience.

Anxiety

One of the most commonly observed psychiatric symptoms in the acute phase of cancer diagnosis and treatment is anxiety. Most of this anxiety is situational and does not meet diagnostic criteria for a specific syndrome. Specific types of anxiety include:

- *Separation anxiety*, defined as a "developmentally inappropriate and excessive anxiety concerning separation from home or from those to whom the individual is attached" [4]. Younger children, children who have not been away from home overnight before, or children with pre-existing anxiety disorders are more likely to develop symptoms of separation anxiety. Common symptoms include nightmares about separation from their parents and home, intrusive thoughts that a loved one (usually parent) is in

Pediatric Psycho-oncology: Psychosocial Aspects and Clinical Interventions, Second Edition.
Edited by Shulamith Kreitler, Myriam Weyl Ben-Arush and Andrés Martin.
© 2012 John Wiley & Sons, Ltd. Published 2012 by John Wiley & Sons, Ltd.

danger, and physical symptoms of anxiety such as headaches, abdominal pain or nausea.

- *Acute Stress Disorder (ASD)* is a physiological and emotional response to an event that involved actual or threatened death or injury, and elicited an immediate response of intense fear, horror, or helplessness [4]. Like Posttraumatic Stress Disorder (PTSD), ASD includes symptoms of hyperarousal (elevated heart rate, amplified startle responses, hypervigilance), avoidance of reminders, and intrusive thoughts of the event that was traumatic. ASD differs from PTSD in three ways: (1) it is time-limited (no less than 2 days, no more than 4 weeks); (2) it is acute (within 4 weeks of the traumatic event); and (3) it involves dissociative amnesia, numbing, depersonalization, derealization, or a feeling of being dazed. In children ASD may be manifested by agitated and disorganized behavior, particularly in response to a perceived threat. Children and adolescents with pre-existing anxiety disorders are at higher risk for both ASD and PTSD. Given the overlap in symptoms, ASD can be mistaken for depression, anxiety or delirium. Indeed, a study comparing 76 medically ill children to 31 otherwise traumatized children found that a commonly used screening tool, the UCLA PTSD Index for DSM-IV [5], was not as effective in diagnosing PTSD in the medically ill children as in the otherwise traumatized children. The study suggested that intrusion symptoms were of most utility when assessing PTSD in medically ill children [6].
- *Phobias* are intense and unreasonable fears of specific objects or situations, even when they do not pose any immediate danger. Most of what people may see as a phobic response in a medical setting is better understood as a conditioned response (such as vomiting in response to the smell of chemotherapy) or a response to traumatic reminders (elevated heart rate and agitation when someone in a white coat enters the room). With children it is also not uncommon for the fear to appear reasonable within the context of their understanding of the world. For example, a 4-year-old who has no concept of blood vessels may truly believe he is exsanguinating when an IV comes out.

Delirium

Delirium is a fluctuating neuropsychiatric disorder due to encephalopathy. This type of brain disturbance often reflects an electrolyte imbalance, drug toxicity, or end-organ failure, and is a bad prognostic sign when seen in hospitalized patients. The symptoms of impaired alertness, apathy, anxiety, disorientation, and hallucinations appear to be similar in adults and children with delirium. However, a recent comparison found that sleep–wake disturbance, fluctuating symptoms, impaired attention, irritability, agitation, affective lability, and confusion were more commonly observed in children, while impaired memory, depressed mood, speech disturbance, delusions, and paranoia were more often seen in adults [7].

Diagnosis of delirium in infants and very young children is particularly challenging [8]. The Pediatric Anesthesia Emergence Delirium Scale (PAED) appears to have promise. A study of 184 patients in the pediatric intensive care unit, aged 1–17 years, monitored over $3\frac{1}{2}$ years, found that the survey could be successfully administered to 93.5% of the patients and had a sensitivity of 91% and a specificity of 98% (AUC 0.99) compared to the "gold standard" clinical interview [9].

Although delirium in the adult is a significant concern, the literature on delirium in children is still quite limited. A review published in 2010 explored the literature from 1980 to March 2009, and found data on only 217 child and adolescent patients with definite delirium and 136 with "probable delirium" [10]. In one of the largest series, 1027 consecutive psychiatric consultations over four years yielded a diagnosis of delirium in 84 patients between the ages of 6 months and 18 years. Mortality among these patients was 20% (high compared to the norm) and length of hospital stay was prolonged. Of the children with delirium, 7% had cancer [11].

Depression

It is surprisingly difficult to determine whether or not a medically ill child is depressed [6]. Common symptoms of depression, such as alterations in sleep or appetite can be attributed to the illness or treatment. Boredom and conservation of energy can be mistaken for anhedonia. Chemotherapy-related fatigue can produce symptoms of decreased energy, lack of interest in previously enjoyed activities, and social withdrawal. Despite these problems, recent studies have found that it is possible to distinguish between chemotherapy-related fatigue and depression, so as to proceed with the appropriate intervention [12]. There is also evidence that self-report measures can be used to identify children who need interventions for depression. In a study of 125 medically ill children aged 8–19 years, the Children's Depression Inventory was compared to semi-structured diagnostic interviews. Using a cutoff of 11 and above correctly identified 80% of those with depression, with a specificity of 70% [6]. This is a lower cutoff score than is commonly used in general populations, which is either 13 or 20, depending on the sensitivity required [13]. A study of 41 adolescents on active cancer treatment who were administered the Beck Youth Inventory II (BYI II) Depression and Anxiety scales found that only three patients were in the moderate or extremely elevated range for depression, and only two in the moderate or extremely elevated range for anxiety, compared to published norms [14].

Long-Term Issues for Survivors

In addition to the acute toxicities of treatment, clinicians have found a number of health problems which emerge five to ten years after successful pediatric cancer treatment ends [15]. These are called "late effects". Two of every three childhood cancer survivors will develop at least one late-onset therapy-related complication. One quarter of these complications are severe or life-threatening [16]. These health risks are related to the age of treatment, and the specific therapeutic modalities used [17]. As a result, the Children's Oncology Group (COG), which coordinates the treatment protocols and outcome data collection for childhood cancer centers across the United States, has organized exposure-based health screening guidelines [16]. These help optimize long-term outcomes by successfully monitoring for and treating the late effects that may occur as a result of previous cancer therapies.

Psychological Distress and Quality of Life

Historically, studies of the quality of life (including psychiatric issues) for long-term childhood cancer survivors have been inconsistent in their findings, due to use of a variety of measures, small samples, and variability in diagnosis and treatment. A review of all studies using quantitative measures and statistical tests to compare health-related quality of life (HRQL) or QOL of childhood cancer survivors with population norms or matched comparison groups found only 13 papers published in English between 2001 and 2008. There were few differences noted, other than in the domain of physical well-being [18]. A review of 1734 studies examining the psychosocial impact of childhood cancer treatment found 19 meeting inclusion criteria. The review found that both positive and negative outcomes were reported. Survivors reported lower psychological well-being, mood, liveliness, self-esteem, and motor and physical functioning, as well as increased anxiety, problem behaviors, and sleeping difficulties. Survivors also reported high self-worth, good behavioral conduct, and improved mental health and social behavior [19].

A recent study comparing 167 childhood cancer survivors to 170 healthy controls found no statistically significant difference between survivors and controls in terms of psychological distress or health-related quality of life, although survivors did endorse less adaptive health beliefs [20]. A study of 73 long-term (mean 20 years off-therapy) survivors of childhood acute lymphoblastic leukemia compared to 146 healthy controls found that the survivors were significantly less likely to report symptoms of depression on the Beck Depression Inventory than controls. There were no significant differences between survivors and controls on a General Health Questionnaire assessment of mental distress [21].

However, there has been some speculation that these comforting findings may reflect a response bias on the part of cancer survivors. A study of 107 adult (mean age 31.85) survivors of childhood cancer found quality of life ratings to be similar to normative groups. However, the survivors scored significantly higher on the Self-Deception Enhancement Scale (SDE) than norms. The SDE was significantly correlated with the scores on the two quality of life measures. This suggests a systematic tendency to under-report difficulties [22].

The Childhood Cancer Survivor Study (CCSS) has attempted to answer some of these questions in a more definitive manner by using a national sample of long-term childhood cancer survivors. The CCSS is a longitudinal cohort study that tracks the health status of survivors of childhood cancer diagnosed between 1970 and 1986 and treated at collaborating centers across the United States and Canada. This study, funded by the National Cancer Institute over the past 15 years, has greatly improved our understanding of long-term survival after childhood cancer. The initial sample included 20,691 long-term survivors of childhood cancer identified for the original cohort. Even with 3,058 (14.8%) lost to follow-up, this has provided data on many issues having to do with survival of childhood cancer [23].

A CCSS study of psychological quality of life, health-related quality of life (HRQOL) and life satisfaction found that a significant proportion of survivors reported more symptoms of global distress and scored lower in the physical but not emotional domains of HRQOL. With the exception of brain tumor survivors, most survivors report both good present and expected future life satisfaction. Psychological distress and poor HRQOL were positively correlated with female sex, lower educational attainment, unmarried status, annual household income less than $20,000, unemployment, lack of health insurance, presence of a major medical condition, and treatment with cranial radiation and/or surgery [24]. Ethnicity does not appear to be significantly predictive of psychological distress. The only difference noted in a comparison of mental health outcomes in the CCSS date was that survivors who self-identified as black were less likely to report adverse mental health outcomes [17].

Posttraumatic Growth, Perceived Positive Impact, and Benefit Finding

Studies like those described above have made clinicians and researchers skeptical about papers reporting that survivors perceived some positive changes after the cancer experience which were associated with a higher perceived positive quality of life. [25]. Survivors reported improvements in the way they treat others and make friends, the way their family and others treat them, the quality of their schoolwork and behavior, and their plans for the future [26]. This kind of positive change out of adversity is sometimes conceptualized as posttraumatic growth, in which a traumatic event changes a person's view of life, resulting in personal growth. It has also been conceptualized as benefit finding. A study of the revised Benefit/Burden Scale for Children (BBSC) with 79 children with cancer found that reported burden of the cancer was orthogonal to reported benefits of the cancer [27].

A recent Japanese study compared 185 survivors of childhood cancer (in remission for at least one year) to 1000 healthy controls in depression, anxiety, posttraumatic stress and posttraumatic growth. The survivors in this study were approximately 8 years old at diagnosis and approximately 23 years old at the time of the survey. There were no significant differences between the survivors and controls in terms of depression and anxiety, but survivors reported significantly both more posttraumatic stress and posttraumatic growth than controls [28].

A study from the Childhood Cancer Survivors Study (CCSS) examined Perceived Positive Impact of the cancer experience on young adult survivors of childhood cancer using self-reports from 6425 survivors and 360 siblings on a modified version of the Post-traumatic Growth Inventory (PTGI). Perceived Positive Impact was reported significantly more commonly by survivors than by siblings, and more often in female and non-white survivors. Medical predictors of Perceived Positive Impact included exposure to at least one intense therapy, a second malignancy or cancer recurrence, diagnosis at an older age, and fewer years since diagnosis [29].

Suicidal Ideation

Despite these positive findings about many survivors having a very positive perspective on their cancer experience, there are some worrisome data. Another CCSS study examined survey data on suicidal ideation from 9126 adult survivors of childhood cancer and 2968 siblings. Survivors were significantly more likely to report suicidal ideation in the past week, (7.8% versus 4.6%, odds ratio = 1.79; 95% CI, 1.4 to 2.4). Suicidal ideation was unrelated to age at time of survey, age at diagnosis, sex, type of cancer therapy, whether or not there had been a recurrence, time since diagnosis, or second malignancy. Positively correlated with suicidal ideation in survivors were: a primary CNS cancer diagnosis, depression, and poor health outcomes including chronic conditions, pain, and poor global health rating. Suicidal ideation was significantly related to poor current physical health even after adjusting for cancer diagnosis and depression [30].

Posttraumatic Stress Disorder

As mentioned above in the discussion of acute responses of children with cancer, the diagnosis and treatment can be experienced as traumatic, with resulting stress responses. The prevalence and risk factors for Posttraumatic Stress Disorder in survivors of childhood cancer have been the focus of a number of studies over the past twenty years [27, 31, 32]. The Childhood Cancer Survivor Study examined self-reports from 6542 survivors and 368 siblings, using the Posttraumatic Stress Diagnostic Scale [33]. Survivors were over four times as likely to have PTSD, with 589 survivors (9%) and 8 siblings (2%) reporting symptoms consistent with the full diagnostic criteria. Demographic correlates of PTSD in survivors included an educational level of high school or less, being unmarried, having an annual income below $20,000, and being unemployed. Intensive treatment was also associated with an increased risk of PTSD (OR: 1.36 [95% CI: 1.06–1.74]) [34].

Families of Pediatric Patients and Survivors

Parents

Families and family functioning are impacted by cancer diagnosis and treatment. In a study of 144 adolescent cancer survivors 1 to 12 years post-cancer treatment (M = 5.3 years) and their parents, 47% of the adolescents, 25% of mothers, and 30% of fathers reported poor family functioning on the Family Device [35]. Adolescents whose families were perceived as functioning poorly were five times as likely to report symptoms consistent with PTSD on a structured diagnostic interview [35]. The impact of the diagnosis and treatment of cancer can also be traumatic for the parents. In a study of 129 mothers and 72 fathers of 138 newly diagnosed children with cancer, 51% of the mothers and 40% of the fathers met DSM-IV diagnostic criteria for Acute Stress Disorder (ASD) [36].

A recent longitudinal study of 107 mothers and 107 fathers of children on active treatment for cancer was conducted by phone, administering the PTSD Checklist (Civilian) at one week, two months and four months after the child's diagnosis. At one week post-diagnosis, 33% of the parents reported symptoms consistent with Acute Stress Disorder. The prevalence decreased to 28% at two months, and 22% at four months. Mothers reported a higher number of symptoms than fathers [37]. Another study which suggests little decrease in distress over time, compared 27 parents of childhood cancer survivors (mean age = 25.6 y) and 28 parents of current pediatric cancer patients (mean age = 10.2 y) on, or within one year of, active treatment. The two groups did not differ significantly in psychological functioning, posttraumatic stress symptoms, and adjustment to the disease experience. Parents of children on active treatment did report more objective and family burden (e.g., financial cost, time off from work, less time with family members), and more anger associated with the illness experience [38].

These findings are consistent with earlier studies. A survey of 63 mothers and 42 fathers of childhood leukemia survivors found that 39.7% of the mothers and 33.3% of the fathers reported symptoms consistent with a severe level of posttraumatic stress [39]. Analysis of surveys of mothers and fathers from 331 families of childhood cancer survivors found that trait anxiety was the strongest predictor of PTSD in the parents. Other significant contributors were perceived life threat, perceived treatment intensity, and social support. Objective medical data about diagnosis or treatment were not a significant independent contributor to posttraumatic stress symptoms [40].

This discrepancy between how the oncologists view the situation and how parents view the situation was also seen in a recent study of parental optimism. Four hundred eleven parents of children on active cancer treatment were surveyed. Parental optimism was associated with an absence of depression, parental education, and the parents' perception of the child's prognosis. Correlations between the parents' and the oncologists' view of the child's prognosis were low. Optimism was hypothesized to be a trait of the parent which predicted resiliency, as trait anxiety had been found to be associated with PTSD [41].

Interventions for parental distress are important not only for the well-being of the parents. A prospective study of 55 childhood cancer survivors and 60 healthy peer controls collected data during the active treatment phase, and then after the subjects urned 18 years old.

Mother and father reports of initial parent distress were associated with their reports of young adult distress at follow-up for both survivors and controls. Intensity of initial treatment and late effects as rated by health care professionals moderated the association between parent and young adult distress in the cancer survivors [42].

Siblings

There are limited data on the siblings of children under active treatment for cancer and childhood cancer survivors. A recent review found 19 published articles that suggested that aspects of psychosocial health were impacted by doubts, worries, and memories. In some cases these were associated with behavioral problems, depression, somatic complaints and PTSD [43]. A survey of parents from 86 families found that parents felt that their healthy children were likely to have problems due to cancer diagnosis of their sibling, and that the current support offered was not adequate [44]. Specific issues identified in another study of parental perception of needs of siblings were losses arising from the illness experience, behavioral challenges and adaptation, and parent–sibling communication [45].

The Childhood Cancer Survivors Study (CCSS) has significantly increased the amount of data available on siblings of young adult survivors from the 1970s and 1980s in the United States and Canada, since it used siblings as a matched control group for their investigations. A review of these studies demonstrated that siblings appeared to be doing quite well, particularly relative to their affected siblings [24]. CCSS studies report that the prevalence of PTSD in siblings of young adult survivors is 2% [34] and that suicidal ideation is reported by 4.6% of siblings [30]. We also know that siblings are less likely to see a perceived positive impact of the cancer experience than survivors [29].

Therapeutic Interventions

Survivors

Individual, group, and camp interventions are the primary types of psychosocial interventions specifically for children under active treatment for cancer or childhood cancer survivors. Preventative interventions with Child Life or Child Development experts are recommended as a part of all childhood cancer centers [1]. There are a limited numbers of studies on the effectiveness of most of the interventions with these children and adolescents. A review of studies specifically with adolescents found only four rigorous studies, and one of these found a significant improvement compared with a waitlist control group. The participating adolescents in that study had an overall decrease in the level of distress, and improvements in body image and anxiety about psychosexual issues [46].

Psycho-educational efforts have been developed for children and families. These include materials for distribution to pediatricians and parents about expected response to cancer treatment, such as the Medical Traumatic Stress Toolkit [47], available through the National Child Traumatic Stress Network website at www.nctsnet@org. However, a pilot study of the use of a Web-based resource for families of children newly diagnosed with cancer found a disappointing level of use. Most of the hits on the site were on the peer discussion groups [48]. This appears to be an avenue deserving more investigation.

Data in the Cochrane Central Register of Controlled Trials found that distraction and hypnosis had the largest impact on self-reported pain, and cognitive behavioral interventions had the largest effect size on other-reported and behavioral measure of distress in children undergoing needle-related procedures [49]. This was supported by a later review of the literature specifically in pediatric oncology, which found 32 research articles suggesting that the use of mind–body interventions such as hypnosis, distraction, and imagery can be helpful for managing procedure-related pain, anxiety and distress [50].

Siblings

A variety of interventions have been used to provide psychosocial support for siblings of children or adolescents who are on active treatment or are survivors of cancer, including groups, camps or individual interventions. The focus in most cases is on enhancing the coping skills and increasing their knowledge and understanding of the medical situation. For example, a study examined the impact of a summer camp on 77 siblings aged 6–17 years old. Using projective measures, the Human Figure Drawing and the Kinetic Family Drawing-Revised, emotional distress scores decreased significantly after camp compared to pre-camp measures [51]. A review of studies of sibling interventions found that there were significant improvements in depressive symptoms, health-related quality of life and medical knowledge [52].

Family-Focused Interventions

Weekend camps and retreats have been used for many years and are still the most frequent types of family-focused interventions. These are designed to reduce the feelings of isolation commonly reported by the families of childhood cancer patients on active treatment, and are well received by families [53]. Family-level interventions based on a posttraumatic stress model have also been used, with apparently beneficial results [54].

However, it is likely that global interventions will be low yield, given the overall resilience of children and families. Targeted interventions are needed, but this requires identifying those at higher risk for problems. A promising screening tool has been developed and evaluated which is designed to identify families at high, moderate or low need for interventions. The Psychosocial Adaptation Tool risk classification was stable over time, with 57–69% of families remaining at the same level of risk across the first four months of cancer treatment. Families classified at higher levels of psychosocial risk at diagnosis had more distress, more family problems, and greater psychosocial service use four months into treatment [35].

Psychopharmacology

There are few studies available to help guide clinicians regarding safe and effective medications for use in psychiatric disturbances in pediatric oncology. One published study used an 8-week, open-label trial to examine the use of fluvoxamine 100 mg/day to treat depression in 15 children and adolescents with cancer. The fluvoxamine was well tolerated and symptoms of anxiety and depression improved significantly [55]. Another study of 46 children and adolescents diagnosed with delirium found that low-dose haloperidol was effective in treating symptoms, such as sleep–wake cycle disturbance, agitation, lability of affect, and impairments of orientation, attention, and short-term memory [56].

Despite this limited data base, oncologists are prescribing psychoactive medications. In a survey of 151 pediatric oncologists from nine children's cancer centers, 71% of the oncologists reported prescribing SSRIs for their patients. Only 28% reported monitoring patients on SSRIs at the intervals recommended by the FDA for children and adolescents, and only 9% reported they assess for suicidal ideation [57]. A previous study at one major pediatric oncology center surveyed 40 oncologists and found that half of the oncologists prescribed SSRIs for their patients. The most common reasons were a perception that the patient was sad, anxious, or had a major depressive disorder. Most of these prescriptions were given during the first year of treatment [58].

Use of psychopharmacology in children under active treatment for cancer requires great care and careful monitoring [59]. There are some guidelines available for use of medication for delirium and for management of procedural pain. A treatment algorithm has been published for the use of medications to treat delirium in pediatric oncology, based on subtypes of delirium which have been identified. Hyperactive and hypoactive/mixed types of delirium appear to have differential response to haloperidol and risperidone [60].

Principles of interventions to deal with the pain and distress of repeated invasive medical procedures have been the same for over 20 years: maximize comfort and minimize pain, use both nonpharmacologic and pharmacologic interventions, include preparation and support of the child and family at a developmentally appropriate level, consider the developmental age of the child [61]. However, the pharmacological recommendations have changed somewhat over the years. Premedication with benzodiazepines, once used routinely for pediatric procedures, has been actively questioned as not being of benefit to all children [62]. Sedation for diagnostic imaging is only used if necessary, and used agents include chloral hydrate, barbiturates, and benzodiazepines. Newer agents being used for this purpose include etomidate, propofol, and dexmedetomidine [63].

Conclusion

Given the enormity of the psychological and physiological insult of a diagnosis and treatment of childhood cancer, survivors, siblings, and parents are remarkably resilient. Pre-existing anxiety and family conflict increase vulnerability to later problems with depression, anxiety, and PTSD. Screening tools are emerging that can allow targeted interventions. Intensity of treatment may be a risk factor for later psychiatric distress, although this appears to be associated with treatments that affect cognitive function. Little specific research has been done on the effectiveness of psychotropic drugs with children or adolescents on active cancer treatment, although SSRIs, haloperidol, and risperidone are commonly used. Progress in cancer survival and in more targeted treatments will result in yet larger numbers of childhood cancers survivors who will require specialized psychiatric understanding.

References

1. American Academy of Pediatrics, Section on, Hematology/Oncology. Guidelines for Pediatric Cancer Centers: Policy Statement. *Pediatrics* 2004;**113**:1833–1835.
2. Linabery AM, Ross JA. Childhood and adolescent cancer survival in the US by race and ethnicity for the diagnostic period 1975–1999. *Cancer* 2008;**113**:2575–2796.
3. Kurtz BP, Abrams AN. Psychiatric aspects of pediatric cancer. *Child and Adolescent Psychiatric Clinics of North America* 2010;**19**:401–421, x–xi.
4. American Psychiatric, Association. *Diagnostic and Statistical Manual.* Washington, DC: APA Press, 1994.
5. Steinberg AM, Brymer MJ, Decker KB, Pynoos RS. The University of California at Los Angeles Post-traumatic Stress Disorder Reaction Index. *Current Psychiatry Reports* 2004;**6**:96–100.
6. Shemesh E, Annunziato RA, Newcorn JH, et al. Assessment of posttraumatic stress symptoms in children who are medically ill and children presenting to a child trauma program. *Annals of the New York Academy of Sciences* 2006;**1071**:472–477.
7. Turkel SB, Trzepacz PT, Tavaré CJ. Comparing symptoms of delirium in adults and children. *Psychosomatics* 2006;**47**:320–324.
8. Silver GH, Kearney JA, Kutko MC, Bartell AS. Infant delirium in pediatric critical care settings. *American Journal of Psychiatry* 2010;**167**:1172–1177.
9. Janssen NJ, Tan EY, Staal M, et al. On the utility of diagnostic instruments for pediatric delirium in critical illness: an evaluation of the Pediatric Anesthesia Emergence Delirium Scale, the Delirium Rating Scale 88, and the Delirium Rating Scale-Revised R-98. *Intensive Care Medicine* 2011; May 13.
10. Hatherill S, Flisher AJ. Delirium in children and adolescents: a systematic review of the literature. *Journal of Psychosomatic Research* 2010;**68**:337–344.
11. Turkel SB, Tavaré CJ. Delirium in children and adolescents. *Journal of Neuropsychiatry and Clinical Neuroscience* 2003;**15**:431–435.
12. Whitsett SF, Gudmundsdottir M, Davies B, et al. Chemotherapy-related fatigue in childhood cancer: Correlates, consequences, and coping strategies. *Journal of Pediatric Oncology Nursing* 2008;**25**:86–96.
13. Matthey S, Petrovski P. The Children's Depression Inventory: error in cutoff scores for screening purposes. *Psychological Assessment* 2002;**14**:146–149.
14. Kersun LS, Rourke MT, Mickley M, Kazak AE. Screening for depression and anxiety in adolescent cancer patients. *Journal of Pediatric Hematology-Oncology* 2009;**31**:835–839.
15. Hudson MM, Mertens AC, Yasui Y, et al. Health status of adult long-term survivors of childhood cancer: a report from the Childhood Cancer Survivor Study. *JAMA* 2003;**290**:1583–1592.
16. American Academy of Pediatrics, Section on Hematology/Oncology, Children's Oncology, Group. Long-term follow-up care for pediatric cancer survivors. *Pediatrics* 2009;**123**:906–915.
17. Castellino SM, Casillas J, Hudson MM, et al. Minority adult survivors of childhood cancer: a comparison of long-term outcomes, health care utilization, and health-related behaviors from the Childhood Cancer Survivor Study. *Journal of Clinical Oncology* 2005;**23**: 6499–6507.
18. McDougall J, Tsonis M. Quality of life in survivors of childhood cancer: a systematic review of the literature (2001–2008). *Support Care Cancer* 2009;**17**:1231–1246.
19. Wakefield CE, McLoone J, Goodenough B, et al. The psychosocial impact of completing childhood cancer treatment: a systematic review of the literature. *Journal of Pediatric Psychology* 2010;**35**:262–274.

20. Kazak AE, Derosa BW, Schwartz LA, *et al.* Psychological outcomes and health beliefs in adolescent and young adult survivors of childhood cancer and controls. *Journal of Clinical Oncology* 2010;**28**:2002–2007.

21. Harila MJ, Niinivirta TI, Winqvist S, Harila-Saari AH. Low depressive symptom and mental distress scores in adult long-term survivors of childhood acute lymphoblastic leukemia. *Journal of Pediatric Hematology-Oncology* 2011;**33**:194–198.

22. O'Leary TE, Diller L, Recklitis CJ. The effects of response bias on self-reported quality of life among childhood cancer survivors. *Quality of Life Research* 2007;**16**:1211–1220. [E-pub 2007 July 11].

23. Robison LL, Armstrong GT, Boice JD, *et al.* The Childhood Cancer Survivor Study: a National Cancer Institute-supported resource for outcome and intervention research. *Journal of Clinical Oncology* 2009;**27**:2308–2318.

24. Zeltzer LK, Recklitis C, Buchbinder D, *et al.* Psychological status in childhood cancer survivors: a report from the Childhood Cancer Survivor Study. *Journal of Clinical Oncology* 2009;**27**:2396–2404.

25. Zebrack BJ, Chesler MA. Quality of life in childhood cancer survivors. *Psychooncology* 2002;**11**:132–141.

26. Kazak AE, Barakat LP, Meeske K, *et al.* Posttraumatic stress symptoms, family functioning, and social support in survivors of childhood leukemia and their mothers and fathers. *Journal of Consulting and Clinical Psychology* 1997;**65**:120–129.

27. Currier JM, Hermes S, Phipps S. Brief report: children's response to serious illness: perceptions of benefit and burden in a pediatric cancer population. *Journal of Pediatric Psychology* 2009;**34**:1129–1134. [E-pub 2009 Apr 2].

28. Kamibeppu K, Sato I, Honda M, *et al.* Mental health among young adult survivors of childhood cancer and their siblings including posttraumatic growth. *Journal of Cancer Survivors* 2010;**4**:303–312.

29. Zebrack BJ, Stuber ML, Meeske KA, *et al.* Perceived positive impact of cancer among long-term survivors of childhood cancer: a report from the Childhood Cancer Survivor Study. *Psychooncology* 2011; Mar 22. DOI: 10.1002/pon.1959.

30. Recklitis CJ, Diller LR, Li X, *et al.* Suicide ideation in adult survivors of childhood cancer: a report from the Childhood Cancer Survivor Study. *Journal of Clinical Oncology* 2010;**28**:655–661.

31. Hobbie WL, Stuber M, Meeske K, *et al.* Symptoms of posttraumatic stress in young adult survivors of childhood cancer. *Journal of Clinical Oncology* 2000;**18**: 4060–4066.

32. Bruce M. A systematic and conceptual review of posttraumatic stress in childhood cancer survivors and their parents. *Clinical Psychology Review* 2006;**26**:233–256.

33. Foa EB. *Posttraumatic Stress Diagnostic Scale: Manual.* Minneapolis, MN: National Computer Systems, 1995.

34. Stuber ML, Meeske KA, Krull KR, *et al.* Prevalence and predictors of posttraumatic stress disorder in adult survivors of childhood cancer. *Pediatrics* 2010;**125**:e1124–1134.

35. Alderfer MA, Mougianis I, Barakat LP, *et al.* Family psychosocial risk, distress, and service utilization in pediatric cancer: predictive validity of the Psychosocial Assessment Tool. *Cancer* 2009;**115** (18 Suppl.): 4339–4349.

36. Patiño-Fernández AM, Pai AL, Alderfer M, *et al.* Acute stress in parents of children newly diagnosed with cancer. *Pediatric Blood & Cancer* 2008;**50**:289–292.

37. Pöder U, Ljungman G, von Essen L. Posttraumatic stress disorder among parents of children on cancer treatment: a longitudinal study. *Psychooncology* 2008;**17**:430–437.

38. Hardy KK, Bonner MJ, Masi R, *et al.* Psychosocial functioning in parents of adult survivors of childhood cancer. *Journal of Pediatric Hematology-Oncology* 2008;**30**: 153–159.

39. Stuber ML, Christakis DA, Houskamp B, Kazak AE. Posttraumatic symptoms in childhood leukemia survivors and their parents. *Psychosomatics.* 1996;**37**:254–261.

40. Kazak AE, Stuber ML, Barakat LP, *et al.* Predicting posttraumatic stress symptoms in mothers and fathers of survivors of childhood cancers. *Journal of American Academy of Child and Adolescent Psychiatry* 1998;**37**:823–831.

41. Fayed N, Klassen AF, Dix D, *et al.* Exploring predictors of optimism among parents of children with cancer. *Psychooncology* 2011;**20**:411–418. doi: 10.1002/pon.1743.

42. Robinson KE, Gerhardt CA, Vannatta K, Noll RB. Survivors of childhood cancer and comparison peers: the influence of early family factors on distress in emerging adulthood. *Journal of Family Psychology* 2009;**23**:23–31.

43. Buchbinder D, Casillas J, Zeltzer L. Meeting the psychosocial needs of childhood survivors: a family systems approach. *Journal of Pediatric Oncology Nursing* 2010; Nov 22.

44. Ballard KL. Meeting the needs of siblings of children with cancer. *Pediatric Nursing* 2004;**30**:394–401.

45. Sidhu R, Passmore A, Baker D. An investigation into parent perceptions of the needs of siblings of children with cancer. *Journal of Pediatric Oncology Nursing* 2005;**22**:276–287.

46. Seitz DC, Besier T, Goldbeck L. Psychosocial interventions for adolescent cancer patients: a systematic review of the literature. *Psychooncology* 2009;**18**:683–690.

47. Stuber ML, Schneider S, Kassam-Adams N, *et al.* The medical traumatic stress toolkit. *CNS Spectrum* 2006;**11**:137–142.

48. Ewing LJ, Long K, Rotondi A, *et al.* Brief report: a pilot study of a web-based resource for families of children with cancer. *Journal of Pediatric Psychology* 2009;**34**:523–529.

49. Uman LS, Chambers CT, McGrath PJ, Kisely S. Psychological interventions for needle-related procedural pain and distress in children and adolescents. *Cochrane Database of Systematic Reviews* 2006;**4**:CD005179.

50. Landier W, Tse AM. Use of complementary and alternative medical interventions for the management of procedure-related pain, anxiety, and distress in pediatric oncology: an integrative review. *Journal of Pediatric Nursing* 2010;**25**:566–579. [E-pub 2010 Mar 12.]

51. Packman W, Mazaheri M, Sporri L, *et al.* Projective drawings as measures of psychosocial functioning in siblings of pediatric cancer patients from the Camp Okizu study. *Journal of Pediatric Oncology Nursing* 2008;**25**: 44–55.

52. Prchal A, Landolt MA. Psychological interventions with siblings of pediatric cancer patients: a systematic review. *Psychooncology* 2009;**18**:1241–1251.

53. Ruffin JE, Creed JM, Jarvis C. A retreat for families of children recently diagnosed with cancer. *Cancer Practice* 1997;**5**:99–104.

54. Pai AL, Kazak AE. Pediatric medical traumatic stress in pediatric oncology: family systems interventions. *Current Opinion in Pediatrics* 2006;**18**:558–562.

55. Gothelf D, Rubinstein M, Shemesh E, *et al.* Pilot study: fluvoxamine treatment for depression and anxiety

disorders in children and adolescents with cancer. *Journal of American Academy of Child and Adolescent Psychiatry* 2005;**44**:1258–1262.

56. Grover S, Malhotra S, Bharadwaj R, *et al.* Delirium in children and adolescents. *International Journal of Psychiatry in Medicine* 2009;**39**:179–187.

57. Phipps S, Buckholdt KE, Fernandez L, *et al.* Pediatric oncologists' practices of prescribing selective serotonin reuptake inhibitors (SSRIs) for children and adolescents with cancer: a multi-site study. *Pediatric Blood & Cancer* 2011; Jan 31. DOI: 10. 1002/pbc.22788.

58. Kersun LS, Kazak AE. Prescribing practices of selective serotonin reuptake inhibitors (SSRIs) among pediatric oncologists: a single institution experience. *Pediatric Blood & Cancer* 2006;**47**:339–342.

59. Kersun LS, Elia J. Depressive symptoms and SSRI use in pediatric oncology patients. *Pediatric Blood & Cancer* 2007;**49**:881–887.

60. Karnik NS, Joshi SV, Paterno C, Shaw R. Subtypes of pediatric delirium: a treatment algorithm. *Psychosomatics* 2007;**48**:253–257.

61. Hockenberry MJ, McCarthy K, Taylor O, *et al.* Managing painful procedures in children with cancer. *Journal of Pediatric Hematology-Oncoogyl* 2011;**33**:119–127.

62. Rosenbaum A, Kain ZN, Larsson P, *et al.* The place of premedication in pediatric practice. *Paediatric Anesthesia* 2009;**19**:817–828.

63. Rutman MS. Sedation for emergent diagnostic imaging studies in pediatric patients. *Current Opinion in Pediatrics* 2009;**21**:306–312.

6

Psychosocial Effects of Hematopoietic Cell Transplantation in Children

Ronit Elhasid, Michal M. Kreitler, Shulamith Kreitler, Myriam Weyl Ben-Arush

Introduction: Outlines of the Procedure

Stem cell transplantation (SCT) is an established treatment of many malignant and non-malignant hematological, hereditary and immunological diseases. The widespread use of SCT in the treatment of a steadily increasing number of life-threatening disorders is the culmination of over four decades of research by a great number of investigators. The first successful allogeneic transplants (i.e., SCT from a donor) of hematopoietic stem cells were done in 1968 in three children with congenital immunodeficiency diseases [1]. Since then, thousands of patients have received SCT to treat life-threatening malignant and non-malignant diseases.

Hematopoietic stem cells are the most important stem cells needed for successful transplantation. These cells can be harvested from the bone marrow as well as from the peripheral blood. Rapid hematopoietic recovery was shown after peripheral blood stem cell transplantation as compared with bone marrow transplantation (BMT) [2]. Stem cells are taken from the patient, in the case of autologous peripheral blood stem cell transplantation (PBSCT), or from a donor, in the case of allogeneic PBSCT. A donor may be found in the patient's close family, usually a matched sibling, and if not, through a search designed to identify an unrelated donor matched in HLA (human leukocyte antigens) system. Genes of the HLA system encode a complex array of histocompatibility molecules that play a central role in immune responsiveness and in determining the outcome of tissue transplantation [3]. Umbilical cord blood stem cells are another alternative source of hematopoietic stem cells in patients lacking a suitable sibling donor.

Advances in histocompatibility testing and development of marrow donor registries, such as the National Marrow Donor Program in the USA, as well as the establishment of cord blood banks have facilitated the use of unrelated donors and thus enabled the expansion of the number of patients who could receive transplants.

The transplant process is often described as consisting of five phases:

(1) *Conditioning,* which typically lasts for 7–10 days and in which chemotherapy and/or radiation are administered to eliminate malignancy, prevent rejection of new stem cells and create space for the new cells.

(2) *Stem cell infusion,* which usually lasts about an hour, whereby the period varies with the volume infused and procedure of stem cell processing.

(3) *The neutropenic phase,* which lasts 2–4 weeks, and in which the patient is highly susceptible to mucositis, infections such as herpes simplex virus and various skin and gut pathogens. This phase is treated mainly by antibiotics, antifungal agents and supportive care.

(4) *The engraftment phase,* which may last for several weeks, and in which the infections start slowly to clear, whereby the greatest challenge becomes the management of graft versus host disease (GVHD) and prevention of viral infections.

(5) *The post-engraftment phase,* which may last for months to years, and is marked by the gradual development of tolerance, weaning off of immunosuppression, management of chronic GVHD, and immune reconstitution.

There are multiple and diverse indications for each type of transplant. Autologous SCT is usually performed in recurrent solid tumors, such as brain tumors

Pediatric Psycho-oncology: Psychosocial Aspects and Clinical Interventions, Second Edition.
Edited by Shulamith Kreitler, Myriam Weyl Ben-Arush and Andrés Martin.
© 2012 John Wiley & Sons, Ltd. Published 2012 by John Wiley & Sons, Ltd.

or Ewing sarcoma, as well as in advanced stage neuro-blastoma. Allogeneic SCT is done in recurrent or high-risk hematological malignancies, immunodeficiency states, metabolic diseases, and hematological diseases, such as thalassemia major or stem cell disorders, such as aplastic anemia.

Diverse complications can arise during and after SCT. Infections remain a major problem due to the myelosuppression caused by the conditioning regimen. Gram-negative as well as gram-positive bacteria are responsible for much of the morbidity [4]. Isolation, use of high-efficiency particulate air filtration systems and hand washing are used to minimize contact of these compromised hosts with infectious agents. In patients undergoing allogeneic SCT, the depressed immunity continues after transplant due to the use of immunosuppression given post-transplant to prevent GVHD. Viral and fungal infections predominate during this period [5].

Veno-occlusive disease of the liver is a common and often fatal complication of high dose chemo-radio-therapy. It consists of the triad of weight gain, painful hepatomegaly and hyper-bilirubinemia. It is now the most common life-threatening complication of prepar-ative regimen-related toxicity of BMT [6].

GVHD results from HLA disparity between the hematopoietic stem cell donor and the transplant recipient. In GVHD the new transplanted immune sys-tem attacks, as it were, the whole body. It generally involves the skin, the gastrointestinal tract and the liver, causing a rash and blistering, diarrhea and hyper-bilirubinemia, respectively. Acute GVHD is usu-ally observed within 30–40 days of marrow infusion, but with the advent of more potent immunosuppressive agents such as cyclosporine, its onset may now be delayed by several months. Chronic GVHD usually occurs more than 100 days after allogeneic stem cell infusion, and the clinical pattern differs somewhat from that observed in acute GVHD. The most com-monly involved organs are skin, liver, salivary glands, mucous membranes and muscles [7].

Acute and chronic GVHD can cause high morbidity and mortality. Immunosuppression administered as prophylaxis treatment for GVHD further decreases the immune status. However, since it involves a delay in immune reconstitution, it may bring about more mor-bidity. Chronic GVHD remains one of the prime deter-minants of late transplant-related morbidity and impaired quality of life (QOL). It includes abnormali-ties of growth and development in children, and prob-lems of employment and functional performance status in the survivors as adults [8].

Isolation and Other Stressors

Length of hospitalization for stem cell transplantation is about one month. To minimize complications, the child is isolated in a room with a high-efficiency partic-ulate air filtration system, and is not allowed to leave the room for the whole period of the transplantation. An early study reported on the psychological responses of children to isolation in a protected environment [9]. The participants in the study were cancer patients with advanced stage solid tumors, treated in a laminar air-flow unit. Behavioral observations of 14 children were carried out over a period of two years, whereby the total number of available observations was 3629. The results referred to perception, sleep, intellectual func-tioning, physical discomfort, mood, management problems, activity patterns, social communicative behavior, and sedation. No changes were observed in intellectual functioning as measured by standard psy-chometric tools. In general, no debilitating or long-term psychological effects related to prolonged treat-ment in a protected environment were noted. No child had to be removed from isolation because of psycho-logical factors. The investigators concluded that chil-dren adapt more easily than adults to protected environments.

Nevertheless, and despite a strong program of psy-chosocial support, some of the children had hallucina-tory experiences and regressive symptoms in mood and communication, mostly after 6 weeks or more in isola-tion. Notably, the average isolation period of the patients in that study was 90 days, which is longer than nowadays.

Another study described factors that affect the cop-ing processes of adolescents with aplastic anemia and infants with severe combined immunodeficiency dis-ease treated in laminar flow isolation rooms [10]. The children in the study stayed in rooms devoid of win-dows. An intercom system was the only means of com-munication between the patient, the family, and the staff. This study was descriptive, presenting examples of coping with the isolation experience, relying on informal observations, without the use of any standard psychological tests. The findings indicate clearly that isolation, with its concomitant drastic reduction in nor-mal emotional supports, enhances appreciably the stress of being ill and of having to undergo BMT.

Nowadays laminar airflow isolation is no longer a must and the protected environments are achieved by using rooms with hepafiltration. Only one study has examined stress reactions and psychic adaptation of 15 children aged 8–12 years after SCT in single-room treatment under such isolation conditions. This prospective longitudinal study was based on free diagnostic interviews, projective tests and self-report questionnaires as well as intelligence tests administered in order to evaluate different adaptation processes in the children [11]. The responses to the self-report questionnaires revealed predominantly the conscious levels of emotional organization. This perspective highlighted the children's strong tendencies to adapt to the situation and to normalize their behavior under the isolation conditions. A comparison of pre- and posttransplant responses showed an "over-normalization" of the scores for anxiety, depression, neuroticism, and extraversion and a relatively undifferentiated perception of one's own body.

In contrast, the psychoanalytic interview, and the projective tests (e.g., Rorschach) tapped deeper levels of emotional responsiveness and exposed a completely different angle on the children's change in emotional adjustment from before to after the transplantation. Of the 15 children, nine dealt much more intensely than before with fears of death, feelings of depression, loneliness, and rage and had fantasies of guilt and punishment. Only two children showed a decreased intensity of their emotions and a more rigid organization of defenses than prior to transplantation. The limitations of this study are mainly the small number of studied children and their restricted age range.

In the Oncology/Hematology Department at Tel Aviv Medical Center, the transplant rooms are equipped with high pressure as well as a high-efficiency particulate air filtration system. The child is not allowed to leave the room but is not alone. Usually, one of the parents stays with the child in the same room for the whole transplant period. Other people who enter the room are limited, including the nurse and the physician in charge. Thus, the physical isolation is not as extreme as it used to be when laminar airflow system was used. However, in the course of transplantation the patient cannot leave the room or meet other family members or friends for a long period. It seems that changes in isolation practices have reduced the difficulties of isolation in general and the emotional burden in particular. Thus, a prevalent impression of health professionals is that isolation per se is less of a problem than it used to be. However, this impression still remains to be tested empirically.

And yet prolonged hospitalization in a protected environment and the enforced isolation both during and subsequent to hospitalization remain serious stressors for patients.

Further BMT-related stressors include the life-threatening nature of the BMT procedure,

disruption and dislocation of the family, acute toxicity of high-dose chemotherapy and radiotherapy used in conditioning regimens, intense physical discomfort involved in the treatment, required compliance with aversive daily routines, and the generally high levels of transient treatment-related morbidity [12]. It is important to note also the stressful impact of the pain that most children undergoing BMT experience. A study with 20 children, aged 5–17, undergoing BMT, showed that despite getting continuous infusion opioid therapy with additional boluses as needed for pain, all children reported pain after one month of treatment [13]. The impact of the stressors is enhanced by the extended period of the treatment, which is long per se and may be further prolonged through frequent complications. Studies show that the parents of children undergoing BMT also experience high levels of stress [14, 15]. This may further enhance the children's distress. Packman et al. [16] reviewed the psychological effects of hematopoietic SCT on pediatric patients, siblings and parents demonstrating that 20%, 56%, and 41% of parents had clinically significant levels of stress pre-transplant, one month post transplant, and 6 months post transplant, respectively. Most studies focused on the mother's psychological well-being [14, 17, 18] demonstrating, for example, that 66% of mothers had clinically significant levels of depression pre-HSCT [17] while 12% of mothers were diagnosed with PTSD 18 months post-HSCT [14]. Not surprisingly, as the mother is usually the main caregiver, she tends to be the one to quit her job, relocate, and assume the care and support of the child, so that the impact of her emotional distress on her child's well-being cannot be over-emphasized [19]. The magnitude of the children's stress is such that the responses of some pediatric BMT patients have been described as representing a variant of posttraumatic stress disorder, with symptoms similar to those observed in children who have been traumatized by violence [20, 21]. Jobe-Shields et al. [22] investigated the interaction between parental depressive symptoms, family environment and child distress at admission for SCT. Some 146 patients and their caregivers were studied with 82% of the parents being mothers. Child symptoms of distress were measured using a modified version of the UCLA Posttraumatic Stress Disorder Index, a measure of posttraumatic stress symptoms. Parental symptoms of depression were assessed with the Center for Epidemiologic Studies Depression Scale. The family environment scale included items of family cohesion, expressiveness and conflict. Parents of younger children reported greater depressive symptoms. There was a positive relationship between child-reported distress and parental depressive symptoms and negative correlation between parental depression and levels of family cohesion and expressiveness. In multiple regression analyses, parental depressive symptomatology was the only factor to explain unique variance in levels of child distress. These findings should promote further studies testing interventions for parents of children before SCT in order to improve child adjustment during the transplant procedure. All those stressors could affect the children's quality of life post-transplant.

One indication of the extremity of the stress involved in BMT is the high incidence of non-compliance noted in pediatric BMT patients. It was found that almost all of these patients had at some point difficulties ingesting oral medication (due to the unpalatable mouth rinses they were required to use), and all but the youngest group had compliance problems, which in over 50% of the cases required intervention [23].

Effects on Quality of Life (QOL)

During the past decades better use of high-dose chemotherapy and improved management of supportive care have resulted in higher survival rates for children with cancer in general and of patients who have undergone BMT in particular. These advances have highlighted the importance of the issue of maintaining a good QOL. Health, as defined by the World Health Organisation as early as 1948, is not only the absence of disease, but also the presence of physical, mental, and social well-being [24]. The terms "quality of life" and more specifically, "health-related quality of life" refer to the effects of health on the physical, psychological and social domains of life, considered as distinct areas that are influenced by a person's perceptions, experiences, expectations, and beliefs (see Chapter 3 in this volume on quality of life).

The impact of health on each of these domains can be measured in terms of two dimensions: objective assessments of functioning or health status; and more subjective perceptions of health. The two dimensions are distinct, since two people with the same health status may have different levels of QOL [25].

Understanding the impact of the BMT on QOL can assist in counseling children and their families who are considering BMT as a treatment option, and may lead to changes in the current medical and nursing protocols across phases of the transplant process to long-term rehabilitation [26].

Two models were proposed for analyzing the relations of SCT to the patient's QOL. Ferrell *et al.* [27, 28] proposed a model that focuses on four identified dimensions of well-being: physical, psychological, social, and spiritual. Each dimension was analyzed according to the patients' responses in interviews. Ford *et al.* [29] presented another model that focuses on examining separately each of the following four specific phases: pre-SCT, day of SCT up to 100 days, post-SCT from 100 days to 1 year, and 1 or more years since SCT.

The four-dimensional model and the four-phase model jointly provide a theoretical framework for assessing QOL after SCT. Notably, each dimension may differ in each phase. For example, physical well-being between the day of SCT up to 100 days is not the same as it is one or more years following SCT. Thus, applying the two models together makes it possible to identify ways for intervention in regard to each dimension at each phase, covering the entire period.

Parsons *et al.* [30] have raised the following important question: Health-related QOL in pediatric BMT survivors: according to whom? In the past, QOL assessments of BMT survivors have been based on proxy reports, provided primarily by the parents. Several studies have shown that maternal distress and depression, marital adjustment and health locus of control influence parents' assessment of the child's functioning and behavior [31–33]. Parsons *et al.* [30] studied 82 patients in the age range of 5–12 years. Forty-seven patients (57%) had received an allogeneic transplant, and 35 patients (43%) received an autologous transplant. The majority (96%) of patients had an underlying malignancy. The time interval between BMT and the assessment of QOL ranged from 24 days to 8.4 years. The perceptions of parents and children's health status following BMT were compared, using the Child Health Rating Inventories (CHRIs) and its companion measure, the Disease Impairment Inventory-BMT (DSII-BMT). The findings showed good agreement between parental reports and child self-assessment with regard to "objective" issues, such as missed school days and utilization of resources (e.g., emergency room visits). Children's scores were correlated highly with physicians' ratings of clinical disease severity and varied within each functional status domain both by transplant type and by time after BMT, in predictable ways. In contrast, parental ratings for disease-specific problems and pain were not significantly correlated with disease severity ratings. Further, little agreement was found between parental and child ratings in regard to the dimensions of mental health or QOL, regardless of the time after BMT, the type of transplant or the presence vs. absence of chronic GVHD. Children who had undergone BMT within the previous 6 months reported doing better in all areas of functioning than their parents reported about them. In the later time periods, the pattern was reversed, with the parents reporting higher scores than the children in regard to physical functioning, role function and energy. It is evident that children and parents base their reports on different considerations, for example, in the first period after SCT parents could be considering the toxicity of the transplant, whereas the children could be focusing on the recent isolation and the fate of other children on the unit. Be that as it may, the results of Parsons et al. [30] suggest that children are capable of providing valid and reliable information about their health-related QOL, information that varies predictably among clinical subgroups.

Phipps et al. [34] used the Behavioral, Affective and Somatic Experiences Scale (BASES) to assess aspects of health-related QOL in children undergoing BMT. There were separate versions for parent, nurse and patient reports. In regard to patients at least 5 years old, BASES data were obtained weekly from parent, patient and nurse. For patients less than 5 years of age data were obtained only from the parent and nurse. Once-weekly observations were obtained through week +6, followed by once-monthly observations through month +6. Nurse observations were stopped when the patient was discharged from the initial BMT hospitalization. Longitudinal data were obtained from a cohort of 105 children (61 had allogeneic BMT and 44 autologous). Yet only 45 children were older than 5 years and completed the patient version of the BASES. Clear patterns of change from one phase to another were found on measures from all respondents. The parental reports showed significant effects over time for all scales. The children's reports showed significant changes on all BASES subscales except Quality of Interaction. The nurses' reports showed significant changes on all subscales except Quality of Interaction and Compliance. All separately checked items of the Somatic Distress Scale (viz. nausea/vomiting, mucositis) and the Mood Disturbance Scale (viz., cheerful/friendly, sad/subdued, fearful/anxious, and angry/irritable) showed significant declines according to the parents' and nurses' reports. Again, in line with parents' and nurses' reports, most somatic distress items showed a high peak in the week after BMT conditioning, followed by a decline to baseline or lower by week +4 or +5. Both parents' and nurses' reports show a difference in line with the type of transplantation: patients undergoing allogeneic BMT experienced significantly higher effects on the subscales of Somatic Distress and Activity, but not on the subscales of Compliance, Mood Disturbance and Quality of Interaction. According to parents and nurses, the lowest degrees of somatic distress were experienced by the youngest children, the highest degrees by adolescents, and intermediate degrees by children in the 6–12 year group. In all subscales of the BASES, younger patients had scores indicating better QOL than adolescents. There were no differences between the genders in any of the subscales, except one (Compliance subscale, in which males were reported by the nurses as having greater difficulties).

A recent study by Phipps et al. [35] focused on assessing the acute effects of BMT on 153 children (age range 51 year to 20), especially in regard to somatic distress and mood disturbances. The instruments (the BASES, parent version and child version for children above 5 years of age) and the observation schedule were similar to those used in a previously reported study [34]. The findings showed that when children enter the hospital for BMT, their QOL is already compromised: they have high levels of somatic and mood disturbance symptoms, and low levels of activity. The situation exacerbates during the BMT procedure and peaks about one week after the transplant. But by the fourth to fifth week post-transplant there is a decline in distress back to the levels at admission, and a further decline in the 4–6 months after the transplant.

Quality of Life of BMT Survivors

Several studies focused on QOL assessments in cancer survivors who have undergone BMT. In a review aiming to evaluate health-related quality of life (HRQL) following pediatric SCT, 15 studies were included [36]. The authors found that 6 months to 8 years post transplant, HRQL was comparable to the normal population. Studies demonstrated that HRQL was already compromised pre transplant, deteriorated immediately following conditioning, only to improve 4–12 months post transplant. Predictors of HRQL included family functioning and child cognitive, behavioral and social functioning. One of the early studies reported observations on 43 children with normal cognitive abilities, 26 of whom were 5–16:8 years old, and 17 were younger than 5 years [20]. They were followed for 12 months post-transplant. Most of the children had leukemia. Three kinds of comparisons were undertaken: first, the status of the BMT children 6 and 12 months post-transplant were compared; second, the BMT children were compared to children who had undergone another kind of serious medical procedure (cardiac surgery); and third, the BMT children were compared to healthy children who had not undergone any stressful procedure. The findings indicated an increase in behavior problems from pre-BMT (15%) to 6 months post-transplant (about 3 months after discharge from the hospital) (40%). The observed rate was higher than in the normal population (15%). The characteristic pattern for the children over 5 years included depressive symptoms, decreased interest in enjoyable activities, fear of disease recurrence, emotional detachment from parents and friends and difficulties in concentration, as well as eating difficulties and temper tantrums. No effects were observed on general cognitive functioning but there were significant declines in scholastic achievement (viz. arithmetic) and difficulties in dealing with academic pressures in general. The characteristic pattern for children under 5 included lethargy, eating problems, and social difficulties, with a tendency for regression in self-help skills. Twelve months after BMT, most of the children (80.8%), regardless of their age, had improved in their psychological state and were already on their way to reintegration into normal life. However, comparisons with the healthy children showed that the BMT survivors manifested more disturbed behavior in the academic, social and emotional domains even 12 months after transplant (35%, as compared with 15% in the controls). However, BMT survivors resembled greatly in their behavior symptoms and rate of disturbance (though not in the deficit in cognitive functioning) another group of children who had undergone cardiac surgery, which also qualifies as a life-threatening stressful medical procedure. It is possible that the serious effects noted in this study are due to the stringent conditions of BMT and the absence of psychosocial awareness of the risks and difficulties for pediatric patients almost 20 years ago.

Another early study of BMT survivors [37] also noted their psychological difficulties, in particular in the social field in the framework of school. A more recent study was done specifically in order to evaluate the behavioral reputation and social acceptance of pediatric BMT survivors [38]. The comparison of peer, teacher and self-report data was done between a group of 48 BMT survivors, aged 8–16, and 48 healthy children in the same classroom, with a similar gender distribution. The study showed that BMT survivors had fewer friends and were described by their peers (though not by the teachers or by themselves) as more socially isolated. The peers also described them as physically less attractive and less skilled in sports, that is to say, as being deficient in

properties that are commonly considered as socially desirable. It is possible that prolonged absenteeism from the school coupled with deficiency in socially desirable characteristics may lay the groundwork for social difficulties that could impair the children's social and emotional QOL. However, not all studies of BMT survivors report difficulties. A study based on 39 patients, who had at least 2 years of follow-up after they had undergone allogeneic BMT (with a median follow-up of 5.7 years), did not reveal any evident impairment in QOL as assessed in terms of psychosocial functioning [39]. Further, another study [40] used a mixed sample of 162 adults and 50 pediatric survivors, who had all been allogeneic marrow recipients. The data were obtained by means of interviews during clinic visits (5%), or over the telephone (95%). The interview referred to three domains of QOL: (1) productive activity and functioning; (2) health status and treatment-related physical symptoms; and (3) qualitative aspects of daily life. The patients graded their overall QOL on a 1–10 scale, to yield a Karnofsky score. The patients were contacted at least one year following their BMT. The majority (90%) of the 40 pediatric transplant recipients, who had attended school full-time before diagnosis, had been able to return to full-time attendance or employment when surveyed. Also those who had not been enrolled in school pre-diagnosis were all enrolled in school or employed full-time when surveyed. All pediatric patients were rated with Karnofsky performance status of 90 or 100 at the time of the survey. A subjective rating of their overall QOL, on a scale running from 0 to 10 (i.e., low to high, respectively), showed that the median score was 9.5. The authors concluded that the younger patients might overcome the treatment-related toxicity more completely than older (adult) persons.

Another study [41] focused on 36 children and adolescents who had been in the age range of 2 to 16 years when transplantation took place. Patients who had undergone BMT at least 6 months before were included. This survey consisted of self-rating questionnaires, for the recipients and for the parents according to the patients' age. The investigators used a self-devised questionnaire for parents, the Busnelli anxiety scale for 17 patients aged 8–15 years, the Children's Depression Scale for 17 patients aged 9–16 years, the Parent Symptoms questionnaire for 13 parents of patients aged 4–9 years, and the Offer self-image questionnaire for 11 adolescent patients. According to the parents, most of the children did not think back about BMT with anxiety, although many preferred not to talk about it with their parents (41%) or friends (50%).

Only 16% of the interviewed patients complained about physical problems. Return to school figured as the cause of most difficulties. Tests that evaluate affective status indicated normal levels of anxiety, while in adolescents a slight depression state was reported, causing a sense of inadequacy. Self-image was substantially normal. Anxiety levels appeared to be higher in pre-school children. The investigators concluded that QOL in their respondents was good. Nevertheless, homogeneous instruments would be more appropriate to identify those at risk of having future difficulties in coping with the BMT procedure.

Notteghem *et al.* [42] evaluated the neuro-psychological and adaptive functioning of children who have undergone autologous BMT without previous cranial irradiation. The major goal of the study was to determine whether high-dose chemotherapy alone might cause cognitive deficits. There were 76 children in the sample. They had all undergone BMT as treatment for an extracranial solid tumor. The BMT conditioning regimen consisted of high-dose chemotherapy with either total body irradiation or supratentorial cranial irradiation. The inclusion criteria were continuous complete remission 5 years or more after BMT, no sign of mental retardation, no developmental delay, and no psychosis prior to diagnosis. Median age at the time of the transplant was 4.5 years, and at neuropsychological examination, 15.7 years. The median interval between transplantation and neuropsychological examination was 9.1 years. Overall, the performance and skills of the participants were in the normal range and their professional and academic outcomes were satisfactory. A deleterious effect of deafness on verbal IQ associated with the previous administration of cisplatin was observed. In addition, reading difficulties had arisen that could be related to absence from kindergarten or primary school during hospitalization. Finally, in the younger subgroup, visual–perceptual skills were found to be more fragile.

Further aspects of the QOL of BMT survivors were highlighted in another study of 73 survivors after allogeneic BMT with an observation time of 1–15 years (median: 5.6 years) [43]. The Karnofsky–Orlansky scale was used to assess functional status. Lack of a more specific tool for assessing in a comprehensive way the QOL of children induced the investigators to design a questionnaire focusing on the practical aspects of daily life. The first part included questions concerning frequency of medical consultation in the last four months prior to the study, school attendance after transplantation and professional career. The second part included 12 items referring to physical and psychological aspects. All but one patient (with severe neurological impairment) had Karnofsky–Orlansky scores over 80. In the case of children younger than 12 years, the QOL questionnaires were completed by the parents. Responses to the questionnaire of QOL revealed that 75% of the patients reported non-physical or psychological impairment. QOL was related inversely with the diagnosis of chronic GVHD. The findings of the study are, however, to be interpreted with caution, first, because its design was cross-sectional with a variable time interval between BMT and self-assessment; and second, because no age-adjusted control group of healthy individuals was used.

An innovative approach to assessing QOL in pediatric patients who have undergone BMT was adopted by Kreitler, Kreitler and Ben-Arush [44]. In contrast to most studies that focus either on comparing BMT patients with themselves in different periods or sometimes with healthy controls, they compared BMT patients (n = 18) with other pediatric cancer patients, matched to the BMT patients in diagnoses and the various demographic variables (n = 56). All patients had terminated their treatment (mean time since end of treatment 3.88 years, SD ¼ 2.27). The major difference between the groups was undergoing BMT or not. There were no significant differences between the groups in disease stage, recurrence, time since diagnosis, time since end of treatment, age (9–17 years), gender distribution, and country of origin. They were administered the CQL questionnaire. Significant differences between the groups were not found in any of the scales or the total QOL score but only in five (of 56) items. However, the trend of the findings is suggestive of the possibility that precisely because of the severe stressful nature of BMT, the patients, their families and the staff invest psychosocial efforts to alleviate and remedy the situation, with the result that overall QOL of BMT survivors can be even better than that of "regular" pediatric cancer patients.

Psychosocial Factors of Children's Adjustment

As may be expected, there are individual differences in the responses of children undergoing BMT [20]. The study of these differences and of the determining factors is of great importance, both in order to identify as early as possible children who may be at risk for enhanced psychological distress and later psychological difficulties, and for providing all children the preparation prior to the treatment that may help them cope as best as possible. Pot-Mees [20] focused on two kinds of determinants: coping styles and social environment. He found that the most effective attitude on the part of the children was a coping style of inner-directedness, withdrawal, waiting, "holding back impulses," seeking distraction even if only temporarily, rather than attempting to get an active solution. Further, the children who were better adjusted post-transplant were those with a resilient personality who responded to the stressful situation with denial and self-protectiveness. Insofar as the social environment is concerned, Pot-Mees noted that the best-adjusted children were those whose parents were emotionally adjusted, experienced marital satisfaction and were able to provide the children social support.

Further studies have focused specifically on identifying psychological factors that could contribute to differential adjustment of children undergoing BMT. For example, Phipps and Mulhern [45] used a prospective longitudinal design in order to examine the psychological adjustment of survivors of pediatric BMT, and to determine predictors of adjustment, particularly by identifying variables that confer protection from, or indicate vulnerability to, the stresses of BMT. Measures of patients' social competence, behavior problems, and self-esteem, as well as perceived family conflict, cohesion and expressiveness, were obtained before hospital admission for BMT and again 6 to 12 months following BMT.

There were significant declines in social competence and overall self-concept after BMT. Before BMT, perceptions of family conflict had a moderate negative correlation with patient adjustment, whereas family cohesion and expressiveness were unrelated or only weakly related with adjustment measures. But all variables of family environment obtained pre-BMT were highly predictive of adjustment post-BMT. By means of a cross-lagged correlation, it was shown that perceived family cohesion and expressiveness act as protective factors, enabling resilience to the stresses of BMT. The findings provide clues for designing programs to improve the QOL of pediatric patients undergoing BMT.

Barrera et al. [18] examined children's QOL and behavioral adjustment pre-BMT and 6 months post-BMT. Their measure was specifically developed for children with cancer and assessed physical well-being, role restriction and emotional well-being. They compared the pre- and 6 months post-BMT QOL (assessed only by parents' reports), behavioral adjustment and severity of medical symptoms of pediatric BMT patients as well as maternal psychological adjustment and family functioning. The participants were 26 children (mean age 8.5 years) and their mothers, 18 with allogeneic transplant and 8 with autologous transplant. The children undergoing BMT improved in their overall QOL at 6 months after BMT and did not present

with symptoms of serious psychological maladjustment at either pre- or 6 months post-BMT, as measured by the Child Behavior Checklist behavioral scores. On the basis of mothers' reports, there was an increase in the children's overall QOL by 6 months post-BMT, as well as specific decrease in the extent of physical discomfort and role restriction, as measured by the Pediatric Oncology Quality of Life scale. They emphasized that these interpretations need to be put to further empirical test using children's self-reports in addition to parental reports of the children's psychological well-being. Of all the child, parent, family, and medical variables assessed at pre-BMT, only family cohesion and child adaptive functioning were significantly related to children's QOL and behavioral adjustment six months following BMT. Higher levels of family cohesion were related with better QOL in survivors. Thus, family connectedness pre-BMT appeared to play the role of a protective factor against the stresses characteristic of the post-BMT period.

Psychosocial Effects on Disease Course and Outcome

In view of studies with adult patients that showed effects of psychosocial factors on disease course in cancer [46], interest arose in studying the effects of psychological variables on medical outcomes after BMT. A retrospective cross-sectional study [47] with 32 pediatric BMT patients found four factors that contributed to so-called "unexpected" severe physical complications (i.e., they accounted for 55% of the variance): the child's functional impairment, family dysfunction, paternal psychopathology, and geographical dislocation. The same study showed that four similar factors contributed to predicting "unexpected" deaths in the patients' sample (accounting for 36% of the variance): the child's functional impairment, parental psychopathology, family dysfunction, and the child's personality. The major limitations of this study are the small size and poor medical state of the sample, and the retrospective nature of the design. A more recent study investigated the hypothesis that in addition to clinical factors, family characteristics would contribute to predicting the physical outcomes of BMT in pediatric patients [48]. This prospective study was done over a 6.5-year period, with 68 pediatric patients who underwent BMT (29.4% autologous, 70.6% allogeneic). At transplant, their mean age was 7.5 years (range 4 months to 18 years). Their initial prognosis was rated by physicians, on the basis of the child's diagnosis, known risk factors, and donor type. Both parents completed two questionnaires assessing family well-being and marital satisfaction. Nurses also rated the children's QOL 120 and 365 days following the BMT on the Play Performance Status scale. The two outcome measures used were medical complications and death of the child. The study found no effect of family stress or marital satisfaction on the child's survival. There were no predictors in the data for medical complications or the Play Performance score. The best predictor of deaths was the initial prognosis. The authors emphasize that in order to get proof for the effect of social support on survival it would have been necessary to check directly the children's perceptions rather than rely only on the parents' reports.

Some Conclusions

In his excellent review paper of BMT, Phipps [49] noted a certain lagging of psychological studies of BMT behind the rapid medical advances in BMT. Although well-designed studies aimed at shedding light on the psychological effects of BMT have been published since then, there is still a gap between the levels of psychological and medical information in regard to the psychosocial effects of BMT. Basically, the studies showed that the BMT procedure has a marked psychosocial impact on the pediatric patient, which may last beyond the medical procedure itself, and which is largely dependent on the physical sequelae of the treatment. However, the studies also show that the effects seem to be reversible and are remediable by proper psychosocial interventions. The social and emotional support the child receives, particularly from the family, seems to be an important beneficial factor in regard to the child's QOL. At present, the pronounced deficit in psychosocial research consists in regard to intervention procedures designed to improve the coping of the children and raise the level of their QOL during and after the treatment.

Acknowledgements

Thanks are due to Jawdat Eid and Rivka Rosenkranz for their help and contributions.

References

1. Bach FH, Albertini RJ, Joo P, et al. Bone marrow transplantation in a patient with the Wiskott–Aldrich syndrome. Lancet 1968;2:1364–1366.
2. Bensinger WI, Martin PJ, Storer B, et al. Transplantation of bone marrow as compared with peripheral-blood cells from HLA identical relatives in patients with hematologic cancers. New England Journal of Medicine 2001;344: 175–181.
3. Bodmer WF. Evolutionary significance of the HLA system. Nature 1972;23:139–145.
4. Meyers JD. Infections in marrow recipients. In: Mandell GL, Douglas RG, Bennett JE (eds.) Principles and Practice of Infectious Diseases. New York: Wiley, 1985; pp. 1674–1676.
5. Peterson PK, McGlave P, Ramsay NKC, et al. A prospective study of infectious diseases following bone marrow transplantation: emergence of aspergillus and cytomegalovirus as the major causes of mortality. Infection Control 1983;4:81–89.
6. Shulman HM, Hinterberger W. Hepatic venoocclusive disease–liver toxicity syndrome after bone marrow transplantation. Bone Marrow Transplantation 1992;10: 197–214.
7. Rowe JM, Ciobanu N, Ascensao J, et al. Recommended guidelines for the management of autologous and allogeneic bone marrow transplantation: a report from the Eastern Cooperative Oncology Group (ECOG). Annals of Internal Medicine 1994;120:143–158.
8. Duell T, van Lint MT, Ljungman P, et al. Health and functional status of long-term survivors of bone marrow transplantation: EBMT Working Party on Late Effects and EULEP Study Group on Late Effects. European Group for Blood and Marrow Transplantation. Annals of Internal Medicine 1997;126:184–192.
9. Kellerman J, Rigler D, Siegel SE. Psychological response of children to isolation in a protected environment. Journal of Behavioral Medicine 1979;2:263–274.
10. Kutsanellou-Meyer M, Christ GH. Factors affecting coping of adolescents and infants on a reverse isolation unit. Social Work in Health Care 1978;4:125–137.
11. Gunter M, Karle M, Werning A, Klingebiel T. Emotional adaptation of children undergoing bone marrow transplantation. Canadian Journal of Psychiatry 1999;44: 77–81.
12. Patenaude AF. Psychologic impact of bone marrow transplantation: current perspective. Yale Journal of Biological Medicine 1990;63:515–519.
13. Pederson C, Parran L, Harbaugh B. Children's perceptions of pain during 3 weeks of bone marrow transplant experience. Journal of Pediatric Oncology Nursing 2000;17:22–32.
14. Manne S, DuHamel K, Nereo N, et al. Predictors of PTSD in mothers of children undergoing bone marrow transplantation: the role of cognitive and social processes. Journal of Pediatric Psychology 2002;27:607–617.
15. Streisand R, Rodrigue JR, Houck C, et al. Brief report. Parents of children undergoing bone marrow transplantation: Documenting stress and piloting a psychological intervention program. Journal of Pediatric Psychology 2000;25:331–337.
16. Packman W, Weber S, Wallace J, Bugescu N. Psychological effects of hematopoietic SCT on pediatric patients, siblings and parents: a review. Bone Marrow Transplantation 2010;45:1134–1146.
17. Nelson AW, Miles MS, Belyea MJ. Coping and support effects on mothers' stress responses to their child's hemopoietic stem cell transplantation. Journal of Pediatric Oncology Nursing 1997;14:202–212.
18. Barrera M, Boyd Pringle L-A, Sumbler K, Saunders F. Quality of life and behavioral adjustment after pediatric bone marrow transplantation. Bone Marrow Transplantation 2000;26:427–435.
19. Rodrigue JR, MacNaughton K, Hoffman RG, et al. Transplantation in children: a longitudinal assessment of

mothers' stress, coping and perceptions of family functioning. *Psychosomatics* 1997;**38**:478–486.

20. Pot-Mees CC. *The Psychological Effects of Bone Marrow Transplantation in Children*. Delft, The Netherlands: Eburon, 1989.

21. Stuber ML, Nader K, Yasuda P, Pynoos RS, Cohen S. Stress response after pediatric bone marrow transplantation: preliminary results of the prospective longitudinal study. *Journal of the American Academy of Child and Adolescent Psychiatry* 1991;**30**:952–957.

22. Jobe-Shields L, Alderfer MA, Barrera M, *et al.* Parental depression and family environment predict distress in children before stem cell transplantation. *Journal of Developmental & Behavioral Pediatrics* 2009;**30**:140–146.

23. Phipps S, DeCuir-Whalley S. Adherence issues in pediatric bone marrow transplantation. *Journal of Pediatric Psychology* 1990;**15**:459–475.

24. World Health Organization. Constitution of the World Health Organization. In: *Handbook of Basic Documents*, 5th edn. Geneva: UN Publications, 1952; pp. 3–20.

25. Testa MA, Simonson DC. Assessment of quality of life outcomes. *New England Journal of Medicine* 1996;**334**:835–840.

26. Grant M. Assessment of quality of life following hematopoietic cell transplantation. In: Thomas ED, Forman SJ, Blume KG. *Hematopoietic Cell Transplantation*, 2nd edn. Oxford: Blackwell, 1999; pp. 407–413.

27. Ferrell B, Grant M, Schmidt GM, *et al.* The meaning of quality of life for bone marrow transplant survivors. Part 1: The impact of bone marrow transplant on quality of life. *Cancer Nursing* 1992a;**15**:153–160.

28. Ferrell B, Grant M, Schmidt GM, *et al.* The meaning of quality of life for bone marrow transplant survivors. Part 2: Improving quality of life for bone marrow transplant survivors. *Cancer Nursing* 1992b;**15**:247–253.

29. Ford R, McDonald J, Mitchell-Supplee KJ, Jagles BA. Marrow transplant and peripheral blood stem cell transplantation. In: McCorkle R, Grant M, Frank-Stromborg M, Baird SB (eds.) *Cancer Nursing: A Comprehensive Textbook*, 2nd edn. Philadelphia, PA: W.B. Saunders, 1996; pp. 504–530.

30. Parsons SK, Barlow SE, Levy SL, Supran SE, Kaplan SH. Health-related quality of life in pediatric bone marrow transplant survivors: according to whom? *International Journal of Cancer*, 1999;**Suppl. 12**:46–51.

31. Mulhern RK, Fairclough DL, Smith B, Douglas SM. Maternal depression, assessment methods, and physical symptoms affect estimates of depressive symptomatology among children with cancer. *Journal of Pediatric Psychology* 1992;**17**:313–326.

32. Renouf AG, Kovacs M. Concordance between mothers' reports and children's self-reports of depressive symptoms: a longitudinal study. *Journal of the American Academy of Child and Adolescent Psychiatry* 1994;**33**:208–216.

33. Sanger MS, Maclean WEJr, Van Slyke DA. Relation between maternal characteristics and child behavior ratings. *Clinical Pediatrics* 1992;**31**:461–466.

34. Phipps S, Dunavant M, Jayawardene D, Srivastava DK. Assessment of health-related quality of life in acute inpatients settings: use of the BASES instrument in children

undergoing bone marrow transplantation. *International Journal of Cancer* 1999;**Suppl. 12;**18–24.

35. Phipps S, Dunavant M, Garvie PA, *et al.* Acute health-related quality of life in children undergoing stem cell transplant: I. Descriptive outcomes. *Bone Marrow Transplantation* 2002;**29**:425–434.

36. Clarke SA, Eiser C, Skinner R. Health-related quality of life in survivors of BMT for paediatric malignancy: a systematic review of the literature. *Bone Marrow Transplantation* 2008;**42**:73–82.

37. Alby N. Difficultés psychologiques de la période postgreffe de moelle osseuse [Psychological problems in the period after bone marrow transplantation.] *Soins Chirurgie* 1986;**38–40**:483–484.

38. Vannatta K, Zeller M, Noll RB, Koontz K. Social functioning of children surviving bone marrow transplantation. *Journal of Pediatric Psychology* 1998;**23**:169–178.

39. Uderzo C, Biagi E, Rovelli A, *et al.* Bone marrow transplantation for childhood hematological disorders: a global pediatric approach in a twelve year single center experience. *Medical and Surgical Pediatrics* 2000;**21**:157–163.

40. Schmidt GM, Niland JC, Forman SJ, *et al.* Extended follow-up in 212 long-term allogeneic bone marrow transplant survivors: issues of quality of life. *Transplantation* 1993;**55**:551–557.

41. Nespoli L, Verri AP, Locatelli F, *et al.* The impact of pediatric bone marrow transplantation on quality of life. *Quality of Life Research* 1995;**4**:233–240.

42. Notteghem P, Soler C, Dellatolas G, *et al.* Neuropsychological outcome in long-term survivors of a childhood extracranial solid tumor who have undergone autologous bone marrow transplantation. *Bone Marrow Transplantation* 2003;**31**:599–606.

43. Matthes-Martin S, Lamche M, Ladenstein R, *et al.* Organ toxicity and quality of life after allogeneic bone marrow transplantation in pediatric patients: a single center retrospective analysis. *Bone Marrow Transplantation* 1999;**23**:1049–1053.

44. Kreitler S, Kreitler MM, Ben Arush, M.The quality of life of children with cancer: a retrospective and prospective study, in press.

45. Phipps S, Mulhern RK. Family cohesion and expressiveness promote resilience to the stress of pediatric bone marrow transplant: a preliminary report. *Journal of Developmental & Behavioral Pediatrics* 1995;**16**:257–263.

46. Fox BH. Psychosocial factors in cancer incidence and prognosis. In: Holland JC (ed.) *Psycho-oncology*. New York: Oxford University Press, 1998; pp. 110–124.

47. McConville BJ, Steichen-Asch P, Harris R, *et al.* Pediatric bone marrow transplants: Psychological aspects. *Canadian Journal of Psychiatry* 1990;**35**:769–775.

48. Dobkin PL, Poirier R-M, Robaey P, *et al.* Predictors of physical outcomes in pediatric bone marrow transplantation. *Bone Marrow Transplantation* 2000;**26**:553–558.

49. Phipps S.Bone marrow transplantation. In: Bearison DJ, Mulhern RK (eds.) *Pediatric Psychooncology: Psychological Perspectives on Children with Cancer*. New York: Oxford University Press, 1994; pp. 143–170.

7

Psychosocial Aspects of Radiotherapy in Pediatric Cancer Patients

Shulamith Kreitler, Elena Krivoy, Amos Toren

Introduction

Radiotherapy (RT) has increasingly become an integral part of the treatment offered to children in a broad range of malignancies, applied to a variety of body parts, including the whole body. RT designates a set of therapeutic procedures in pediatric oncology including conventional RT, proton therapy, or intensity-modulated RT, which may have an adjunct therapeutic role in combination with chemotherapy or surgery for the disease or local tumor control, a preventive role of CNS prophylaxis for high-risk ALL, a central role in brain tumors, and a palliative role for metastatic disease [1].

The treatment is usually given in a hospital RT department as a series of short daily sessions, lasting 10–15 minutes, over a few weeks. The procedures of applying RT as well as the duration of the treatment may vary with the child's age, the treated body site, and the type of tumor.

The basic procedure includes a preparatory stage with a simulator machine designed to establish the precise sites and dosages of the RT, often accompanied by specific skin marks. The treatment itself is not painful but requires the child to stay alone in the room in the course of the treatment, without moving for at least several minutes. In the case of specific body sites the procedure may include the use of further instruments, such as a protective mask for the face in the case of treatment of the head or neck.

In the case of young children, mostly under the age of 4 years, who are unable or find it difficult to cooperate with the treatment requirements, sedation or general anesthesia is applied so that the children may be able to sleep all through the therapy without impairing

the precision required by the treatment or suffering any undue distress.

RT may have various effects and side effects, some of which appear in the course of the treatment itself and in conjunction with it, immediately or soon afterwards as a cumulative effect of the radiation, whereas others are delayed and appear months or even years after termination of the treatment.

Short-term and Immediate Psychological Effects of RT

Children's Distress in the Course of RT

There are several obvious reasons why it may be expected that distress reactions occur frequently in children in the course of RT [2, 3]. The treatment is given under special unfamiliar conditions to the child, that differ from those of chemotherapy. Further, the RT equipment may produce sights and sounds that may be experienced as frightening. Most importantly, during the treatment, the child is separated from parents and caregivers and has to stay alone in the room. An additional stress-evoking factor is the requirement that the child stay immobilized in a fixed position for the duration of the treatment. An early review [4] showed that 50–60% of pediatric cancer patients undergoing RT were sedated or anesthesized so as to get them to cooperate with the treatment. Since then the percentages seem to have increased although precise numbers are not available. Anesthesia and high doses of sedation may reduce anxiety but they are time-consuming and also have various shortcomings mainly in terms of eating and drinking restrictions preceding sedation, increased risks for medical complications involved in anesthesia, and financial costs.

Pediatric Psycho-oncology: Psychosocial Aspects and Clinical Interventions, Second Edition.
Edited by Shulamith Kreitler, Myriam Weyl Ben-Arush and Andrés Martin.
© 2012 John Wiley & Sons, Ltd. Published 2012 by John Wiley & Sons, Ltd.

One study focused on the distress of children prior to their first RT experience which was to be a simulation session in which no RT was administered but the situation resembled actual RT [2]. The participants were 80 children, 2–7 years old, with various cancer diagnoses, with no or mild degrees of functional impairment, about to receive RT in an outpatient clinic. After explaining to them the study, and before the RT simulation was introduced, the children's distress was assessed through a behavioral observational checklist and by examining their heart rate, as well as through questionnaires administered to the parents. The findings showed that 65% of children manifested at least some degree of anticipatory behavioral distress while 16.3% manifested high distress both in their behavior and heart rate. The major factors that predicted the child's high level of distress were younger age of the child and higher expectations of the parents that the child would experience distress, which in turn was at least partly a function of the child's young age. However, the parents' anxiety levels proved to be unrelated to their expectations of the child's distress reactions.

In a similar sample of 79 children [3], the need for anesthesia prior to the simulation session was used as a measure of distress in addition to the above-mentioned measures of Observation Scale of Behavioral Distress and heart rate. At simulation, 62% of the children required pharmacological intervention to complete the procedure. Further, younger age and higher behavioral distress predicted the use of anesthesia for the simulation. Higher baseline heart rate predicted lower behavioral distress. Notably, a prone position (as opposed to a sitting position) during simulation was related to increased behavioral distress and higher heart rate.

A detailed recording of 4232 procedures involving RT or simulation in regard to 198 children with cancer showed that 37% required sedation for a total of 1033 procedures (a mean of 14 sedations each). These children were 9 months to 14 years old (median 3.8 years), and 96% had a mold (85% of the head and neck). Notably, 37% of the children required sedation at the start of RT but 15% required it even after 30 fractions. Of all sedations, 93% were completed satisfactorily, 5% with some difficulty, and 2% could not be completed. General anesthetic resulted more often in satisfactory sedation (97%) than conscious sedation (68%).The median time from start of medication to the end of RT was 10 min. for general anesthetic and 30 min. for conscious sedation [5].

The described studies demonstrate that pediatric cancer patients tend to experience distress prior to the simulation session, in the simulation session, and in the course of RT proper. However, the more specific reasons for the distress were revealed in a study in which 30 pediatric patients and 30 parents (of a different sample of pediatric patients) in two major medical centers in Israel were interviewed about the difficulties they experienced in regard to RT [6]. The pediatric patients were children 7–18 years old, with various cancer diagnoses, who were either in the last phase of RT or had terminated the treatment up to 14 days earlier. The main sites of RT were the head (55%), neck (15%), the chest (5%), the abdomen (15%) and the limbs (10%). They had 5–35 RT sessions. The parents of the second sample had children who were undergoing RT or who had terminated the treatment a few days earlier, with RT administered to the head (35%), face (10%), neck (10%), abdomen (15%), chest (10%), back (5%), and limbs (15%). In the interviews, which were conducted in individual sessions, the children and parents were asked about the RT (e.g., duration, involved body parts); short-term and long-term effects of RT; difficulties concerning RT and their comparison to those of other treatments and to the expectations; specific behaviors of the children during the RT; and suggestions for facilitating RT.

Most of the parents (80%) mentioned the immediate or short-term effects of RT, which included nausea, diarrhoea, reddening of the skin and loss of hair in the treated area, tiredness, somnolence, headaches, and changes in gustatory and olfactory sensations. The majority (85%) also mentioned possible long-term effects, primarily cognitive impairment (40%), fertility difficulties (30%), problems in regard to growing and overall development (40%), and the risk of a secondary cancer (20%).

Concerning difficulties of RT, the parents mentioned the emotional difficulty (50%) and the difficulty they had to get to the hospital every day for the treatment (60%). Concerning the difficulties of the children, the parents mentioned mainly the difficulty of staying in a waiting room shared by children and adults, the unpleasantness of getting the treatment in the radiation unit which is not the regular ward familiar to the children, the fear evoked by the noise of the instruments, the anxiety of staying alone in the treatment room, the pressures attending the need to come to the hospital every day, and the fatigue in the course of the treatment. All parents (100%) noted that RT was easier than chemotherapy, but as compared to the expectations beforehand, it was easier (45%), more difficult (20%) or in conformity with the expectations (35%).

The major suggestions of the parents for rendering RT easier referred to the necessity of providing continuous psychosocial support to the parents (85%) and to the children (75%) prior to the treatment and in the course of it, in order to reduce anxiety, and improve cooperation. The parents also emphasized the desirability of using treatment rooms and waiting spaces designed specifically only for children, with toys, pictures, music and other objects to distract and relax the children before the treatment. Most importantly, the parents (85%) dwelt on the need to improve the provision of information about the treatment and its effects beforehand as well as in the course of the RT itself to the parents and to the children, using verbal materials implemented by films, videos and modelling, so as to improve comprehension and recall. The emphasis on the need for more information coincides with the results of a recent study that shows that, although the parents feel knowledgeable about neurocognitive late effects of RT, they continue to have a need for further information, and those who reported high emotional distress wanted the information even earlier than the others [7].

Most of the interviewed children (70%) listed several short-term side effects of RT, mainly feeling sick, losing hair, feeling tired, difficulty in concentrating, pain, nausea, no appetite, feeling sad, and feeling lonely. The majority (90%) knew about long-term effects, and mentioned specifically fertility problems (90%); body image deformities (90%, e.g., irregularities in the skin, brown dirty-looking skin, too short neck, remaining small and not growing up tall as other children, shorter limb, baldness forever); various physical disorders (malignancies, heart problems, endocrine disorders, remaining in general "weak" or vulnerable in regard to diseases) (75%); and various social and interpersonal issues (35%, e.g., being rejected by other kids, not finding friends or partners because of physical deformities or esthetic appearance). An important set of side effects emphasized by the children focused on changes in body image, specifically, changes in limbs, skin, stature, body symmetry, scalp and hair that might affect the functioning of their body and change their physical appearance. These changes may affect the children's functioning also in other domains. The children themselves mentioned that a damaged physical appearance may affect the attitude of peers to them in the present and perhaps also in the future and thus alienate them at school and negatively affect their academic achievements.

Concerning difficulties of the treatment itself, the children emphasized the need to come every day to the hospital for the treatment (80%) and the unpleasantness (i.e., anxiety, fear, tension, sense of being abandoned) the word of staying alone in the RT room (85%). For example, an 8-year-old child said, "I feel as if all the world recedes far away and gets smaller and smaller, and I am the last dot in that increasing emptiness." Another 12-year old said, "When I get into the room I am afraid that when I get out, there will be no one to meet me and I will be alone outside too." Some children (30%) mentioned the unpleasantness of getting the treatment in an unfamiliar setting. Many (60%) said RT was easier than chemotherapy, while 40% said it was equally difficult. Further, 20% claimed RT was easier than they had expected, 20% claimed it was as they had expected, but 60% claimed it was more difficult than they had expected, mostly because of misleading information they had received concerning RT.

Most of the improvement suggestions given by the children focused on decreasing the feeling of loneliness in the RT room, for example, by enabling the child to hear the voice of the parents or nurse outside, by listening to music, or by seeing projected pictures. Other suggestions referred to being able to discuss what went on in RT with someone from the staff or the family every day. Both sets of interviews indicate that the parents and the children identify RT as a distinct phase of the treatment marked by emotional distress and suffering of the children due to characteristic features of RT.

Intervention Procedures for Reducing Distress During RT

As noted earlier, the use of anesthesia to reduce distress is frequent in pediatric cancer patients. Despite its safety record, at least some health professionals feel discomfort about applying it repeatedly in multiple sessions of RT with the children. Hence, there have been various attempts to develop psychosocial procedures to minimize the use of anesthesia or sedation for the administration of RT in children.

Several intervention procedures focus on behavioral and emotional coping skills. Thus, one study reported the results of applying a behavioral procedure designed to teach cooperation and motion control to children 3–7 years old with special needs [8]. Of 10 children, 8 benefited from the behavioral program and did not need sedation or anesthesia. Bucholtz [9] emphasized the desirability of developing skills in nurses designed to provide comfort to the children and their parents in the RT set-up. Applying an effective play preparation program markedly minimized sedation in children 2–5 years old who are commonly assumed to require sedation. In a pediatric oncology center over a five-year period, of 1030 treatment days, only in 111 days (10.8%) sedation was required, for the whole age range. No general anesthetics were given. Only 6 patients were sedated for the whole treatment (9.5%), with 52 patients requiring no sedation at all (82.5%) [10].

The use of musical instruments prior to meeting the radiologist may also have beneficial effects [11]. The children who were waiting in an outpatient clinic for treatment or consultation were given the opportunity to explore the sounds, play with the instruments or produce music. This enabled increased communication with the parents and self-expression of fears which resulted in reduced anxiety.

Some programs focused on testing the effects of providing the children and their families with coping strategies based on preparing the children and the parents for the procedure, while attending flexibly to the needs of each particular child [12]. The program applied to 55 children showed increases in satisfaction with care among the child, family, and the staff.

An interactive intervention program for reducing RT distress among pediatric cancer patients was tested with 79 children in a simulation session [13]. The intervention included a 7-minute filmed modeling of the procedure, exposure to an interactive Barney character, and passive auditory distraction by use of a noninteractive Barney character (so as to emphasize the need for immobility in the simulation room). The control group children were exposed to a cartoon-video, a noninteractive children's control character, and stories on a cassette in the simulation room. Children in the intervention group differed from the control participants in having a lower heart rate but not in reduced distress manifested in behavior.

A comprehensive psychoeducationally-based intervention was tested with 223 consecutive pediatric cancer patients treated with RT over a period of six years [14]. The experimental group had 90 RT courses corresponding with 1561 RT fractions; the control group had 154 RT courses corresponding with 2580 RT fractions. The intervention included talks with the patients and the parents about practical aspects of the upcoming RT and an age-appropriate explanation of the RT treatment and procedure, implemented by picture books, playful inclusion of toys, and a reward system using beads as tokens for every accomplished RT session. Attendance by one of two specially trained nurses at least to prepare for the CT, RT simulation and the first RT session and as weekly visits during the RT itself was accomplished, so that each patient was met on average five times for the duration of 5–7.5 hours. The groups did not differ in age at RT, gender, diagnosis, localization of RT and positioning during RT. The intervention resulted in a reduction in the need to use anesthesia: in the experimental group, 8.9% of the children needed anesthesia as compared to 21.4% in the control group, and the median age of cooperating patients without anesthesia decreased from 3.2 to 2.7 years.

The major means used in the various interventions are giving information about the treatment, adjusted to the child's developmental level [15]; providing support, including encouragement and comfort; and diverting the child's attention away from the stressful situation by means of games, music and toys. LeBaron and Zeltzer [16, 17] have pioneered the use of guided imagery and hypnotherapy to reduce pain and anxiety in children with cancer. Other means of overcoming the anxiety of children evoked by RT may be based on art therapy, play therapy, role playing, drama, and production of stories (see Chapter 13 in this volume). Developing, applying and evaluating programs of this kind would render it possible to select in each case the best program in line with the needs of the child, the utility of the intervention, and the resources of the clinic or hospital.

Long-Term and or Delayed Psychological Effects of RT

Cognitive Effects of RT

A large number of studies deal with investigating the cognitive effects of RT, especially cranial radiotherapy (CRT) [18]. The studies have led to an increase in information about the kind of cognitive effects of RT as well as the relations between these effects and various characteristics of RT. However, the findings need to be considered with caution for several reasons. First, despite our attempts to focus only on the effects of RT, it is likely that in at least some of the studies the participating children underwent not only RT but also surgery and chemotherapy that could have impacted cognition; in addition to the RT second, many of the children treated with RT received the treatment for brain tumors, which could have affected cognition independently of the RT; and third, over 40% of brain tumor survivors, especially those with pituitary, hypothalamic and optic pathway tumors, or those who received CRT of at least 2400 cGy, are at risk of significant neuroendocrine deficiencies, which may also impact neurocognitive function [19]. Finally, the cognitive functioning of survivors who received RT may be negatively affected by neurologic deficits from strokes, seizures, ataxia and neuropathies as well as vision or hearing loss that are side effects of the disease or treatments they received [20, 21].

The effects of radiation on the brain are usually described in terms of three stages: (1) the acute phase, often associated with a sudden neurological deterioration; (2) the subacute phase (2–6 weeks after RT), when the "somnolence syndrome" may occur together with fatigue and a transient exaggeration of the neurological signs; and (3) the late phase in which various gradual neurocognitive deficits show up [22]. Most of the reported findings refer to the third phase.

Effects of RT on Intelligence

A large number of studies report the effects of RT on intelligence. One review showed that in 12 of the 18 reviewed studies, patients who received RT had IQ levels 12–14 points lower than those who did not receive RT [23]. In a Japanese sample of 30 children aged 3–16 at diagnosis, treated in the course of seven years, 1.7 years after RT, the level of IQ was almost 20 points lower than in healthy controls [24]. A comparison of children with ALL who received RT with children with ALL treated with chemotherapy and with healthy controls showed that the group who received RT had deficits in IQ that were at least partly independent of other cognitive impairments [25]. The decline in IQ is more severe in those treated with CRT than in those who underwent surgery alone for medulloblastoma [26].There was less decline in those who received a reduced dose CRT (23.4 Gy vs 36 Gy) and were older (above 8.8 yrs) at the time of treatment [27] (see also [28]). Further evidence about the deleterious effects of RT on general intelligence comes from a study which showed declines in IQ in CRT-treated groups [29]. Comparing 16 children with brain tumor, treated with CRT or local RT, with 15 nonirradiated children with ALL showed that on the full scale of the IQ, the mean standard scores were significantly decreased in the brain tumor group [30] (see also [31]). A review [32] found that children treated with CRT may manifest significant drops in IQ scores especially when they are young. In younger patients the decline starts earlier, in the course of the first year, and increases more as time from treatment increases [33], even when there is no tumor recurrence or hydrocephalus [24]. Similarly, in 31 patients (with medulloblastoma or ependymoma) treated with standard dose or reduced dose RT, there was a 2- to 4-point decline per year in intelligence scores. In the younger subjects, intellectual function declined quickly in the first few years after treatment, and then more gradually [34]. The cognitive deficits following RT persist over time, as found in a study of 138 survivors (73 with acute leukemia and 65 with solid tumors), diagnosed before the age of 15 years, with therapy duration over two years, who had been evaluated at least 10 years after diagnosis. The IQ scores of solid tumor survivors were higher than those of leukemia survivors who had CRT at dosages $> = 24$ Gy

(Mean IQ scores 108 vs 98; $p = 0.03$), and resembled those of leukemia survivors with CRT at lower dosages (Mean IQ score 102) or who had no CRT (Mean IQ score 109). Normal IQ was found to be correlated positively with age at diagnosis and negatively with CRT. Survivors of acute leukemia who relapsed scored 14 points less than those who had not relapsed [35]. It seems that the decline in IQ may be due partly to a decreased rate of acquiring new information [36].

Effects of RT on Specific Cognitive Functions

Up to 40% of childhood cancer survivors who were exposed to CRT may experience neurocognitive impairment in one or more specific domains [37]. Deficits in cognitive functioning following CRT are evident in attention, executive functioning, processing speed, working memory, and memory, all of which contribute to declines in intellectual and academic abilities [38]. Monje [39] reported that CRT is associated with a progressive decline in cognitive function, prominently memory function, whereby impairment of hippocampal neurogenesis is thought to be an important mechanism. Children with ALL, who had been treated with RT, had deficits in working memory and processing speed relative to healthy controls. It is likely that deficits in processing speed and working memory following CRT may underlie the frequently reported declines in IQ [25].

A review of pediatric cancer survivors treated with RT [32] showed that affected children tend to have problems with receptive and expressive language, attention span, and visual and perceptual motor skills, as well as academic difficulties in reading, language, and mathematics. A follow-up of 59.6 months after termination of therapy [40] showed a small but significant decline in reading scores, while math and spelling performance remained stable. The decline in the reading decoding and spelling skills seems to be independent of the risk level of the disease [41]. The deficits in the cognitive skills required in academic frameworks contribute to the frequently reported school problems and poor academic performance of children who have undergone CRT [42].

Accordingly, many long-term survivors of medulloblastoma treated with RT had significant school problems (72%), impairments of attention and processing speed (79%), learning and memory difficulties (88%), language disabilities (56%), and deficits in visual perception (50%), or executive functions (64%) [43]. Similarly, in 31 patients (with medulloblastoma or ependymoma), treated with standard dose or reduced dose RT, there were significant declines in visual-motor integration, visual memory, verbal fluency, and executive functioning but there was no decline in verbal memory and receptive vocabulary [34].

An earlier study with pediatric cancer survivors from various diagnostic groups showed that CRT was associated with deficits in several nondominant hemispheric neuropsychological functions, most likely to be reflected in nonverbal intelligence, perceptual abilities and distractibility [44]. Further evidence about the effects of CRT on cognition is provided by findings indicating that academic achievement, verbal knowledge and reasoning, and perceptual-motor abilities were significantly lower among CRT-treated groups of patients and that there were significant negative associations between CRT dose estimates for cortical regions and perceptual-motor abilities [29]. In another group of 138 survivors (with acute leukemia or solid tumors), who had been diagnosed before the age of 15 years, had been treated over two years, and were evaluated at least 10 years after diagnosis, assessment of cognitive functioning showed that the most affected cognitive areas were comprehension, arithmetic ability, attention, visual and verbal memory, causative reasoning and visual-motor coordination. No relationship was found between sensory sequelae (that were mostly mild) and cognitive capacities [35].

In a group of pediatric patients with malignant posterior fossa tumors, tested one year after treatment and at several time points later, no significant differences in cognitive performance were found between those treated with reduced dose CRT and those who received the standard dose. Their performance declined for spelling, mathematics and reading according to achievement tests and ratings by parents and teachers. However, further analyses revealed that there was no loss of skills but a reduced rate of skill acquisition [42]. Further, according to the assessment of parents on a visual analog scale, children with brain tumors, who had been treated with CRT or local RT, functioned with a significantly slower tempo than children diagnosed with ALL who did not receive RT. Low speed and hypoactivity seemed to limit the majority of these children in school and daily life activities [30].

Special emphasis has been placed on memory and attention, both because deficits in these functions showed up in a great number of studies and because they may be responsible for further cognitive difficulties and thus for lower academic achievements in general. Memory deficits following CRT are a recurrent finding. Thus, a study with 60 children diagnosed with acute lymphoblastic leukemia, who were in full remission for at least two years after terminating treatment, showed that all those who received CRT had memory impairment as compared with those who did not receive CRT [45]. Another study showed that children treated with CRT for medulloblastoma had verbal memory deficits in retrieval and recognition verbal memory following RT [47].

Attention deficits are common following RT in pediatric cancer patients (e.g., [19, 27, 47]). Assessments of attention in 120 patients with primary brain tumors (ages 2–24.4 years) showed that before CRT the patients had only mild inattentiveness, during CRT, their impulsivity declined (which indicates the absence of early radiation-related cognitive sequelae), and after CRT their inattentiveness increased markedly, whereby global attention disorders were associated with different types of brain tumors [48].

A study on attention with 22 children (mean age at diagnosis 7.62 years) about 2.5 years after treatment termination, showed that attention span mediated the relationship between time since the initiation of RT and daily living skills. Since the findings were specific to attention, they suggest that attention decreases with time since RT and that poor attention in turn may be associated with lower adaptive functioning on daily life tasks [49].

In sum, CRT brings about decline in a whole range of specific cognitive functions, both verbal and nonverbal, especially memory, attention, and processing speed, as well as global intellectual functioning as manifested in IQ scores, school performance and academic achievement. The impairment shows up within 1–2 years after treatment termination and appears to worsen over time [38, 50]. Impairment in some functions is likely to affect further functions. Factors responsible for increased severity of impairments are younger age when RT is applied (especially younger than 5 yrs) and high dose RT (at least standard dose).

In recent years there have been increased attempts to develop cognitive intervention methods to improve the cognitive functioning of pediatric patients and reduce neurocognitive deficits in the course of their treatment or afterwards [38, 51–54]. Programs of this kind have great potential in counteracting cognitive deficits following RT or sometimes perhaps even preventing them. In sometimes early diagnosis of the difficulties may help in minimizing the damage and reducing the effect of specific deficits on other domains of cognitive functioning.

Further Factors Involved in Cognitive Functioning

Some studies identified nonmedical factors likely to affect cognitive functioning in children who received RT. Thus, in children in remission, evaluated 9–11 months after diagnosis with ALL, IQ and achievement were related to parental social class but not to history of somnolence syndrome, age at irradiation, irradiation-examination interval, and radiation dosages. The strongest predictor of IQ and achievement was parental social class [55]. Similarly, in ALL survivors with complete remission for 3.5 years, parental education levels accounted for more neuropsychologic variability than factors, such as age at diagnosis, or type of therapy [56]. In another group of survivors with cognitive impairment, absence from school during treatment and age at diagnosis were more predictive of reading and spelling academic achievement than having received CRT [44]. Findings of this kind suggest that the child's environment is a factor whose importance for the cognitive functioning of the pediatric patients in remission who received RT must not be underrated.

Social and Behavioral Effects of RT

Difficulties in behavioral adjustment may be expected in survivors of pediatric cancer. Some early studies with heterogeneous samples of pediatric cancer patients who underwent RT found that the survivors manifested mood problems and withdrawal [57–61]. However, stress in the family and coping of the parents were also found to affect the child's behavioral adjustment [62].

A more recent study showed that higher scores on the index of CNS treatment intensity were associated with poorer peer acceptance, fewer friendships, greater social sensitivity-isolation, and diminished leadership-popularity based on peer-report. These associations were stronger for boys and children who were younger than 10 years at diagnosis. In contrast, CNS treatment intensity was related only to teacher perceptions of aggressive-disruptive behavior but it was unrelated to social self-perceptions [63].

A comparison of survivors of brain tumors with those who have been treated with RT, in the age range of 18–30 years, showed that the latter group achieved significantly fewer milestones in the psychosexual and social domains than the other survivors, and accordingly also scored lower on quality of life [64]. Long-term survivors of medullobastoma treated with RT rated social functioning more than healthy controls as the most affected dimension of quality of life. Of 12 survivors over 18 years, none had a boyfriend or girlfriend. The ratings of the patients' social

behavior by their parents were even lower than those by the patients [43].

Mood disorders were evaluated 10 years after diagnosis in a sample of survivors diagnosed with acute leukemia or solid tumors before the age of 15 years, and who underwent therapy of over two years. Compared to healthy controls, they scored higher on depression but not on anxiety [35].

Comparing the adjustment of 16 children diagnosed with brain tumor, who had been treated with CRT or local RT, with a group of 15 nonirradiated children diagnosed with ALL, showed that those who received RT were rated by mothers and teachers as lower on overall adjustment. The difficulties of these children in daily life activities were mostly related to their slowness (low speed) and overall hypoactivity [30]. Children with medulloblastoma treated with low-dose RT functioned socially better after RT than those who received standard dose RT [28].

The performance of children, diagnosed with malignant posterior fossa tumors, who had been treated with reduced or standard dose CRT, was assessed one year after treatment and at several time points later. The parents' ratings showed that the children had medium problems in social withdrawal, depression and anxiety, and those who received reduced CRT dose had fewer problems in aggressiveness and oppositional behavior. Social problems increased with increasing time since termination of treatment, reaching after 12 yrs the clinically significant range [42].

Highly optimistic results were found in a sample of ALL survivors, some of whom have been treated 20 years earlier with CRT, whereas others had not. The whole group of adults had achieved good physical, cognitive, emotional and behavioral development and adjustment. Further, the two groups did not differ significantly from each other and from corresponding national figures in education and occupational level as well as in marriage and fertility [45].

It seems that pediatric cancer survivors may be at risk of having problems in social adjustment and interpersonal relations in general. Since poor peer relations tend to persist and also to affect academic achievement and overall adjustment, it is of special importance to diagnose social adjustment difficulties of pediatric cancer patients as early as possible and launch projects for their minimization. The recommendation for early diagnosis and application of remedial interventions holds in regard to social adjustment no less than in regard to cognitive functioning. Awareness of the need for both may help to improve the functioning and quality of life of the survivors of pediatric cancer who have undergone RT.

References

1. Gibbs IC, Tuamokumo N, Yock TI. Role of radiation therapy in pediatric cancer. *Hematology Oncology Clinics of North America* 2006;**20**:455–470.

2. Tyc VL, Klosky JL, Kronenberg M, *et al.* Children's distress in anticipation of radiation therapy procedures. *Child Health* 2002;**31**:11–27.

3. Klosky JL, Tyc VL, Tong X, *et al.* Predicting pediatric distress during radiation therapy procedures: the role of medical, psychosocial, and demographic factors. *Pediatrics* 2007;**119**:1159–1166.

4. Lew CC. Special needs of children. In: Dow KH, Hilderly LJ (eds.) *Nursing Care in Radiation Oncology.* Philadelphia, PA: Saunders, 1992; pp. 177–202.

5. Seiler G, De Vol E, Khafaga Y. Evaluation of the safety and efficacy of repeated sedations for the radiotherapy of young children with cancer: a prospective study of 1033 consecutive sedations. *International Journal of Radiation Oncology Biology Physics* 2001;**49**:771–783.

6. Kreitler S, Ben Arush M, Krivoy E, *et al.* Psychosocial aspects of radiotherapy for the child and family with cancer. In: Halperin EC, Constine LS, Tarbell NJ, Kun LE (eds.) *Handbook of Pediatric Radiation Oncology*, 5th edn. Philadelphia, PA: Lippincott, Williams & Wilkin, 2010; pp. 449–457.

7. Trask CL, Welch JJ, Manley P, *et al.* Parental needs for information related to neurocognitive late effects from pediatric cancer and its treatment. *Pediatric Blood & Cancer* 2009;**52**:273–279.

8. Slifer KJ, Bucholtz JD, Cataldo MD Behavioral training of motion control in young children undergoing radiation treatment without sedation. *Journal of Pediatric Oncology Nursing* 1994;**11**:55–63.

9. Bucholtz JD Comforting children during radiotherapy. *Oncology Forum* 1994;**21**:987–994.

10. Scott L, Langton F, O'Donoghue J. Minimising the use of sedation/anaesthesia in young children receiving radiotherapy through an effective play preparation programme. *European Journal of Oncology Nursing* 2002;**6**:15–22.

11. O'Callaghan C, Sexton M, Wheeler G. Music therapy as a non-pharmacological anxiolytic for paediatric radiotherapy patients. *Australian Radiology* 2007;**51**:159–162.

12. Filin A. Radiation therapy preparation by a multidisciplinary team for childhood cancer patients aged $3\frac{1}{2}$ to 6 years. *Journal of Pediatric Oncology Nursing* 2009;**26**:81–85.

13. Klosky JL, Tyc VL, Srivastava DK, *et al.* Brief report: Evaluation of an interactive intervention designed to reduce pediatric distress during radiation therapy procedures. *Journal of Pediatric Psychology* 2004;**29**:621–626.

14. Haeberli S, Grotzer MA, Niggli FK, *et al.* A psychoeducational intervention reduces the need for anesthesia during radiotherapy for young childhood cancer patients. *Radiation Oncology* 2008;**3**:17–23.

15. Rasnake LK, Linscheid TR Anxiety reduction in children receiving medical care: developmental considerations. *Journal of Developmental & Behavioral Pediatrics* 1989;**10**:169–175.

16. LeBaron S, Zeltzer LK Research on hypnotherapy for the relief of pain, anxiety, nausea and vomiting in children with cancer. *Texas Psychology* 1985a;**37**:12–14.

17. LeBaron S, Zeltzer LK. The role of imagery in the treatment of dying children and adolescents. *Journal of Developmental & Behavioral Pediatrics* 1985b;**6**:252–258.

18. Ris MD Lessons in pediatric neuropsycho-oncology: what we have learned since Johnny Gunther. *Journal of Pediatric Psychology* 2007;**32**:1029–1037.

19. Turner CD, Rey-Casserly C, Liptak CC, *et al.* Late effects of therapy for pediatric brain tumor survivors. *Journal of Child Neurology* 2009;**24**:1455–1463.

20. Oeffinger KC, Nathan PC, Kremer LC. Challenges after curative treatment for childhood cancer and long-term follow up of survivors. *Hematology/Oncology Clinics of North America* 2010;**24**:129–149.

21. Armstrong GT, Liu Q, Yasui Y, *et al.* Long-term outcomes among adult survivors of childhood central nervous system malignancies in the Childhood Cancer Survivor Study. *Journal of the National Cancer Institute* 2009;**101**:946–958.

22. Moore BD. Neurocognitive outcomes in survivors of childhood cancer. *Journal of Pediatric Psychology* 2005;**30**:51–63.

23. Mulhern RK, Hancock J, Fairclough D, *et al.* Neuropsychological status of children treated for brain tumors: a critical review and integrative analysis. *Medical and Pediatric Oncology* 1992;**20**:181–191.

24. Sugita Y, Kobayashi S, Uegaki M, *et al.* Assessment of functional status in children with brain tumors. *Progress in Neurological Surgery* 1987;**15**:643–649.

25. Schatz J, Kramer JH, Ablin A. Processing speed, working memory, and IQ: a developmental model of cognitive deficits following cranial radiation therapy. *Neuropsychology* 2000;**14**:189–200.

26. Mulhern RK, Merchant TE, Gajjar A, *et al.* Late neurocognitive sequelae in survivors of brain tumors in childhood. *Lancet Oncology* 2004;**5**:399–408.

27. Mulhern RK, Kepner JL, Thomas PR, *et al.* Neuropsychologic functioning of survivors of childhood medulloblastoma randomized to receive conventional or reduced craniospinal irradiation: A Pediatric Oncology Group study. *Journal of Clinical Oncology* 1998;**16**:1723–1728.

28. Halberg FE, Wara WM, Fippin LF, *et al.* Low-dose craniospinal radiation therapy for medulloblastoma. *International Journal of Radiation Oncology, Biology, Physics* 1991;**20**:651–654.

29. Dowell RE, Copeland DR, Francis DJ, *et al.* Absence of synergistic effects of CNS treatments on neuropsychologic test performance among children. *Journal of Clinical Oncology* 1991;**9**:1029–1036.

30. Fossen A, Abrahamsen TG, Storm-Mathisen I. Psychological outcome in children treated for brain tumor. *Pediatric Hematology-Oncology* 1998;**15**:479–488.

31. Roger J, Packer, Leslie N, *et al.* A prospective study of cognitive function in children receiving whole-brain radiotherapy and chemotherapy: 2-year results. *Journal of Neurosurgery* 1989;**70**:707–713.

32. Bhatia S, Landler W. Evaluating survivors of pediatric cancer. *Cancer* 2005;**1**:340–354.

33. Palmer S, Gajjar A, Reddick W, *et al.* Predicting intellectual outcome among children treated with 35–40 Gy craniospinal irradiation for medulloblastoma. *Neuropsychology* 2003;**17**:548–555.

34. Spiegler BJ, Bouffet E, Greenberg ML, *et al.* Change in neurocognitive functioning after treatment with cranial

radiation in childhood. *Journal of Clinical Oncology* 2004;**22**:706–713.

35. Monleon BMC, Andreu LJA, Estelles SII, *et al.* Psychological sequelae in long term cancer survivors. *Annales Españoles de Pediatróa*, 2000;**53**:553–560.

36. Palmer SL, Goloubeva O, Reddick WE. Patterns of intellectual development in long term survivors of pediatric medulloblastoma: a longitudinal analysis. *Journal of Clinical Oncology* 2001;**19**:2302–2308.

37. Krull KR, Gioia G, Ness KK, *et al.* Reliability and validity of the Childhood Cancer Survivor Study neurocognitive questionnaire. *Cancer* 2008;**113**:2188–2197.

38. Askins MA, Moore BD. Preventing neurocognitive late effects in childhood cancer survivors. *Journal of Child Neurology* 2008;**23**:1160–1171.

39. Monje M. Cranial radiation therapy and damage to hippocampal neurogenesis. *Developmental Disabilities Research Review* 2008;**14**:238–242.

40. Conklin HM, Li C, Xiong X, *et al.* Predicting change in academic abilities after conformal radiation therapy for localized ependymoma. *Journal of Clinical Oncology* 200;**26**:3965–3970.

41. Raymond K. Mulhern RK, Shawna L, *et al.* Neurocognitive consequences of risk-adapted therapy for childhood medulloblastoma. *Journal of Clinical Oncology* 2005;**24**:5511–5519.

42. Mabbott DJ, Spiegler BJ, Greenberg ML, *et al.* Serial evaluation of academic and behavioral outcome after treatment with cranial radiation in childhood. *Journal of Clinical Oncology* 2005;**23**:2256–2263.

43. Ribi K, Relly C, Landolt MA, *et al.* Outcome of medulloblastoma in children: long-term complications and quality of life. *Neuropediatrics* 2005;**36**:357–365.

44. Butler RW, Hill JM, Steinherz PG, *et al.* Neuropsychologic effects of cranial irradiation, intrathecal methotrexate, and systemic methotrexate in childhood cancer. *Journal of Clinical Oncology* 1994;**12**:2621–2629.

45. Massimo LM, Wiley TJ, Bonassi S, *et al.* Longitudinal psychosocial outcomes in two cohorts of adult survivors from childhood acute leukemia treated with or without cranial radiation. *Minerva Pediatrics* 2006;**58**:1–7.

46. Copeland DR, DeMoor C, Moore BD, *et al.* Neurocognitive development of children after a cerebellar tumor in infancy: a longitudinal study. *Journal of Clinical Oncology* 1999;**17**:3476–3486.

47. Reeves CB, Palmer SL, Reddick WE, *et al.* Attention and memory functioning among pediatric patients with medulloblastoma. *Journal of Pediatric Psychology* 2006;**31**:272–280.

48. Kiehna EN, Mulhern RK, Li C, *et al.* Changes in attentional performance of children and young adults with localized primary brain tumors after conformal radiation therapy. *Journal of Clinical Oncology* 2006;**24**:5283–5290.

49. Papazoglou A, King TZ, Morris RD, *et al.* Attention mediates radiation's impact on daily living skills in children treated for brain tumors. *Pediatric Blood & Cancer* 2008;**50**:1253–1257.

50. Harila MJ, Winqvist S, Lanning M, *et al.* Progressive neurocognitive impairment in young adult survivors of childhood acute lymphoblastic leukemia. *Pediatric Blood & Cancer* 2009;**53**:156–161.

51. Butler RW, Sahler OJ, Askins MA, *et al.* Interventions to improve neuropsychological functioning in childhood cancer survivors. *Developmental Disabilities Research Review* 2008;**14**:251–258.

52. Butler RW, Copeland DR, Fairclough DL, *et al.* A multicenter, randomized clinical trial of a cognitive remediation program for childhood survivors of a pediatric malignancy. *Journal of Consulting and Clinical Psychology* 2008;**76**:367–378.

53. Hardy K, Willard V, Bonner M. Computerized cognitive training in survivors of childhood cancer: a pilot study. *Journal of Pediatric Oncology Nursing* 2011;**28**:27–33.

54. Butler RW, Mulhern RK. Neurocognitive interventions for children and adolescents surviving cancer. *Journal of Pediatric Psychology* 2005;**30**:65–78.

55. Trautman PD, Erickson C, Shaffer D. Prediction of intellectual deficits in children with acute lymphoblastic leukemia. *Journal of Developmental & Behavioral Pediatrics* 1988;**9**:22–128.

56. Whitt JK, Wells RJ, Lauria MM, *et al.* Cranial radiation in childhood acute lymphocytic leukemia: neuropsychologic sequelae. *American Journal of Diseases of Children* 1984;**138**:730–736.

57. Carpentieri SC, Mulhern RK, Douglas S, *et al.* Behavioral resiliency among children surviving brain tumors: a longitudinal study. *Journal of Clinical Child Psychology* 1993;**22**:236–246.

58. LeBaron S, Zeltzer PM, Zeltzer LK, *et al.* Assessment of quality of survival in children with medulloblastoma and cerebellar astrocytoma. *Cancer* 1988;**62**:179–185.

59. Mulhern RK, Carpentieri S, Shema S, *et al.* Factors associated with social and behavioral problems among children recently diagnosed with brain tumor. *Journal of Pediatric Psychology* 1993;**18**:339–350.

60. Radcliffe J, Bennett D, Kazak AE, *et al.* Adjustment in childhood brain tumor survival: child, mother, and teacher report. *Journal of Pediatric Psychology* 1996;**21**:529–539.

61. Seaver E, Geyer R, Sulzbacher S, *et al.* Psychosocial adjustment in long-term survivors of childhood medulloblastoma and ependymoma treated with craniospinal irradiation. *Pediatric Neurosurgery* 1994;**20**:248–253.

62. Carlson-Green B, Morris RD, Krawiecki N. Family and illness predictors of outcome in pediatric brain tumors. *Journal of Pediatric Psychology* 1995;**20**:769–784.

63. Vannatta K, Gerhardt CA, Wells RJ, *et al.* Intensity of CNS treatment for pediatric cancer: prediction of social outcomes in survivors. *Pediatric Blood & Cancer* 2007;**49**:716–722.

64. Maurice-Stam H, Grootenhuis MA, Caron HN, *et al.* Course of life of survivors of childhood cancer is related to quality of life in young adulthood. *Journal of Psychosomatic Oncology* 2007;**25**:4358.

8

Communicating with Children: their Understanding, Information Needs, and Processes

M. Louise Webster, Jane E. Skeen

Speak, speak. When the time comes
do not be silent but know the time.
(Helen Shaw, *I Listen: Reflections and Meditations.*
Auckland: Puriri Press, 1995)

Introduction

In the past, communication with seriously ill children about their disease, treatment and prognosis was often overlooked or actively avoided, and the majority of pediatric oncology patients were not told their diagnosis, in the belief that this would spare them anxiety and distress. The past two decades have seen a significant change in pediatric medical practice such that the importance of open and honest communication with children and adolescents is regarded as a central tenet in North American, European and United Kingdom child health policies and pediatric oncology Management Guidelines [1]. Studies in this area still reveal, however, that up to a third of pre-adolescent children have not been told that they have cancer by either their parents or treating teams, mainly because their parents continue to fear that disclosure of such information will be detrimental to their child [2–4]. These fears are even more prevalent among the parents of terminally ill children, with studies suggesting that less than a third of families acknowledge the child's impending death with their child, and families either assume that the child is unaware of the situation, or actively block discussion [5, 6]. There still remains for many adults the mistaken belief that children are not able to understand the seriousness of their condition and are best spared the burden of such knowledge. Cultural and societal

beliefs also influence medical and parent practices: in the United States, 65% of pediatricians state that they "always tell" children their diagnosis and only 4% "rarely or never tell" the child; in Japan, the widespread belief that telling a child of a life-threatening illness will prevent their recovery results in only 9.5% of Japanese pediatric oncologists "always telling" and 34.5% "rarely or never telling" children of their diagnosis [7]. Even when health professionals and parents believe in principle that they should communicate with children about the illness, they can be inhibited in doing so by the grief and feelings of impotence of having to acknowledge the unthinkable and deal with life-threatening or terminal illness in a child.

Failure of treating teams and parents to provide such information to children does not mean, however, that the child never finds out that they have cancer; children are resourceful, they overhear conversations, read their own case notes, and talk to fellow patients. Today's children are flooded with media stories about cancer through magazines, talk shows, televised hospital dramas, movies and documentaries. Social networking and the internet provide children with fingertip access to a vast array of information about cancer, much of it frightening and inaccurate.

The child who learns of his or her cancer in such a manner rather than hearing it directly from parents and treating team, learns that this is a matter that cannot be discussed, even with trusted adults, but which must be endured alone in secrecy and silence.

For the child or young person who develops cancer and their family there are many issues that require explanation, discussion, and wherever possible, active

Pediatric Psycho-oncology: Psychosocial Aspects and Clinical Interventions, Second Edition.
Edited by Shulamith Kreitler, Myriam Weyl Ben-Arush and Andrés Martin.
© 2012 John Wiley & Sons, Ltd. Published 2012 by John Wiley & Sons, Ltd.

involvement of the young person in decision-making. These issues include diagnosis, prognosis, treatment regimes, side-effects, invasive procedures, body image alteration, limb salvage procedures and amputation, major surgery, stem-cell transplantation, fertility preservation, loss and late effects of treatment.

The involvement of many young people in large multi-center treatment trials places explicit requirements on treating teams to inform older children of diagnosis and the treatment options when obtaining their assent or consent [1].

Even with the best treatments currently available, 15–20% of children and adolescents diagnosed with cancer will die from their malignancy. These young people need to know that further curative treatment is not possible, but that palliative care and support will continue. They need the opportunity to talk about death and about their own death, and to be involved, where possible, in decisions about how they will live the life they still have.

This chapter will first review the evidence base for a practice of being open and honest with children about cancer, the factors that make it hard for parents to talk to their children about serious matters, children's understanding of illness and of death, and child and family preference regarding how information is given. In the second part of the chapter we present practical strategies in speaking with children. In our consideration of all of these matters it is important to remember that children and adolescents cannot be considered in isolation, but must always be seen in the context of their family, the family's cultural affiliation and spiritual beliefs, and the wider societal systems. In approaching communication about serious illness with children we need to include the important people in the child's world: their parents, siblings, extended family, and often friends and classmates.

Literature Review

Information Given to Children and Psychological Outcomes

In the era when the majority of children with cancer died from their disease and standard practice was to "protect" children from full knowledge of the disease, early observational studies revealed that most did nevertheless find out about their disease and prognosis from other children [8]. The isolation and distrust that resulted from the secrecy surrounding them left many children unable to communicate with family or hospital staff about their fears or their situation [9].

Subsequent studies involving standardized assessment of psychological symptoms in children and adolescents with cancer have explored the relationship between information given to the child about diagnosis and prognosis by the parents or doctor, and subsequent psychological adjustment. Findings have been remarkably uniform; better information leads to lower levels of general distress and negative behavior change [3], lower levels of depressive and anxiety symptoms [10, 2], and better psychosocial adjustment many years later in young adulthood [11].

Type of cancer and prognosis does not influence depressive or anxiety scores [2]. Children who are not given any explanation or rationalization for treatments and procedures are just as likely to experience treatment side-effects as children who are given information [10].

These findings are consistent with those from studies of communication between parents who themselves have cancer and their children. Children and adolescents who are not informed openly about their parents' disease report more anxiety and psychological distress than those who are well informed [12]. While some have questioned whether such findings reflect general family functioning and mental health, of which open communication is just one of many markers [11], in families in which some children have been told and some have not been told, the children who are better informed are less anxious than their siblings [13].

In summary, studies looking at the relationship between timing and specificity of information given to children with cancer by their parents or physicians and the emotional well-being of such children have not demonstrated any "protective effect" of withholding information from children. Instead the studies have shown that children who are not given information about their diagnosis and treatments early in the course of their illness are more vulnerable to anxiety and depression during cancer treatment, and to long-term psychosocial adjustment problems following treatment. Moreover, it seems to be important that such information is given openly by trusted adults in the child's life such as parents and physicians, rather than being covertly acquired from peers or other sources.

Information Given to Children and Physical Health Outcomes

Good communication is at the heart of the life-long relationship that a young person with cancer has with health care services. It is critical to treatment adherence during the acute illness and also to the young person's willingness to engage with subsequent late-effects follow-up care. Both short- and long-term treatment outcomes may be jeopardized when a young person is not adequately informed about their cancer, or does not have an open and trusting relationship with their parents and medical team. Treatment adherence in adolescence is known to be a problematic area, and there are studies that have found oral medication non-adherence rates of over 50% in adolescent oncology outpatients. While there are many factors that influence treatment adherence, adolescents and parents who are in agreement, both about information given by the medical team regarding the cancer and treatments and about chemotherapy dosage and timing, have been shown to be more likely to achieve good adherence to chemotherapy [14, 15]. For the long-term survivors of childhood cancer who are at risk of late effects of treatment including growth and hormonal deficiencies, cardiac complications, infertility, and secondary malignancies, a good therapeutic relationship with treating teams and good information about their own diagnosis and treatment are essential in order to be able to access follow-up clinics and to seek medical help if problems arise in adult life. However, studies of adults attending childhood cancer late-effects clinics show that many patients know very little about their previous diagnosis or the treatments they received [16–18].

Factors Influencing Parental Choice to Give Information to Children

There are a number of studies that have examined the factors influencing choices parents make to either give or withhold information from their children. While most health professionals advocate an open approach in giving children information about their cancer, the actual job of talking to children is often left to parents, either because parents request this, or because staff believe that parents "know their child best" and are therefore the most appropriate people to talk about such matters. This can leave parents feeling overwhelmed, unsupported, and that they are in some way failing their child by giving bad news and not being able to prevent or protect them from what is happening. Staff have been found to seriously overestimate how often parents have actually discussed serious matters with their children, and this suggests that staff themselves sometimes avoid the issue and tend to underestimate how difficult it is for parents to talk about such matters [5].

Parents of children with cancer are more likely to talk to their child about the cancer if the child is older [2–4, 9, 10], and if there are older siblings in the house [9]. Parents are less likely to give information about diagnosis and treatment if they perceive their child to be more emotional, and if they themselves hold the belief that cancer is not curable [4]. Type of cancer, prognosis, relapse status and serious complications do not appear to influence parents' decisions to talk to their child.

A number of reasons for withholding information from children have been given by parents of children with cancer and by mothers who themselves have cancer [2, 19]. Parents may believe that their child is too young to burden with frightening serious facts, that their child is too young to understand, may wish to avoid questions about cancer and death, may wish to prevent child distress, and may wish to avoid disrupting special family events. Some parents also fear that their child will "give up" if told the diagnosis, or that the child's distress will impair the body's ability to fight against the cancer.

On the other hand, parents who have chosen to talk about the cancer believe that by doing so they will preserve their child's trust, and promote the child's acceptance of the illness and treatment. Such parents also share a belief that communicating about such matters will decrease their child's distress, and that their child has a right to be informed. Many parents who have chosen not to tell their children the diagnosis later identify this "lack of candor" as a source of stress or other difficulty both during and after the treatment period [11], and in a study of parents' communication with children who died from cancer, at least a quarter of parents who chose not to tell their children that they were dying subsequently regretted that decision [6].

Parents have identified things that would help them to talk about serious matters to their children, including assistance from health professionals with information about child development, discussion of age appropriate strategies for telling children about cancer [19] and having the healthcare provider give information about the diagnosis and treatment to parents and child simultaneously [4].

Developmental Changes in Children's Understanding of Illness and of Death

Research into this area has attempted to link children's understanding of illness and death to Piaget's theory of cognitive development, and to examine the influences of other factors such as culture, illness experience, and health education on level of understanding. The majority of studies have found that children's concepts of health, illness and death are broadly linked to the child's cognitive and developmental stage, and that these schemata develop and evolve over time in a predictable fashion [20–24].

There is less agreement about the impact of personal illness on understanding, and no consistent evidence that having a chronic illness or being hospitalized increases the child's level of understanding of either experience-specific illness or general illness causality [24–27]. A previous experience of the death of someone close does not necessarily result in a more accurate understanding of death by children [24, 28]. These findings are perhaps to be expected, given the lack of information provided to many children who have serious illnesses, and in particular to younger children. There is, however, evidence that when children are provided with an explanation and education about illness that is targeted to their developmental stage, they demonstrate significant increases in understanding [29–31].

Children's Understanding of Illness

A knowledge of the conceptual stages of illness understanding is important for those attempting to talk with children about illness-related issues. However, it is equally important to remember that a wide variability in the level and stage of understanding may be found in the individual child at any given age, hence the need to check first with the child what he/she understands about a particular situation or condition.

In the sensorimotor period (age 0–2 years) the young infant is unable to distinguish between self and the external physical world, and is dependent on caregivers and the developing attachment relationship for security and soothing. Preverbal infants learn to associate certain events with environmental cues and can develop conditioned responses and learn coping strategies for stressful events, but are still dependent on the caregiver for integration and interpretation of here and now experiences. The development of a cognitive schema to explain illness requires the development of explicit or verbal memory, that is, the conscious recollection of previous experiences, and the development of semantic or declarative knowledge. These developmental processes are linked to evolving language skills and cognitive development, and occur in the third and fourth years of life [32]. Refer to Example 1.

EXAMPLE 1

A 2-year-old became distressed when the nurse entered her room wearing a purple over-gown but not when wearing a yellow gown; purple was worn when chemotherapy was given and yellow for protective isolation.

EXAMPLES 2–4

A 4-year-old girl said that she "got leukemia" when she came to hospital, because coming to hospital was the event that was associated with being declared "sick" and with being subjected to unpleasant treatments and procedures.

A 3-year-old became distressed when he saw his nurse with a nasogastric tube under her arm, assuming that it was about to be inserted into him (he already had one in situ). He had also assumed that his nurse looked after no other children.

A 6-year-old was experiencing expected side effects of his leukemia treatment and asked why. When told that the symptoms related to his treatment, he replied, "I thought the leukemia treatment was meant to make me better."

The pre-operational period (age 2–7 years) is generally associated with thinking that is concrete and egocentric, and children may have difficulty distinguishing between reality and representation. Interpretation of words is often literal. They may utilize magical thinking and will often focus on one part of an event or experience, without being able to register the wider context. Illness concepts and beliefs at this stage include phenomenism—illness is caused by events or sensory stimuli that are closely temporally associated—and contagion—illness is caused by objects or environments close to the child's body at the onset of the illness. Young children may also see painful procedures as being "punishment" by parents and staff for some imagined wrongdoing. Refer Examples 2–4.

The concrete operational period (age 7–11 years) is characterized by an increasing capacity to think logically and to understand wider contexts for events or experiences. Children can keep track of time, number, and sequence of events, and can differentiate between self and the outside world. They are able to appreciate that other people may hold differing points of view. Children at this stage understand that illness can be caused by contamination—contact with germs or dirt, or by exposure to cold weather without appropriate clothing—but do not appreciate the complex inter-relationship of multiple variables that might lead to illness. They believe that illness can be cured by simple measures such as taking the right medicines and staying in bed, and that medication taken by mouth has an effect on internal organs and processes (internalization). Refer example 5.

EXAMPLE 5

A 7-year-old boy whose younger brother had died of disseminated abdominal neuroblastoma believed that he had caused his brother's illness because he had patted a dirty dog and then touched his brother. He was now presenting with recurrent abdominal pain and was worried that he had "caught" cancer from his brother.

EXAMPLE 8

After a 2-year-old boy died at home, the family were choosing which of his toys to put in his coffin. His sister aged 5, who had been kept involved throughout his illness and death, was insistent that a hammer be included as he would need it to "hammer the coffin lid off when he got to heaven."

The formal operational period (age 11+ years) is associated with the capacity for abstract reasoning, deductive logic, and the ability to explore hypothetical situations. Young people at this stage can "understand that there might be many interrelated causes of illness, that the body might respond variably to any or a combination of agents, and that illness might be caused and cured as a result of a complex interaction between host and agent factors" [21]. They can conceptualize on both a physiological and psycho-physiological level [20].

It is not uncommon for cognitively competent people of all ages to make magical attributions regarding the causes of childhood cancer. This may be in part because the causes of childhood cancer are so poorly understood. Refer examples 6 and 7.

Children's Understanding of Death

Studies examining children's beliefs about death show that these center around evolving concepts of irreversibility, non-functionality, universality, and causality [22, 28]. For infants up to the age of 3 years, the primary focus is on attachment relationships and separation from close adults, so that death cannot be distinguished from separation or abandonment. By the age of 3 years children know that death occurs, but see death as temporary and reversible. They may show magical thinking about causes of death, and understand death as a separation from loved ones and as "going to another place." Refer example 8.

From 6 years onwards, children develop the understanding that everyone dies at some stage including they themselves, that death is irreversible, and learn about possible causes of death. While the concept of non-functionality also develops, children of this age can struggle still with worrying, for example, that someone who has died might be feeling cold after being buried.

From 12 years onwards in the stage of formal operational thinking, adolescents have an adult understanding of death. However, the sense of invulnerability that can accompany evolving adolescent individuation and autonomy may make it difficult for some adolescents to acknowledge that they themselves might die from cancer. Refer example 9.

How Do Children and Families Want Information to Be Given?

There is little empirical research evaluating strategies for talking with children (or indeed adults) about their

EXAMPLES 6–7

A 12-year-old boy who had relapsed leukemia said to a doctor: "I was playing rugby and someone knee-ed me in the chest and then someone kicked me in the head and then I wasn't feeling well. And that's why I got cancer. Mum thinks so too."

A Chinese family had become Christians a year before their daughter developed cancer. They believed at the time of diagnosis that the cancer had occurred because, as part of their move to Christianity, they had destroyed their traditional Chinese statues of Gods, including the one that protects children.

EXAMPLE 9

A 16-year-old girl developed widespread metastases from a relapsed abdominal rhabdomyosarcoma and was admitted to a hospice for palliative care and pain management. She had been kept well informed about her diagnosis and her prognosis, and had actively participated in the decision to stop chemotherapy. Several weeks after admission to the hospice she told her therapist that she had "only just realized" that she was going to die.

illness. Awareness of the importance of this area has led to practical guidelines for health care professionals on how to break bad news to adults [33, 34], and how to talk to children about death [35–37]. There are also uncontrolled studies describing positive outcomes of various information-giving practices, such as the use of an analogy of weeds in a flower garden as a way of telling young children about their diagnosis of leukemia [38], and the use of a "final stage conference" to discuss therapeutic choices with children who have end-stage cancer [39].

The guidelines for adult patients developed by Baile and Buckman stress the importance of good listening and communication skills on the part of the health care professional, and recommend a stepwise progression that starts with ensuring that the physical setting is appropriate and that the right people are present. This is followed by finding out how much the patient knows, finding out how much the patient wants to know, sharing information, responding to the patient's emotions, and jointly planning follow-up. Empathy on the part of the health care provider is one of the most important factors for children and for their parents during such discussions [4].

Parents whose children have cancer have been shown to have a high level of agreement with their pediatricians regarding the content of what needs to be discussed when a child is first diagnosed with cancer [40]. Parents seek advice on "what to tell the child" as ranking closely in importance to discussion about diagnosis, prognosis, and therapy, and many parents prefer that the information be given to them and their child simultaneously [4].

Studies investigating the preferences of children and adolescents suggest that the majority of young people want their parents to be involved in any communication about their illness [41, 42] and want to share end-of-life decision-making if they should become very ill [43]. However, parents may also constrain the process of communication, restricting the amount of information given [42], and it is easy for young people to become marginalized during three-way consultations between doctors, parents and the young person [44].

Practical Strategies in Speaking with Children

The following guidelines are based on the authors' personal experiences working with children and adolescents with cancer, and in the light of the body of literature reviewed above. In this section we cover general guidelines in speaking with children and adolescents about their illness and treatment, specific clinical

---

EXAMPLE 10

A 12-year-old girl found it difficult to verbally communicate with family or staff her fears about forthcoming high-risk surgery, or to engage in any discussions about the surgery. However, while playing with her old doll, she was able to tell her doctor how frightened her doll was and have a discussion about what information "the doll might like."

---

situations, other issues that may need addressing, and speaking with children and adolescents about death. We acknowledge that there are many different ways of approaching such matters, and it is important that clinicians develop an approach that they personally feel comfortable with.

There are two important prerequisites to speaking with children. The first is learning to listen to what children say and how they say it. Only then can we understand their concerns and needs, and start to provide appropriate information and support. Good listening is essential both in formal settings where we sit down with children and speak with them about their illness, and in the unexpected moments when children indicate their thoughts and their anxieties through direct questions, conversational talk, play and drawings, or through their silence. Refer examples 10 and 11.

The second prerequisite is the provision of support to staff. Working with seriously ill children and children who die places unavoidable emotional demands on staff. To listen to and talk with children about the difficult issues that arise when they have cancer requires a willingness to enter the child's world, to see their reality as they see it, and to hear their fears and their losses as they feel them. This is not easy, for children often cut through the defenses, rationalizing and

---

EXAMPLE 11

A 9-year-old boy whose parents wished to shield him from any possibility that he might not recover from his leukemia, drew a picture of his family and carefully included the family dog, explaining that the dog had died recently. His parents were shocked as they had told him that the dog had "gone to live with another family." However, they then realized that they needed to talk more openly with their son about his illness.

pretense that many adults use when faced by life-threatening illness in children. Children expect honest answers to honest questions. Staff may work with young patients who overwhelmingly remind them of their own children at home. Staff may also struggle to acknowledge or express their own grief and anger when children with whom they have had daily contact relapse, experience devastating disease or treatment outcomes, or die.

For staff to be able to continue to hear children and speak with children, we need systems of support for staff to ensure that they can do this work without becoming too overwhelmed by, or distanced from their patients' worlds. We need a pediatric oncology team culture that acknowledges the emotional impacts of such work on staff, and the routine provision of staff supervision and support that focuses on these issues. It is only when these structures are in place that staff can safely listen to children and speak with them about serious matters.

General Guidelines

1 Before Talking with Children, Talk to the Parents to Plan with Them How Best to Talk with Their Child

When a child has cancer, parents or primary caregivers are facing two challenging tasks simultaneously. They have to learn about and integrate new and often over-whelming information about their child's diagnosis, prognosis and treatments, and cope with their own emotional response to the situation. At the same time they are having to support and parent as best they can, a child whose life is under threat and who is dependent on them for physical and emotional support and containment. Talking to parents first gives them an opportunity to process the information and ask questions, and space to openly express their emotions or distress, before having to focus on their child's needs. Parents are the best source of information about their child—they know what terms or words their child uses, what sorts of experiences with illness or hospital systems the child has had previously, and how their child has coped in the past with stressful situations. They also provide important information on family spiritual and cultural beliefs that are relevant to what is said to the child and how it is framed. It is then possible to plan with the parents what is to be communicated to the child, and for what purpose.

2 Ways that Meeting with a Child Might Then Proceed

- Meeting the child together with the parents/primary caregivers.

> **EXAMPLE 12**
>
> An 8-year-old boy and his parents met with the doctor to hear the diagnosis of osteogenic sarcoma and to discuss the treatment plan for chemotherapy and surgery.
>
> After his parents left the room, the boy turned to his nurse and asked if "children died from what he had." The nurse told him that most children got better with the medicines and surgery, but that some children did die. She went on to tell him that everyone hoped that the treatments would make his cancer go away, but that no matter what happened, his parents and his doctors and nurses would look after him.

- Meeting with the child without parents; this is sometimes the preference of older adolescents, who might prefer another support person such as a friend or partner to be present.
- Meeting with the child and parents after the parents have talked to their child.

It may be important to give children the opportunity to talk to the doctor/nurse by themselves. Some children attempt to protect their parents from knowing how much information they have acquired, and the extent to which they understand their illness and prognosis. The child may wish to ask questions or discuss subjects that they feel unable to raise in front of their parents. This is the first step towards allowing the family to discuss openly matters that have been avoided, and to move beyond the "mutual pretense" identified by Bluebond-Langner [8] in children with cancer and their families. Refer example 12.

3 Ensure that the Setting Is Appropriate

A place that is private, child-friendly and safe is a necessity. Arrange to have everyone seated, and if the child is confined to bed, ensure that adults are not standing over the child. Children will not feel safe if the procedures room, where invasive or unpleasant tests and treatments take place, is used for discussions.

4 Ask the Child What He/She Knows of the Illness and/or Treatments to Date

This helps to know what the child understands and what terms to use. It also allows correction of any misunderstandings that the child may have. Children invariably know from the reactions of those around them that something serious has happened, even if they are unsure of what exactly it is. Refer example 13.

EXAMPLE 13

A young man of 17 wrote about coming to the hospital when he was diagnosed with leukemia 7 years earlier: "I remember my first time. My mum sat there not doing anything. My dad came along. He looked haggard."

5 Check with the Child How Much He/She Wants to Know

Some children may not want to know details about their cancer or treatments, or may not want to know about more than the immediate plans. Younger children may not be able to comprehend the time scale of extended and sequential treatment regimes. Children with marked anticipatory anxiety may need information presented in manageable sections prior to each stage, with enough time to prepare adequately for new treatments but not so far in advance that they become overwhelmed with anxiety. Refer example 14.

6 Explain in Terms that Are Appropriate to the Child's Level of Understanding

Use simple language, avoiding complex medical terms and abbreviations. Be aware that words which have more than one meaning may be interpreted very literally by children according to their past experiences. Children also overhear information given to their parents or to other patients, and may misinterpret what they hear or place it out of context. Refer examples 15 and 16.

In the following examples, children needed to have technical terms explained to them in simple language so that they could understand what was happening. Refer examples 17–19.

When treatment is provided in a language other than the child's native tongue, it is important to use an interpreter, and to ensure that the interpreter has an

EXAMPLE 14

A boy aged 8 had several relapses of his leukemia and required intensive treatment regimes. His mother subsequently recalled how her son coped best when he was given information openly and honestly. However, she and his treating team found that he needed to be told the immediate treatment plan only, because if they discussed all of the future options in his presence, he became confused and agitated and stopped listening.

EXAMPLE 15

Mark, aged 4, came back from the operating room with a surgical drain in place. He asked the play specialist for a specific book which told the story of a mechanical digger, digging a drain in the ground and had appropriate illustrations. After the story was read he said, "I've got a drain. That's what I have got. Why have I got a drain—what's my one?"

He was told that the drains that the digger put in the ground were pipes to take away water. His drain was a little pipe or tube that the doctor had put there to take away water from his chest and help him to get better.

EXAMPLE 16

An 8-year-old girl became anxious about going to the operating room and being "put to sleep" by the anesthesiologist. Recently her pet cat had become sick and had been "put to sleep" by the vet before being returned home and buried in the garden.

understanding of developmentally appropriate concepts and language for the child. Simple pictures or diagrams may also be useful. Proceeding without an interpreter can lead to serious misunderstandings and distress. Refer example 20.

EXAMPLE 17

Vela, aged 4, with newly diagnosed leukemia, asked the mother of another patient why they couldn't play together, and was told that the other child was "neutropaenic." Indignantly she demanded: "Why's she got new peanuts and I haven't?"

EXAMPLE 18

Hearing the words "bone marrow," a child became agitated as she thought staff were talking about using a "bow and arrow."

EXAMPLE 19

A 7-year-old boy whose intravenous line pump gave the alarm signal asked, "What's that beeping? Is my confusion complete?"

EXAMPLE 20

A 2-year-old Indian girl came to a new, English-speaking country for medical treatment of her brain tumor, and required radiotherapy before returning home. She saw a thick cable of black electrical cords crossing the back wall of the room and attached to the radiation machine. She cried repeatedly "Snake, snake" in Hindi.

There was no common language between the child and her family and the radiation therapist, and she and her family had not had an opportunity to view the room and become familiar with the equipment before the treatment began.

EXAMPLE 22

A boy, aged 5, while playing with the hospital Playmobile medical play figures, described his double lumen central line to the play specialist.

"My person's got a Hickman—Hickman means two. I'll show you mine, see the two [holding up his line and displaying it], they go into this one. I've got cancer medicine and other medicine."

The boy clearly understood what his central line was for, and that different medicines went down each of the two parts of the line.

EXAMPLE 23

The mother of a child with Aplastic Anaemia told everyone that her child had ALL—the recognized abbreviation for Acute Lymphoblastic Leukemia. She knew in fact that her daughter did not have leukemia, but had heard people talk of ALL and assumed that this was the abbreviation for Aplastic Anaemia.

There may be difficulties when the interpreter's own cultural beliefs are in conflict with the information they are being asked to convey to the child and family. Difficulties can also arise when the interpreter has a pre-existing relationship with the family, which is another reason why professional interpreters, rather than family members, especially older siblings, be used. An ongoing working relationship between the service and interpreter, and opportunity to discuss such issues with the interpreter prior to meeting with the child and family is helpful. Refer example 21.

Many younger children may only be able to understand complex procedures through the use of play. Using dolls to show where central lines, cannulae, or post-operative drains will be placed, or to rehearse the steps of a procedure helps the child to understand what is about to happen. Child Life Specialists or Play Specialists are trained to assist children in this manner, and the inclusion of such professionals in pediatric oncology teams is now standard practice [45]. Refer example 22.

Parents are the source of daily information for the child regarding what is happening and why. If parents are not well informed, they may misinterpret what they have been told. Abbreviations are used freely in a medical setting and parents hear these and may repeat them in the context of their own understanding. Refer example 23.

Earlier findings about adolescents' disregard of pamphlets notwithstanding, providing written information in the form of handouts, pamphlets, and books for children and their parents is one way of reducing the confusion of disease names and abbreviations. Advice on helpful websites is also valuable as many young people and families will turn to the internet as their preferred source of information.

7 Existing Understandings

Check back with the child about their understanding of the previous discussion and ask if they have any questions. Refer example 24.

EXAMPLE 21

A clinician was explaining a difficult situation to a family with the assistance of an interpreter. Also present was a support worker of the same ethnicity as the interpreter and family. Halfway through the meeting the support worker interrupted and said, "Please interpret what the Doctor is saying." The interpreter responded that "It was such bad news she wanted to protect the family from hearing it."

EXAMPLE 24

A 5-year-old girl who had been given an explanation about leukemia asked, "Why are they called white cells when your blood is red?"

EXAMPLE 25

A young boy displayed a range of somatic and anxious responses after being told about plans for him to be the bone-marrow donor for his sibling's transplant. When asked directly what was wrong, he replied, "I don't want to do that bone-marrow." It was then possible to explore with him his concerns, and the reasons for his reluctance.

---

8 Check with the Child How He/She is Feeling and if He/She has any Specific Worries

Children may feel unable to spontaneously volunteer concerns they have, especially if they think that their concerns or feelings will upset others. They need to be asked directly about how they are feeling. Refer example 25.

9 Outline What Is Going to Happen Next, and Indicate Your Availability for Further Discussions

This should include making sure that the child can identify someone that they feel able to talk to if they feel upset or have any questions.

Specific situations

Limb Salvage Procedures and Limb Amputation

Amputation of a limb represents a sudden and irrevocable alteration in body appearance and integrity, and parents and adolescents in particular may feel intense distress and repugnance at the thought of what will happen in surgery. Younger children may not be so concerned about changes in body appearance, or may not realize that the loss is irreversible. Fortunately limb salvage procedures have reduced the need for amputation in many cases. Refer example 26.

EXAMPLE 26

A 4-year-old boy whose toe had been amputated asked his father if his toe would grow back again. He was told that his toe would not grow back, and that he would always have four toes on that foot. He needed reassuring that no other parts of his body were going to be removed. He was also told that he would still be able to walk and run like before.

EXAMPLE 27

A father, when the surgeon explained about limb-salvage surgery to his son's upper arm, was extremely concerned as to whether his 8-year-old son would be able to fulfill his potential as a cricketer. He needed support to be able to acknowledge the loss of some of the hopes and dreams that he, as a father, had for his son, and to separate those from the more immediate issues that his son was worried about.

Children need permission to grieve for the loss of such a tangible part of themselves by way of acknowledgment and acceptance from the adults around them of their anger or sadness.

Some of the potential losses may be a more immediate concern to the parent than to the child. Refer example 27.

When mutilating surgery such as amputation is required, special care is needed in preparing the child/adolescent for the post-operative appearance of the limb. For younger children, play preparation may be invaluable in conveying to them some understanding of what will happen. Children who are not told or adequately prepared for amputation are likely to feel angry and betrayed by the adults involved. Refer example 28.

Limb salvage procedures pose particular challenges when discussing what will happen with children and their families. Surgery such as a rotation plasty involves both loss of part of the limb, and a marked alteration in orientation or appearance of other parts of the limb in a manner that is visually and conceptually difficult to adjust to. However, when children are adequately prepared for surgery, they adapt more easily. Refer example 29.

EXAMPLE 28

The parents of a 9-year-old boy with an osteosarcoma of the radius were unable to bring themselves to tell their son that he was to have his lower arm amputated. The boy was devastated to wake up from surgery to find his arm gone, and subsequently as an adolescent became estranged from his family, blaming his father and the surgeon for the loss of his arm.

EXAMPLE 29

An 8-year-old girl with an osteosarcoma of the femur was to have a Van Ness rotation plasty to allow her ankle to take the place of her knee. There was much anxiety about how to present the information about the forthcoming surgery to her. However, after viewing a videotape showing other children who had undergone the same procedure, she commented, "I won't have to reach so far to smell my foot."

Her parents had stressed to her that her survival was the main priority and that was why she needed the surgery. After the surgery she would get a prosthetic (artificial) leg fitted and she would once again have two legs to stand on.

Children may want to know what happens to the amputated limb and may wish to choose what is done with the limb. Refer examples 30 and 31.

Adolescents may use humor as a way of coping with loss or with challenging situations. While this can be a useful defense and coping strategy, it is important that

EXAMPLE 30

An 11-year-old girl with an osteogenic sarcoma of the humerus underwent an amputation of her arm following thorough discussion of treatment options with her and her parents. Shortly after the amputation she asked what had happened to her amputated arm and expressed a wish to see it. Her doctor undertook to investigate where the arm was, and to view the arm first prior to the girl seeing it. The girl was informed by her doctor that her arm was still in the pathology department, whereupon she then decided that she no longer wished to see it and consented to it being disposed of. When the cancer returned several years later, she asked to visit the pathology department to see the original pathological slides of the tumor. Being able to do this helped her to acknowledge and reconcile what had happened previously with what was happening now.

EXAMPLE 31

An adolescent boy chose to have his amputated leg cremated, and the ashes returned to him, giving him some sense of control and ownership of his leg.

EXAMPLE 32

A 15-year-old boy used "black" humor to overcome awkward situations following amputation of his leg. Soon after discharge from hospital while he was still on crutches and awaiting a prosthesis, he visited the supermarket with his mother. When people stared at him, he responded, "I seem to have lost my leg, have you seen it?—Perhaps I should try the meat department."

such humor be initiated by the adolescent rather than by others. It is also important not to ignore the underlying feelings of loss. Refer example 32.

Stem Cell Transplantation

When stem cell transplantation is planned, good explanation and communication are essential, and this is particularly so when the marrow donor is a sibling. There are many misunderstandings that can arise if this is not done carefully—siblings may not have received much information from parents or staff about cancer, and often will not have the knowledge that is obtained by children with cancer from the peer group on the ward and at special camps [8].

The actual procedure may be seen by the sibling donor as involving removal of one of their bones or of all of their bone marrow to give to the recipient, and they may worry about how they will manage without it. Siblings may also have difficulty understanding the concept of Human Leukocyte Antigen (HLA) matching. Refer examples 33 and 34.

EXAMPLE 33

A 4-year-old girl was a perfect HLA match to her 6-year-old sister with relapsed leukemia. Prior to the transplant she began to worry about exactly when she would get sick, need medicines and lose her hair, because she had been told that she had the "same blood" as her sister. She was reassured that her blood was strong and healthy, and that she was not going to get sick like her sister because she didn't have the sick leukemia blood. She was also told that she couldn't "catch" leukemia from her sister. She was then told that the medicines were making her sister's sick leukemia blood go away, and that her healthy blood would help her sister to grow strong healthy blood like hers.

EXAMPLE 34

A 7-year-old boy was to be the marrow donor for his older sister who had leukemia. He had heard numbers being discussed and knew that this was important, but did not understand what the numbers referred to. While playing with the hospital Playmobile medical dolls he said, "That's me doing the bone marrow thing for my big sister. I'm 100 out of 100—that's why I'm doing the bone marrow. My little sister is 20 out of 10 and Mum is 60 . . . What do I do when I do the bone marrow?"

As in the previous example, he needed a careful explanation of what was to happen.

Where there are several siblings who have compatible marrow, there may be sibling rivalry as to who is the preferred donor, and when a sibling is found to not be a match, he/she may feel that they have failed to help. Children may also feel coerced and resentful at the prospect of being a donor, especially if there is not an opportunity to talk openly about their fear of the procedure, or their feelings towards their sibling. Refer example 35.

There are obvious implications for the donor if the transplant fails because of non-engraftment, infection, graft versus host disease (GVHD) or relapse of the cancer. The sibling may feel personally responsible for the outcome, and fear that his or her marrow was not "good enough."

Advances in assisted reproductive technology make it possible to selectively conceive a "savior" infant who

EXAMPLE 35

A teenage boy, who had been in conflict with his parents over many matters, was found to be a compatible marrow donor for his younger brother. The older boy angrily told his parents that "They only wanted him for his marrow." An urgent family meeting was held with him and his parents at which his current distress was acknowledged, and his parents were able to tell him that they loved him. Additional extended family supports were put in place for the boy over the transplant period when the parents would not be very available, and he and his parents were encouraged to look at other ways of resolving conflict.

is a good HLA match for an older sibling requiring a cord-blood stem-cell transplant. The complex ethical issues raised by this situation have been debated in bioethics circles and in popular literature [46], and the risk that such a sibling might later feel valued only for their "donor potential" has been highlighted. It is important therefore, that as they grow older, sibling donors are explicitly reassured by parents that they were and are, loved and wanted "for themselves."

Fertility

The impact of certain cancer treatments on fertility is an area that should be routinely discussed in some detail with adolescents shortly after diagnosis, and with preadolescent children at some stage during their cancer treatment. All patients attending Late Effects Clinics require information about fertility and the offer of further investigation and treatment. Adolescents also need to be reassured that infertility is not synonymous with impotence.

In some adolescent boys, the issue of sperm collection and storage needs to be discussed prior to commencement of chemotherapy. This can be an extremely difficult area for the young adolescent with emerging sexuality and sexual identity to discuss, especially if they have just learned that they have cancer, and needs to be approached with great sensitivity. While some parents of adolescents will have previously established open and honest communication about sexuality with their adolescent, other parents will have no communication pathways established, and thus have little idea of how best to approach this topic. As with any other discussion of serious matters, this needs to take place in a private setting, and with acknowledgment that this may be an issue that the adolescent finds difficult to discuss. It is important that the health professional who raises this issue is comfortable with discussing such a sensitive subject and with answering broader questions regarding sexual function and sexuality should they arise. It is helpful to find out how much the adolescent already understands about sexual reproduction and physiology, and the words they use to describe this. After careful explanation of the impact of treatment on fertility, the adolescent needs to be told about the possibility of storing sperm so that when he is older he can have children should he wish, and be offered the opportunity to discuss ways that sperm collection can be undertaken. Research continues into strategies and techniques for fertility preservation in young women: oophoropexy, ovarian/ovarian strip storage for pre-pubertal girls, harvesting of eggs in the pubertal girl, and storage of embryos are also possibilities, but involve more invasive

---

EXAMPLE 36

A 19-year-old leukemia survivor said that he was prepared to provide a semen sample, but not yet; he was still not ready for working through the issues that would arise should the sample show that he was in fact sterile.

EXAMPLE 37

A 15-year-old boy who had completed cancer treatment stated that he thought he might be the father of his pregnant friend's unborn child. The oncology staff knew that he was highly unlikely to be the biological father. However, he did not wish to pursue blood testing to prove paternity, and chose to maintain the hope that the child could be his.

EXAMPLE 38

The parents of a 13-year-old girl who developed leukemia decided to treat her as an adult, allowing her a large say in the treatment decisions on the basis that it was better to have her as an active participant. This led to many disagreements in which the girl became anxious and angry, and culminated in the girl informing her parents that she would not have cranial irradiation and would not complete the consolidation phase of treatment. The family then moved to another city where the new medical team, mindful of what had already occurred, was able to work with the parents to set the ground rules for the girl's ongoing management. These were based on the notion that while her assent would be sought for treatment, she was not able to give or withhold consent because she was too young to be able to make the major treatment decisions. The girl completed treatment satisfactorily and was less anxious and distressed.

---

procedures and time. Appropriate ethics approval is also more challenging.

If parents are reluctant to even consider such issues with respect to their young person on the basis of cultural and religious beliefs, there may still be an ethical and legal obligation to inform the adolescent of the options and consequences.

While infertility is relatively common in the general population and affects one in six couples, most people with infertility do not have to acknowledge or address these issues until they are older adults in a stable relationship. An understandable reluctance to face definite confirmation of infertility and the inherent loss for the future may result in fertility testing being declined by adolescents attending late-effects clinics. Refer examples 36 and 37.

Adolescents who have impaired fertility may feel angry that their parents gave consent to treatment that was known to impair fertility when the adolescent was younger. They may need to have the original treatment dilemmas and decisions explained to them, and acknowledge the loss involved for them.

Contextual Issues

Informed Consent/Assent

The type of information given to a child or adolescent may be influenced by the need for informed consent versus assent. While it is important where possible to have a child's assent to treatment and procedures, there are many situations where treatments will proceed even without this, as long as parents are giving consent. However, in the case of older cognitively competent adolescents, most services expect both the adolescent and their parents to give informed consent before proceeding with treatment. This requires active discussion of the advantages and disadvantages of the possible courses of action and outcomes, including the likely outcome of not treating. Such information would not be routinely given to younger children unless they were requesting it, as they can become overwhelmed and confused by the multiple possibilities and complex decision-making. It is important that the adults presenting information to children or adolescents are clear before they start whether they are seeking the young person's assent or their consent, and that they make this explicit to the young person also [47]. Refer example 38.

Situations where adolescents and parents disagree on treatment consent are rare and can usually be resolved by careful exploration of the issues and concerns with the adolescent and with the parents. It is helpful to see the parties both alone and together, take time for discussion, and make sure that good supports are in place for the adolescent and for the parents. It may be necessary to formally assess the adolescent's level of decision-making competence, and to request legal advice. Situations where consensus is not reached are distressing for everyone, particularly if this results in a widening rift between the adolescent and parents. Refer example 39.

EXAMPLE 39

A young man who had been 5 years old at diagnosis with leukemia, died at age 15 after multiple relapses. Prior to his death when conventional therapies had been exhausted, his parents were engaged in a bitter discussion about alternative therapies for their son. One parent was in favor and the other vehemently opposed.

In an attempt to resolve the conflict, an extended family meeting was called with appropriate cultural supports present. In the meeting the boy told his parents and extended family, "No way am I taking any more pills—end of story!"

This served as the catalyst to bring his parents together so that they could support him in the time he had left, and no further treatment was sought.

Siblings

Inadequate knowledge and poor parent–sibling communication about the illness have been identified as risk factors for poor emotional adjustment in the siblings of children who have cancer [48]. It is easy for healthy siblings to become almost invisible to the health care team, and for parents to attempt to shield them from distressing information. If the healthy sibling does not have much contact with the hospital, they also do not develop a context into which information they are given or which they overhear can be put. This highlights the need for siblings to receive ongoing information about their brother's or sister's illness, and to have their anxieties and concerns listened to and addressed. Refer example 40.

Community Peers

The friends and classmates of children who have cancer are part of the network of support for the

EXAMPLE 40

The 11-year-old sister of a child who was dying with a rhabdomyosarcoma told the nurse, "My sister has cancer in some muscle thing—I don't know where, Mum doesn't tell me." Her mother was subsequently encouraged to sit down with her daughter and a staff member and tell her more about her sister's cancer and treatments.

EXAMPLE 41

A young man aged 15 was reluctant to tell friends when his treatment-resistant cancer recurred, wanted to continue "living" as normal a life as possible—attending school, playing rugby, and being with his friends. His friends, who could see how unwell he was becoming, shielded him on the rugby field while he could still play, and spent time with him. Eventually the friends' mothers decided to tell their sons about the cancer, thus enabling their sons to continue to provide unconditional support to their dying friend. He chose not to talk about his illness or his death with friends or family. Shortly before his death, the school sought advice on how to prepare the school community for his impending death, and his funeral was subsequently held at the school. The friends "included" him in subsequent school events, organizing an annual fundraising fashion parade for child cancer support and talking about their sadness and their positive memories of him at their final school dinner two years later.

sick child, and can at times carry a heavy emotional load if a sick child or adolescent chooses to confide hopes, fears, and stark realities to close friends. Other adolescents choose not to tell friends about their illness, preferring to maintain what "normality" they can for as long as possible. This also is hard for friends, who must maintain the pretense that all is well despite obvious signs that the ill friend is deteriorating. Such situations raise issues of confidentiality and respect for the ill adolescent's autonomy, versus the information needs of peers to enable them to cope with their distress and grief. For many children and adolescents, this may be the first experience they have had of serious illness or death in someone close to them. Refer example 41.

Ward Peers

Treatment for a child with cancer is not something that requires one visit, one operation or a single course of chemotherapy. A treatment regimen may last many months or years; some delivered solely as an inpatient, others as a combination of inpatient and outpatient visits. Ward and clinic friendships develop, not just between the parents but the children as well, especially when the children are the same age, have the same diagnosis, or have similar treatment schedules.

Families tend to link in with those families whose children were diagnosed around the same time, and families from particular ethnic groups congregate together to communicate in their own language. When treatment is not going well with a child, there are ramifications beyond the family unit, and the relapse or death of a child is felt keenly by other children and families. In the ward setting, children are acutely aware of what is happening with other patients, but often do not have permission to discuss this with the adults. In some instances it may be necessary to meet with the other inpatient children to talk about their anxieties and answer their questions directly. This requires delicate balancing between open acknowledgment of what is common unspoken knowledge, and protection of the privacy and confidentiality of the index child and family.

Speaking with Children about Death

Speaking with children about death should be part of normal living, because children rapidly learn that everyone will die at some stage. Healthy children not infrequently ask parents if the parents will die, or ask if they themselves could die as a consequence of certain events. Children need honest replies to such questions to the effect that everyone, including parents, will die some day, usually when they are old and have lived a full life. Children also need the reassurance that if anything did happen to their parent that they would be cared for.

When a child who has cancer asks, "Am I going to die?" they need to have acknowledged that death is a possibility with any child with cancer, and that they could die. They also need to be told about the treatments that are planned, and the hope and expectation that those treatments will make the cancer go away. However, the most important thing to reassure the child about is that no matter what happens, they will be looked after, loved, and kept comfortable.

Children seem to ask this question at times when parents and hospital staff least expect it, such as in the middle of the night, or in the car in busy motorway traffic. Adults need to be prepared to answer, no matter when the question is asked. They also need to be prepared to say "I don't know" and acknowledge that they may not have answers for every question, but will endeavor to find answers for their child.

Sometimes in talking with children about death, it takes time to sort out exactly what the child is asking about, especially with young children who are concrete in their thinking. Refer example 42.

EXAMPLE 42

A boy aged 4 had never known his grandfather, but stated that he would like to see his grandfather's body. His parents were concerned that their son had a "morbid obsession with death." They subsequently realized that their son wanted was to see a full-length photo of his grandfather, as all the photographs on display showed only head and shoulders: he wanted to see that his grandfather had a torso, arms, and legs.

When a Child Has Relapsed or Has an Incurable Disease

(1) When a child is expected to die, how they are informed about this must take into account their age, level of understanding, previous experiences of death in the family, and cultural and religious beliefs.

(2) Reinforce how hard the child and parents and medical team have worked to 'overcome' the illness/cancer. Explain that the illness hasn't gone away and that the treatments are not able to cure the cancer. Everyone's "job" is now to keep the child feeling comfortable and able to spend time with their family and friends. Refer example 43.

(3) Check for questions and ask how the child is feeling now. Children often realize that they may die, and already know the implications of their medical condition. This allows them to voice their concerns, and ask directly. Refer example 44.

(4) Explain that when someone gets very sick with this illness they die, and that this is what the doctors think will happen. Incorporate the family's spiritual and cultural beliefs about death if appropriate. Avoid using euphemisms to describe death as younger children may interpret these in a literal and concrete manner. Refer example 45.

(5) Reassure the child that, no matter what, they will be cared for, loved, and not abandoned, and that

---

EXAMPLE 43

A boy aged 5 with relapsed leukemia was playing with medical play equipment while he talked to the play specialist. He said to her: "Mummy says this doesn't work anymore. We're going home to see what love can do. Mummy says no more treatment, lots of love."

EXAMPLE 44

A girl aged 11 years had been sick since infancy with a slow growing tumor and had a poor prognosis. Her younger siblings, who had been given little information about her illness, met with the doctor at their parents' request, to talk about her cancer and likely outcome. After the doctor had told the siblings that sometimes cancers could not be cured and would not get better, the brother aged 8 said, "Is that what is happening with my sister? Do children die from that, is my sister going to die?" The doctor explained to the boy and his brother that their sister was very sick and that her cancer was not going to get better, and that this was not anyone's fault. They were told that their sister was going to die sometime soon from the cancer. Both children were then able to talk with their mother and the doctor about their sadness and their parents' sadness, and to check with their parents that they would not get cancer from their sister.

EXAMPLE 45

A boy who had died of cancer was laid out on his bed at home. A young neighborhood friend came with his parents to say goodbye. He was keen to see the dead boy's back, as he had been told that "when someone dies they become an angel" and he wanted to see if the wings were growing yet.

they will always part of their family. While this may seem self-evident, many children may fear that they will be left alone or abandoned, and need concrete reassurance to the contrary. Refer example 46.

EXAMPLE 46

A 7-year-old boy who was dying at home became extremely anxious after his parents talked about him "going to be with his grandmother in heaven" and did not want his parents to leave his bedroom. Once they reassured him that they would be with him "no matter what happened," he became settled and let them come and go from the room.

EXAMPLE 47

The nursing staff caring for a 16-year-old boy who was dying with a Ewings Sarcoma became concerned that he was "denying his impending death" and needed reassurance. The young man had acknowledged that he was dying, but sometimes talked about attending university in the future. The nursing staff were encouraged to acknowledge his hopes without challenging them, while at the same time not actively planning with him a future that was unrealistic. This enabled them to support him as he held both his loss and his hope.

EXAMPLE 48

A girl developed leukemia at 7 years, and died aged 12 after a relapse. When the doctor told her that she had relapsed, she responded with outrage and shouted abuse at the doctor (a person she knew well and trusted). She had to have someone to blame. She was then able to move on from her anger and plan her own funeral, choosing the dress her mother was to wear, the music and words for the funeral, and writing her will leaving her prized personal possessions to family and friends.

(6) Allow for hope for a different outcome if this is important to the child or family. Refer example 47.
(7) Explain that children and parents are often sad or angry at times like this and that this is a normal reaction. Refer examples 48 and 49.

EXAMPLE 49

An 18-year-old with poor prognosis relapsed leukemia was fully informed and involved in decisions regarding what active treatments he would be willing to receive. He was very keen to participate with his peer group in a day of parachuting, remarked as he left the clinic "Hope my parachute doesn't open." He was neither depressed nor actively suicidal, but keen not to die in hospital or in discomfort.

EXAMPLE 50

An adolescent girl who was dying became very agitated; it was only at the point when she was told that the hospital staff would support her distressed parents that she visibly relaxed and died peacefully.

EXAMPLE 51

A 12-year-old boy had multiple surgical treatments and therapies for recurrent cancer. He was reluctant to tell his family that he no longer wanted treatment because he felt that "stopping fighting" was letting the family down, and they would be distressed if he died.

(8) Outline ongoing supports for the child and family. Children and adolescents often worry about how their parents will cope after their death. This may make it difficult for children to openly voice their feelings, or allow themselves to relinquish the struggle to stay alive. Refer examples 50 and 51.

David's Story

The following extract was written by the mother of a 5-year-old boy who died of leukemia, and illustrates some of the issues discussed above.

How do you explain to a 5-year-old child that he is not going to get better?

How do you tell him that he is going to die? Do you in fact tell a child so young that he is going to die? This was the agonising choice I was faced with just before my son David died.

When it became clear that David would not survive, I talked to our nurse who had been assigned to help us at home. She reassured me that, despite his age, David needed to know. Nevertheless I was apprehensive about telling him.

We were sitting on the floor one afternoon playing when I felt I could broach the subject. I began by asking what he thought would happen if he didn't get better. His reply was, "I'll be in a wheelchair for the rest of my life." I replied that that wouldn't be the case and then explained gently that he would die and go to Heaven. He thought carefully about this for a moment or two and then said, "Oh! Then I'll be able to say hello to the astronauts."

His next response was "Am I going to die today?"

When I reassured him that he wasn't, he said, "That's okay then."

David left the house once in the last six weeks of his life. He did not want to go anywhere else. He was happy sleeping, playing with his train set and Lego when he felt able to do so, being read to, watching the occasional comedy on TV with his Dad and laughing heartily, celebrating his sixth birthday lying in bed smiling at a helium balloon floating up to the ceiling of his bedroom and trying to cope physically with his failing body.

It was a bittersweet time for all of us, but those last few weeks of David's life were very special.

He died very peacefully and quickly late in the afternoon.

He had time to ask me to hold him and intimated that I was to get his Dad, who then held him in his arms as he died and both of us knew at the moment of his death that something very special had happened to him. I knew in that instance that David was well at last and it was the most profound and comforting feeling.

I cannot advise other people about what they should or should not say if they know their child is dying, but I wanted to share my experience in the hope that it may help others.

When Parents Are Reluctant to Have a Child Told about the Diagnosis or Prognosis

Some parents do not want their child to be told anything about the diagnosis of cancer or the prognosis. This wish may derive from the parents' fears that honest information will damage their child emotionally and make them "give up fighting the cancer," or may arise from strongly held cultural and spiritual beliefs and practices. Many parents, given the opportunity to talk about their fears or beliefs with the medical team will then be able to join with the staff in planning how best to proceed. It is helpful for parents to be given information about both the benefits of being open with their child, and the risks to the child's emotional well-being if secrecy is maintained. Refer example 52.

In the situation where parents continue to decline permission to give the child or adolescent any information, the rights of the child to information need to be balanced against the rights of the family to choose how they manage their child during a life- threatening illness. Debate on this topic has not resolved the question of how to proceed [49, 50]; some pediatric oncology teams have a policy of talking openly with the child from the initial point of diagnosis, others will accommodate parental views and wishes with the proviso that if the child asks staff members a direct question about their disease or prognosis, the child will be given an honest answer.

EXAMPLE 52

After an 8-year-old girl was diagnosed with metastatic cancer, a trial of chemotherapy showed the tumor to be unresponsive and aggressive. Staff were concerned that her parents had not informed her about her diagnosis and its prognosis. The family were recent immigrants, and informed the staff that it was culturally inappropriate for Chinese children to be told about a diagnosis of cancer, and that dying was never mentioned as they believed that talk of dying leads to "a loss of interest" which hastens the death.

The parents were, however, persuaded by staff that it would be helpful for their daughter to know that the treatment for her cancer was not working. They requested that her nurse, who spoke their dialect of Chinese and had established a rapport with their daughter, do the talking, and that they (the parents and older siblings) would be available but not present in the room.

The girl told her nurse that she already knew exactly what her diagnosis was, and that her cancer was unresponsive and progressive. She knew that she was dying, despite no direct discussions having taken place about such matters.

What she then wanted conveyed to her parents was the fact that "she knew what they knew." Although further open discussions did not occur, the family was then able to provide love and support until she died.

She made her will, requested that her birthday be celebrated early and her friends come to visit, and the family visit the snow (a new experience).

Ten years on, her parents told their doctor that they believed it was worth telling their daughter her diagnosis, that she had the right to know that she was dying, but that they hadn't wanted to be the ones to tell her. Knowing openly what was happening and removing the "mutual pretense" [8] allowed her to plan her remaining life. However, 20 years after their daughter's death, they returned to their original belief that, from a cultural perspective, it had been the wrong decision to tell her.

When Adolescents Choose Not to Talk about Dying

Some children and adolescents choose to not discuss their advancing disease or death, despite open information and opportunity to talk. In such instances, the young person's choice must be respected. Expressions of fear and loss, if they do occur, may be indirect or non-verbal. Refer example 53.

EXAMPLE 53

A young man who was 14 when he was diagnosed with a brain tumor, died four years later aged 18. Throughout his illness, communication with his medical care-givers was difficult as he never established eye contact and would sit with his cap pulled down around his eyes during clinic visits. Despite having a close family and an excellent relationship with his parents, he did not wish to discuss dying.

Days before he died, when his vision had failed, he dictated a letter to a friend, expressing his thanks to the friend for being there and for visiting, and hoped he would remember him after his death. He described in the letter how scared he felt, and spoke of his fear of dying. His mother was writing down the words for him; it was the first time that she had really heard how her son felt.

Importance of Cultural and Spiritual Issues

For many families, their spiritual beliefs and cultural practice are the foundations on which their lives are based. Communication with the child and with the family regarding illness and death needs to be done in a manner that is congruent with and respectful of the family beliefs. Staff should if necessary seek advice and guidance from cultural workers and spiritual leaders in order to be able to work appropriately with the child and family. They do not, however, have to share the same faith themselves to be able to communicate well and provide good care. Refer example 54.

EXAMPLE 54

Mary was 14 years when diagnosed with an osteosarcoma. Treatment involved surgery (amputation) and chemotherapy. Five years later a local recurrence with metastatic spread was diagnosed. She declined palliative chemotherapy, but accepted, after extensive family meetings, radiotherapy. Even though at 19 she was legally an adult, she needed approval from her father as head of the family before agreeing to the radiotherapy. This provided temporary shrinkage of the rapidly expanding tumor recurrence.

Her devout Christian faith and close community of family and friends provided her with strength and support during her terminal illness.

After her death, her social worker wrote:

Mary and her family had a profound and sincere faith and they never really gave up hope that Jesus would save Mary. She talked about her very strong belief that Jesus would make the right decisions for her and that her parents wanted her to put the utmost faith in him. Mary and her parents (particularly her father) prayed for hours every day. Mary had a goal–to go to her parents' homeland to see their religious leader. Initially it was for her and her father, then for her and her mother and then towards the end just for her mother. Acknowledging that she would not be going was the final acceptance that her death was now inevitable.

Mary talked about her beliefs so openly because she had trust in her medical team, borne out of long association. Throughout those last months of her life, although the tumor moved rapidly at its own pace, Mary always talked at her pace–sometimes about her faith, often about her hopes of visiting her parents' homeland and of attending university. Her valedictory at school was that she had made it to university, the first to do so in her extended family.

The things that were important for Mary and her family were their trust, the preservation of her and her parents' dignity, caring for her family and community, acceptance of her faith, and moving at her pace. These all came together to enable a "conversation" with a terminally ill young woman that often didn't need words.

Talking about Funerals

Some children and adolescents, confronted by the knowledge that they are dying, choose to plan their own funeral. They may want to discuss in great detail the issues of service format, cremation vs. burial, and giving away their possessions. Such discussion can be difficult for the adults involved, who might hold different views about what should happen after death, and who may have difficulty facing the child's stark view of reality.

However, for young people this process can give them a sense of control over one part of their existence, while still having to deal with advancing disease over which they have no control.

Attendance of children at funerals varies according to cultural, religious, and family tradition and practice. Included in these traditions are beliefs about whether children should be encouraged to visit and spend time with the body of the dead person prior to the funeral, whether children will attend open casket funerals, and inclusion or exclusion of children from religious ceremony and rituals.

When a child with cancer dies, fellow patients and their families often choose to attend the funeral but may not have much knowledge of the funeral customs that they will witness or be expected to participate in. Older children and adolescents often make a conscious decision to attend or not attend a particular funeral, whereas younger children may attend because their parents wish to show support to the family, but may have even less understanding of what is going to happen. Children need an explanation of what will happen at the funeral, what they will see and hear, and how other people might react emotionally. It will also help if they understand a little about the religious beliefs and rituals practiced by the dead child's family. Refer example 55.

> **EXAMPLE 55**
>
> At the graveside of a classmate, a group of 5-year-olds were peering into the grave as the coffin was lowered into the ground. The officiating priest told them not to look into the ground but up at the sky, because their friend had become an angel. The children, fascinated, looked upwards but were extremely bewildered and disappointed when they saw nothing—no angel flying.

Conclusion

In this chapter we have tried to suggest ways in which the important issues for children and adolescents with cancer can be talked about. It is by listening to children and speaking with them truthfully about their illness, their treatment, and for some their death, that we give them the solid ground from which they and their families can find a way through whatever lies ahead.

Acknowledgments

Our thanks to the children and their families encountered while working in Pediatric Oncology for the lessons we have learned from them.

We would also like to thank our colleagues in the multidisciplinary pediatric oncology and consultation liaison teams at Starship Children's Hospital for their constructive comments on this chapter and for their support, and in particular to thank Barbara Mackay for allowing us to use some case illustrations drawn from her paper [51] and her ongoing clinical work.

The names of children in the case examples have been changed to protect their privacy.

References

1. Levetown M and the Committee on Bioethics. Communicating with children and families: from everyday interactions to skill in conveying distressing information. *Pediatrics* 2008;**121**:1441–1460.
2. Last BF, van Veldhuizen AM. Information about diagnosis and prognosis related to anxiety and depression in children with cancer aged 8–16 years. *European Journal of Cancer* 1996;**32A**:290–294.
3. Clarke S, Davies H, Jenney M, *et al.* Parental communication and children's behaviour following diagnosis of childhood leukaemia. *Psycho-oncology* 2005;**14**:274–281.
4. Zwaanswijk M, Tates K, van Dulmen S, *et al.* Communicating with child patients in pediatric oncology consultations: a vignette study on child patients', parents', and survivors' communication preferences. *Psycho-oncology* 2011;**20**:269–277.
5. Goldman A, Christie D. Children with cancer talking about their own death, with their families. *Pediatric Hematology and Oncology* 1993;**10**:223–231.
6. Kreicbergs U, Valdimarsdottir U, Onelov E, *et al.* Talking about death with children who have severe malignant disease. *New England Journal of Medicine* 2004;**351**: 1175–1186.
7. Parsons S, Saiki-Craighill S, Mayer D, *et al.* Telling children and adolescents about their cancer diagnosis: cross-cultural comparisons between pediatric oncologists in the US and Japan. *Psycho-oncology* 2007;**16**:60–68.
8. Bluebond-Langner M. *The Private Worlds of Dying Children.* Princeton, NJ: Princeton University Press, 1978.
9. Chesler MA, Paris J, Barbarin OA. "Telling" the child with cancer: parental choices to share information with ill children. *Journal of Pediatric Psychology* 1986;**11**: 497–516.
10. Claflin CJ, Barbarin OA. Does "telling" less protect more? Relationships among age, information disclosure, and what children with cancer see and feel. *Journal of Pediatric Psychology* 1990;**16**:169–191.
11. Slavin L, O'Malley J, Koocher G, *et al.* Communication of the cancer diagnosis to pediatric patients: impacts on long-term adjustments. *American Journal of Psychiatry*, 1982;**139**:179–183.
12. Kroll L, Barnes J, Jones AL, *et al.* Cancer in parents: telling children. *British Medical Journal*, 1998;**316**:880.
13. Rosenheim E, Reicher R. Informing children about a parent's terminal illness. *Journal of Child Psychology and Psychiatry* 1985;**26**:995–998.
14. Tebbi CK. Treatment compliance in childhood and adolescence. *CANCER Supplement* 1993;**71**:3441–3449.
15. Tebbi CK, Cummings KM, Zevon MA, *et al.* Compliance of pediatric and adolescent cancer patients. *Cancer* 1986;**58**:1179–1184.
16. Blackley A, Eiser C, Ellis A, *et al.* Development and evaluation of an information booklet for adult survivors of cancer in childhood. *Archives of Disease in Childhood,* 1998;**78**:340–344.
17. Byrne J, Lewis MES, Halamek L, *et al.* Childhood cancer survivors' knowledge of their diagnosis and treatment. *Annals of Internal Medicine* 1989;**110**:400–403.
18. Eiser C, Levitt G, Leiper A, *et al.* Clinic audit for long-term survivors of childhood cancer. *Archives of Disease in Childhood* 1996;**75**:405–409.
19. Barnes J, Kroll L, Burke O, *et al.* Qualitative interview study of communication between parents and children about maternal breast cancer. *British Medical Journal* 2000;**321**:479–482.
20. Bibace R, Walsh ME. Developmental stages in children's conceptions of illness. In: Stone GC, Cohen F, Adler NE (eds.) *Health Psychology.* San Francisco: Jossey-Bass, 1979; pp. 285–301.
21. Perrin EC, Gerrity PS. There's a demon in your belly: Children's understanding of illness. *Pediatrics* 1981;**67**: 841–849.
22. Koocher GP. Talking with children about death. *American Journal of Orthopsychiatry* 1974;**44**:404–410.
23. Hansdottir I, Malcarne VL. Concepts of illness in Icelandic children. *Journal of Pediatric Psychology* 1998;**23**: 187–195.
24. Thompson RJ, Gustafson KE. Developmental changes in conceptualizations of health, illness, pain, and death. *Adaption to Chronic Illness in Children.* Washington, DC: American Psychological Association, 1996; pp. 181–195.
25. Burbach DJ, Peterson L. Children's concepts of illness: a review and critique of the cognitive-developmental literature. *Health Psychology* 1986;**5**:307–325.
26. Crisp J, Goodnow JJ, Ungerer JA. The impact of experience on children's understanding of illness. *Journal of Pediatric Psychology* 1996;**21**:57–72.
27. Sherman M, Koch D, Giardina P, *et al.* Thalassemic children's understanding of illness: a study of cognitive and emotional factors. *Annals of the New York Academy of Sciences.* 1985;**445**:327–336.
28. Cotton CR, Range LM. Children's death concepts: relationship to cognitive functioning, age, experience with death, fear of death, and helplessness. *Journal of Clinical Child Psychology* 1990;**19**:123–127.
29. Potter PC, Roberts MC. Children's perceptions of chronic illness: the roles of disease symptoms, cognitive development, and information. *Journal of Pediatric Psychology* 1984;**9**:13–27.
30. Schonfeld DJ, O'Hare LL, Perrin EC, Quackenbush M, Showalter DR, Cicchetti DV. A randomised, controlled trial of a school-based, multifaceted AIDS education program in the elementary grades: the impact on comprehension, knowledge and fears. *Pediatrics* 1995;**95**:480–486.
31. Rushforth H. Practitioner review: communicating with hospitalized children: review and application of research pertaining to children's understanding of health and illness. *Journal of Child Psychology & Psychiatry* 1999;**40**:683–691.
32. Fundudis T. Young children's memory: how good is it? How much do we know about it? *Child Psychology & Psychiatry Review* 1997;**2**:4.
33. Baile WF, Buckman R, Lenzi R, *et al.* SPIKES: A six-step protocol for delivering bad news: application for the patient with cancer. *The Oncologist* 2000;**5**:302–311.

34. Shields CE. Giving patients bad news. *Primary Care* 1998;**25**:381–390.
35. Grollman EA. *Talking About Death: A Dialogue Between Parent and Child*, rev. edn. Boston: Beacon, 1976.
36. Spinetta JJ, Swarner JA, Sheposh JP. Effective parental coping following the death of a child from cancer. *Journal of Pediatric Psychology* 1981;**6**:251–263.
37. Faulkner KW. Children's understanding of death. In: Armstrong-Dailey A, Goltzer SZ (eds.) *Hospice Care for Children*. New York: Oxford University Press, 1993; pp. 9–21.
38. Jankovic M, Loiacono NB, Spinetta JJ, *et al*. Telling young children with leukemia their diagnosis: the flower garden as analogy. *Pediatric Hematology and Oncology* 1994;**11**:75–81.
39. Nitschke R, Humphrey GB, Sexauer CL, *et al*. Therapeutic choices made by patients with end-stage cancer. *The Journal of Pediatrics* 1982;**101**:471–476.
40. Greenberg LW, Jewett LS, Gluck RS, *et al*. Giving information for a life-threatening diagnosis. *American Journal of Diseases of Children*, 1984;**138**:649–653.
41. Levenson PM, Pfefferbaum BJ, Copeland DR, *et al*. Information preferences of cancer patients ages 11–20. *Journal of Adolescent Health Care* 1982;**3**:9–13.
42. Young B, Dixon-Woods M, Windridge K, Heney D. Managing communication with young people who have a potentially life threatening chronic illness: qualitative study of patients and parents. *British Medical Journal*, February 2003; 326.
43. Lyon M, McCabe M, Patel K, D'Angelo L. What do adolescents want? An exploratory study regarding end-of-life decision-making. *Journal of Adolescent Health* 2004;**35**:6, el–529. e6.
44. Tates K, Elbers E, Meeuwesen L, Bensing J. Doctor–parent–child relationships: a '*pas de trois*'. *Patient Education and Counseling* 2002;**48**:5–14.
45. United Kingdom Children's Cancer Study Group (UKCCSG). Requirements of a children's cancer treatment centre wishing to participate within the UKCCSG. May 1997.
46. Picoult J. *My Sister's Keeper*. New York: Simon and Schuster, 2004.
47. Leikin SL. The role of adolescents in decisions concerning their cancer therapy. *CANCER Supplement* 1993;**71**:3342–3346.
48. Murray JS. Social support for school-aged siblings of children with cancer: a comparison between parent and sibling perceptions. *Journal of Pediatric Oncology Nursing* 2001;**18**:90–104.
49. Higgs R. A father says "Don't tell my son the truth." *Journal of Medical Ethics* 1985;**11**:53–158.
50. Hilden J.M., Watterson J., Chrastek J. Tell the children. *Journal of Clinical Oncology*. 2000;**18**:3193–3195.
51. Mackay B.When your brother or sister has cancer: supporting siblings' rights to know. Paper presented at the Children's Issues Centre's 3rd Child and Family Policy Conference, July 1999, Dunedin, New Zealand, 1999.

9

Psychosocial Interventions: a Cognitive Behavioral Approach

Bob F. Last, Martha A. Grootenhuis

Introduction

Childhood cancer in the family is an obviously stressful situation. A great deal of research has been conducted to investigate the emotional reactions and coping strategies of children with cancer and their parents. Different findings are reported for both children with cancer and their parents. Several studies that investigated the psychological and social adaptation of children with cancer found that they did not differ significantly from healthy controls, but subsets of more vulnerable children have been identified [1]. In a review on young childhood cancer survivors it is also shown that overall emotional adjustment of the survivors as a group was within normal limits [2]. However, one-third of the adolescent survivors met the criteria for lifetime posttraumatic stress disorder (PTSD), which is a higher percentage than in the general population [3, 4]. Moreover, research on specific areas of psychosocial adjustment has found that about one-third of survivors and their family members have experienced personal, family or social difficulties that have affected their academic achievement, employment, interpersonal relationships or self-esteem [5]. Many studies have been conducted among parents of children with cancer and different reactions have been reported for different periods of treatment [6]. Researchers who focused on parents of newly diagnosed children with cancer, or children who are in treatment, report increased emotional distress such as anxiety or depression, when compared to parents of healthy children. Some studies have found that parents continue to experience psychological distress over time [7], while others have found that the elevated levels of distress decline, within a few years to comparable levels in the general population [8, 9].

Contradictory findings among children and parents can partly be attributed to the inappropriateness of instruments to measure the impact of childhood cancer. Studies focusing on illness-related psychosocial consequences instead of depression and anxiety, found that problems for parents concerned uncertainty and loneliness [10, 11], or anxiety about the child's future, health and relapse [12]. Other explanations for the scarcity of serious adjustment problems are children's and parents' capacities to develop strengths and abilities to "bounce back" [13]. Another possible explanation could be "response shift," which means that the experience with cancer has changed the children's conceptualization of problems. As a result of this response shift, problems are being underreported. Response shift has also been described in adults with cancer [14]. In other words, the reliance on different coping strategies such as avoidance, social support, and open communication play an important role in the emotional adjustment of children with cancer and their parents.

Several intervention studies showed the possibilities of improving coping strategies and reducing feelings of distress in children with cancer [15]. Empirical evaluations of intervention programs for parents are, however, rare and report limited significant effects on adjustment [16]. The aim of this chapter is to provide an understanding of the emotions and coping strategies, and behavioral reactions of children with cancer and their parents. First, the cognitive approach will be outlined, with the theoretical background of cognitions and emotions. This will include a description of emotions in the light of different situational meaning structures which determine the appraisal of the situation for children with cancer and their parents. Situational

Pediatric Psycho-oncology: Psychosocial Aspects and Clinical Interventions, Second Edition.
Edited by Shulamith Kreitler, Myriam Weyl Ben-Arush and Andrés Martin.
© 2012 John Wiley & Sons, Ltd. Published 2012 by John Wiley & Sons, Ltd.

meaning structures which are important for children and parents are, for example, uncertainty about the outcome of the disease, responsibility for the cause and the course of the illness, and the uncontrollability of the situation. Thereafter, the process of coping is discussed and a conceptual framework is presented as a tool to comprehend children's and parental reactions to childhood cancer. Because the coping process of children with cancer and their parents is greatly influenced by the uncontrollability of the situation, we chose the model developed by Rothbaum, Weisz and Snyder [17] in addition to the traditional approach. Their model describes control strategies which can be used to understand the coping behaviors of children with cancer and their parents. The traditional approach of learned stimulus–response relationships is outlined with examples of behavioral therapeutic techniques. Based on the concepts of the cognitive and behavioral approach of emotions, we suggest an integrated model for psychosocial intervention. Three cases will be presented to show how the psychosocial intervention model can be applied in pediatric oncology.

Cognition and Emotions

Appraisal

Through cognitive appraisal processes, people evaluate the significance of events for their well-being. Lazarus and Folkman [18] distinguish three kinds of cognitive appraisal: primary, secondary, and reappraisal. Primary appraisal is the first assessment of the situation. If the situation is considered stressful, it can take three forms: harm/loss, threat, and challenge. At this moment, the person decides whether the situation is an emotional one or not [19]. This results in a number of emotions, or psychological reactions to events, depending on the relevance for the concerns of a person [19]. Positive emotions are evoked by events which correspond to what a person desires (safety, absence of pain). Negative emotions are evoked by events, which do not correspond to the needs or desires of a person (uncertainty, fear of loss, pain). In recent emotion theory, cognition is a determinant of emotional response through processes of "appraisal" or "meaning-analysis" [19]. Each specific emotion corresponds to a different appraisal, a different situational meaning structure. Every situation consists of different components. The component which is dominant for a person determines which emotion will arise. Shifts in dominance within the situational meaning structure lead to shifts in emotional experience. The negative outcome of medical examinations will raise uncertainty in a cancer patient followed by feelings of fear, while focusing on the progress in cancer treatment evokes subsequently feelings of hope. In the cognitive approach of emotions, the appraisal process not only refers to actual stimulus conditions but also to the associations of a person with the actual situation [20]. These associations are the cognitive representations that refer to the component that dominates in the situational meaning structure. For instance, a cancer patient who has experienced the death of a fellow patient after he or she was removed to a certain room may easily feel fear remembering this event when moved to this room some time later. This associative process can be understood in terms of classic conditioning. Associative learning is conceived as a basic principle in contemporary classical conditioning. For instance, empirical study on the acquisition of phobic fears revealed that cognitive representation of a conditioned stimulus (CS) with an unconditioned stimulus (UCS) evokes a conditioned response (CR)—not only in a sequential relationship (an event predicts the occurrence of an other event) but also as a referential relationship (an event activates the memory of an earlier event) [21, 22]. Therefore, analysis of the cognitive representations present in the appraisal of the situational meaning structure of a person is of importance in psychodiagnostics, prior to psychosocial and/or psychotherapeutic interventions [21, 23].

Appraisal by Children with Cancer and their Parents

The components, which are important in the appraisal of the situation for children with cancer and their parents, are uncertainty, uncontrollability of the situation, responsibility, the restriction of freedom, and the long duration of the situation [24]. In the case of children, the appraisal of the situation is highly dependent on the rapidly changing developmental level. Uncertainty about the course and the outcome of the disease is a condition related to hope and fear. Indications pointing to a remission of the disease contribute to a feeling of hope and trust, while indications of a relapse or recurrence of the disease evoke feelings of fear that all efforts to find a cure will be unsuccessful. Feelings of uncertainty about the future and fear of a relapse are often reported by parents of children with cancer [12]. In the first major study on surviving childhood cancer [25], it was shown that the uncertainty of parents was one of the major concerns. Parents of childhood cancer survivors were mainly uncertain about the long-term effects of the treatment and the possibilities of a relapse. Being confronted with cancer means being in a situation of uncontrollability, which easily evokes feelings of helplessness. Children and parents cannot influence the disease or the treatment process very much. This is in the hands of doctors and nurses. The child has to undergo painful medical procedures while parents stand by helplessly. In reaction, children can easily develop avoidant and/or resistant behavior in order to "flee" from the noxious stimuli [26]. Moreover, young children in particular are subject to cognitive distortions that can influence the appraisal [27]. In the case of medical procedures, children can have immature conceptualizations about bodily processes, such as fear that one's blood will leak out during a venepuncture [28]. Another example of a cognitive distortion is children's idea that the disease is contagious. Distress in children of all ages undergoing medical procedures has been documented repeatedly [27]. Determination of the controllability of the situation determines whether individuals feel insecure or confident. Parents of children with cancer with lower survival perspectives, that is, children with cancer who have had a relapse, reported more feelings of helplessness [11]. The child is frequently not able to attend school, to participate in sports, and/or to play with friends. Parents have to make arrangements for work, housekeeping, holidays, support for siblings, and so on. These limitations on freedom of action evoke feelings of frustration and anger. Families with a child with cancer also often have financial problems due to additional costs such as travel and extra meals [29]. These additional problems further restrict families. The answer to the question who or what is responsible for the situation is related to feelings of guilt if the person feels he/she is to blame, or anger if someone else is to blame. Eiser, Havermans and Eiser [30] investigated feelings of responsibility of parents of children with cancer. Both mothers and fathers frequently blamed the general practitioner. Pride may play a role if the child or parent feels they are able to hold on in spite of all difficulties. This is an example of a positive emotional consequence. Positive psychosocial consequences should not be overlooked because the ability of children and parents to have an improved outlook on life or enhanced relationships is also part of the illness experience. Greenberg and Meadows [31] reported that children and parents often express gratitude for the child's survival. The long duration of the threatening situation is associated with feelings of exhaustion and depression if the child or parent does not perceive an end to the suffering. High levels of depression have been reported for mothers of children in relapse [11]. Besides the actual conditions, associative cognitive representations are also central in the appraisal process of children with cancer and their parents. For instance, for a child

with cancer, the stimulus "take your medicine" can easily be associated with traumatic memories of a "struggle" with an impatient nurse in the hospital and may evoke anxiety originally emanating from uncontrollability.

For parents, seeing their seriously ill child with symptoms comparable to a fellow patient can be associated with images about a fellow patient dying and evoke thoughts about the possible death of their own child.

Coping

Emotions are not only evoked by appraisal of what a situation may do to a person, but also by the appraisal of what a person can do to change that situation. Cognitive appraisal and reappraisal are the first stage in coping; how a person deals with a stressful situation. One's perceptions, or cognitive appraisals, are an important element in regulating distress (emotion-focused coping) or managing the problem causing the distress (problem-focused coping). Problem-focused coping involves direct efforts to ameliorate the problem causing the distress, whereas emotion-focused coping is directed towards regulating affects surrounding a stressful experience [18]. Coping should not be equated with mastery over the environment: many sources of stress cannot be mastered, and effective coping under these conditions is that which allows the person to tolerate, minimize, accept, or ignore what cannot be mastered. It should also be recognized that coping is, to some extent, a temporally and situation-specific process. Consequently, coping is defined by Lazarus and Folkman [18], as "constantly changing cognitive and behavioral efforts to manage specific external and/or internal demands that are appraised as taxing or exceeding the resources of a person" (p. 141). The definition is process-oriented: the efforts and strategies are constantly changing. Considering the situation-specific process, it may also be presumed that coping is susceptible to changes and sensible to interventions. Frijda [19] stresses the importance of regulation. People not only have emotions, they also handle them. Regulations refer to all processes that have the function of modifying other processes induced by a given stimulus situation. Parents of children with cancer have few possibilities to regulate events, but they have the ability to regulate appraisal. The appraisal of a situation can be regulated by selective attention and self-serving cognitive activities. These appraisal regulations are comparable to emotion-focused coping strategies. Appraisal regulations are part of the emotion process. One of the best-known appraisal regulations is the use of denial. Individuals facing a life-threatening illness often go through a phase of denial; they try to protect themselves from painful or frightening information related to external reality [32]. Whether denial is a negative force or can be considered as adaptive is a point of controversy. Denial can be useful, but in the long run, denial can also lead a patient to conceal serious physical complaints. This is the difference between denial of facts and denial of implications [33]. In patients who are able to function effectively and are able to maintain a high degree of optimism, behavior which may be viewed as denial can also be viewed, from a cognitive viewpoint, as "selective information processing" or can be considered as healthy denial [34]. The term "resilience" has been introduced to bridge the gap between the differing viewpoints. It describes the strengths and abilities of patients and families who can "bounce back" from the stress and challenges they face and eliminate, or minimize, negative outcomes [34, 35]. Many health care providers know that patients or families show the ability to adapt to stress and to be able to cope with a threatening situation. This capacity to keep on going is what is meant by "being resilient." In relation to this, Folkman and Moskowitz [36] stress the importance of positive affect which co-occurs with distress. Especially positive appraisal (cognitive strategies for reframing a situation to see it in a positive light) appears to be an important kind of coping that determines positive affect.

Another area which has received considerable attention in the research on coping with cancer is the importance of turning to others for social support. Social support affects coping in several ways. Social resources can reinterpret the meaning of the situation so it seems less threatening, or it may influence the use of other coping strategies, e.g., provide distraction. Social support is therefore considered a coping resource by several researchers [37, 38].

Control Strategies

Rothbaum, Weisz and Snyder [17] emphasize the concept of uncontrollability in their two-process model of perceived control, separating primary and secondary control strategies. Primary control strategies are classified as attempts to gain control by bringing the environment into line with their wishes (e.g., seeking treatment, changing one's own and other people's behavior). Secondary control strategies are attempts to gain control by bringing themselves into line with environmental forces (e.g., seeking explanations and changing expectations or attitudes). This is similar to the classification of problem- and emotion-focused coping strategies [18]. Rothbaum, Weisz and Snyder [17], however, further classified control into four strategies: (1) predictive; (2) vicarious; (3) illusory; and (4) interpretative, all possibly used in primary or secondary form (Figure 9.1). These four control strategies well describe the frequently occurring reactions of children with cancer and their parents.

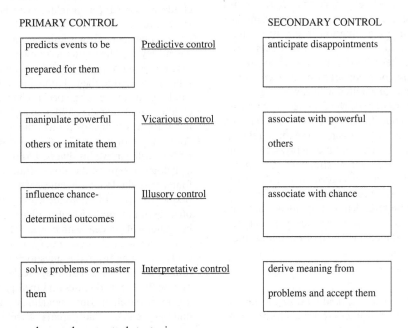

Figure 9.1 Primary and secondary control strategies.

Predictive Control

Strategies of primary predictive control include gaining knowledge about the expected course of the disease, of the treatment schedule, and the side effects of treatment. The gaining of knowledge in the case of primary predictive control focuses on everything that can contribute to prediction and can satisfy the need to know what to expect. In predicting events, a feeling of control over the situation is created. Secondary predictive control involves attempts by a child or the parents to predict events to avoid disappointment. Most striking in this way of coping with the threatening situation are parents who react with "anticipatory mourning" while the treatment of their child is still curative. By predicting and grieving about a "certain" loss, they prevent themselves from feeling the shock and pain related to the possibility of the death of their child. This type of parental coping is regularly found in clinical encounters, but was not representative of the group of parents of children with cancer participating in our own study [39], in which the parents protected themselves more by being optimistic than by preparing themselves for disappointment. Secondary predictive control can apparently manifest itself in two ways. On the one hand, parents can protect themselves against disappointment by expecting the worst, but, on the other hand, they can also protect themselves by having positive expectations. By living day to day and by being optimistic, children and parents may try to control their emotions. Such manifestations of secondary predictive control can also be considered as forms of healthy denial or attempts to reframe the situation in a positive light [36]. In our own study [40], we found that persistence in being hopeful, that is having positive expectations, proved to be the major predictor of positive emotional outcome for parents of children with cancer.

The same findings were shown for children with cancer [41]. We found no differences between children with different prognosis (in remission or with a relapse) either on measures of anxiety and depression, or on measures of cognitive control strategies. Emotional adjustment of the children was predicted by defensiveness and by positive expectations about the course of the illness. These findings demonstrate again that having positive expectations about the course of the illness are of major importance for the emotional adjustment of children with cancer.

Vicarious Control

Vicarious control can be exercised by trying to imitate or manipulate powerful others (primary form) or by attempts to associate with them (secondary form).

Children with cancer and their parents are highly dependent on doctors. Their attempts to influence the doctors' choices can especially be seen when treatment is not successful and the survival perspective is reduced. Trying to avoid the possibility of death, parents may try to convince the doctor not to terminate treatment, or to use experimental therapies. The secondary manifestation of vicarious control is demonstrated by attributing special power to the doctor, on whom all hope is focused. In this case, a sense of control is derived from the perception that others, such as the medical caregivers, can exert control. We know from clinical experiences and written diaries how important medical caregivers are to parents and children. An example of this is found in the diary of a girl treated for leukemia [42] who wrote, after hearing the diagnosis: "I am in the best hospital now, with the best professor in the Netherlands" (p. 15).

Illusory Control

Illusory control is used to attempt to influence chance-determined outcomes or as a secondary process, to associate with chance. Attempts to influence the chance-determined outcome of the illness can be sought in changes in lifestyle, eating habits, or alternative healthcare. These actions offer children and parents the possibility to do something themselves, and thus promote a sense of control. Our finding of increased use of alternative treatment by families of children with cancer in relapse can be considered as indicative of the use of this type of control [43]. Secondary illusory control is found in children and parents when they put their situation down to fate, admitting that fate is more powerful, but create the illusion that fate will be kind to them. Hoping for a miracle, wishful thinking, or attributing special characteristics to the child as proof that the child is one of the survivors are illustrations of illusory control in its secondary form. An example of this is a mother who says: "I am sure my son will survive his illness. I know this because his astrological sign is the lion." Bull and Drotar [44] found that children with cancer who are off-treatment frequently used intrapsychic coping strategies. They often used praying, wishful thinking, or self-encouraging statements to deal with cancer-related stress, which can be considered as secondary illusory control. In a study, we administered a questionnaire measuring all four cognitive control strategy scales to several children with chronic diseases and their parents participating in research in our department. Based on these findings we know that parents of children with cancer rely more on illusory control than parents of children with other chronic illnesses [41]. Reliance on wishful thinking appears to be very important to them. By attributing positive characteristics to their child, parents create an image of the child as being full of life, hence fostering the illusion that fate will be kind to them. The parents need to believe that the child is strong, because if the child can handle the situation, it increases their confidence that the child will survive. We found support for parents' attribution of positive characteristics to their children with cancer. We discovered that parents of children with cancer attributed more cheerful behavior to their children than parents of children with asthma and healthy children do [45].

Interpretative Control

Primary interpretative control is focused on understanding problems so as to able to solve them or otherwise master them. Gaining information about the disease and the different treatment modalities is often seen in children and parents and is obvious around the time of diagnosis. Empirical research confirms that the majority of older children prefer to be informed about their disease and treatment [46]. Secondary interpretative control refers to the search for meaning and understanding. Finding an answer to questions like "What caused cancer in my child?" and "Why did this happen to me?" serves the process of acceptance and helps children and parents to find meaning in the cancer experience. Attempts by parents to search for information on the internet is also an example of interpretative control. In our study on the use of the four secondary control strategies by parents of children with cancer, we found that all the parents [39] used secondary interpretative control most frequently. The use of interpretative control appears to be important, regardless of educational level and survival perspective. Although mothers of children with cancer relied more on interpretative control than fathers, interpretative control seemed to be meaningful for all parents. The cognitive approach of emotional reactions is in addition to the traditional behavioral approach. In the behavioral approach, all behavior is conceived as learned stimulus–response relationships. The process of learning is governed by principles of classic conditioning [47], operant conditioning [48] and imitation [49]. In classical conditioning, a reflexive response to a stimulus is brought under control of another stimulus by the contiguity of both stimuli. An example in pediatric oncology of this principle is found in the child already vomiting at home when he has to go to the hospital to get a chemotherapeutic cure with nausea-evoking drugs. In operant conditioning a specific stimulus is brought under control by consistent reinforcement of a response that follows the specific stimulus. In operant conditioning, behavior is determined by its consequence, using the principle of contingency. This principle is working in the example of the child having learned that he will hear his favorite story after taking his medicine. Observation of behavioral sequences in others can also establish behavior. The observer learns to associate certain responses with the observed conditions, providing a basis for imitation when the observer is in a similar position as the model. Children with cancer learn a lot from their fellow patients. Observing another child in the ward during chemotherapy can serve as a role model in a positive but also in a negative way.

Application of Behavioral Therapeutic Techniques

The use of the learning principles underlying the behavioral approach has been shown to be beneficial to the child with cancer, in particular in handling anxiety- and pain-provoking treatment procedures (e.g. venepuncture, bone marrow aspiration, lumbar-puncture, infusion of chemotherapeutic drugs and/or operations). Besides improvements in using anesthetics and nausea-reducing drugs, the application of behavior therapeutic techniques remains important in many cases. The possibilities of the behavioral approach have been extensively described (e.g. [50, 51]). The main techniques used are summarized in Figure 9.2.

Pre-exposure prevents the child from aversive conditioning through exposure to possible anxiety-provoking stimuli at a moment when the child is quiet and relaxed. This technique is useful as a method of preparation and only applicable in situations with a high probability of occurrence and low stress intensity, as for instance in children who will undergo radiotherapy or general anesthesia. Showing a book of photographs of a medical procedure and/or showing the room and apparatus for examination or treatment are supportive

---

Pre-exposure
Positive reinforcement
Relaxation and breathing exercises
Modelling
Systematic desensitization
Guided imagery

Figure 9.2 Anxiety- and pain-reducing techniques.

in using this type of intervention. With positive reinforcement, parents and medical caregivers can encourage cooperative behavior. Social reinforcement through approval can be completed with material reinforcers after undergoing medical examination or treatment. Relaxation and breathing exercises are useful in decreasing the activity of the sympathetic and motor nervous system in tense situations. In learning and encouraging the child to use these techniques during medical procedures, the level of experienced anxiety and pain can be reduced. Modeling videos are used to inform the child about a stressful medical procedure and also to teach the child techniques (such as relaxation or self-distraction) to remain in control during the event. When watching the video the child is encouraged to imitate the behavior of the model child shown in the video. Systematic desensitization (SD) is used in the case of a child reacting with extreme avoidant behavior. SD involves the composition of a hierarchy of increasingly anxiety-provoking stimuli. Step-by-step exposure to these stimuli, together with a corresponding response such as relaxation, reduces the level of anxiety and the tendency to react with avoidance. With guided imagery the child's attention is distracted from the aversive medical procedure by a fantasy story unrelated to the painful event. This technique has proved to be successful in children and adolescents who are sensitive to suggestions. It is preferable to agree with the child on a story he or she likes. If a child likes Superman, invite him to identify with Superman in solving problems and challenges. In practice, the above-mentioned techniques are often used in combination [52]. For instance, pre-exposure to the radiotherapy room is often followed by instructions on how to relax. When doing so, it can be agreed with the child that a distracting story will be told during therapy and then to positively reinforce the child after treatment. Kazak *et al.* [53] integrated the above-mentioned stress reactions and interventions in a model to assess so-called pediatric medical traumatic stress (PMTS). In this model, for each phase of the treatment, guidelines for recognition of PMTS and suggestions for using materials and cognitive-behavioral techniques aimed at reduction of PMTS are described.

The Psychosocial Intervention Model

Framework

The main characteristics of the situation, the different emotions, the types of primary and secondary control and the history of learned behavior are brought together in a model for psychosocial intervention (see Figure 9.3).

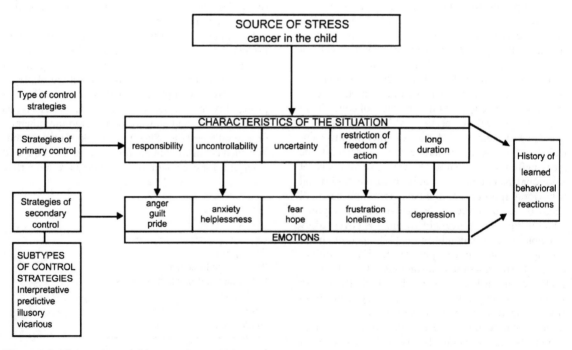

Figure 9.3 The psychosocial intervention model.

This framework addresses the main features of the situation, the related emotions, the role of primary and secondary control, and also the history of learned behavior. In coping with a stressful situation, children and parents use the various control strategies in their specific way. Psychosocial intervention is indicated if control fails and subsequently, child and/or parents need support in rebuilding their defenses or to reduce or eliminate unpleasant behavioral reactions. Using this scheme, we can analyze and understand the emotional reactions of the child and his/her parents and use it as a guide to psychosocial interventions. In working with this model, we ask the following questions: (1) What situational components and emotions are dominant for the child and the parents?; (2) Which control strategies are especially used by the child and by the parents?; (3) What is the history of learned behavioral reactions related to the disease and the treatment?; (4) To what extent do the child and parents use their control strategies effectively? If, for instance, child and/or parents are anxious about the course of the disease and mainly attempt to use interpretative control to reduce uncertainty, we have to look critically at the information they have been given about the disease and the treatment. If child and/parents fear a negative outcome of the disease and show little confidence in the medical doctor, it may be necessary to enhance their vicarious control. And, also, if the child remains anxious about a treatment procedure, it makes sense to look at his history of learned behavioral reactions and use specific behavioral therapeutic techniques to overcome this fear (as is shown in the Jim's case study below).

Case Studies

EXAMPLE: MARIA

Maria is a 7-year-old girl and has been treated for osteosarcoma. She has had an operation and has had post-surgical chemotherapy. She lost her hair due to chemotherapy. The tumor was removed and she is in remission. She only comes to the hospital for check-ups and whether the disease will remain in remission is uncertain. Maria is bald, but very full of life. She goes to school with pleasure. Her parents came to the Pediatric Psycho-Social Department with the complaint that Maria has trouble sleeping. She calls for her parents from her bed, and ends up sleeping with her parents. Her parents are not able to sleep well, and especially her father is exhausted. In Maria's case we wondered why

she was afraid to be alone in her bed. We wondered what associations the parents may have had when Maria went to bed, and what associations when Maria called them at night.

Situational Components

Because Maria is young, her feelings of certainty are very dependent on her parents. After inquiry, it turns out that Maria woke up from her operation earlier than expected and that her parents found her very upset. Consequently, when she is alone in her bed, she feels uncertain. The appraisal of the situation as uncertain concurs with Maria's association of being alone in her bed and the uncertainty about whether her parents are available. Maria's father appraises the situation as uncertain. Would Maria survive her illness? Because her illness started with pain in her belly, before going to bed, father urges Maria to call them if she feels something in her belly. Maria's mother has confidence in Maria's treatment and her uncertainties mainly relate to her husband's worries and Maria's sleeping problems.

Control Strategies and Effectiveness

Maria does not know whether her parents are available, and she is not sure about her illness. It seems that she has little possibility of relying on interpretative control. Maria's mother is confident (secondary predictive control: positive expectations) that Maria will survive her illness. She says that Maria is an optimistic and strong girl who will be able to survive her illness (secondary illusory control: attribution of positive characteristics). Maria's father worries about her illness and he is anticipating a negative outcome. He thinks Maria will not survive (secondary predictive control: negative expectations). After inquiry, it turns out that his father (Maria's grandfather) died of cancer 6 months earlier and that Maria's father has not come to terms with this. There also appears to be an important association influencing the appraisal for the father: "When I see Maria sleeping, it is like seeing my father on his death-bed." For the father, Maria's going to sleep appears to be a conditioned stimulus triggering anxiety arising originally from uncertainty about the outcome of the disease. Maria's father appears to be wanting Maria to get out of her bed; it reassures him temporarily.

Intervention

Having analyzed the situation, we now know more about the cognitive representations and emotional reactions of Maria and her parents. In the first place, Maria should be helped to increase her feeling of safety, and it should be explained that she is in remission and not ill right now (increasing her interpretative control). She should know more about her illness. The main psychosocial support should be directed at the father. His mourning for his father should be discussed and supported to break the association between his dying father and his sick daughter. Maria's symptoms should no longer be negatively predicted by the father.

EXAMPLE: MICHAEL

Michael is a 12-year-old boy suffering from a non-Hodgkin lymphoma. He is tall for his age and looks older. His cancer is being treated with intensive chemotherapy over a long period of 53 weeks. At the moment of referral to the Psycho-Social Department he was in the 22nd week. Michael is rebellious in the hospital and is non-compliant with protective rules of his therapy (e.g., brushing his teeth and rinsing his mouth). He is also abusive to his mother and the nurses in the ward. His parents feel helpless and are tired of all the quarrels.

Situational Components and Emotions

Michael is a popular teenager who feels very frustrated by the restriction imposed on his freedom by his illness. He is directing his frustration and anger especially at his mother. His mother believes she cannot control the situation and feels helpless. She also feels responsible towards the nurses for Michael's behavior, which causes her to experience guilt, together with being angry at Michael. Michael's father admits that he is very uncertain about Michael's survival chances and the father admits he only cries when he is alone.

Control Strategies and Effectiveness

Because Michael seems older than he is, it is easy to assume he understands his illness and treatment. Michael does not really know the consequences of his disease (little interpretative control) and he relies little on vicarious control, resulting in rebellious behavior against the hospital staff. Because Michael is non-compliant with his treatment schedule, his treatment protocol cannot be followed as well as it should be. Little primary predictive control is therefore possible for his mother. His mother has a great deal of confidence in the hospital (secondary vicarious control). That Michael's father is the most pessimistic of the family shows that he is anticipating disappointment (secondary predictive control).

Intervention

The family needs a better understanding of the treatment, survival chances, and consequences of non-compliance. Therefore, a meeting with the physician was organized. This enhances the interpretative control and vicarious control of all family members. In this round-table discussion, the effects of the medication Michael is taking were also discussed. The use of dexametason is known to cause mood disturbances. Because Michael has difficulties with the restriction of his freedom he was supported in finding an alternative to playing football. He is being supported in doing something together with his father.

EXAMPLE: JIM

Jim is a 6-year-old boy highly anxious and angry about undergoing his chemotherapy. "I don't want it," he cried. The doctors gave Jim sedative medicines before the infusion was installed. Nevertheless he remained very upset and frequently tried to eliminate the infusion. Psychological intervention was requested. In discussion with Jim and his parents it became clear that Jim had experienced a traumatic sequence with his first chemotherapy. His mother was late arriving at the ward because of a traffic jam, the doctors had already started Jim's first infusion. A nurse and a play therapist had prepared Jim as well as possible, but Jim was angry and felt alone. When his mother arrived, he was very upset and shouted at her.

Situational Components

It seemed that as a consequence of his first traumatic experience in the hospital Jim appraises every hospitalization as highly uncertain and uncontrollable. He experienced associated memories to the event of staying alone and undergoing a sudden painful procedure. A high level of arousal motivated by separation anxiety blocked any information needed to build up a certain sense of control in the situation.

Response and Consequences

Jim reacted with crying and shouting and attempts to escape from the situation. This behavior resulted in a struggle and the anger of the nurses and his parents to get the job done in the end. Sometimes the procedure was postponed which reinforced his rebellious behavior.

Intervention

An intervention was designed aimed at enhancing Jim's feeling of self-control and reduction of stress in the short period of time, before the next chemotherapy. The first session was focused on a ventilation of feelings about the traumatic event using talking and painting. Moreover, a hierarchy of low, middle and highly anxiety-provoking stimuli was composed. His mother took part in the sessions. As an antagonistic response Jim learned breathing exercises by blowing at a little kite and learned muscle relaxation by getting weak as a pudding. Jim enjoyed the training and played with hospital materials. Together we looked at a model film in which a 7-year-old boy used the exercise when getting a venipuncture. In this film the boy also uses distraction by counting little stars in the eyes of his mother while the doctor inserts a needle in a blood vessel. Jim was encouraged to do the same. In the final session Jim practiced the instruction in a simulated infusion procedure. He was encouraged for his efforts and improvements. Mother rewarded him with an ice cream in the main hall of the hospital. On the day of the next cure Jim

arrived more relaxed. Also his mother showed more confidence knowing how she could support her son. Jim cried for a short while but was cooperative.

Conclusion

The model for psychosocial intervention presented in this chapter is meant to be a helpful instrument in arranging and analyzing the findings from previous diagnostic efforts. The model presented, emphasizes the importance of the characteristics of the situation, the main primary and secondary control strategies, and the history of learned behavioral reactions. These aspects are involved in analyzing the emotional and behavioral reactions of children with cancer and their parents. It is important that health care providers understand emotional and behavioral reactions, and coping strategies, because with this knowledge they can respond more appropriately. If health care providers respond adequately, this will be beneficial to the children's and parents' emotional adjustment. The focus on the described control strategies is not meant as an exclusive point of view. Children and parents also rely on other coping strategies (e.g. classical defense mechanisms) or other coping resources (social and financial support). To understand emotional and behavioral reactions, careful diagnostics are necessary. In many cases the child's and/or the parents' emotional problems or problems of adjustment cannot easily be attributed to cause and consequence. We also have to keep in mind that parents and children may rely on more than one control strategy at the same time and that the same person or situation may generate different feelings of control. This is also important to realize when arranging interventions. The model serves as a guideline to hypothesize about the occurrence and origins of psychosocial adjustment problems of the child with cancer and his parents. Based on these hypotheses, focused interventions can be initiated.

References

1. Patenaude AF, Kupst MJ. Psychosocial functioning in pediatric cancer. *Journal of Pediatric Psychology* 2005; **30**:9–27. Review.
2. Stam H, Grootenhuis MA, Last BF. Social and emotional adjustment in young survivors of childhood cancer. *Supportive Care Cancer*, 2001;**9**:489–513.
3. Spirito A, Stark LJ, Cobiella C, *et al.* Social adjustment of children successfully treated for cancer. *Journal of Pediatric Psychology* 1990;**15**:359–371.

4. Kazak E, Alderfer M, Rourke MT, *et al.* Posttraumatic stress disorder (PTSD) and posttraumatic stress symptoms in families of adolescent childhood cancer survivors. *Journal of Pediatric Psychology* 2004;**18**: 493–504.

5. Friedman DL, Freyer DR, Levitt GA. Models of care for survivors of childhood cancer. *Pediatric Blood & Cancer*, 2006;**46**:159–168.

6. Grootenhuis MA, Last BF. Adjustment and coping by parents of children with cancer: a review of the literature. *Supportive Care in Cancer* 1997c;**5**:466–484.

7. Norberg AL, Lindblad F, Boman KK. Parental traumatic stress during and after paediatric cancer treatment. *Acta Oncol*, 2005;**44**:382–388.

8. Sawyer M, Antoniou G, Toogood I, *et al.* Childhood cancer: a 4-year prospective study of the psychological adjustment of children and parents. *Journal of Pediatric Hematology Oncology*, 2000;**22**:214–220.

9. Wijnberg-Williams BJ, Kamps WA, Klip EC, Hoekstra-Weeber JE. Psychological adjustment of pediatric cancer patients revisited: five years later. *Psycho-oncology*, 2006; **15**:1–8.

10. Van Dongen-Melman, JEWM, Pruyn JFA, De Groot A, *et al.* Late psychosocial consequences for parents of children who survived cancer. *Journal of Pediatric Psychology* 1995;**20**:567–586.

11. Grootenhuis MA, Last BF. Parents' emotional reactions related to different prospects for the survival of their children with cancer. *Journal of Psychosocial Oncology* 1997a;**15**:43–62.

12. Leventhal-Belfer L, Bakker AM, Russo CL. Parents of childhood cancer survivors: a descriptive look at their concerns and needs. *Journal of Psychosocial Oncology* 1993;**11**:19–41.

13. Gudmundsdottir E, Schirren M, Boman KK. Psychological resilience and long-term distress in Swedish and Icelandic parents' adjustment to childhood cancer. *Acta Oncologica* 2011;**50**:373–380.

14. Sprangers MAG, Schwartz CE. Integrating response shift into health-related quality of life research: a theoretical model. *Social Science Medicine* 1999;**48**:1507–1515.

15. Kazak AE. Evidence-based interventions for survivors of childhood cancer and their families. *Journal of Pediatric Psychology* 2005;**30**:29–35.

16. Pai AL, Drotar D, Zebracki K, *et al.* A meta-analysis of the effects of psychological interventions in pediatric oncology on outcomes of psychological distress and adjustment. *Journal of Pediatric Psychology* 2006;**31**: 978–988.

17. Rothbaum F, Weisz JR, Snyder SS. Changing the world and changing the self: a two-process model of perceived control. *Journal of Personality and Social Psychology* 1982;**42**:5–37.

18. Lazarus RS, Folkman S. *Stress, Appraisal, and Coping.* New York: Springer, 1984.

19. Frijda NH. *The Emotions.* Cambridge: Cambridge University Press, 1986.

20. Davey GCL. Classical conditioning and the acquisition of human fears andphobias: a review and synthesis of the literature. *Advising Behavioural Research Therapy* 1992;**14**: 29–66.

21. Davey GCL. UCS revaluation and conditioning models of acquired fears. *Behavioural Research Therapy* 1989;**27**: 521–528.

22. Field AP. Is conditioning a useful framework for understanding the development and treatment of phobias? *Clinical Psychology Review* 2006;**26**:857–875.

23. Korrelboom CWK, Kernkamp JHB. *Gedragstherapie.* Muiderberg: Dick Coutinho, 1993.

24. Van Veldhuizen AM, Last BF. *Children with Cancer: Communication and Emotions.* Amsterdam: Swets & Zeitlinger, 1991.

25. Koocher GP, O'Malley JE. *The Damocles Syndrome: Psychosocial Consequences of Surviving Childhood Cancer.* New York: McGraw-Hill, 1981.

26. Humphrey GB, Van de Iel HB, Boon CM, Van den Heuvel CF. Stress reduction interventions in pediatric oncology: could coping strategies play a role? In: Last BF, Van Veldhuizen AM. (eds.) *Developments in Pediatric Psychosocial Oncology.* Lisse: Swets & Zeitlinger, 1992.

27. Manne SL, Andersen BL. Pain and pain-related distress in children with cancer. In: Bush JP, Olson AL, Boyle WE, *et al.* (eds.) Overall function in rural childhood cancer survivors. *Clinical Pediatrics* 1991;**32**:334–342.

28. Peterson L. Coping by children undergoing stressful medical procedures: some conceptual, methodological, and therapeutic issues. *Journal of Consulting and Clinical Psychology* 1989;**57**:380–387.

29. Eiser C, Upton P. Costs of caring for a child with cancer: a questionnaire survey. *Child Care Health and Development* 2007;**33**:455–459.

30. Eiser C, Havermans T, Eiser JR. Parents' attributions about childhood cancer: implications for relationships with medical staff. *Child Care, Health and Development* 1995;**21**:31–42.

31. Greenberg HS, Meadows AT. Psychosocial impact of cancer survival on school-age children and their parents. *Journal of Psychosocial Oncology* 1991;**9**:43–56.

32. Breznitz S.The seven kinds of denial. In: Breznitz S (ed.) *The Denial of Stress.* New York: International University Press, 1983; pp. 257–280.

33. Lazarus RS. The costs and benefits of denial. In: Breznitz S (ed.) *The Denial of Stress.* New York: International University Press, 1983; pp. 1–30.

34. Druss RG, Douglas CJ. Adaptive responses to illness and disability: healthy denial. *General Hospital Psychiatry* 1988;**10**:163–168.

35. Patterson JM. Promoting resilience in families experiencing stress. *Pediatric Clinics of North America* 1995;**42**: 47–63.

36. Folkman S, Moskowitz JT. Positive affect and the other side of coping. *American Psychologist* 2000;**55**:647–654.

37. Suzuki LK, Kato PM. Psychosocial support for patients in pediatric oncology: the influences of parents, schools, peers, and technology. *Journal of Pediatric Oncology Nursing* 2003;**20**:159–174.

38. Woodgate RL. The importance of being there: perspectives of social support by adolescents with cancer. *Journal of Pediatric Oncology Nursing* 2006;**23**:122–134.

39. Grootenhuis MA, Last BF, De Graaf-Nijkerk JH, Van Der Wel M. Secondary control strategies used by parents of children with cancer. *Psycho-oncology* 1996;**5**:91–102.

40. Grootenhuis MA, Last BF. Predictors of parental adjustment to childhood cancer. *Psycho-oncology* 1997b;**6**: 115–128.

41. Grootenhuis MA, Last BF. Children with cancer with different survival perspectives: defensiveness, control

strategies, and psychological adjustment. *Psycho-oncology, Special Issue* 2001;**4**:305–314.

42. Peneder F. *Het dagboek van Floortje Peneder*. Amsterdam: Nijgh and Van Ditmar, 1994.
43. Grootenhuis MA, Last BF, De Graaf-Nijkerk JH, Van der Wel M. Use of alternative treatment in pediatric oncology. *Cancer Nursing* 1998a;**21**:282–288.
44. Bull BA, Drotar D. Coping with cancer in remission: stressors and strategies reported by children and adolescents. *Journal of Pediatric Psychology* 1991;**16**: 767–782.
45. Grootenhuis MA, Last BF, Van Der Wel M, De Graaf-Nijkerk JH. Parents' attributions of positive characteristics to their children with cancer. *Psychology and Health* 1998b;**13**:67–81.
46. Last BF, Van Veldhuizen AMH. Information about diagnosis and prognosis related to anxiety and depression in children with cancer aged 8–16 years. *European Journal of Cancer* 1996;**32A**:290–294.
47. Pavlov IP. *Conditioned Reflexes*. New York: Oxford University Press, 1927.
48. Skinner BF. *Contingencies of Reinforcement*. New York: Appleton-Century-Crofts, 1969.
49. Bandura A. *Principles of Behavior Therapy*. New York: Holt, Rinehart & Winston, 1969.
50. Van Broeck NGA. Behavioral therapeutic techniques as preparation for aversive medical procedures. In: Last BF, Van Veldhuizen AM. (eds.) *Developments in Pediatric Psychosocial Oncology*. Lisse: Swets & Zeitlinger, 1992; pp. 117–136.
51. LeBaron S. The use of images and suggestion in the treatment of pain in children. In: Last BF, Van Veldhuizen AM (eds.) *Developments in Pediatric Psychosocial Oncology*. Lisse: Swets & Zeitlinger, 1992; pp. 137–146.
52. Rudolph KD, Dennig MD, Weisz JR. Determinants and consequences of children's coping in the medical setting: conceptualization, review, and critique. *Psychological Bulletin* 1995;**118**:328–357.
53. Kazak AE, Kassam-Adams N, Schneider S, *et al.* An integrative model of Pediatric Medical Traumatic Stress. *Journal of Pediatric Psychology* 2006;**31**:343–355.

10

Education in Pediatric Oncology: Learning and Reintegration into School

Ciporah S. Tadmor, Rivka Rosenkranz, Myriam Weyl Ben-Arush

Introduction: The Rationale for Preventive Intervention in the School

Risk Factors that Endanger the Mental Health of Children with Cancer

School Absenteeism

The underlying rationale for preventive intervention is derived from empirical and clinical studies that report excessive absenteeism from school for pediatric cancer patients. In spite of a general consensus with respect to the significance of school in a child's life, it is well reported in the literature that cancer creates educationally related barriers for children with cancer, which may contribute to school problems [1], to school absenteeism [2], and even to school phobia [3]. Research has shown for at least 30 years that children with chronic diseases are likely to have 50% more school absences a year than other children. Among these, children diagnosed with cancer have three to six times more school absences a year than do chronic or orthopedic conditions (91, 29, and 15 days per year, respectively). Indeed, the only significant factor associated with the number of absences caused by treatment was the type of illness, namely cancer [4]. Pediatric cancer patients appear to have very high absence rates, even after their return to school [5–7]. The absence rate decreases but still remains considerably high for two [8] or three years after diagnosis, not necessarily related to treatment [9]. As early as 1979, Lansky and Cairns [2] reported that the average school absence after diagnosis was 41 days, 35 days in the first year post-diagnosis, 29 days in the second year, and 28 days in the third year. Fourteen years later, the absence rate is strikingly similar at 45–21 days per year [10]. Concern regarding the academic achievement and psychological

adjustment of children with cancer is advanced by findings that suggest that children who miss 20 or more days per year are liable not to maintain their pre-illness academic level of achievement. School absenteeism of 20 days or more a year is associated with other significant school difficulties, such as a decline in grades, behavioral problems, inattention, acting out [2], and repeating a grade [11]. These problems are serious obstacles that interfere with rehabilitation and reintegration into the school setting.

School Phobia

School phobia is seen in 1% of the general population and was reported in 10% of school-aged children with cancer [3]. School phobia is characterized by a refusal to attend school due to fear of separation and somatic complaints [12], and fear of social rejection and teasing due to altered physical appearance [13]. The latter holds true in particular for adolescents whose impaired self-image and loss of autonomy and control, coupled with fear of peer reactions and loss of academic work, may lead to absenteeism and, consequently, to social isolation [12]. Even in children who are not school phobic, absenteeism is a significant problem. In a study conducted in 1975 in Kansas, the authors found that 67% of their large study population were absent from school for more than four weeks per year for no apparent reason [3].

Academic Achievement of Survivors of Childhood Cancer

Further support for the significance of preventive intervention designed to facilitate the re-entry of children with cancer into the school is derived from studies that

Pediatric Psycho-oncology: Psychosocial Aspects and Clinical Interventions, Second Edition.
Edited by Shulamith Kreitler, Myriam Weyl Ben-Arush and Andrés Martin.
© 2012 John Wiley & Sons, Ltd. Published 2012 by John Wiley & Sons, Ltd.

investigate the academic achievement of survivors of childhood cancer. Although, in general, findings are quite optimistic and suggest that there are no overall differences in self-esteem of young adult survivors of childhood cancer as compared to their siblings [14] and matched controls [15], and although, in general, the survivors of childhood cancer were coping well in their adult life, 75% of survivors of childhood cancer reported that their education had suffered as a result of their illness. Some traced the difficulties of their re-entry into the school to the lack of communication between teachers, parents and the medical staff [14]. Furthermore, survivors of childhood cancer were significantly less likely to go on to higher education (16 years plus) than their siblings [14] and were more likely to be placed in special education classes than their siblings [16].

Factors that Interfere with the Successful Return to School of Children with Cancer

There are many factors that interfere with the child's successful return to school. Some of the problems are associated with parents, teachers, peers and the child [17].

Problems Associated with Parents

Problems associated with parents stem from their own fears about separation and about the child's safety and health [18]. Some parents have a tendency to ignore problems related to the child's absenteeism and may even encourage it. Others are very concerned about the child's poor school attendance, but have difficulty in enforcing discipline. They feel helpless, frustrated and in constant conflict with the child due to their own unresolved guilt feelings about the child's disease [18]. Other parents are reluctant to share information about the nature of the disease with school personnel and the child's classmates [17]. They may fear that exposing the child's disease may evoke negative reactions from peers and teachers [19]. Parents, overwhelmed and burdened by the illness, its treatment and the threat to the child's life in the present, may not at times focus on the child's potential to achieve in the future. Children sense their parents' lack of confidence in their ability and react with disillusionment, helplessness and anger [20]. The end result is overprotection by the parents and a discriminatory or preferential attitude by school personnel [19].

Problems Associated with Teachers

Problems associated with teachers may derive from misconceptions, lack of knowledge about childhood cancer, and their own personal biases. The teacher is expected to share responsibility for the child's care upon his return to school; however, teachers may be neither trained nor emotionally prepared to deal with this responsibility. In many cases, a teacher may have little knowledge about childhood cancer, its treatment and prognosis, and may neither understand nor accept the frequent absences and changes in physical appearance of the child [21]. Teachers may struggle with their own personal biases and experiences with cancer, which, at times may evoke images of death and the futility of treatment. This pessimistic outlook may affect the teacher's ability to successfully manage the child's return to school, becoming overly lenient with the child's academic performance, sending the message that he or she does not have to make an effort, lowering expectations and performance, and reinforcing the already impaired self-image. The teacher, burdened by the responsibility of caring for the child and insecure about how to deal with medical emergencies, may feel trapped and overwhelmed. The teacher's lack of knowledge of what to expect of the child physically and academically may lead to the child's exclusion from class activities, leading to social isolation [17].

Problems Associated with Peers

Problems associated with peer reactions stem from their lack of knowledge about their classmate's illness. They often have myths and misconceptions about cancer, which can affect their reactions to their sick friend [22]. Data suggest that children and adolescents with cancer are more likely to be perceived by their peers as more socially isolated, sick, fatigued, and often absent from school even after treatment has ended [23–25].

A teacher, unable to deal with his/her own insecurities and misconceptions, may be unable to reassure the classmates, to help them to understand the long absences from school and the changes in physical appearance. If the teacher is lenient with the child with cancer, peers may react negatively, isolating and alienating the child even further [17].

Problems Associated with the Child

There are also difficulties associated with the child, which may interfere with a smooth return to school. Firstly, there are medical factors that contribute to absenteeism, such as: (1) chemotherapy regimens; (2) hospitalization; (3) routine follow-up; (4) stage of the disease; (5) infection; and (6) chickenpox in the classroom [17]. Other factors are associated with invisible side effects of chemotherapy, such as nausea, fatigue and neutropenia, visible side effects, such as hair loss or weight fluctuations [26, 27], or treatment-induced learning disabilities, such as a reduced level of concentration or memory deficits [28]. In addition, there are psychosocial factors that contribute to the child's refusal to attend school. The child may feel burdened by the threat of a recently diagnosed cancer, heightened by an impaired self-image. The low self-image may derive from the side effects of chemotherapy, which alters physical appearance, such as hair loss, weight fluctuations or loss of limb through amputation. These emotional difficulties are aggravated by a fear of being rejected and teased by peers [13] and by a loss of academic work and fears that he or she cannot keep up with schoolmates [17].

The possible stigma associated with children with cancer highlights the risk of a self-fulfilling prophecy placing them at risk for social isolation and alienation even after treatment has ended [29]. In line with concerns that children with cancer are perceived by their peers as having psychological problems and of being socially isolated, children with cancer, especially those who have a higher level of behavioral problems, are more likely to view themselves as having lower levels of scholastic competence, lower levels of close, confiding friendships and lower levels of social acceptance from peers [15], perceiving themselves as more socially isolated and exhibiting more shy and anxious behavior patterns [25]. The end result is that the child may dislike school, resort to absenteeism [2] or drop out of school to avoid situations that heighten feelings of insecurity. All these misconceptions may lead to negative personality changes, low motivation, underachievement, social isolation, negative attitudes toward school, excessive absenteeism and, eventually, school phobia [3, 12].

Protective Factors that Enhance Mental Health

Recent studies investigating the psychosocial adjustment of pediatric cancer patients have resulted in mixed findings. Some studies suggest that these children are at high risk for psychosocial problems both during and after treatment [29], while other studies have reported no such effect [30]. Discrepant findings among studies addressing the adaptation of youth with cancer may be the result of methodological and design variables: (1) source of information—self, teacher or peers; and (2) the specific instrument employed—questionnaires or clinical interviews. While self-reporting questionnaires are likely to yield a remarkable positive picture [31] due to social desirability and/or defensive denial [32], clinical interviews suggest impairments in the psychological well-being of survivors of childhood

cancer [33]. Another interpretation that may explain the observed variability in the individual adaptation of pediatric cancer patients is mediating or protective factors, such as self-esteem and social support [27, 34, 35].

Peer Support

Empirical findings identify mainly two protective factors related to school that buffer children from the negative emotional sequelae of cancer. The first and most consistent factor is perceived classmate support. Peer support was consistently and significantly associated with psychological adjustment measures at a greater magnitude than other perceived social support domains, namely that of parents and teachers. Higher perceived social support was associated with fewer depressive symptoms, lower state, trait and social anxiety, higher general self-esteem, and lower acting-out behavior [27], and a lower perception of stressors associated with cancer and the side effects of chemotherapy, yielding a lower negative affectivity score [35]. These empirical findings are in line with theoretical works that identify peer relations as playing a central role in children's social and emotional development [36]. Peer relations are viewed as fundamental for the development of adequate social skills and for the emergence of a healthy self-concept [37]. These notions hold true for children and adolescents in general and for pediatric cancer patients in particular. The ability to maintain social relationships during the illness was identified as an important factor in the long-term adjustment of survivors of childhood cancer [38].

School Attendance

The second protective factor identified by empirical findings as an excellent predictor for psychological adjustment of children with cancer is school attendance. Children who missed more school days had a lower adjustment rate and more stressors associated with cancer. The more integrated into the school setting the child with cancer is, the more likely that he or she will perceive as less stressful cancer-related stressors, such as hair loss, nausea, fatigue, pain, and weight fluctuations, and the more likely to keep up with school assignments, have more friends, share feelings, be happy and content, and display positive thinking and enhanced self-image [39]. Recent complementary findings [40] suggest that children's adjustment is a predictor of school attendance.

These findings highlight the significance of interventions designed to facilitate the return of children with cancer to school to prevent psychological maladjustment. School represents the work of children and the opportunity for socialization and social support. For the child newly diagnosed with cancer, continuation of social and academic activities as early as is medically feasible provides an important opportunity to normalize as much as possible an ongoing stressful experience by focusing on the healthy aspects of life. These findings suggest that peer support is not only critical in the psychosocial adjustment of the child but also facilitates return to school. When the perceived social support of the classmates is low, not only may the child feel depressed and exhibit low self-esteem, but she/he may also avoid school altogether. Children who are poorly accepted by their peers are more likely to manifest school adjustment problems and are at a greater risk for long-term maladjustment [41].

The implications of these findings cannot be overstated. Peer support and school attendance are the two most important facets of preventive intervention since they are crucial for the child's normal socialization and positive adaptation. In this context, preventive intervention designed to facilitate the smooth return of pediatric cancer patients to school and the opening of channels of communication between children with cancer, and their classmates and teachers is of the utmost importance.

Preventive intervention for pediatric cancer patients in the school falls into the realm of primary prevention designed to promote emotional well-being and psychological adjustment [42, 43], and to promote their mental health and quality of life. Implications of these findings are twofold: (1) the significance of intervention in the school to promote academic and psychosocial adjustment of children with cancer is highlighted; and (2) preventive intervention designed to facilitate the return to school must be comprehensive and address the concerns of children with cancer, their parents, teachers and classmates.

Survey of School Intervention Programs for Children with Cancer

School is an important facet of children's lives. It is a critical psychological goal for children in general and for children with cancer in particular. Consequently, school is a crucial area of concern in the comprehensive treatment of children with cancer for many reasons. Firstly, it is important for these children to maintain their pre-illness level of academic achievement to become productive adults. Secondly, children with cancer, like all children, need normal peer contacts and a social life to help them become mature adults [37]. Finally, regular school attendance and participation in regular intellectual and social activities counterbalance

anxiety and depression in children diagnosed with cancer [24].

Regular school attendance by children with cancer is considered to be the primary measurable parameter of rehabilitation [39]. It is an anchor emphasizing the healthy aspects of children's lives; it instills hope and enables planning for the future. Klopovich et al. [12] enumerated the following contributions of school attendance to the well-being of children with cancer: (1) provides social contacts with peers; (2) boosts morale; (3) counterbalances boredom; (4) maintains dignity; and (5) normalizes life. All these assets are facilitating factors which promote the quality of life of children with cancer and enhance their mental health. Children who are denied continued school participation are denied a major opportunity to engage in age-appropriate goal-oriented behavior, which may lead to hopelessness, learned helplessness and despair [7, 44, 45]. The accompanying social isolation experienced by children with cancer has been related to problems in adaptation to the disease [26, 39, 46, 47].

In the 1980s, realizing the significance of regular school attendance by children with cancer, the American Cancer Society funded research projects designed to develop school intervention programs to ease the return of children with cancer to school and to identify cognitive dysfunction that might be due to treatment. This explains the abundance of school intervention programs, each with its unique characteristics, throughout the USA and Europe [48]. However, in 1997, realizing that return to school of children with cancer could not be taken for granted, the Leukemia Society of America made the development of school re-entry programs a top priority [18].

Survey of School Intervention Programs

The objectives of most school intervention programs are: (1) to open channels of communication between the child, parents, hospital staff, school personnel and peers; (2) to safeguard academic progress and peer relations; (3) to facilitate a smooth return to school; and (4) to prevent delayed psychosocial difficulties. Table 10.1 presents a representative sample of school programs to date.

As soon as the child is diagnosed with cancer, the child's teacher is contacted and a school conference is scheduled with school personnel, either in the hospital [12, 14, 17, 48–50] or in the school [18, 26, 51–53]. The scheduled school conference is conducted, in general, between a hospital interdisciplinary team, such as the hospital teacher, pediatric oncology

Table 10.1 School intervention programs for pediatric cancer patients in the USA, Canada and Europe.

Authors	Mode of intervention			Focus of intervention				Location of intervention		Liaison personnel	Evaluation
	School conference	Class presentation	Day seminar	Child	Parent	School personnel	Peers	Hospital	School		
Lansky and Cairns (1979)	x			x	x	x					
Sach (1980)			x							Educational counselor	
Klopovich et al. (1981)	x					x	x	x		School nurse, nurse clinician	Overall improvement in school attendance
Ross and Scarvalone (1982)			x			x		x		Social worker	Increased knowledge, dispelled fears, increased confidence, positive feedback
Katz et al. (1992)	x	x		x	x	x	x		x	Hospital pediatric psychologist	Positive feedback from children, parents and teachers
Deasy-Spinetta (1993); Adamoli et al. (1997)	x	x		x	x	x	x	x	x	School teacher, counselor or psychologist	Regular school attendance
Baysinger et al. (1993)	x			x	x	x	x		x	Pediatric oncology nurse	Positive feedback from children, parents, peers, and teachers
Gregory, Parker and Craft (1994)			x		x	x		x		Community nurses and social workers	Smooth reintegration into the school
Häcker, Klemm, and Böpple (1995)		x		x	x	x	x		x	Hospital teacher	Enhanced confidence and knowledge of teachers and peers

Larcombe and Charlton (1996)		x		x	x	Enhanced knowledge and confidence
Cleave and Charlton (1997)		x		x	(University) x	Enhanced teacher confidence
McCarthy, Williams and Plumer (1998)	x	x	x	x	x Pediatric oncology nurse x	Positive feedback, some original concerns resolved, new emerged
Whitsett, Pelletier and Scott-Lane (1999)		x	x	x	x	

nurse and team psychologist, and school personnel, such as the school nurse, teacher counselor and principal [14]. The pediatric oncology nurse [18] or the pediatric hematologist [48] provides information about the child's specific disease, treatment options, expected side effects and realistic prognosis. The hospital psychologist suggests how to deal with peer reactions and encourages maintaining contact with the child during prolonged absences [14].

Some school intervention programs identified liaison professionals to play a central role in the implementation of school intervention. Deasy-Spinetta [48] identified the classroom teacher, the school psychologist and the school counselor as playing a pivotal role in facilitating the school intervention program. Klopovich et al. [12] preferred the school nurse to play a valuable role in the reintegration of the child with cancer into the school for three reasons: (1) the school nurse is the source of information for health-related issues; (2) the authors report findings that suggest that the school nurse is the most pessimistic with respect to the child's prognosis; and (3) the school nurse is the best trained to deal with medical problems that may occur, such as bleeding, fever and chickenpox exposure. Other authors have designated the hospital teacher as the liaison between the hospital and the school [52]. The liaison person is in charge of setting up the school conference and periodic follow-up visits to the school. Katz et al. [26] identified the hospital pediatric psychologist as the one to open channels of communication between the hospital and the school. He or she is in charge of setting up the conference in the child's school with the teacher, focusing on the child's medical and psychosocial concerns, such as school attendance, grades and discipline. Other authors delegated this role to the pediatric oncology nurse [18, 51], while still others identified the teacher counselor [22, 48] or the social worker [17] as the one to implement school intervention, whether at home or in the school. Some school intervention programs focus not only on the child and school personnel but also on the concerns of parents and siblings. A school re-entry program implemented in Alberta Children's Hospital in Alberta, Canada, includes, in addition to school conferences with teachers, workshops for parents and siblings to facilitate the return of the child with cancer to school [53].

Some comprehensive school intervention programs not only address the concerns of the child, parents and teachers, but also focus on the needs of the child's classmates [1, 18, 26, 51–53]. The presentation in the child's classroom begins with discussing the classmates'

experiences with cancer, followed by information about childhood cancer according to the developmental phase of the children. Emphasis is placed on some basic facts, such as that the disease is treatable and not contagious. The peers are encouraged to keep in touch and support their sick friend [26]. Häcker, Klemm and Böpple [52] and Adamoli et al. [1] reported that a physician visits the child's school and provides information about childhood cancer to the classmates. Whitsett, Pelletier and Scott-Lane [53] relate that, because of recent budget constraints, their visits to schools have been discontinued and, instead, a handbook entitled Childhood Cancer, School Re-Entry is sent to each school to assist teachers in managing the child with cancer safely back to school.

All school intervention programs are implemented after permission is received from the parents and the child with cancer. The child with cancer is involved in some intervention programs [26] and, although they are encouraged to attend the class presentation, most abstain [18]. Instead of a school conference, a few school intervention programs entail a one-day seminar conducted for school personnel in the hospital. One such program was initiated as early as 1978 by Ross and Scarvalone [17]. The authors identified the social worker to play a principal role in the implementation of the one-day seminar. The objectives of the seminar were: (1) to increase the participants' knowledge about childhood cancer; (2) to increase their confidence to deal with the child with cancer upon his/her return to school; and (3) to increase their ability to share information with classmates. The one-day seminar consisted of frontal lectures followed by small-group discussions and a tour of the pediatric cancer facility. Larcombe and Charlton [50], like Ross and Scarvalone [17], have conducted study days for teachers. The first part of the seminar consisted of information about childhood cancer provided by hospital staff, and the second part consisted of small-group discussions on either the teachers' personal experiences with cancer or on relevant topics dealing with prevention of cancer, such as smoking, sun exposure, etc.

In the past few years, school re-entry programs have been initiated by parents, teachers and hospitals. Sample class presentations appropriate to different age levels [54] and other materials including videos are available through resources such as the Leukemia and Lymphoma Society [55]. In an environment of financial concerns, this trend is understandable; however, it cannot replace the comprehensive school reintegration program initiated and applied by the hospital-based interdisciplinary team in coordination with parents, child and school personnel.

Evaluation of School Reintegration Programs

All the authors conducting school intervention programs report favorable outcomes. Some studies report positive feedback from parents, children and teachers [18, 26, 51]. Other studies suggest an increase in the teacher's confidence [52, 56] and knowledge [17, 50], and increased optimism and alleviation of fears [17]. The most significant finding of school intervention programs is the smooth reintegration of the child with cancer back into the school [49] and improved school attendance [1, 12].

School reintegration programs involving children and adolescents with cancer have not been widely or rigorously assessed, primarily due to methodological limitations. In 2008, in a review of the recent literature, Ranmal and colleagues [57] identified only two well-designed studies. The first, conducted by Katz and colleagues [58] employed a before and after design as compared to a retrospective standard care control group, and the second, conducted by Varni and colleagues [59], used a multicenter randomized controlled clinical trial design. Both attested to the success and high social validity of a comprehensive school reintegration intervention. Findings of the former suggest that, in pre and post comparisons as well as in comparison to a retrospective standard care control group, children in the school reintegration group had reduced depression, increased self-esteem, and enhanced interpersonal, scholastic and behavioral functioning. The latter compared a group of children who received social skills training in addition to school reintegration intervention with a group of children who received only the school reintegration intervention. The parents of the first group reported fewer behavioral problems, greater school competence and enhanced social supports at 9 months. However, these initial findings were demonstrated with low statistical power, leading the authors to conclude that these initial findings did not demonstrate superiority of social skills training when added to the school reintegration intervention. Consequently, in an environment of financial concerns, it may be more efficacious to identify those children who are at risk for social skills deficits and provide them with social skills training, rather than allocating limited resources across all children.

Preventive Intervention in the School for Children with Cancer: The Perceived Personal Control (PPC) Crisis Model

Theoretical Background

Preventive intervention is based on a theoretical model of crisis that has received empirical and theoretical verification [60–62]. The theoretical crisis model is a synthesis derived from Lazarus' [63] notion of idiosyncratic perception of the stressor and Caplan's [42] notion of availability of a coping response that mediates between the individual's appraisal of the event and his response to it. The theoretical crisis model, denoted as the Perceived Personal Control (PPC) Crisis Model, explains the locus and intensity of crisis as a function of the PPC of the individual. It is assumed that the potential benefit of the PPC is derived from a combination of perceived control on the emotional, cognitive, and behavioral levels.

The PPC model has significant implications for crisis intervention. It calls for manipulation of situational variables, such as natural and organized support systems, information, anticipatory guidance, and the person's share in the decision-making process, as well as task-oriented activity geared to enhancing emotional, cognitive and behavioral control of the individual, respectively. The PPC model adheres to the goals of primary prevention, namely preventing emotional dysfunction in a population free of psychiatric symptomatology, and implies intervention on two distinct but complementary levels: (1) preventive intervention administered by a network of natural and organized support systems, denoted as Personal Interaction; and (2) introduction of changes in policies, structures and allocation of resources and services in the relevant departments conducive to positive mental health, referred to as Social Action [42].

The PPC Preventive Intervention Model has been implemented at Rambam Medical Center in Haifa, Israel, since 1980, and has been successfully applied, for example, to the following populations at risk from a mental health point of view: (1) caesarean birth mothers [60–62, 64]; (2) children undergoing elective surgery and their parents [65]; (3) changes in policies designed to promote mental health for children with leukemia [66]; (4) children with leukemia [67]; (5) changes in policies designed to enhance quality of life for children with cancer at the end-of- life [68]; and (6) children with cancer at the end of life [69]. In 1986, the PPC Preventive Intervention Model for the caesarean birth population and pediatric surgery patients was selected by the American Psychological Association (APA) Task Force on Promotion, Prevention and Intervention Alternatives in Psychology as an exemplary model with another 13 primary prevention models and was published by the APA in 1988 in a book entitled *14 Ounces of Prevention: A Casebook for Practitioners* [70].

Preventive Intervention Based on the PPC Model for Children with Cancer and their Parents

Preventive intervention based on the PPC model is one of the emerging preventive technologies [71, 72]. It empowers people by increasing control over their lives by either competence building or by modifying institutional practices that contribute to dysfunctional outcomes for the target population that is the focus of the preventive intervention. Thus, the PPC preventive intervention is both preventive and empowering, since mental health promotion activities are clearly empowering as well as preventive [72]. In this chapter, a comprehensive preventive intervention on both counts for pediatric cancer patients is presented, with particular emphasis on preventive intervention in the school. Preventive intervention is implemented by an interdisciplinary staff designed to answer the specific concerns of children with cancer, their parents, siblings, teachers and peers. The interdisciplinary staff consists of psychologists, social workers, art and music therapists, hospital teachers, teacher counselor and volunteers who empower the child and parents, each in his/her area of expertise to deal with the threatening disease and its emotional sequelae.

The content of preventive intervention is to enhance emotional, cognitive and behavioral control of pediatric cancer patients. Emotional control is achieved by convening a network of support systems around the pediatric cancer patient, consisting of natural supports, such as the parents and peers, and organized supports, including an interdisciplinary staff and survivors of childhood cancer. Cognitive control is achieved by the provision of information with respect to diagnosis, treatment options and medical tests, anticipatory guidance with respect to expected side effects of chemotherapy and a share in the decision-making process with respect to timing medical tests, starting treatment, preferred ways of induction of anesthesia, etc. Behavioral control is attained by task-oriented activities, making the child an active participant in his/her treatment and recovery process. Activities include caring for the Broviac catheter, taking the medication, patient-controlled analgesia, employing relaxation, guided imagery and problem-solving techniques, and reintegration into the school system as soon as is medically feasible.

Mental health services consist of crisis intervention and supportive counseling. In most instances, the hospital-based medical psychologist attends the session when the pediatric hemato-oncologist imparts the diagnosis to the child. In the initial phase of diagnosis, a considerable amount of time is spent with the parents and the child and siblings to assist them in assimilating and coping with the threatening situation. In addition, a series of 6–8 workshops are conducted for parents and children by an interdisciplinary staff on relevant topics such as: (1) childhood cancer and treatment options; (2) expected side effects of chemotherapy; (3) psychological coping with cancer; (4) siblings' coping; (5) significance of school attendance; (6) nutrition; (7) innovative treatments, such as bone marrow transplantation, and (8) meetings with pediatric cancer survivors.

Follow-up of the child and his/her parents is conducted during hospitalization and day-care treatment, as well as during the maintenance phase and the medical follow-up in the outpatient clinic. Psychological intervention is more intensive during the initial phase of diagnosis and the induction phase, and as needed during continuation of treatment. At times of crises, relapse or the terminal phase, psychological intervention is considerably more intensive.

Preventive intervention is complemented by a series of changes in policies in the Department of Pediatric Hematology Oncology, designed to promote the mental health of pediatric cancer patients. Great care is taken to differentiate between necessary pain and unnecessarily painful procedures. In order to reduce pain and ameliorate fears associated with invasive medical procedures, such as bone marrow aspiration (BMA), bone biopsy (BB) and lumbar puncture (LP), a combination of psychological preparation and pharmacological agents is employed. The psychological preparation consists of anticipatory guidance coupled with relaxation and guided imagery techniques and parental presence. The pharmacological preparation employed consists of conscious sedation by administration of midazolam through the Broviac or Port catheter by the pediatric hemato-oncologist for LP, and deep sedation administered by a pediatric anesthesiologist for BMA and BB. Changes in the policies of the departments catering to pediatric cancer patients to foster positive mental health are discussed elsewhere [67].

Preventive Intervention in the School

Historical Perspective

Preventive intervention in the school is one facet of a comprehensive preventive intervention approach for pediatric cancer patients. The general objective of preventive intervention in the school is to open channels of communication between hospital staff, parents, children, school personnel and classmates. As early as 1982, a school conference was scheduled in the hematology outpatient clinic between an interdisciplinary hospital staff consisting of a pediatric oncology nurse, a hospital-based medical psychologist, a social worker, and school personnel, which included the child's teacher, school nurse and guidance counselor. The conference was initiated with the permission of the parents and the child. The purpose of the school conference was to exchange information about the child. The school personnel updated the hospital staff about the child's academic and social status, while the hospital team imparted information about leukemia, its treatment and side effects. School personnel were made aware that the child would be absent from school for some six to seven months because of the side effects of chemotherapy, such as immunosuppression and aggressive treatment regimens. In light of these constraints, a coordinated plan of action was set in motion to care for the child's academic and psychosocial needs. Subsidized interim tutoring at home or in the hospital was initiated. This service was enabled by a series of laws enacted to safeguard the scholastic achievements of pediatric cancer patients. The Ministry of Education makes it mandatory for each school to provide from three to four hours weekly of homebound instruction. A personal computer is provided to the children by volunteer organizations and access to the internet in the Department of Pediatric Hematology Oncology enables the children to participate in class lectures in real time via Skype. Additional interim instruction in computers is provided by a private organization subsidized by the Ministry of Education, and an additional six weekly hours of tutoring are supplemented by the Israel Cancer Association. The teachers are encouraged to reinforce continuous peer contact and support while the hospital staff see to it that the child attends class as soon as medically feasible. An ongoing follow-up system was established, keeping channels of communication open between the hospital staff and school personnel.

Until 1986, the hospital-based medical psychologist conducted occasional presentations in the class of the sick child. However, in 1995, when an educational counselor joined the pediatric hemato-oncology department, preventive intervention in the school became institutionalized and systematic, benefiting every pediatric cancer patient.

Preventive Intervention for School Personnel

When the child is initially diagnosed as having cancer, his/her teacher is contacted by the educational counselor and a meeting is scheduled in the pediatric hemato-oncology department. The conference is attended by the pediatric hemato-oncologist, the hospital-based medical psychologist, the social worker and the educational counselor. The school personnel include the child's teacher, school counselor, school nurse and, occasionally, the school principal.

The school conference focuses on an exchange of information about the child's academic, medical and psychological status. Topics such as childhood cancer, treatment options and expected side effects are discussed. Teachers are made aware of the realistic challenges associated with the child's reintegration process, as well as the dangers entailed in school absenteeism for the mental health of the child with cancer. Issues such as discipline, grading, peer reactions and management of typical situations that may be encountered when the child returns to school are raised. Furthermore, a realistic expectation about the child's progress is provided. This issue is particularly important since teachers who have a pessimistic outlook about the child's chances to survive are likely to refrain from making any demands on attendance and performance. This attitude will be internalized by the child, impairing his/her chances for continued academic progress. In this context, teachers are encouraged to be aware of their own biases, to treat the child as a regular child and to have realistic expectations about academic performance. Teachers are encouraged to maintain ongoing contact between the child and the classmates, and emphasis is placed on the significance of continuous peer support and regular school attendance, not only on the academic aspects of the child's life but also on his/her psychosocial adjustment in the long run. At the same time, we impress upon teachers that children should be reintegrated into their original classes. At the end of the conference, the school personnel receive written material about relevant topics and a date is set for a class presentation in the school. The duration of the school conference is about an hour and a half.

Preventive Intervention for Classmates

At the scheduled date, the interdisciplinary hospital team, consisting of a pediatric hemato-oncologist, a pediatric oncology nurse, a hospital-based medical psychologist and the educational counselor arrive at the child's school for a class presentation. The child is involved in the class presentation and encouraged to attend with his/her parents and siblings. The class discussion begins with an airing some of the peer concerns about childhood cancer, allowing the peers to express their feelings and to ask relevant questions. The pediatrician provides information about childhood cancer, differentiating it from adult cancer. Topics such as treatment procedures and expected side effects such as hair loss, weight fluctuations, immunosuppression, and the Broviac catheter are discussed. The mental health expert deals with the children's death fears, and dispels rumors and misconceptions associated with cancer, such as it being contagious, and the threat of imminent death. The children are encouraged to express their concern and are encouraged to keep in touch with the sick child by frequent visits and telephone calls. At times, the child him/herself will express concerns, such as infrequent visits by friends and the fear of being abandoned. She/he may be willing to show his/her Broviac catheter to friends and answer some of their questions. A videotape on the experiences of a childhood cancer survivor is screened. In the last session of the class presentation, the educational counselor asks the classmates to organize into groups and to draw pictures or write poems for their friend to take home. The sick child is also involved in this informal creative endeavor. At the end of the session, she/he receives the finished products made by her/his friends. The duration of the class presentation is about two hours. The educational counselor who serves as a liaison between the hospital and the school maintains periodic follow-up concerning the child's school attendance record and scholastic progress.

Evaluation of Preventive Intervention in the School for Children with Cancer

In the past five years, we have conducted 213 systematic school conferences and class presentations, from kindergarten to high school. We have received positive feedback from everyone involved—children, parents, school personnel and classmates. Moreover, class presentations are perceived as a positive and rewarding experience by the hospital staff involved in their implementation. Systematic follow-up conducted by the educational counselor who serves as a liaison between the hospital and the school reveals regular school attendance by all children with cancer who can attend school.

We have witnessed a remarkable evolutionary process in which various segments of the Israeli community have opened up and are willing to deal with cancer facts, thereby reducing the stigma associated with cancer and fostering more positive attitudes toward survivors of childhood cancer. We have reached Arab and

orthodox Jewish populations who, traditionally, were reluctant to disclose issues that were considered secret and private. This openness in the Israeli community facilitates a smoother reintegration of children with cancer back into the school system and gradually fosters more positive and optimistic cancer-related attitudes.

Conclusion

Paradoxically, the improved survival of children with cancer has brought into focus new problems affecting their psychosocial adjustment, problems such as absenteeism, school performance, school anxiety, social isolation and the misconceptions of teachers and peers. Consequently, it is becoming increasingly evident that successful rehabilitation of the child with cancer demands comprehensive preventive intervention, focusing on all aspects of the child's life and not only on medical control of the disease as she/he moves on the continuum from diagnosis to subsequent school reintegration and rehabilitation. Recent studies have suggested that school attendance, participation in school activities and peer support are mediating, buffering factors that affect the perception of the stressors associated with cancer and the child's psychosocial adjustment. The implications of these studies cannot be overstated. The more integrated the child is in the school setting, the more friends she/he has, the more likely that her/his quality of life and mental health will be enhanced. These findings hold true not only in the short run but, indeed, in the long run; the adjustment of survivors of childhood cancer is affected by the extent to which the child was able to maintain social relationships during the illness [38]. These data make preventive intervention in the school an important facet of comprehensive preventive intervention designed to promote the mental health of children with cancer. School re-entry programs are, thus, cost-effective preventive interventions because they can prevent future scholastic and psychosocial problems for children with cancer. Consequently, it is recommended that preventive intervention in the school should be an integral part of the comprehensive treatment plan of pediatric hemato-oncology centers and should be provided to all newly diagnosed children with cancer. The preventive intervention program must be initiated as early as possible in the treatment. Clinical and empirical findings indicate that children who do not return to school early in their treatment find it increasingly difficult to be reintegrated at a later date [47]. This holds true for pediatric oncology patients in general. Special consideration should be given to children who are at risk for poor academic outcomes and children treated for central nervous system [CNS] tumors and leukemia, especially if they received CNS direct treatment or intrathecal methotrexate [73].

Regular school attendance is a vital, normal developmental task for children in general and for children with cancer in particular. Consequently, school reintegration intervention serves as an important rehabilitative goal for children and adolescents with cancer and acts as a moderator of children's adjustment, especially in educational and occupational domains.

It is possible to differentiate two kinds of preventive intervention programs in the school for newly diagnosed children with cancer: (1) programs such as annual seminars and workshops designed to enhance communication skills for school personnel to deal more effectively with cancer-related crises [56]; and (2) school reintegration interventions targeted specifically for teachers and peers who currently have a child with cancer in the classroom [47]. Although the former generic intervention may have a valuable educational purpose within a primary prevention realm, it may not be as effective as more individualized, targeted presentations to teachers and students who currently have in the classroom a child recently diagnosed with cancer [74]. Given limited resources, targeted interventions are more feasible and cost-effective. Yet, incorporating systematic presentations on cancer facts into the regular curriculum may increase cancer knowledge among all children and may facilitate the acceptance of a specific child with cancer [75] as well as alleviate fears associated with cancer in the community. Both kinds of preventive interventions are complementary and examples of primary intervention at its best.

Acknowledgments

The authors express their thanks and appreciation to the interdisciplinary staff members of the Miri Shitrit Department of Pediatric Hematology Oncology for their dedication and active involvement in the implementation of preventive intervention in the school for children with cancer: Dr R. Elhasid and Dr A. Ben-Barak, Nurse L. Sweetat, Clinical Psychologist E. Krivoy, Social Workers J. Eid and N. Perets-Salton, Art Therapist A. Magen and Music Therapist O. Levanoni. The authors also thank Mrs M. Perlmutter for her assistance in the preparation of this chapter.

References

1. Adamoli L, Deasy-Spinetta P, Corbetta A, *et al.* School functioning for the child with leukemia in continuous first remission: screening high-risk children. *Pediatric Hematology/Oncology* 1997;**14**:121–131.
2. Lansky SB, Cairns NU. Poor school attendance in children with malignancies. *Proceedings of the American Association for Cancer Research* 1979;**20**:390.
3. Lansky SB, Lowman JT, Vats T, *et al.* School phobia in children with malignant neoplasms. *American Journal of Diseases of Children* 1975;**129**:42–46.
4. Charlton A, Larcombe IJ, Meller ST, *et al.* Absence from school related to cancer and other chronic conditions. *Archives of Disease in Childhood* 1991;**66**:1217–1222.
5. Lansky SB, Cairns NU. The family of the child with cancer. In: *Proceedings of the American Cancer Society National Conference on the Care of the Child with Cancer.* New York: American Cancer Society, 1979; pp. 156–162.
6. Cairns NU, Klopovich P, Hearne E, *et al.* School attendance of children with cancer. *Journal of School Health* 1982;**52**:152–155.
7. Lansky SB, Cairns NU, Zwartjes W. School attendance among children with cancer: a report from two centers. *Journal of Psychosocial Oncology* 1983;**12**:75–82.
8. Stehbens JA, Kisker CT, Wilson BK. School behavior and attendance during the first year of treatment for childhood cancer. *Psychology School* 1983;**20**:223–228.
9. Eiser C. How leukemia affects a child's schooling. *British Journal of Social and Clinical Psychology* 1980;**19**:365–368.
10. Brown RT, Madan-Swain A. Cognitive, neuropsychological and academic sequelae in children with leukemia. *Journal of Learning Disabilities* 1993;**26**:74–90.
11. Gerhardt CA, Miller MD, Vannatta K, *et al.* Educational and occupational outcomes among survivors of childhood cancer during the transition to emerging adulthood. *Journal of Developmental & Behavioral Pediatrics* 2007;**28**:448–455.
12. Klopovich P, Vats TS, Butterfield G, *et al.* School phobia: interventions in childhood cancer. *Journal of Kansas Medical Society* 1981;**82**:125–127.
13. Ross DM, Ross SA. Teaching the child with leukemia to cope with teasing. *Issues in Comprehensive Pediatric Nursing* 1984;**7**:59–66.
14. Evans SE, Radford M. Psychological adjustment and achievements of survivors of childhood cancer. *Archives of Disease in Childhood* 1995;**72**:423–426.
15. Sloper J, Larcombe IJ, Charlton A. Psychological adjustment of five-year survivors of childhood cancer. *Journal of Cancer Education* 1994;**9**:163–169.
16. Haupt R, Fears TR, Robison LL, *et al.* Educational attainment of long-term survivors of childhood acute lymphoblastic leukemia. *JAMA* 1994;**272**:1427–1432.
17. Ross JW, Scarvalone SA. Facilitating the pediatric cancer patient's return to school. *Social Work* 1982;**27**:256–261.
18. McCarthy AM, Williams J, Plumer C. Evaluation of school re-entry nursing intervention for children with cancer. *Journal of Pediatric Oncology Nursing* 1998;**15**:143–152.
19. McCollum AT. *Coping with Prolonged Health Impairment in Your Child.* Boston: Little Brown, 1975.

20. Katz ER, Kellerman J, Rigler D, *et al.* School intervention with pediatric cancer patients. *Journal of Pediatric Psychology* 1977;**2**:72–76.

21. Kaplan DM, Smith A, Grobstein R. School management of the seriously ill child. *Journal of School Health* 1974;**44**:250–254.

22. Sach MB. Helping the child with cancer go back to school. *Journal of School Health* 1980;**50**:328–331.

23. Noll RB, Bukowski WM, Rogosch FA, *et al.* Social interactions between children with cancer and their peers: teacher ratings. *Journal of Pediatric Psychology* 1990;**15**:43–53.

24. Noll RB, LeRoy S, Bukowski WM, *et al.* Peer relationships and adjustment in children with cancer. *Journal of Pediatric Psychology* 1991;**16**:307–326.

25. Noll RB, Bukowski WM, Davies WH, *et al.* Adjustment in the peer system of adolescents with cancer: a two-year study. *Journal of Pediatric Psychology* 1993;**18**:351–364.

26. Katz ER, Varni JW, Rubenstein CL, *et al.* Teacher, parent and child evaluative ratings of school reintegration intervention for children with newly diagnosed cancer. *Child Health Care* 1992;**21**:69–75.

27. Varni JW, Katz ER, Colgrove RJr, *et al.* Perceived social support and adjustment of children with newly diagnosed cancer. *Journal of Developmental & Behavioral Pediatrics* 1994;**15**:6–20.

28. Rubenstein CL, Varni JW, Katz ER. Cognitive functioning in long-term survivors of childhood cancer: a prospective analysis. *Journal of Developmental & Behavioral Pediatrics* 1990;**11**:301–305.

29. Vannatta K, Garstein MA, Short A, *et al.* A controlled study of peer relationships of children surviving brain tumors: teachers, peer and self-ratings. *Journal of Pediatric Psychology* 1998;**23**:279–287.

30. Kazak AE, Meadows AT. Family of young adolescents who have survived cancer: social-emotional adjustment, adaptability and social support. *Journal of Pediatric Psychology* 1989;**14**:175–191.

31. Puukko LR, Sammallahti PR, Siimes MA, *et al.* Childhood leukemia and body image: interview reveals impairment not found with a questionnaire. *Journal of Clinical Psychology* 1997;**53**:133–137.

32. Gray RE, Doan BD, Shermer MA, *et al.* Psychological adaptation of survivors of childhood cancer. *Cancer* 1992;**70**:2713–2721.

33. Fritz GK, Williams Jr., Issues of adolescent development for survivors of childhood cancer. *Journal of American Academy of Child and Adolescent Psychiatry* 1988;**27**:712–715.

34. Varni JW, Wallander JL.Pediatric chronic disabilities. In: Routh DK (ed.) *Handbook of Pediatric Psychology.* New York: Guilford Press, 1988; pp. 190–221.

35. Varni JW, Katz ER. Stress, social support and negative affectivity with newly diagnosed cancer: a prospective transactional analysis. *Psychooncology* 1997;**6**:267–278.

36. Sullivan HS. *The Interpersonal Theory of Psychiatry.* New York: WW Norton, 1953.

37. Bukowski WM, Hoza B. Popularity and friendship: issues in theory, measurement, and outcomes. In: Berndt T, Ladd G (eds.) *Contributions of Peer Relations to Children's Development.* New York: Wiley, 1989; pp. 15–45.

38. O'Malley JE, Koocher G, Foster D, *et al.* Psychiatric sequelae of surviving childhood cancer. *American Journal of Orthopsychiatry* 1979;**137**:94–96.

39. Hockenberry-Eaton M, Manteuffel B, Bottomley S. Development of two instruments examining stress and adjustment in children with cancer. *Journal of Pediatric Oncology Nursing* 1997;**14**:178–185.

40. Harris MS. Psychosocial predictors of child adjustment and school reintegration outcome in pediatric cancer survivors. Doctoral dissertation. University of Houston, Texas, 2009.

41. Parker JG, Asher SR. Peer relations and later personal adjustment: are low accepted children at risk? *Psychology Bulletin* 1987;**102**:357–389.

42. Caplan G. *Principles of Preventive Psychiatry.* New York: Basic Books, 1964.

43. Joint Commission on Mental Illness and Health. *Action for Mental Health.* New York: Basic Books, 1961.

44. Katz ER. Illness impact and social reintegration. In: Kellerman J (ed.) *Psychological Aspects of Cancer in Children.* Springfield, IL: Thomas, 1980; pp. 14–45.

45. Deasy-Spinetta P, Spinetta JJ. Educational issues in the rehabilitation of longterm survivors. In: Pizzo PA, Poplack DG (eds.) *Principles and Practice of Pediatric Oncology*, 2nd edn. Philadelphia, PA, Lippincott, 1981.

46. Varni JW, Katz ER. Psychological aspects of cancer in children: a review of research. *Journal of Psychosocial Oncology* 1987;**5**:93–119.

47. Katz ER, Dolgin MJ, Varni JW. Cancer in children and adolescents. In: Gross AM, Drabman RS (eds.) *Handbook of Clinical Behavioral Pediatrics.* New York: Plenum, 1990; pp. 129–146.

48. Deasy-Spinetta P. School issues and the child with cancer. *Cancer* 1993;**71**:3261–3264.

49. Gregory K, Parker L, Craft AW. Returning to primary school after treatment for cancer. *Pediatric Hematology-Oncology* 1994;**11**:105–109.

50. Larcombe I, Charlton A. Children return to school after treatment for cancer: study days for teachers. *Journal of Cancer Education* 1996;**11**:102–105.

51. Baysinger M, Heiney SP, Creed JM, *et al.* A trajectomy approach for education of the child/adolescent with cancer. *Journal of Pediatric Oncology Nursing* 1993;**10**:133–138.

52. Häcker W, Klemm M, Böpple E. Heimatschulbesuche bei krebskranken Schulerinnen und Schulern während und nach der Therapie (Local school attendance by students with cancer during and after therapy). *Klinische Padiatrie* 1995;**207**:181–185.

53. Whitsett SF, Pelletier W, Scott-Lane L. Meeting impossible psychosocial demands in pediatric oncology: creative solutions to universal challenges. *Medical and Pediatric Oncology* 1999;**32**:289–291.

54. Keeney SN, Katz ER. *Cancervive Parents' and Teacher's Guide for Kids with Cancer.* Los Angeles Cancervive, 2005.

55. Leukemia and Lymphoma Society. *Learning and Living with Cancer: Advocating for Your Child's Educational Needs.* (Brochure) White Plains, NY, 2005.

56. Cleave H, Charlton A. Evaluation of a cancer-based coping and caring course used in three different settings. *Child Care Health and Development* 1997;**23**:399–413.

57. Ranmal R, Prictor M, Scott JT. *Intervention for Improving Communication with Children and Adolescents about Their Cancer.* The Cochrane Collaboration. John Wiley & Sons Ltd. http//www.thecochranelibrary.com, 2008.

58. Katz ER, Rubenstein CL, Hubert N, *et al.* School and social reintegration of children with cancer. *Journal of Psychosocial Oncology* 1988;**6**:123–140.

59. Varni JW, Katz ER, Colegrove R Jr, *et al.* The impact of social skills training on adjustment of children with newly diagnosed cancer. *Journal of Pediatric Psychology* 1993;**18**:751–767.

60. Tadmor CS. The perceived personal control crisis intervention model: training of an application by physicians and nurses to a high risk population of Caesarean birth in a hospital setting. Doctoral dissertation, Hebrew University, Jerusalem, 1984.

61. Tadmor CS, Brandes JM. The perceived personal control crisis intervention model in the prevention of emotional dysfunction for a high risk population of Caesarean birth. *Journal of Primary Prevention* 1984;**4**:240–251.

62. Tadmor CS, Brandes JM, Hofman JE. Preventive intervention for a Caesarean birth population. *Journal of Preventive Psychiatry* 1987;**3**:343–364.

63. Lazarus RS. Emotions and adaptations conceptual and empirical relations. In: Arnold WJ (ed.) *Nebraska Symposium on Motivation.* Lincoln, NE: University of Nebraska Press, 1968.

64. Tadmor CS. The perceived personal control preventive intervention for a caesarean birth population. In: Price RH, Cowen EL, Lorion RP, Ramos-McKay J (eds.) *14 Ounces of Prevention: A Casebook for Practitioners.* Washington, DC: American Psychological Association, 1988; pp. 141–152.

65. Tadmor CS, Bar-Maor JA, Birkhan J, *et al.* Pediatric surgery: a preventive intervention approach to enhance mastery of stress. *Journal of Preventive Psychiatry* 1987;**3**:365–392.

66. Tadmor CS, Weyl Ben-Arush M. Changes in the policies of the department of hematology, 1982-1998, designed to promote the mental health of children with leukemia and enhance their quality of life. *Pediatric Hematology-Oncology* 2000;**17**:67–76.

67. Tadmor CS. Perceived personal control. In: Gullotta TP, Bloom M (eds.) *Encyclopedia of Primary Prevention and Health Promotion.* New York: Kluwer Academic/Plenum Press, 2003; pp. 812–821.

68. Tadmor CS, Weyl Ben Arush M, Postovsky S, *et al.* Policies designed to enhance the quality of life of children with cancer at the end-of-life. *Pediatric Hematology-Oncology* 2003;**20**:43–54.

69. Tadmor CS. Preventive intervention for children with cancer and their families at the end-of-life. *Journal of Primary Prevention* 2004;**24**:311–323.

70. Price RH, Cowen EL, Lorion RP, *et al.* (eds.) *14 Ounces of Prevention: A Casebook for Practitioners.* Washington, DC: American Psychological Association, 1988.

71. Gullotta TP. Prevention's technology. *Journal of Primary Prevention* 1987;**8**:4–24.

72. Swift C, Levin G. Empowerment: an emerging mental health technology. *Journal of Primary Prevention* 1987;**8**:71–94.

73. Lancashire ER, Frobisher C, Reulen RC, *et al.* Educational attainment among adult survivors of childhood cancer in Great Britain: a population-based cohort study. *Journal of National Cancer Institute* 2010;**102**:254–270.

74. Chekryn J, Deegan M, Reid J. Impact on teachers when a child with cancer returns to school. *Children and Health Care* 1987;**15**:161–165.

75. Mabe PA, Riley WT, Treiber FA Cancer knowledge and acceptance of children with cancer. *Journal of School Health* 1987;**57**:59–63.

11

Psychopharmacology in Pediatric Oncology

Elizabeth G. Pinsky, Annah N. Abrams

Introduction

The last decades have brought increasing recognition of mental illness in all populations of children. There has been a concurrent increased recognition of the impact that mental illness can have on the health and well-being of children with medical illness and the impact that medical illness can have on a child's mental health. While pediatric psychopharmacology in the medically ill child lags behind evidence-based adult practices, there are nevertheless an expanding number of treatment options. Here we will explore pharmacologic considerations for children with cancer; these include psychiatric side effects of common non-psychoactive medications, psychoactive medications by indication, and pharmacologic interactions and adverse effects at the intersection of oncology and psychiatry.

Medications with Adverse Psychiatric Effects

Some children with malignancies will have new psychiatric symptoms while in treatment; others will experience exacerbation of preexisting difficulties, most often with anxiety or mood. For some of these children, symptoms may be related to anti-neoplastic or other medications used as part of their treatment regimen. The treatment team and families should be familiar with the neuropsychiatric sequelae of common medications, in order that psychiatric side effects can be promptly detected if they do occur, parents can be guided and reassured about mild effects, and treatment can be instituted early when appropriate.

Corticosteroids

Corticosteroids are frequently used for treatment of childhood cancers, including standard chemotherapy protocols for leukemias and lymphomas. They are also used for management of adverse effects and sequelae of treatment, including those associated with the treatment of solid tumors (i.e., swelling and inflammation). Corticosteroids are also associated with an array of psychiatric adverse effects. In adult patients, the most common psychiatric side effects include mild or moderate changes in mood, sleep, and appetite [1]. Less often corticosteroids may cause significant changes in mental status including delirium and psychosis, or severe disturbance of mood including depression and mania. Effects are dose-dependent, with delirium and psychosis more common for patients receiving high-dose corticosteroids [2]. There is generally resolution of symptoms after cessation of steroid treatment; however, it is important to monitor for a few days following discontinuation as the side effects often linger.

While the psychiatric sequelae of steroids in pediatric patients are less studied, there is data in children with hematologic malignancies [3, 4], as well as renal and pulmonary disease that demonstrates a similar pattern of adverse events [5, 6]. Common adverse effects include irritability, labile mood, sleep disturbance, anxiety and fatigue. Younger children tend to be more affected [4].

Most steroid-induced symptoms, including mild hyperactivity and irritability, are transient and can often be managed with behavioral or environmental intervention. The more significant psychiatric symptoms associated with corticosteroids can be successfully treated with medications targeted at symptom clusters. There is evidence for use of antipsychotics (e.g., risperidone) for steroid-induced mood disturbance and psychosis in children [7–9]. Sleep difficulties and increased anxiety can be treated with benzodiazepines. Rarely, severe psychiatric symptoms, including depressed mood with suicidality, mania or refractory psychosis, may require adjustment in dose or even discontinuation of corticosteroid therapy. For children who do experience mood disturbances on steroids, it

Pediatric Psycho-oncology: Psychosocial Aspects and Clinical Interventions, Second Edition.
Edited by Shulamith Kreitler, Myriam Weyl Ben-Arush and Andrés Martin.

can be helpful during ongoing treatment to prophylax with an atypical antipsychotic prior to administration of steroids [7].

Interferon

In pediatric oncology, Interferon-alfa (IFN) is used for the treatment of malignant melanoma and giant cell tumors. Data from adult populations who received INF for viral hepatitis or malignancies demonstrate significant and common psychiatric sequelae, most frequently depressed mood, fatigue and anxiety [10, 11]. Adult data have also demonstrated that the depressive syndrome associated with IFN can be successfully prevented and treated with standard antidepressant therapy, most commonly the selective serotonin reuptake inhibitors (SSRIs) [12, 13]. While there is no data in pediatric populations, clinical experience suggests that children with IFN-induced depressed mood can also be treated with standard depression treatment, including psychotherapy for mild symptoms and antidepressants for children with more significant symptoms. It is helpful to perform baseline depression screening on all children prior to treatment with INF and follow their mood symptoms throughout the course of treatment.

Decision to Use Psychoactive Medications

When children with cancer present with psychiatric symptoms, medications may be an important part of their overall treatment. The scope of this chapter is limited to psychopharmacology; however, medications are rarely (if ever) used as monotherapy, and adjunctive non-pharmacologic treatment modalities are almost always employed to boost efficacy, increase adherence, and sustain response to pharmacologic management. Options for non-pharmacologic treatment for depressed mood and anxiety include traditional individual therapy as well as family therapy and cognitive behavioral therapy (CBT). Hypnosis, distraction, guided relaxation, and other behavioral techniques can be useful for procedural anxiety and for anticipatory anxiety and nausea. Even in delirium, non-pharmacologic environmental interventions including frequent reorienting, early mobilization, exposure to natural light and prevention of dehydration, are important treatment modalities. Finally, psychoeducation of patients and families is essential for all symptom clusters and syndromes, including psychotic illness.

There are some psychiatric urgencies common in medically ill children where prompt pharmacologic intervention is essential. These foremost include acute agitation or aggression, though the acute mental status changes seen in delirium, psychosis and mania also require emergent pharmacologic intervention, whether or not agitation is present. Substance withdrawal also requires emergent treatment, including both the syndromes with high mortality (i.e., alcohol and benzodiazepine withdrawal) and those that are severely uncomfortable though not life-threatening (e.g., opiate withdrawal). We also argue for prompt psychopharmacologic treatment of children with dense symptoms and suffering associated with clinical depression and anxiety. These children may be unable to fully engage in non-pharmacologic treatments, and require prompt alleviation of symptoms. Psychopharmacologic treatment at the outset for these children acknowledges the Herculean effort required to engage in therapy when immobilized by depressed mood or anxiety.

Similarly, there is compelling reason to consider prompt medication evaluation for a child who has significant functional impairment, even if he or she is able to concurrently engage in therapy. Pharmacologic intervention should also be considered for children who have partial response to other interventions. Finally, pharmacology is a reasonable choice for children or families who simply prefer to start with medications as primary treatment, or for whom there are barriers to other types of care. Common barriers to therapy include time, cost, and availability; in many parts of the world, including the United States, there is a remarkable dearth of child mental health providers.

Commonly Used Psychoactive Medications in Pediatric Oncology by Indication

For children with cancer who do require pharmacologic management, treatment is often directed at symptom clusters as opposed to formal psychiatric diagnoses. Children will often, for example, present with situational anxiety and will benefit from anxiolytic medications, but do not meet criteria for a generalized anxiety disorder. Similarly, children may have depressed mood and benefit from antidepressants during treatment without meeting criteria for major depressive disorder (i.e., symptoms lasting greater than two weeks, multiple neuro-vegetative symptoms, etc.). Finally, there is a great deal of symptom overlap for individual children, medically ill or not, and symptom-targeted treatments are often of greatest benefit. Therefore medications are described here according to symptom cluster: delirium and agitation, depressed mood, anxiety and insomnia, and neuro-cognition (including long-term survivors).

Delirium and Acute Agitation

Delirium, also known as acute confusional state, is a syndrome characterized by: (1) an acute onset and a waxing and waning course; (2) disturbance of arousal; and (3) cognitive impairment or confusion. These symptoms occur either in the setting of an underlying general medical illness or secondary to substances including medicines or toxins [14], which are commonly encountered in pediatric oncology (see Table 11.1). There is a growing body of literature demonstrating that pediatric delirium is common, but under-recognized, and that the symptoms of pediatric delirium are similar to those seen in adult delirium [15–19].

In addition to confusion, other common symptoms of pediatric delirium include hallucinations, delusions, disorganized behavior, disorientation and disruptions in memory, mood, affect, and the sleep–wake cycle [19]. The quality of the disturbance of arousal in delirium may vary. Hyperactive delirium may be associated with combativeness and agitation, which can interfere with care and endanger the patient or the care providers (e.g., a patient who pulls at lines or who tries to get out of bed). Hypoactive delirium is a state of quiet confusion, and as a result is often overlooked by care providers since the symptoms do not interfere with a child's care. The underlying mechanisms of delirium remain poorly understood, but it is thought to represent derangements in multiple neurotransmitter systems, particularly dysregulation of acetylcholine and a state of excess dopamine in the central nervous system. Delirium is not a disease but a cluster of symptoms,

and has a broad array of potential underlying causes. It may be caused by systemic illness (e.g., infection, electrolyte derangement), by central nervous system processes (e.g., intracranial mass, stroke), or by exposure to medications or other toxins. Medications that are regularly used in pediatric oncology are a frequent cause of delirium, including anticholingergic agents like benzodiazepines and opiates and many chemotherapeutic agents (see Table 11.1).

While definitive treatment for the delirious patient must be identification and treatment of the underlying cause of the syndrome, it is important to treat the delirium while the etiology is being determined in order to ensure safety for patients and staff. Environmental interventions, including reassurance and frequent reorienting to place and familiar people, can ameliorate some of the stress and behaviors associated with delirium. Pharmacologic interventions can ease distressing symptoms including psychosis and fear as well as decrease agitation. While staff will readily treat the agitated patient, we also advocate treating the hypoactive delirious patient, who may not interfere with care or endanger themselves, but who nevertheless may be suffering.

Dopamine blockade is the mainstay of pharmacologic management, and for adult patients haloperidol delivered intravenously is the traditional treatment of choice [20]. IV haloperidol has minimal anticholinergic activity, is calming but not sedating, and has little or no risk of hypotension or respiratory depression. Haloperidol does carry a risk of cardiac arrhythmia related to QTc prolongation, and caution should be used for patients with electrolyte derangement, with underlying cardiac conduction abnormalities, or for those on other QT prolonging agents (reviewed in greater depth later in this chapter). While delirium in young children has historically been under-recognized or treated with environmental interventions only (i.e., restraint), there is evidence for the use of IV haloperidol even in young infants [16, 21]. Atypical antipsychotics have become increasingly first-line agents for delirious patients who are able to take oral medications. Olanzapine, risperidone and quetiapine are all good oral agents for treatment of the delirious patient, with some evidence for use in the pediatric oncology population [22].

Benzodiazepines should almost always be avoided in the delirious patient (with the notable exception of delirium caused by alcohol or benzodiazepine withdrawal). Benzodiazepines are likely to exacerbate anticholinergic effects, and compound the core symptoms of confusion and disorientation. Diphenhydramine can also exacerbate confusional states.

Table 11.1 Common oncologic medications associated with delirium.

Amphotercin-B
Benzodiazepines
Cyclosporine
Cytarabine
Diphenhydramine
Glucocorticoids
Interleukin-II
L-aspariginase
Methotrexate
Opiate pain medications
Tacrolimus

Sources: [2, 86–89].

Depressed Mood

As reviewed in Chapter 9 on the psychiatric impact of childhood cancer, the majority of children with malignancies do not develop significant long-term psychological distress, and overall children with cancer are similar to their peers in terms of their emotional health [23–25]. That said, depression is a common illness in all populations of children and adolescents, with an estimated incidence by the end of adolescence of 20% [26], and there is evidence that some subgroups of children with cancer may be at increased risk [27].

Children with cancer who do present with clinically significant depression and who require psychopharmacologic intervention are, for the most part, treated similarly to their well peers. The treatment is most distinguished by the challenges involved in diagnosing depression and monitoring the response to treatment in the setting of active medical illness. The neurovegetative signs and symptoms of depression, including changes in sleep, appetite, energy and cognition, may all be impacted by both cancer and cancer treatments. Therefore, when assessing response to treatment, it is important to consider improvement in the symptoms of depression that are more independent of physical illness, including apathy, hopelessness and anhedonia, than the symptoms of sleep, energy and appetite.

Data on antidepressant treatment specific to children with malignancies is lacking, though there are some small studies demonstrating that SSRIs are well tolerated and efficacious in children with cancer [28]. Moreover, there is evidence that pediatric oncologists frequently prescribe SSRIs for treatment of depression and anxiety [29, 30]. It is similarly our clinical experience that SSRIs are frequently used and safe treatments for the pediatric oncology population. Most important, there is strong data supporting the use of the SSRIs as first line pharmacologic treatment for healthy children and adolescents with depression [31].

The SSRIs are a class of compounds that act in the central nervous system primarily by increasing the concentration of the neurotransmitter serotonin—initially through potent inhibition of serotonin reuptake at the synaptic cleft, and then by a more gradual process of re-equilibration of the neurotransmitter system. To date, the largest study of SSRIs in children is the Treatment for Adolescents with Depression Study (TADS). TADS was a large-scale, randomized controlled trial (RCT) that showed favorable results for the use of combination treatment with SRRIs and psychotherapy. In TADS, 439 adolescents aged 12 to 17 with moderate to severe depression were randomized to treatment with: (1) fluoxetine alone; (2) cognitive behavioral therapy (CBT) alone; (3) a combination of fluoxetine and CBT; or (4) placebo only. After 12 weeks, 71% of children responded to the combination treatment of fluoxetine and CBT, 61% responded to the fluoxetine-only treatment, 43% responded to the CBT only treatment, and 35% responded to placebo only [32].

In addition to evidence regarding their efficacy, the SSRIs are generally well tolerated and do not require cardiovascular or ECG monitoring or blood work, which is particularly important when attempting to minimize invasive procedures for pediatric cancer patients. The most common side effects of the SSRIs are headache and gastrointestinal symptoms including nausea and diarrhea, which often improve within 5–7 days of initiating treatment. Other common adverse effects include sleep disturbance (insomnia or somnolence), restlessness, changes in appetite (increase or decrease), and sweating. Sexual dysfunction is another common side effect of the SSRIs, and it is important to be honest with adolescent patients about this risk. There is also some risk of mood destabilization when treating children with SSRIs. Some children, particularly younger children, may develop disinhibition with silliness, impulsivity, agitation, and behavioral activation within days or even hours of initiating treatment with an antidepressant [33]. These symptoms of activation resolve with discontinuation of the medication, and are distinct from symptoms of mania or hypomania that may develop weeks after initiation of antidepressant therapy. These later symptoms, sometimes referred to as "bipolar switching," can indicate an underlying bipolar diathesis. Additional adverse effects that are rare but that have particular relevance to the pediatric oncologist, including serotonin syndrome and hematologic effects, are discussed at greater length later in this chapter.

While medications within the class of SSRIs all act with one putative mechanism, they are in fact a chemically heterogeneous class of compounds with different pharmacokinetic and pharmacodynamic properties and different side-effect profiles (see Table 11.2). Although the SSRIs have similar efficacy overall, many children and adults will respond to one SSRI but not to another, with no clear pattern to responders and non-responders. There are a variety of factors to consider when selecting a specific SSRI for first-line treatment. These include side-effect profile, anticipated drug interactions, and pharmacokinetic considerations including half-life. Many of these properties are

Table 11.2 Characteristics of antidepressant medications used in pediatric patients.

	Elimination half-life (hr)	Starting dose (mg)	Adult target dose (range)	Notes
SSRIs				
Citalopram	33	5–10	20 (20–80)	Fewest drug-drug interactions
Escitalopram	22	2.5–5	10 (10–20)	FDA approved for depression ages ≥12
Fluoxetine	87	5–10	20 (40–80)	Most studied in children with MDD, FDA approved for depression ages ≥7
Fluvoxamine	19	12.5–25	200 (50-300)	Pediatric data for anxiety, approved for OCD ages ≥8. Sedating.
Paroxetine	21	5–10	20 (20–60)	Not first-line, use in children <18 prohibited in Europe
Sertraline	26	12.5–25	50 (50–200)	Approved for OCD ages ≥6
Other				
Bupropion	15	37.5	300 (75–450)	Demonstrated efficacy in ADHD
Duloxetine	12	20	40 (40–120)	Evidence for use in chronic pain for adults
Mirtazapine	30	7.5	15 (15–45)	Prominent weight gain, sedation
Venlafaxine	3.6	18.75–37.5	300 (75–375)	Significant discontinuation syndrome, associated with tachycardia and hypertension

Sources: [90, 91].

summarized in Table 11.2; specific notable qualities relevant to for the pediatric oncology patient of the individual SSRIs are discussed here.

Among the SSRIs, fluoxetine is distinguished by a particularly long half-life and by the presence of an active metabolite, norfluoxetine, which has an elimination half-life of 7–14 days. This characteristic makes fluoxetine a good choice for children or families who struggle with medication adherence. However, this may be problematic for children who develop adverse mood-related effects, including disinhibition or bipolar switch. For these children, behavioral or mood symptoms may persist for weeks while fluoxetine and its metabolites are gradually eliminated. Citalopram and its s-enantiomer, escitalopram, have the lowest rate of drug–drug interactions, which makes them a good choice for the child with cancer who is likely taking many concurrent medications. While the SSRIs as a class overall are likely to cause some activation, fluvoxamine is more likely to cause sedation and can be helpful for children with sleep-onset difficulties. The majority of existing data on fluvoxamine is in children with anxiety, however, and there are no controlled trials of fluvoxamine in children or adolescents with depression. Paroxetine has the shortest half-life and is most likely to cause an uncomfortable discontinuation syndrome, requiring a long taper. In our experience, paroxetine is also the

most likely to cause activation and akathisia. Of note, in December 2004, the European Medicines Agency prohibited the use of paroxetine in children under 18 because of data around risk of suicidality, which is discussed at greater depth later in this section.

Government regulation of medications is an additional consideration, and the status of individual SSRIs varies internationally. In the United States, only two SSRIs are approved for use in treating depression in children and adolescents: fluoxetine for children 7 and older, and escitalopram for children 12 and older. In practice, both citalopram and sertraline are commonly prescribed "off label" to children with depression, and have data supporting their efficacy and tolerability for this indication. Fluvoxamine and sertraline are both approved by the United States Federal Drug Agency (FDA) for use in children with obsessive-compulsive disorder.

Once an SSRI is selected, it should be started at a low dose and gradually titrated upwards (see Table 11.2). This is particularly important to minimize common side effects such as nausea and diarrhea. All SSRIs take 4–6 weeks to reach full efficacy; improvement should be assessed and dosages adjusted upwards as appropriate in 2–4 week intervals. Children who have no response at 8 weeks are likely to need alternative treatment, with a goal of remission of symptoms by 12 weeks. Pediatric depression is an illness with high rates of relapse. A randomized, controlled fluoxetine discontinuation trial showed that continued treatment with SSRIs is associated with lower rates of relapse (40%) compared to continued treatment with placebo (69%) [34]. While there is no consensus about the ideal length of treatment, antidepressant therapy should generally be continued for a minimum of an additional 6–12 months after full remission of symptoms has been achieved. Once the decision to discontinue the antidepressant has been reached, both clinician and parents should closely monitor for signs of re-emerging depression. With the exception of fluoxetine, all SSRIs must be tapered to avoid an uncomfortable discontinuation syndrome that may include nausea, diarrhea, headache, cognitive dulling and mild electric shock-like or "zinging" sensations in the extremities. Paroxetine is the most likely to cause discontinuation syndrome, and requires particular care when tapering.

Approximately 60% of healthy children and adolescents will respond to initial treatment with an SSRI [35]. For those who do not respond to first-line treatment, a number of second-line options exist. Switching within class to another SSRI is a reasonable first step with demonstrated efficacy and safety in both children and adolescents. The Treatment of Resistant Depression in Adolescents (TORDIA) study evaluated 334 adolescents ages 12–18 with residual depressive symptoms after initial treatment of adequate duration with an SSRI at adequate dose [36]. The adolescents were randomized to: (1) a medication switch alone or (2) a medication switch in combination with CBT. Patients were further randomized to medication switch to either (1) venlafaxine, a selective noradrenergic reuptake inhibitor (SNRI) with serotonergic and noradrenergic activity, or (2) an SSRI other than that used in their initial treatment. A switch to either medication in combination with CBT was more effective than a medication switch alone (54.8% v. 40.5%). Remission rates were similar for SSRIs and venlafaxine, but SSRIs had fewer side effects. Venlafaxine was also associated with a higher rate of suicidal thoughts.

Few trials have evaluated the effects of other classes of antidepressants for the treatment of depressed youths. Mirtazapine is a serotonin and adrenergic receptor blocker that has showed efficacy for treatment of depression in adults; there are no randomized control trials in children and adolescents, though there is some data demonstrating safety [37]. That said, mirtazapine has a side-effect profile characterized by weight gain and somnolence, which can be useful for treating weight loss and insomnia in adolescents with cancer. Bupropion is a novel antidepressant with dopaminergic and noradrenergic effects through an unclear mechanism of action. It may be used as monotherapy for depression, as an agent to augment partial response to an SSRI, or as a second-line agent for ADHD. There is evidence from ADHD studies supporting its safety in the pediatric population [38, 39]. There is some data associating bupropion with reduced seizure threshold; especially in patients with bulimia and history of seizures or head trauma [40, 41]. Therefore, in children with intracerebral malignancies, those receiving high dose methotrexate and those who are experiencing frequent vomiting, caution should be used.

As described above, venlafaxine showed some efficacy in the TORDIA study, but was associated with side effects and increased risk of suicidality. In other controlled studies venlafaxine has demonstrated superiority to placebo for depressed adolescents, but not depressed children [42]. Duloxetine is another SNRI with similar mechanism of action. There are no controlled studies of duloxetine for the treatment of children or adolescents with depression. However, because it is used to treat chronic and complex pain, it is often prescribed by the pain service to our oncology patients. Theoretically it should also be effective for depressed mood, but should not be used as a first-line agent for the treatment of depression in children. Similar to duloxetine, tricyclic antidepressants are used for treatment of chronic pain including syndromes commonly encountered in pediatric oncology such as neuropathic pain and migraine. Individual controlled trials as well as a meta-analysis have shown that tricyclic antidepressants are no better than placebo for the treatment of child and adolescent depression [43]. Tricyclics are also associated with more side effects than the SSRIs, including anticholinergic and cardiac side effects, and they can be fatal after an overdose. Although tricyclics cannot be recommended for treatment of depression alone, when used in consultation with a pain management team and similar to duloxetine, they may have a role for the depressed child with cancer.

Depression is a serious and, at times, life-threatening illness. Whether or not they receive pharmacologic treatment, some depressed children and adolescents will experience thoughts of suicide or exhibit suicidal behaviors during the course of their illness. There is ongoing controversy about whether treatment with anti-depressants increases the risk of emerging or worsening suicidal thoughts. In 2004, an FDA meta-analysis of 4100 children in 24 randomized controlled trials examining nine antidepressants showed a two-fold increase in emergence or worsening of suicidality (from 2 per 100 on placebo to 4 per 100 on antidepressants). There were no completed suicides. In response to this meta-analysis, in October 2004, the FDA issued a black-box warning on the use of all antidepressants in children. In May 2007, in response to two additional meta-analyses showing increased suicidality, this warning was expanded to include young adults up to age 24. On the other hand, an epidemiological population-based study published in 2003 showed an inverse correlation between rates of antidepressant use in 10–19-year-olds and completed suicides [44], suggesting a protective effect of pharmacologic treatment.

The controversy surrounding this data continues. The most clear and consistent message is that children and adolescents with depression are at risk of self-harm and should be monitored closely, regardless of treatment strategy. The risks associated with treatment should be carefully weighed against the risks of non-treatment (which, of course, also include suicide). Clinicians should ask about suicidal thoughts regularly, and monitor especially closely in the weeks after initiating antidepressant medications and after any dosage increase. Parents should be fully informed about the data surrounding antidepressants and suicide, and whether they elect to use medications or not, they should understand two essential points: first, that worsening mood or suicidality may emerge, and, second, what they should do if either symptom does occur.

Anxiety and Insomnia

Anxiety disorders are common in childhood, with a reported prevalence between 6% and 20%; they are among the earliest psychiatric disorders to emerge [45, 46]. The child with cancer most frequently presents with procedural anxiety and anticipatory anxiety, even in those who do not formally meet criteria for an anxiety disorder. This is not unanticipated, given the numerous anxiety-provoking events that they encounter, including blood draws, lumbar punctures, chemotherapy administrations, and hospital admissions. These symptoms can be effectively treated with pharmacologic agents, usually used in concert with behavioral interventions. Children with cancer may also suffer from acute stress disorder (ASD) or, if symptoms persist, post-traumatic stress disorder (PTSD), as reviewed in Chapter 9.

The SSRIs, reviewed at length in the preceding section on depression, are also first-line treatment for the pharmacologic management of childhood generalized anxiety and for the long-term management of panic disorders [47]. The most studied agents are fluoxetine, fluvoxamine, and sertraline, though in practice all the SSRIs are prescribed for this indication. SSRIs used for anxiety are, in general, also given at similar doses as those used in depression (see Table 11.2). Side effects of the SSRIs (including the controversial data around increased risk of suicidal thoughts) are also reviewed in the above section on depressed mood.

Whether they are used for anxiety or depression, SSRIs generally do not reach full efficacy until the fourth to sixth week of treatment. Depending on the severity of symptoms and the success of non-pharmacologic interventions, many children and adolescents require more immediate relief of anxiety during the weeks while an SSRI is reaching full effect. The benzodiazepines are safe and effective for this short-term control of generalized symptoms, and can also be used for rapid relief of acute anxiety (including pre-procedural, anticipatory and panic).

The benzodiazepines are chemically related compounds that potentiate GABA, the main inhibitory neurotransmitter in the brain. They are distinguished from each other by their pharmacokinetic profiles, including rapidity of onset, duration of effect and presence or absence of active metabolites (summarized in Table 11.3). Lorazepam possesses the added benefit of acting as an anti-emetic—this mechanism of action remains unclear. The main side effect of the benzodiazepines is sedation. Some children, however, will experience paradoxical reactions with disinhibition, aggression and agitation. In our experience, paradoxical reactions are seen more often in young children and in those who have underlying cognitive and behavioral disabilities. For this reason, we recommend caution when using shorter-acting benzodiazepines in younger children. The benzodiazepines also carry a risk of physiologic dependence with chronic use through up-regulation of GABA receptors.

In addition to temporary symptomatic relief of generalized anxiety and panic, benzodiazepines are also the mainstay of treatment for intermittent or context-specific anxiety, including pre-procedural anxiety. Studies have demonstrated efficacy and safety of low-dose oral midazolam in children with cancer undergoing needle-sticks [48], and oral agents including lorazepam are used with great frequency in both inpatient and outpatient settings. Other non-psychoactive pharmacologic interventions prior to procedures include the use of mixed local anesthetic cream (EMLA) and local anesthetics by superficial injection. There is also a growing body of evidence around complementary management of procedural anxiety and pain, including hypnosis and guided imagery [49]. Ideally, minimizing pain and discomfort associated with procedures or treatments can prevent sensitization. These are often unavoidable, however, and anticipatory anxiety and nausea can emerge as a conditioned response [50].

Table 11.3 Commonly used benzodiazepines.

Drug	Half-life (hrs) [active metabolite]	Dosage equivalent (mg)	Onset	Route of admin	Comments
Midazolam	1–12	2	Very fast	IV, IM	Rapid tachyphylaxis
Oxazepam	5–15	15	Slow	PO	Extrahepatic metabolism
Lorazepam	15–20	1	Fast	IV, IM, PO	Anti-emetic
Alprazolam	12–15	0.5	Fast - Intermediate	PO	
Chlordiazepoxide	5–30 [36–200]	10	Intermediate	IV, PO	Frequent agent of choice for alcohol withdrawal
Clonazepam	15–50	0.25	Intermediate	PO	
Diazepam	20–100 [36–200]	5	Fast	IV, PO	

Sources: [92, 93] Devlin JW, Roberts RJ. Pharmacology of commonly used analgesics and sedatives in the ICU: benzodiazepines, propofol, and opioids. Crit Care Clin 2009 vii; Jul;25(3):431–449, Copyright Elsevier, 2009. Reproduced with permission.

Some children, for example, will develop anxiety with nausea or vomiting on the way to the clinic or hospital. For these children, aggressive and proactive treatment of anticipatory symptoms with benzodiazepines (especially lorazepam) can both ameliorate current discomfort and break the cycle of escalating anticipation leading to escalating symptoms.

Insomnia may also emerge during cancer treatment, and may represent a symptom of generalized underlying anxiety or a manifestation of an acute stress response. Insomnia in children with cancer may also be related to medications (e.g., steroids, as reviewed earlier in this chapter), other forms of treatment (e.g., frequent awakenings to void for children receiving large amounts of IV hydration), to the loss of routines or, for hospitalized children, simply the experience of a strange bed, new caregivers, multiple interruptions or a roommate [51]. Some children can be adequately treated with non-pharmacologic interventions including sleep hygiene. Many others will benefit from pharmacologic treatments when hospitalized or when the insomnia is interfering with their daily functioning. Choice of agent should be based on drug interactions, side effect profile, and quality of the insomnia. Agents that decrease sleep-onset latency are appropriate for children who have difficulty falling asleep, and longer-acting agents should be used for children who have difficulty staying asleep. Commonly used agents are summarized in Table 11.4.

The benzodiazepines are often first-line agents for intermittent or time-limited treatment of insomnia in children with cancer, because of their tolerability and the added benefit of nausea control. The choice of benzodiazepine should be based on duration of effect; shorter acting agents such as lorazepam are appropriate for children with delayed sleep-onset, and medium-acting agents such as clonazepam are appropriate for children who also have early awakening or difficulty sustaining sleep. Some children will experience morning sedation, in which case a shorter-acting benzodiazepine or alternative agent should be considered. As when they are used for anxiety, tolerance to benzodiazepines will develop over time, necessitating higher doses to achieve similar results.

In the general pediatric population, over-the-counter (diphenhydramine) and prescription (hydroxyzine) antihistamines are commonly administered to children for insomnia. Anti-histamines act by blocking H1 receptors in the central nervous system, and decrease sleep-onset latency with minimal effect on sleep architecture [52]. The H1 blockers are potent anticholinergic agents. Common anticholinergic side effects—including dry mouth, urinary retention, and constipation—may be particularly unacceptable in pediatric oncology patients, where similar side effects of some chemotherapy agents may be compounded. Antihistamines should always be avoided in children with known or suspected delirium. Similar to the benzodiazepines, some children will experience a paradoxical reaction and develop agitation after administration of antihistamines and younger children are similarly at higher risk for a paradoxical reaction.

Melatonin is a hormone secreted by the pineal gland that regulates a variety of biological functions,

Table 11.4 Medications commonly used for insomnia.

Class	Mechanism of action	Drugs	Adult dose (mg) [pediatric dose]	Half-life (hrs) [peak plasma]	Comments
Benzodiazepines	GABA receptor agonist	Alprazolam	0.125–0.5	12–15	Risk of physiologic dependence
		Clonazepam	0.25–1	15–50 [1–4]	
		Lorazepam	0.5–2	15–20	
Hormone analogs	Suprachiasmatic nucleus	Melatonin	2.5–5 [0.05 mg/kg]	0.5–1 [0.5–1]	Weak hypnotic
Antihistamines	Histamine receptor agonist	Diphenhydramine (Benadryl)	25–100 [0.5 mg/kg]	4–6 [2–4]	Significant anti-cholinergic effects, risk of paradoxical reaction
		Hydroxyzine	25–100 [0.6 mg/kg]	6–24 [2–4]	Significant anti-cholinergic effects, risk of paradoxical reaction
Antidepressants	5-HT, serotonin agonist	Mirtazapine	7.5–15		May have benefit in co-morbid depression
		Trazodone	25–50	[0.5–2]	May have benefit in co-morbid depression
Alpha agonists	α-adrenergic agonists	Clonidine	0.01–0.03	6–24 [2–4]	Narrow therapeutic index, hypotension and bradycardia
Atypical antipsychotics	DA blockade	Olanzapine	1.25–5		Generally acute setting, co-morbid delirium or psychosis
		Quetiapine	12.5–50		
Non-benzdiazepine GABA agonists	Selective GABA type A agonists	Eszopliclone	1–3	5–6 [1]	Class-wide there is minimal data in children
		Zaleplon	5–20	1 [1]	
		Zolpidem	5–10 (IR) 6.25–12.5 (XR)	2.5–3 [1.5]	

Sources: [52, 54, 55, 93, 94].

including the sleep–wake cycle. Melatonin delivered orally augments naturally occurring serum levels. Melatonin is only a mild hypnotic, and is therefore most useful in children with a wide range of circadian rhythm disturbances (including jet lag, blindness, central nervous system pathology, and, interestingly, ADHD) [52]. Melatonin has been studied in pediatric populations and has demonstrated safety and efficacy at shortening sleep-onset latency [53–55]. It is important to note that melatonin is a naturally occurring compound and in the United States is therefore not regulated by the FDA. The quality and consistency of the commercially available preparations vary.

Clonidine is a centrally acting α_2 adrenergic agonist that is widely used for treatment of ADHD in children. It is also commonly used for insomnia. Clonidine acts by decreasing adrenergic tone and has efficacy in decreasing sleep-onset latency. Clonidine has a short half-life, however, and may be less effective for sustaining sleep in children with frequent awakenings. Clonidine was initially developed as an anti-hypertensive, and side effects can include hypotension, bradycardia and rebound hypertension with rapid discontinuation.

Other medications used for insomnia include the sedating antidepressants, trazodone and mirtazapine. Both act centrally on the 5-HT(2) receptor. Trazodone is an older antidepressant that has *not* shown efficacy above placebo in the treatment of depression for children, but can be useful in treating insomnia with co-morbid depression. Trazodone has the rare but notable side effect of priapism in boys, and this risk should be communicated to patients. As described above, there is no data to support use of the newer antidepressant, mirtazapine, in children or adolescents with depression, but given prominent side effects of sedation and weight gain, it can be a good choice for adolescents with insomnia and co-morbid depression with weight loss related to illness or treatment. In the child with delirium or agitation, sedating anti-psychotic medications such as quetiapine and olanzipine may be useful to treat insomnia. At low doses, quetiapine acts as a sedative through blockade of histamine and α-1 adrenergic receptors. As discussed above in reference to their use in delirium, long-term use of these agents is associated with weight gain and metabolic syndrome. They are generally recommended for short-term use, often in an acute setting.

There are a number of newer hypnotic agents used for insomnia in adults, including zolpidem, zaleplon and eszopliclone. These agents interact with the GABA receptor but are chemically unrelated to benzodiazepines, and are more selective in their GABA binding sites. While they are increasingly widely used in adult psychiatry, there is minimal data on their use in children or adolescents [56, 57].

As reviewed in the previous chapter, a small subset of children and adolescents with cancer will go on to develop symptoms of PTSD related to their experiences during diagnosis or treatment [58, 59]. These children are generally treated identically to peers with PTSD resulting from non-medical trauma. While CBT is the mainstay of PTSD treatment for children, there is data supporting the use of SSRIs in adult populations [60]. Antidepressants are frequently used in the pediatric post-trauma population as well as antiadrenergic medications and antipsychotics [61]. Children are otherwise treated symptomatically, with pharmacotherapy targeted at insomnia or anxiety as described in this section.

Neurocognition Long-Term Survivors

There is mounting evidence about, and recommended treatments for, the long-term neurocognitive sequelae of pediatric cancer and cancer treatment. Children with central nervous system (CNS) malignancies are at particular risk of neurocognitive effects of treatment. When compared with well siblings and with matched survivors of *non*-CNS malignancies, children with brain tumors are at significantly increased risk of neurocognitive impairment as adults, as well as lower socioeconomic status and educational attainment [62]. Effects are due to both primary effects of tumor or surgical tumor resection, and to radiation to healthy tissue. Risk factors for cognitive impairment include younger age at diagnosis, female sex, and total dose of radiation [63]. Children with hematologic malignancies may also receive cranial radiation for prevention or treatment of CNS disease, including many children with acute lymphoblastic leukemia (ALL). Children with ALL who are treated with cranial radiation show similar difficulties with cognitive function and attention when compared with healthy siblings and children with Wilms' tumor [64].

In children with non-CNS malignancies who do *not* receive brain irradiation, long-term neuropsychiatric effects of chemotherapy are most common for those treated with methotrexate (MTX), and in particular in children treated with intrathecal MTX. Moreover, there is data that intrathecal MTX has an additive effect when combined with cranial radiation [65]. Intrathecal MTX is standard in many protocols for treatment of ALL for prevention or treatment of CNS disease. Compared to children with primary CNS malignancy there is relative sparing of overall IQ, with sequelae preferentially impacting attention and executive function [66].

There is mounting evidence for the efficacy of stimulant medications in treating cognitive impairment among these childhood cancer survivors. In a placebo-controlled RCT of 106 survivors of CNS malignancy or ALL, ages 6–18, almost half of the children (45.28%) showed response to moderate-dose methylphenidate over three weeks [67]. Children who had more symptoms reported by parents and teachers prior to treatment had greatest response. A follow-up study of long-term methyphenidate use showed improvement in attention and behavior problems in survivors of both acute lymphoblastic leukemia and brain tumors [68].

The stimulant medications have excellent safety data, and have been safely used since the 1940s. While there has been controversy related to case reports of sudden cardiac death, there is no data indicating an association between the use of stimulants and increased sudden cardiac death [69, 70]. The American Academy of Pediatrics and the American Academy of Child and Adolescent Psychiatry do not recommend routine ECG monitoring prior to or during stimulant treatment [71, 72]. However, stimulants are sympathomimetic agents, and can raise blood pressure and heart rate. For this reason, package inserts do recommend monitoring for children with known structural heart disease or with family history of sudden death. In the pediatric oncology and the childhood cancer survivor population one must be cognizant of the prior treatments they received and the impact this may have on their cardiac function. We therefore recommend that children who have received cardiotoxic medications (e.g., adriamycin) or cardiac radiation (e.g., mantlefield) should have ECG screening prior to the administration of stimulant medications. Furthermore if there is concern of cardiac function in addition to conduction, an echocardiogram may be indicated.

Similarly, it is important to remember that long-term survivors of pediatric cancer may present with psychiatric symptoms months or years after completing treatment, either later in childhood or as adults. These same adults may have underlying neurcognitive effects, may have been treated with adriamycin or chest radiation, and may require special surveillance when starting medications that carry risk of conduction abnormalities or other cardiac effects.

Interactions and Adverse Effects of Psychiatric Medications

Interactions

As with all drugs, the administration of psychotropic medications requires consideration of pharmacokinetics,

pharmacodynamics and interactions. These considerations are especially important for medically ill children who are often taking multiple concurrent medications. Here we will present a brief overview of pharmacokinetics and pharmacodynamics, and discuss some of the specific drug–drug interactions and adverse effects of psychoactive medications that are most relevant to the pediatric oncology population.

Pharmaco*kinetics* can be thought of as the study of how the body impacts administered drugs. Pharmacokinetic properties of a medication include the route of administration (e.g., oral, intravenous, etc.), the route of absorption and distribution (e.g., plasma, adipose tissue, etc.), the location of drug metabolism (e.g., plasma, hepatic, etc.) and the route of excretion (e.g., renal, biliary, etc.). Pharmacokinetic interactions occur when the presence of one drug in the body changes the absorption, distribution, metabolism or excretion of another drug. Many pharmacokinetic interactions involve effects on the first-pass metabolism of drugs by the enzymes within the large cytochrome P450 (CYP450) system located within the liver. While a few psychoactive medications are excreted un-metabolized (e.g., lithium), most will pass through the CYP450 system. Drugs that are broken down by a given enzyme within the CYP450 system are referred to as "substrates" of that enzyme. Drugs that increase the activity of a given CYP450 enzyme are called "inducers." These drugs will speed the breakdown of any other drug metabolized by that enzyme, and can lead to lower serum levels of that substrate. Similarly, some drugs decrease the activity of a given enzyme and are known as "inhibitors." These drugs will slow the breakdown of any other drug metabolized by that enzyme, and can lead to higher serum levels of that substrate. These interactions should be considered when prescribing psychoactive medications, and when considering whether to adjust dosages of them or of other medications. For example, both tacrolimus and cyclosporine are substrates of CYP450 3A, which is inhibited by fluoxetine. Administration of fluoxetine may therefore result in higher than expected serum levels of tacrolimus or cyclosporine, which may then require a downward dosage adjustment. A selected group of CYP450 enzymes with their substrates, inhibitors, and inducers are listed in Table 11.5. Note that, for some isoenzymes, a given drug may act as a substrate as well as an inhibitor or inducer (thereby increasing or decreasing the rate of its own metabolism).

Pharmaco*dynamics* can be thought of as the study of how the drug impacts the body. Pharmacodynamic properties of a medication may include mechanism of action, target receptor, receptor binding properties and the dose–response relationship. Pharmacodynamic, or

Table 11.5 Selected relevant CYP450 isoenzyme substrates, inhibitors and inducers.

Isoenzyme	Inhibitors	Inducers	Substrates
1A2	Cimetidine, flouroquinolones, fluvoxamine, grapefruit juice	Cigarettes, modafinil, omeprazole	Acetaminophen, fluvoxamine, haloperidol, mirtazapine, olanzapine, TCAs
2C	Fluoxetine, fluvoxamine, modafinil, omeprazole, oxcarbazepine, sertraline	Carbamazepine, prednisone	Barbituates, diazepam, NSAIDs, PPIs, THC
2D6	Bupropion, cimetidine, citalopram, duloxetine, escitalopram, fluoxetine, methadone, paroxetine, sertraline, TCAs	Dexamethasone	Aripiprazole, atomoxetine, codeine, duloxetine, haloperidol, hydroxycodeine, odansetron, risperidone, SSRIs, TCAs, tramadol, trazodone, venlafaxine
3A3, 3A4, 3A5	Antifungals, cimetidine, fluoxetine, fluvoxamine, grapefruit juice, macrolide antibiotics, voriconazole	Alprazolam, carbamazepine, modafinil, oxcarbazepine, ritonavir	Alprazolam, aripiprazole, caffeine, carbamazepine, cyclosporine, dapsone, diazepam, methadone, midazolam, prednisone, quetiapine, tacrolimus, vinblastine, zolpidem

Notes: NSAIDS = non-steroidal anti-inflammatory agents; PPI = proton pump inhibitor; SSRI = selective serotonin reuptake inhibitor; TCA = tricyclic antidepressant; THC = tetrahydrocannabinol (cannabis).
Sources: [92, 95–97].

"drug–drug," interactions occur when two medications act on the same receptors or systems within the body and cause alterations in the action of one or both drugs. These interactions can be synergistically beneficial or deleterious (and even life-threatening), and can often be predicted and, if needed, prevented with knowledge of the medications' pharmacodynamics.

One specific complication of drug–drug interactions to consider when prescribing psychotropic medications is serotonin syndrome. Serotonin syndrome results when serotonergic activity is abnormally high at both central and peripheral serotonin receptors. Serotonin syndrome is often characterized by the triad of (1) altered mental status; (2) neuromuscular abnormalities; and (3) instability of the autonomic nervous system [73]. Symptoms are variable, but, in addition to mental status changes, include hypertension, tachycardia, hyperreflexia, diaphoresis, and hyperthermia. At its most severe, serotonin syndrome can be life-threatening. Serotonin syndrome is most commonly associated with the interaction between SSRIs and the oldest class of antidepressants, monoamine oxidase inhibitors (MAOIs). MAOIs inhibit enzymatic breakdown of serotonin as well as the other monoamine neurotransmitters (including norepinephrine and dopamine). Use of the MAOI antidepressants with other serotonergic

agents is strictly contraindicated, and the recommendation is generally for a two-week "wash-out" period between the administration of an MAOI and, for example, an SSRI. Serotonin syndrome has also been reported to occur when serotonin medications are used in combination or in overdose, in both children and adults [74, 75]. Most relevant to the pediatric oncology population is the use of the 5-HT3 antagonist antiemetics (e.g., ondansetron and granisetron), as there are a few case reports of serotonin syndrome associated with the use of these 5-HT3 antagonists in combination with antidepressants or fentanyl [76]. However, serotonin syndrome in this situation is very rare and these medications are routinely and safely used in combination. Weak MAOIs pose a similar but less profound risk, and include linezolid and Procarbazine. Linezolid is an oxazolidinone antibiotic used to treat resistant gram-positive organisms, including those commonly seen in children with cancer and hospital-acquired infections (e.g., methicillin-resistant staph aureus, vancomycin-resistant enterococci). Linezolid is also a weak MAOI, and used in combination with antidepressants has been associated with over 20 case reports of serotonin syndrome in the literature [77, 78], including in children [79]. There are no prospective studies or randomized controlled studies, but more recent retrospective case series of patients have revealed low rates of serotonin syndrome in patients treated with linezolid and SSRIs. These have included rates of 3% in a study with n = 72 and 1.8% in a study with n = 53 [78, 80]. For this reason, depending on the severity of illness and with careful monitoring, it is often reasonable to continue a previously prescribed SSRI, even when linezolid therapy is started. Children should be monitored closely for signs of mental status or vital sign instability.

Adverse Effects of Psychiatric Medications

In addition to the pharmacokinetic and pharmacodynamic considerations, psychotropic medications may have adverse effects with particular relevance to pediatric oncology. These adverse effects are approached here according to organ system affected: hematologic, cardiopulmonary and neurologic.

The hematologic adverse effects of psychoactive medications are of particular relevance to the pediatric oncology population. Clinically, the SSRIs have been implicated in increased bleeding and bruising, including in children [81, 82]. Pharmacologically, the actions of the SSRIs are not specific to neurons or to the central nervous system, and they also inhibit reuptake into platelets peripherally. Placebo-controlled trials have shown paroxetine to decrease intra-platelet serotonin concentration, which leads to decrease in serotonin-mediated platelet aggregation [83]. While the SSRIs are frequently used in this group, children with platelet defects or those who are at risk for thrombocytopenia should be closely monitored. In our experience most children with von Willebrands disease can be safely treated with SSRIs; however, one should monitor for

an increase in bruising. Lithium, while less commonly prescribed to children with cancer, is important to mention because of its association with a predictable leukocytosis, which is mediated by both proliferation and demargination from bone marrow [84]. Carbemazepine, an anticonvulsant that is also used as a mood stabilizer, is associated with a transient reduction in peripheral white blood cells in 10% of patients, especially in the first weeks after initiating treatment. It is rarely associated with aplastic anemia.

A number of the psychoactive medications commonly used in medically ill children can be pro-arrhythmic through prolongation of the QTc. The antipsychotics are the psychoactive medications most commonly associated with QTc prolongation. While less commonly prescribed to children for psychiatric indications, tricyclic antidepressants are also implicated in prolonged QTc [85], and may be prescribed to children with cancer and pain syndromes. Special attention is needed for the pediatric oncology population, where other commonly used medications are similarly known to prolong the QTc, including antimicrobial agents (e.g., quinolone and macrolide antibiotics as well as azole antifungals) and methadone. For most children, these medications can be used safely, but when any of these agents are used in combination, the QTc should be monitored at baseline and after initiation of treatment. In the inpatient setting, serum electrolytes, specifically magnesium and potassium, should be closely monitored and repleted to stabilize the myocardium. Clinicians should consider dosage adjustments, alternative agents or more careful monitoring if a child's QTc increases to >450 or to >20% above their pre-treatment baseline. Common QTc prolonging agents are listed in Table 11.6.

Table 11.6 Selected commonly encountered medications with possible QTc prolongation.

Psychoactive medications	Antibiotics	Other
Haloperidol	Clarithromycin	Methadone
Olanzapine	Erythromycin	
Risperidone	Levofloxacin	
Geodon	Fluconazole	
Seroquel		
TCAs		
Sertraline		
Venlafaxine		

Note: TCA = tricyclic antidepressants.
Source: [98].

In addition to serotonin syndrome (discussed above), neurologic adverse effects of the psychoactive medications include the extra-pyramidal symptoms (EPS), a range of movement disorders that are most commonly associated with typical antipsychotics but can be caused by a range of anti-dopaminergic drugs. EPS can include akathisia (severe restlessness) or the acute dystonias. Acute dystonias are spasmodic or sustained muscle contractions that can affect a variety of parts of the body, commonly including the neck, eyes, and jaw. When they are caused by medications, dystonias most often occur within minutes of administration (though some will occur hours or even days later). Acute dystonias are not life-threatening, and will eventually resolve without treatment, but they can be extremely frightening and uncomfortable. They are effectively treated with rapid administration of anticholinergic medications, generally benztropine or diphenhydramine. Akathisia is less commonly encountered, but can also be seen after administration of antipsychotics, stimulants, and antidepressants. Akathisia is described as an inner sense of restlessness and inability to stay still; similar to the dystonias, it is not life-threatening but is extremely distressing. First-line treatment for akathisia is beta blockade, typically with propanolol.

References

1. Warrington TP, Bostwick JM. Psychiatric adverse effects of corticosteroids. *Mayo Clinic Proceedings* 2006;**81**:1361–1367.
2. Patten SB, Neutel CI. Corticosteroid-induced adverse psychiatric effects: incidence, diagnosis and management. *Drug Safety* 2000;**22**:111–122.
3. Felder-Puig R, Scherzer C, Baumgartner M, et al. Glucocorticoids in the treatment of children with acute lymphoblastic leukemia and Hodgkin's disease: a pilot study on the adverse psychological reactions and possible associations with neurobiological, endocrine, and genetic markers. *Clinical Cancer Research* 2007;**13**:7093–7100.
4. Harris JC, Carel CA, Rosenberg LA, et al. Intermittent high dose corticosteroid treatment in childhood cancer: behavioral and emotional consequences. *Journal of American Academy of Child Psychiatry* 1986;**25**:120–124.
5. Stuart FA, Segal TY, Keady S. Adverse psychological effects of corticosteroids in children and adolescents. *Archives of Disease in Childhood* 2005;**90**:500–506.
6. Kayani S, Shannon DC. Adverse behavioral effects of treatment for acute exacerbation of asthma in children: a comparison of two doses of oral steroids. *Chest* 2002;**122**:624–628.
7. Ularntinon S, Tzuang D, Dahl G, Shaw RJ. Concurrent treatment of steroid-related mood and psychotic symptoms with risperidone. *Pediatrics* 2010;**125**:e1241–1245.
8. Pelletier G, Lacroix Y, Moghrabi A, Robaey P. Double-blind crossover study of chlorpromazine and lorazepam in the treatment of behavioral problems during treatment of children with acute lymphoblastic Leukemia receiving glucocorticoids. *Medical and Pediatric Oncology* 2000;**34**:276–277.
9. Ducore JM, Waller DA, Emslie G, Bertolone SJ. Acute psychosis complicating induction therapy for acute lymphoblastic leukemia. *Journal of Pediatrics* 1983;**103**:477–480.
10. Trask PC, Esper P, Riba M, Redman B. Psychiatric side effects of interferon therapy: prevalence, proposed mechanisms, and future directions. *J Clin Oncol* 2000;**18**:2316–2326.
11. Dieperink E, Willenbring M, Ho SB. Neuropsychiatric symptoms associated with hepatitis C and interferon alpha: a review. *American Journal of Psychiatry* 2000;**157**:867–876.
12. Musselman DL, Lawson DH, Gumnick JF, et al. Paroxetine for the prevention of depression induced by high-dose interferon alfa. *New England Journal of Medicine* 2001;**344**:961–966.
13. Kraus MR, Schafer A, Faller H, et al. Paroxetine for the treatment of interferon-alpha-induced depression in chronic hepatitis C. *Alimentary Pharmacology and Therapeutics* 2002;**16**:1091–1099.
14. American Psychiatric Association. *Diagnostic and Statistical Manual of Mental Disorders DSM-IV-TR*. 4th edn. Washington, DC: American Psychiatric Association Publishing, Inc., 2000.
15. Schieveld JN. On pediatric delirium and the use of the Pediatric Confusion Assessment Method for the Intensive Care Unit. *Critical Care Medicine* 2011;**39**:220–221.
16. Silver GH, Kearney JA, Kutko MC, Bartell AS. Infant delirium in pediatric critical care settings. *American Journal of Psychiatry* 2010;**167**:1172–1177.
17. Schieveld JN, van der Valk JA, Smeets I, et al. Diagnostic considerations regarding pediatric delirium: a review and a proposal for an algorithm for pediatric intensive care units. *Intensive Care Medicine* 2009;**35**:1843–1849.
18. Leentjens AF, Schieveld JN, Leonard M, et al. A comparison of the phenomenology of pediatric, adult, and geriatric delirium. *Journal of Psychosomatic Research* 2008;**64**:219–223.
19. Turkel SB, Trzepacz PT, Tavare CJ. Comparing symptoms of delirium in adults and children. *Psychosomatics* 2006;**47**:320–324.
20. Jacobi J, Fraser GL, Coursin DB, et al. Task Force of the American College of Critical Care Medicine (ACCM) of the Society of Critical Care Medicine (SCCM), American Society of Health-System Pharmacists (ASHP), American College of Chest Physicians. Clinical practice guidelines for the sustained use of sedatives and analgesics in the critically ill adult. *Critical Care Medicine* 2002;**30**:119–141.
21. Schieveld JN, Staal M, Voogd L, Fincken J, Vos G, van Os J. Refractory agitation as a marker for pediatric delirium in very young infants at a pediatric intensive care unit. *Intensive Care Medicine* 2010;**36**:1982–1983.
22. Karnik NS, Joshi SV, Paterno C, Shaw R. Subtypes of pediatric delirium: a treatment algorithm. *Psychosomatics* 2007;**48**:253–257.
23. Pai AL, Drotar D, Zebracki K, Moore M, Youngstrom E. A meta-analysis of the effects of psychological interventions in pediatric oncology on outcomes of psychological distress and adjustment. *Journal of Pediatric Psychology* 2006;**31**:978–988.

24. Patenaude AF, Kupst MJ. Psychosocial functioning in pediatric cancer. *Journal of Pediatric Psychology* 2005;**30**:9–27.

25. Gartstein MA, Short AD, Vannatta K, Noll RB. Psychosocial adjustment of children with chronic illness: an evaluation of three models. *Journal of Developmental & Behavioral Pediatrics* 1999;**20**:157–163.

26. Lewinsohn PM, Rohde P, Seeley JR., Major depressive disorder in older adolescents: prevalence, risk factors, and clinical implications. *Clinical Psychology Review* 1998;**18**:765–794.

27. Zeltzer LK, Recklitis C, Buchbinder D, *et al.* Psychological status in childhood cancer survivors: a report from the Childhood Cancer Survivor Study. *Journal of Clinical Oncology* 2009;**10**:2396–2404.

28. Gothelf D, Rubinstein M, Shemesh E, *et al.* Pilot study: fluvoxamine treatment for depression and anxiety disorders in children and adolescents with cancer. *Journal of American Academy of Child and Adolescent Psychiatry* 2005;**44**:1258–1262.

29. Kersun LS, Elia J. Depressive symptoms and SSRI use in pediatric oncology patients. *Pediatric Blood & Cancer* 2007;**49**:881–887.

30. Kersun LS, Kazak AE. Prescribing practices of selective serotonin reuptake inhibitors (SSRIs) among pediatric oncologists: a single institution experience. *Pediatric Blood & Cancer* 2006;**47**:339–342.

31. Practice parameters for the assessment and treatment of children and adolescents with depressive, disorders., AACAP. *Journal of American Academy of Child and Adolescent Psychiatry* 1998;**37**:63S–83S.

32. March J, Silva S, Petrycki S, Curry J, Wells K, Fairbank J, *et al.* Fluoxetine, cognitive-behavioral therapy, and their combination for adolescents with depression: Treatment for Adolescents with Depression Study (TADS) randomized controlled trial. *JAMA* 2004;**292**:807–820.

33. Wilens TE, Wyatt D, Spencer TJ. Disentangling disinhibition. *Journal of American Academy of Child and Adolescent Psychiatry* 1998;**37**:1225–1227.

34. Emslie GJ, Heiligenstein JH, Hoog SL, Wagner KD, Findling RL, McCracken JT, *et al.* Fluoxetine treatment for prevention of relapse of depression in children and adolescents: a double-blind, placebo-controlled study. *Journal of American Academy of Child and Adolescent Psychiatry* 2004;**43**:1397–1405.

35. Emslie GJ, Heiligenstein JH, Wagner KD, Hoog SL, Ernest DE, Brown E, *et al.* Fluoxetine for acute treatment of depression in children and adolescents: a placebo-controlled, randomized clinical trial. *Journal of American Academy of Child and Adolescent Psychiatry* 2002;**41**:1205–1215.

36. Emslie GJ, Mayes T, Porta G, Vitiello B, Clarke G, Wagner KD, *et al.* Treatment of Resistant Depression in Adolescents (TORDIA): week 24 outcomes. *American Journal of Psychiatry* 2010;**167**:782–791.

37. Haapasalo-Pesu KM, Vuola T, Lahelma L, Marttunen M. Mirtazapine in the treatment of adolescents with major depression: an open-label, multicenter pilot study. *Journal of Child and Adolescent Psychopharmacology* 2004;**14**:175–184.

38. Conners CK, Casat CD, Gualtieri CT, Weller E, Reader M, Reiss A, *et al.* Bupropion hydrochloride in attention deficit disorder with hyperactivity. *Journal of American Academy of Child and Adolescent Psychiatry* 1996;**35**:1314–1321.

39. Daviss WB, Perel JM, Birmaher B, Rudolph GR, Melhem I, Axelson DA, *et al.* Steady-state clinical pharmacokinetics of bupropion extended-release in youths. *Journal of American Academy of Child and Adolescent Psychiatry* 2006;**45**:1503–1509.

40. Horne RL, Ferguson JM, Pope HG Jr, Hudson JI, Lineberry CG, Ascher J, *et al.* Treatment of bulimia with bupropion: a multicenter controlled trial. *Journal of Clinical Psychiatry* 1988;**49**:262–266.

41. Johnston JA, Lineberry CG, Ascher JA, Davidson J, Khayrallah MA, Feighner JP, *et al.* A 102-center prospective study of seizure in association with bupropion. *Journal of Clinical Psychiatry* 1991;**52**:450–456.

42. Emslie GJ, Findling RL, Yeung PP, Kunz NR, Li Y. Venlafaxine ER for the treatment of pediatric subjects with depression: results of two placebo-controlled trials. *Journal of American Academy of Child and Adolescent Psychiatry* 2007;**46**:479–488.

43. Hughes CW, Emslie GJ, Crismon ML, Wagner KD, Birmaher B, Geller B, *et al.* The Texas Children's Medication Algorithm Project: report of the Texas Consensus Conference Panel on Medication Treatment of Childhood Major Depressive Disorder. *Journal of American Academy of Child and Adolescent Psychiatry* 1999;**38**:1442–1454.

44. Olfson M, Shaffer D, Marcus SC, Greenberg T. Relationship between antidepressant medication treatment and suicide in adolescents. *Archives of General Psychiatry* 2003;**60**:978–982.

45. Ramsawh HJ, Chavira DA, Stein MB. Burden of anxiety disorders in pediatric medical settings: prevalence, phenomenology, and a research agenda. *Archives of Pediatric and Adolescent Medicine* 2010;**164**:965–972.

46. Costello EJ, Mustillo S, Erkanli A, Keeler G, Angold A. Prevalence and development of psychiatric disorders in childhood and adolescence. *Archives of General Psychiatry* 2003;**60**:837–844.

47. Gleason MM, Egger HL, Emslie GJ, Greenhill LL, Kowatch RA, Lieberman AF, *et al.* Psychopharmacological treatment for very young children: contexts and guidelines. *Journal of American Academy of Child and Adolescent Psychiatry* 2007;**46**:1532–1572.

48. Heden L, von Essen L, Frykholm P, Ljungman G. Low-dose oral midazolam reduces fear and distress during needle procedures in children with cancer. *Pediatric Blood & Cancer* 2009;**53**:1200–1204.

49. Liossi C, White P, Hatira P. A randomized clinical trial of a brief hypnosis intervention to control venepuncture-related pain of paediatric cancer patients. *Pain* 2009;**142**:255–263.

50. Stockhorst U, Spennes-Saleh S, Korholz D, Gobel U, Schneider ME, Steingruber HJ, *et al.* Anticipatory symptoms and anticipatory immune responses in pediatric cancer patients receiving chemotherapy: features of a classically conditioned response? *Brain, Behavior and Immunity* 2000;**14**:198–218.

51. Rosen GM, Shor AC, Geller TJ. Sleep in children with cancer. *Current Opinion in Pediatrics* 2008;**20**:676–681.

52. Owens JA. Pharmacotherapy of pediatric insomnia. *Journal of American Academy of Child and Adolescent Psychiatry* 2009;**48**:99–107.

53. Weiss SK, Garbutt A. Pharmacotherapy in pediatric sleep disorders. *Adolescent Medicine: State of the Art Reviews* 2010;**21**:508–521.

54. van Geijlswijk IM, van der Heijden KB, Egberts AC, Korzilius HP, Smits MG. Dose finding of melatonin for chronic idiopathic childhood sleep onset insomnia: an RCT. *Psychopharmacology* (Berl) 2010;**212**:379–391.

55. Smits MG, Nagtegaal EE, van der Heijden J, Coenen AM, Kerkhof GA. Melatonin for chronic sleep onset insomnia in children: a randomized placebo-controlled trial. *Journal of Child Neurology* 2001;**16**:86–92.

56. Armour A, Gottschlich MM, Khoury J, Warden GD, Kagan RJ. A randomized, controlled prospective trial of zolpidem and haloperidol for use as sleeping agents in pediatric burn patients. *Journal of Burn Care Research* 2008;**29**:238–247.

57. Blumer JL, Findling RL, Shih WJ, Soubrane C, Reed MD. Controlled clinical trial of zolpidem for the treatment of insomnia associated with attention-deficit/hyperactivity disorder in children 6 to 17 years of age. *Pediatrics* 2009;**123**:e770–6.

58. Kazak AE, Barakat LP, Meeske K, Christakis D, Meadows AT, Casey R, et al. Posttraumatic stress, family functioning, and social support in survivors of childhood leukemia and their mothers and fathers. *Journal of Consulting and Clinical Psychology* 1997;**65**:120–129.

59. Stuber ML, Kazak AE, Meeske K, Barakat L, Guthrie D, Garnier H, et al. Predictors of posttraumatic stress symptoms in childhood cancer survivors. *Pediatrics* 1997;**100**:958–964.

60. Davidson JR, Rothbaum BO, van der Kolk BA, Sikes CR, Farfel GM. Multicenter, double-blind comparison of sertraline and placebo in the treatment of posttraumatic stress disorder. *Archives of General Psychiatry* 2001;**58**:485–492.

61. Strawn JR, Keeshin BR, DelBello MP, Geracioti TD, Jr, Putnam FW. Psychopharmacologic treatment of posttraumatic stress disorder in children and adolescents: a review. *Journal of Clinical Psychiatry* 2010;**71**:932–941.

62. Ellenberg L, Liu Q, Gioia G, Yasui Y, Packer RJ, Mertens A, et al. Neurocognitive status in long-term survivors of childhood CNS malignancies: a report from the Childhood Cancer Survivor Study. *Neuropsychology* 2009;**23**:705–717.

63. Mulhern RK, Merchant TE, Gajjar A, Reddick WE, Kun LE. Late neurocognitive sequelae in survivors of brain Tumors in childhood. *Lancet Oncology* 2004;**5**:399–408.

64. Buizer AI, de Sonneville LM, van den Heuvel-Eibrink MM, Veerman AJ. Behavioral and educational limitations after chemotherapy for childhood acute lymphoblastic leukemia or Wilms tumor. *Cancer* 2006;**106**:2067–2075.

65. Butler RW, Hill JM, Steinherz PG, Meyers PA, Finlay JL. Neuropsychologic effects of cranial irradiation, intrathecal methotrexate, and systemic methotrexate in childhood cancer. *Journal of Clinical Oncology* 1994;**12**:2621–2629.

66. Buizer AI, de Sonneville LM, Veerman AJ. Effects of chemotherapy on neurocognitive function in children with acute lymphoblastic leukemia: a critical review of the literature. *Pediatric Blood & Cancer* 2009;**52**:447–454.

67. Conklin HM, Helton S, Ashford J, et al. Predicting methylphenidate response in long-term survivors of childhood cancer: a randomized, double-blind, placebo-controlled, crossover trial. *Journal of Pediatric Psychol* 2010;**35**:144–155.

68. Conklin HM, Reddick WE, Ashford J, et al. Long-term efficacy of methylphenidate in enhancing attention regulation, social skills, and academic abilities of childhood cancer survivors. *Journal of Clinical Oncology* 2010;**28**:4465–4472.

69. Winterstein AG, Gerhard T, Shuster J, et al. Cardiac safety of central nervous system stimulants in children and adolescents with attention-deficit/hyperactivity disorder. *Pediatrics* 2007;**120**:e1494–501.

70. Knight M. Stimulant-drug therapy for attention-deficit disorder (with or without hyperactivity) and sudden cardiac death. *Pediatrics* 2007;**119**:154–155.

71. American Academy of Pediatrics., Subcommittee on Attention-Deficit/Hyperactivity Disorder and Committee on Quality, Improvement. Clinical practice guideline: treatment of the school-aged child with attention-deficit/hyperactivity disorder. *Pediatrics* 2001;**108**: 1033–1044.

72. Dulcan MK, Benson RS. AACAP Official Action. Summary of the practice parameters for the assessment and treatment of children, adolescents, and adults with ADHD. *Journal of American Academy of Child and Adolescent Psychiatry* 1997;**36**:1311–1317.

73. Boyer EW, Shannon M. The serotonin syndrome. [Review] [Erratum appears in *N Engl J Med* 2007 Jun 7;356(23):2437]. *New England Journal of Medicine* 2005;**352**:1112–1120.

74. Soldin OP, Tonning JM, Obstetric-Fetal Pharmacology Research Unit N. Serotonin syndrome associated with triptan monotherapy. *New England Journal of Medicine* 2008;**358**:2185–2186.

75. Phan H, Casavant MJ, Crockett S, et al. Serotonin syndrome following a single 50 mg dose of sertraline in a child. *Clinical Toxicology* (Phila) 2008;**46**:845–849.

76. Turkel SB, Nadala JG, Wincor MZ. Possible serotonin syndrome in association with 5-HT(3) antagonist agents. *Psychosomatics* 2001;**42**:258–260.

77. Quinn DK, Stern TA. Linezolid and serotonin syndrome. *Primary Care Companion Journal of Clinical Psychiatry* 2009;**11**:353–356.

78. Lorenz RA, Vandenberg AM, Canepa EA. Serotonergic antidepressants and linezolid: a retrospective chart review and presentation of cases. *International Journal of Psychiatry and Medicine* 2008;**38**:81–90.

79. Thomas CR, Rosenberg M, Blythe V, Meyer WJ, 3rd. Serotonin syndrome and linezolid. *Journal of American Academy of Child and Adolescent Psychiatry* 2004;**43**:790.

80. Taylor JJ, Wilson JW, Estes LL. Linezolid and serotonergic drug interactions: a retrospective survey. *Clinical Infectious Diseases* 2006;**43**:180–187.

81. Skop BP, Brown TM. Potential vascular and bleeding complications of treatment with selective serotonin reuptake inhibitors. *Psychosomatics* 1996;**37**:12–16.

82. Lake MB, Birmaher B, Wassick S, Mathos K, Yelovich AK. Bleeding and selective serotonin reuptake inhibitors in childhood and adolescence. *Journal of Child and Adolescent Psychopharmacology* 2000;**10**:35–38.

83. Hergovich N, Aigner M, Eichler HG, et al. Paroxetine decreases platelet serotonin storage and platelet function in human beings. *Clinical Pharmacology & Therapeutics* 2000;**68**:435–442.

84. Oyesanmi O, Kunkel EJ, Monti DA, Field HL. Hematologic side effects of psychotropics. *Psychosomatics* 1999;**40**:414–421.

85. van Noord C, Straus SM, Sturkenboom MC, *et al.* Psychotropic drugs associated with corrected QT interval prolongation. *Journal of Clinical Psychopharmacol* 2009;**29**:9–15.

86. Denicoff KD, Rubinow DR, Papa MZ, *et al.* The neuropsychiatric effects of treatment with interleukin-2 and lymphokine-activated killer cells. *Annals of International Medicine* 1987;**107**:293–300.

87. Walker RW, Allen JC, Rosen G, Caparros B. Transient cerebral dysfunction secondary to high-dose methotrexate. *Journal of Clinical Oncology* 1986;**4**:1845–1850.

88. Lazarus HM, Herzig RH, Herzig GP, *et al.* Central nervous system toxicity of high-dose systemic cytosine arabinoside. *Cancer* 198;**48**:2577–2582.

89. Holland J, Fasanello S, Onuma T. Psychiatric symptoms associated with L-asparaginase administration. *Journal of Psychiatric Research* 1974;**10**:105–113.

90. Hiemke C, Hartter S. Pharmacokinetics of selective serotonin reuptake inhibitors. *Pharmacology & Therapeutics* 2000;**85**:11–28.

91. Smiga SM, Elliott GR. Psychopharmacology of depression in children and adolescents. *Pediatric Clinics of North America* 2011;**58**:155–171.

92. Stern TA, Fricchione GL, Cassem NH, Jellinek MS, Rosenbaum JF. *Massachusetts General Hospital: Handbook of General Hospital Psychiatry.* 6th ed. Philadelphia, PA: Saunders, 2010.

93. Devlin JW, Roberts RJ. Pharmacology of commonly used analgesics and sedatives in the ICU: benzodiazepines, propofol, and opioids. *Critical Care Clinics* 2009;**25**:431–449.

94. Pelayo R, Chen W, Monzon S, Guilleminault C. Pediatric sleep pharmacology: you want to give my kid sleeping pills? *Pediatric Clinics of North America* 2004;**51**:117–134.

95. Lynch T, Price A. The effect of cytochrome P450 metabolism on drug response, interactions, and adverse effects. *American Family Physician* 2007;**76**:391–396.

96. Michalets EL. Update: clinically significant cytochrome P-450 drug interactions. *Pharmacotherapy* 1998;**18**: 84–112.

97. Nemeroff CB, DeVane CL, Pollock BG. Newer antidepressants and the cytochrome P450 system. *American Journal of Psychiatry* 1996;**153**:311–320.

98. Al-Khatib SM, LaPointe NM, Kramer JM, Califf RM. What clinicians should know about the QT interval. *JAMA* 2003;**289**:2120–2127.

12

Complementary and Alternative Medicine Use in Children with Cancer

Subhadra Evans, Laura Cousins, Lonnie Zeltzer

Introduction

Population studies in the United States and abroad have shown that the use of complementary and alternative medicine (CAM) is common among adults and children for cancer prevention, slowing of cancer progression, and the palliation of symptoms and side effects of cancer treatment. The aim of the current chapter is to inform health care professionals about the use of CAM for pediatric cancer by, firstly, defining CAM; secondly, reviewing the literature on the prevalence of CAM use for pediatric cancer; thirdly, compiling reports of clinical trials of CAM modalities for pediatric cancer; and lastly, describing the clinical use of hypnosis as one example of how a CAM modality can be used in pediatric oncology.

What Is CAM?

CAM is described by the National Center for Complementary and Alternative Medicine (NCCAM) at the US Department of National Institutes of Health as "a group of diverse medical and health care systems, practices, and products that are not presently considered to be part of conventional medicine" [1]. "Conventional medicine" in this context is defined as "medicine as practiced by holders of M.D. (medical doctor) and D.O. (doctor of osteopathy) degrees and by allied health professionals, such as physical therapists, psychologists, and registered nurses." What is considered to be CAM often changes as therapies that are proven to be safe and effective become integrated into conventional health care.

NCCAM groups CAM therapies into four broad domains. The first is "Natural Products," which includes use of substances found in nature, such as herbal medicines that employ plant preparations for therapeutic effects, vitamins, minerals, other dietary supplements, and foods and special dietary modifications (including probiotics).

The second domain is "Mind–Body Medicine," which consists of a variety of techniques designed to enhance the mind's capacity to affect bodily function and symptoms. Examples include meditation, yoga, acupuncture, deep-breathing exercises, progressive relaxation, guided imagery, qi gong, tai chi, and hypnotherapy. Acupuncture illustrates the way in which the field of CAM changes over time. Whereas acupuncture was once considered unorthodox in Western medicine, scientific evidence has accumulated to support its safety and effectiveness, and it has been assimilated broadly into Western medical practice for specific indications such as managing chronic pain and nausea associated with chemotherapy.

The third domain comprises "Manipulative and Body-Based Practices," including spinal manipulation performed by chiropractors, physical therapists, and osteopaths and massage therapy. These therapies target body structures and systems.

The final domain "Other CAM Practices," include "Movement Therapies," "Traditional Healers," "Energy Therapies," and "Whole Medical Systems." "Movement Therapies" promote physical, mental, emotional, and spiritual well-being using Eastern and Western practices such as Feldenkrais method, the Alexander technique and Pilates. "Energy Therapies" include Reiki and other as yet unproven therapies that intend to manipulate energy biofields within and around the human body; and electromagnetic-based therapies involving the unconventional use of

Pediatric Psycho-oncology: Psychosocial Aspects and Clinical Interventions, Second Edition.
Edited by Shulamith Kreitler, Myriam Weyl Ben-Arush and Andrés Martin.
© 2012 John Wiley & Sons, Ltd. Published 2012 by John Wiley & Sons, Ltd.

electromagnetic fields, such as magnet therapy and light therapy. "Whole Medical Systems" are built upon complete systems of theory and practice and include homeopathic medicine, naturopathic medicine, Ayurveda, and traditional Chinese medicine.

Pediatric CAM Use

According to the 2007 National Health Interview Survey (NHIS) collected by the Centers for Disease Control and Prevention's National Center for Health Statistics in the United States, one in nine children (11.8%) had used CAM therapy in the past year [2]. Children were most likely to have used biologically based therapies (4.7%) and mind–body therapies (4.3%). Children with a parent who used CAM were almost five times as likely (23.9%) to use CAM compared to those whose parent did not (5.1%). Children were also more likely to use CAM when their parent expressed concern about the cost of conventional care. CAM use positively correlated with the number of health conditions and doctor visits children reported over the past 12 months. Sociodemographic factors associated with CAM use among children include being an adolescent, non-Hispanic white, having a college-educated parent, and living in households earning more than $65,000 annually. CAM use was greater in those with private insurance, living in the West, Northeast, or Midwest, reporting difficulty with access to medical care, and missing more school days due to illness. Higher CAM use was also found in prescription medication users, those who have anxiety or stress, and individuals with dermatologic conditions, musculoskeletal conditions, and sinusitis [2].

CAM Use for Pediatric Cancer

In the United States, between 46–85% of children with cancer use CAM therapies. Such therapies are typically used to mitigate symptoms, enhance coping skills, and improve well-being [3]. In most cases, CAM has been used to complement rather than replace traditional treatment. Controversial exceptions do exist wherein parents discontinue their child's conventional treatment in favor of unproven alternative therapies [4].

Bishop *et al.* [5] conducted a systematic review to summarize the prevalence of CAM use in the pediatric cancer population. Twenty-eight studies using survey data between 1975 and 2005 from 3,526 children were assessed. In 20 studies, the prevalence of CAM use since cancer diagnosis ranged from 6–91%. The most popular form of CAM was herbal remedies followed by diet modifications, nutrition-related therapies, and

faith-healing. Patients used CAM therapies to help cure or fight their cancer, alleviate symptoms, and support ongoing conventional treatment.

Post-White *et al.* [6] compared the frequency and factors affecting CAM use between general and specialty pediatrics in Minnesota. As indicated from 281 surveys completed by parents, pediatric oncology patients used the greatest number of CAM therapies with prayer being the most commonly reported CAM therapy used (60.5%) followed by massage. These patients used CAM therapies to manage side effects, particularly from chemotherapy treatment, cope with the emotional impact of their illness, and enhance hopefulness. This study confirmed that children with chronic or life-threatening illnesses use more CAM therapies than children seen in primary care clinics.

Despite inconclusive evidence as to their safety or efficacy, many pediatric cancer patients use nutrition-related therapies. According to surveys completed in the United States, 35–50% of children with cancer use dietary supplements. Of note, many patients fail to discuss this use with their health care providers. Preliminary studies reveal that antioxidant supplements may enhance chemotherapy tolerance and an array of other supplements may reduce GI toxicities from chemotherapy and radiation. Further research is needed to provide more definitive evidence regarding the safety and efficacy of nutrition-related therapies as well as potential interactions with chemotherapy and radiation treatments [7].

An anonymous cross-sectional survey administered to 274 parents of children treated at a combined Nemours oncology practice in Florida and Delaware for leukemia, lymphomas, brain tumors or solid tumors found that parental intensity of CAM use and geographic region were significantly associated with CAM use in children. These surveys revealed that prevalence of CAM use was 24.5% among children (mean age of 9.9 years; 50.8% male), with mind–body interventions the most frequently used. Regionally, children in Florida were more likely to use CAM compared to those in Delaware [8].

Tomlinson *et al.* [9] examined the frequency, types, and determinants of CAM use among children in the palliative phase of cancer. Twenty-two children (29%) had received some type of CAM therapy and 42 parents (55%) considered using CAM for their child. Whole medical systems were the most frequently used CAM, while whole medical systems and biologically based therapies were the most frequently considered types of CAM. Family and disease variables were not highly correlated with CAM use, however, parents with higher education levels and those with a family member with cancer were more likely to consider CAM. Future studies should attempt to discern why a gap exists between CAM consideration and CAM use in the palliative stage of the disease.

CAM treatment for pediatric oncology patients is also popular outside the United States. Forms of CAM therapies used differ globally due to cultural habits, religious beliefs, and availability [10]. In Lebanon, a cross-sectional study by Naja *et al.* [11] examined the frequency, types, and modes of CAM use among pediatric leukemia patients. Out of the 125 caregivers surveyed, 15.2% indicated using at least one CAM therapy for their child. The most prevalent CAM therapies included dietary supplements, prayer/spiritual healing, and unconventional cultural practices (i.e. ingesting bone ashes).

Homeopathy appears to be a popular treatment across parts of Europe. Längler *et al.* [12] compared the responses of homeopathy users to users of other CAM therapies within Germany's pediatric oncology population. From a total of 1063 families who completed the survey, 367 reported using CAM at some point during their child's illness. Approximately 45% of the 367 CAM users surveyed tried homeopathy. Homeopathy remains the most frequently used CAM treatment for pediatric oncology in Germany with high patient satisfaction. A study on the prevalence and reasons for CAM use in an Italian pediatric oncology unit also revealed interest in homeopathy [13]. Twelve parents (12.4%) reported using at least one type of CAM therapy for their child with homeopathy being the most frequently used. Half of the parents surveyed did not discuss their child's CAM use with a health care provider. Although this study was the first to assess the prevalence of CAM use among children suffering from neoplastic disease in Italy, the small, ethnically homogenous, and widely-aged sample size and incomplete questionnaire items limit findings.

Genc *et al.* [14] examined types of CAM therapies used and sociodemographic and medical variables associated with CAM use, among pediatric cancer patients at a large hospital in western Turkey. Parents of 112 pediatric cancer patients (aged 1–18 years) who had been diagnosed with cancer within the past 5 years completed a 22-item questionnaire. Eighty-six of the 112 patients (77%) used at least one CAM therapy with herbs being the most common type of CAM therapy used, particularly nettle and *Salvia officinalis*. Parents expected CAM therapies to enhance their child's immune functioning, purify blood, and cure the illness. Only 29 (26%) parents discussed CAM use with their oncologists. No statistically significant differences emerged between CAM use and sociodemographic and medical variables. This study

indicates that CAM is widely used among pediatric cancer patients in western Turkey.

At a pediatric oncology center in Kuala Lumpur, Malaysia, interviews from 97 parents of children with cancer, aged 0–18 years, were analyzed to investigate the prevalence and types of CAM use [10]. The majority of patients (53%) had acute lymphoblastic leukemia and received chemotherapy treatment or a combination of chemotherapy, radiotherapy, and surgery. Eighty-two children (84.5%) used at least one type of CAM therapy and 62% used more than one CAM therapy. Overall, water therapy, where patients consumed spring water, was the most commonly reported CAM therapy (78% of patients) followed by the nutritional supplement, Spirulina (33% of patients). Other CAM treatments used included vitamin C, multivitamins, traditional healers, sea cucumber, and Chinese traditional medicine. Ultimately, CAM use is common among Malaysian children with cancer and is viewed as a complementary form of treatment that enhances immune functioning.

A common theme across these studies is that many pediatric oncology patients and their families do not disclose CAM use to health care providers. On the flip side, only half of general pediatricians report discussing CAM with their patients. Roth *et al.* [15] examined barriers to CAM communication among pediatric oncologists. Almost all responded that it is important to know what CAM therapies patients are using, but less than half routinely ask their patients about CAM due to time constraints and lack of knowledge. The majority of physicians reported a belief that massage therapy and yoga may improve patient quality of life, while dietary supplements, herbal medicine, dietary modifications, vitamins, and chiropractic therapies might be harmful for patients.

CAM for Pediatric Cancer: The Evidence

Reports of clinical trials of CAM therapies in relation to pediatric oncology were sought in the PUBMED and the CINAHL electronic databases. CAM search terms were gleaned from prevalence studies and paired with "child," "pediatric," and "cancer." Results will be presented using the organizing framework provided by the four domains of CAM delineated by NCCAM. Reports still remain nonexistent for some categories.

Natural Products

The search terms "cartilage," "diet," "herbal," "Laetrile," "megavitamin," "melatonin," "mistletoe," "phytotreatment," and "vitamin" did not lead to records of clinical trials of biologically based therapies in pediatric oncology samples. The search term "plant" led to two clinical trials: one for milk thistle and another for ginger powder.

Since ginger serves as an anti-emetic supplement for women during pregnancy and has been shown to significantly reduce nausea in adults during the first day of chemotherapy, Pillai *et al.* [16] evaluated the efficacy of ginger powder in lowering chemotherapy-induced nausea and vomiting among children and young adults. Sixty patients (aged 9–21 years) undergoing chemotherapy for newly diagnosed bone sarcomas enrolled in the double-blind study. Patients were either randomly assigned to a group that received ginger root powder capsules in addition to standard treatment or a group that received placebo capsules made of starch powder in addition to standard treatment during the first three days of their chemotherapy cycle. Capsule dosage differed according to participant weight. Patients/guardians completed a diary about the child's nausea and vomiting. Analyses indicated that ginger root powder was effective in decreasing the severity of acute and delayed chemotherapy-induced nausea and vomiting in patients receiving high emetogenic chemotherapy.

Ladas *et al.* [17] designed a randomized, controlled, double-blind, multi-center pilot study to evaluate the safety and feasibility of milk thistle in the treatment of hepatotoxicity in children (aged 1–19 years) with acute lymphoblastic leukemia during maintenance-phase chemotherapy. Fifty patients completed the study, with 23 randomly assigned to receive milk thistle for 28 days and 26 patients randomly assigned to receive a placebo for the same length of time. The first dose began one day after administration of the intravenous chemotherapy. Patient adherence was monitored through weekly phone interviews and requesting that patients return medication containers (medication completion was operationally defined as finishing at least 80% of the assigned drug or placebo). Hepatic toxicity was measured at days 0, 28, and 56. Patients receiving milk thistle showed a trend toward significant reductions in liver toxicity by Day 56 and did not experience any antagonizing effects with their chemotherapy treatment. No significant differences in frequency of side effects, toxicity incidence/severity, or infections emerged between both groups. The small sample size ultimately produced insufficient power to detect any treatment effects and the lower compliance rate within the intervention group also impacted outcomes.

Mind–Body Interventions

Several clinical trials for symptom control in pediatric samples were located with the search terms "imagery,"

"hypnosis," and "acupuncture," and one clinical trial was found when using the search terms "yoga," "prayer," and "religion." No clinical trials were located with the search terms "faith," "meditation," or "spirituality."

Using a mixed-methods, within-subject, repeated measures design, Thygeson *et al.* [18] examined the feasibility of a single yoga session for children and adolescents hospitalized with cancer or other blood disorders and their parents to determine whether patients and parents report significant reductions in anxiety from baseline to completion of yoga. Fifteen 6–18-year-old children and their parents completed the study and were recruited from two inpatient hematology/oncology units. Participants completed the child or adult version of the Spielberger State Trait Anxiety Inventory before and after the 45-minute yoga session and responded to an open-ended survey administered after the yoga class. The yoga session was held in the inpatient unit playroom and included meditation and yoga poses. Although younger children's pre to post anxiety scores did not significantly differ, adolescent and parent anxiety scores significantly decreased after the yoga session. Qualitative data revealed that all participants provided positive feedback. Children indicated that the yoga session was "fun," "relaxing," and helped them feel calm. Adolescents had similar responses and added that the yoga served as a self-care strategy. Parents commented on the benefits of exercise and movement and found the yoga relaxing, calming, a useful self-care strategy for stress relief and an ideal opportunity to bond with their child. These preliminary results indicate that yoga is a feasible intervention for a hematology/oncology population. Despite these encouraging results, larger sample sizes and a controlled multi-session intervention are required to test the efficacy of yoga for hematology/oncology patients.

A recent study investigated acupuncture's efficacy as a supportive antiemetic approach in minimizing the need for antiemetic rescue medication during chemotherapy [19]. Twenty-three children (mean age of 13.6 years) undergoing highly emetogenic chemotherapy for solid malignant tumors in Germany were randomized into one of two groups. The first group (12 patients) received acupuncture in addition to antiemetic medications during their second chemotherapy course and only antiemetic medications in their third chemotherapy course, while the second group (11 patients) received treatments in the opposite order. The primary outcome measure—the amount of additional antiemetic medication used during chemotherapy—was significantly lower in the acupuncture group. Episodes of vomiting were also significantly lower after acupuncture. In addition to the high patient acceptance of acupuncture, no side effects or adverse events were reported except 4 out of 23 patients were affected by pain from needling. Given that nausea and vomiting are common chemotherapy-induced side effects and antiemetic medications only alleviate symptoms in a limited number of patients, results from this pilot trial are promising.

An earlier study provides support for the use of hypnosis. Liossi, White, and Hatira [20] conducted a randomized clinical trial to compare the efficacy of local anesthetic to a combination of local anesthetic and hypnosis in the minimization of lumbar puncture-induced pain and anxiety among pediatric cancer patients. This trial additionally assessed whether patients can use hypnosis independently and if level of hypnotizability enhanced the therapy's benefits. Forty-five children (23 boys and 22 girls aged 6–16 years) undergoing lumbar puncture with leukemia or non-Hodgkin's lymphoma participated. Patients were randomized to a group that received a local anesthetic, a local anesthetic combined with hypnosis, or a local anesthetic and attention. The local anesthetic cream was applied to skin approximately 60 minutes prior to the procedure. Baseline measures of pain, anticipatory anxiety, and pain-related anxiety were collected after patients experienced five or six lumbar punctures using the Wong-Baker FACES Pain Rating Scale and the Procedure Behavior Checklist. During a hypnosis session, patients completed a measure of hypnotizability, the Stanford Hypnotic Clinical Scale for Children. Patients in the local anesthesia and hypnosis group reported the least anticipatory anxiety, procedure-related pain and anxiety and displayed the least distress. Level of hypnotizability positively correlated with the extent of treatment benefit and such benefit persisted when patients used hypnosis independently.

Manipulative and Body-Based Practices

Searching the terms "chiropractic," "osteopath," "manipulation," and "massage" led to several clinical trials of massage therapy. Phipps et al. [21] compared the efficacy of a child-targeted health promotion intervention or combined parent- and child-targeted health promotion to standard care in improving well-being and affecting short-term medical outcomes during the acute phase of bone marrow transplantation. One hundred and seventy-one families with children from 6–18 years of age undergoing transplant were recruited from four pediatric transplant centers. Families were randomized to the child-targeted health promotion intervention group, combined parent- and child-targeted

health promotion intervention group, or a standard care group, stratified by site, patient age, and type of transplant. The child intervention consisted of massage and humor therapy, while the parent intervention included massage and relaxation/imagery. Primary outcomes included parent and child responses to the Behavioral, Affective, and Somatic Experiences Scales, collected each week from admission for transplant until six weeks post-transplant. Secondary outcome measures included short-term medical variables such as the number of days spent in the hospital, time to engraftment, medication use (narcotic, analgesic, antiemetic, etc.), and specific toxicities. No significant differences between treatment groups were found on primary or secondary outcomes. The low levels of distress in the patient sample overall, and the diverse combination of therapies may have contributed to the null findings.

Post-White et al. [22] designed a pilot study to assess whether four weekly massage sessions as compared to four quiet-time control conditions lowered anxiety, cortisol levels, fatigue, nausea, and pain in children undergoing chemotherapy for their cancer. This pilot study also examined whether massage reduced anxiety, fatigue, and mood disturbance among patients' parents. In this crossover design, children and their parent were first randomized to a massage therapy or quiet-time group and then to the other condition at the same time point in the subsequent chemotherapy cycle. Follow-up assessments were administered during each condition and a final follow-up two to four weeks after the final session consisted of an audiotape-recorded structured interview with each parent and child. During each session, children's pre- and post-heart rate, respiratory rate, blood pressure, and self-report of pain, nausea, and anxiety were measured. Parents responded to questionnaires assessing anxiety, fatigue, and mood. Twenty-five children completed the study, with 12 children randomized to the massage therapy condition first and 13 children randomized to the quiet-time condition first. Diagnoses included acute lymphoblastic leukemia, brain tumors, lymphoma, rhabdomyosarcoma, Wilms' tumor, and Ewing sarcoma. Although no significant differences in blood pressure, cortisol, pain, nausea, or fatigue emerged, massage therapy lowered heart rate in children, anxiety in children younger than 14, and parent anxiety. Children reported that the massage sessions reduced their anxiety and worries, and had longer-lasting effects compared to the quiet-time condition. The findings remain limited by the small sample size, but indicate preliminary support for the use of massage to treat pediatric therapy-related anxiety.

Movement Therapies

No clinical trials for the pediatric population were located using the search terms "movement," "Feldenkrais method," "Alexander technique," "Pilates," "Rolfing," and "Trager."

Traditional Healers

The term "healer" did not lead to records of clinical trials using traditional healers for pediatric cancer.

Energy Therapies

Searching the terms "energy," "healing," "magnetic," and "Reiki" led to no clinical trials of energy therapies in pediatric oncology samples.

Whole Medical Systems

The search terms "Ayurvedic," "homeopath," and "naturopath" did not produce any records of clinical trials using Whole Medical Systems in pediatric oncology samples.

Summary

Evaluating the effectiveness of CAM for the pediatric cancer population remains difficult given the sparse state of the current empirical literature. The greatest limitation derives from the lack of randomized controlled trials testing the safety and efficacy of most CAM treatments. Even therapies that have been systematically examined are often limited by small sample sizes and unreplicated findings. For studies assessing natural products, difficulties also lie in extrapolating dosage and toxicity data from adult studies. Age differences may moderate responses to CAM therapies. For example, children may experience more anxiety when interacting with a CAM practitioner, while adolescents exhibit unique preferences and coping styles that affect participation. Consent rates (~30–50%) and attrition rates (~20–30%) pose another challenge when enrolling patients in CAM interventions. It remains imperative to design interventions for children and their families at convenient time points, as families may experience heightened stress when enrolled in a study and still taking their child to medical appointments. Future research is also needed to examine the efficacy of CAM on physiological and immune outcomes related to stress and the minimization or prevention of late effects from treatment in pediatric cancer survivors. Overall, individualizing CAM interventions to children's developmental stages, family dynamics, and coping styles may prove more effective [3].

Clinical Application: Hypnotherapy as an Example

Hypnotherapy is often used as a mind–body therapy embedded within a psychological framework. The goals of any psychological intervention for children with pain are fourfold: (1) instill a new paradigm regarding reasons for the pain; (2) reduce focus on self; (3) enhance perceptions of controllability of the pain; and (4) facilitate increased functionality. Before beginning to use hypnotherapy, it is helpful to reframe the pain in terms of pain mechanisms. A simple age-appropriate overview of pain transmission and inhibition, including the impact of emotions and beliefs on this neural system, can be readily accomplished, sometimes with the aid of a schematic diagram (e.g., the affected body part, connections to spinal cord, and brain). This neural definition can then be applied to the child's particular pain problem. The goal of hypnotherapy then, as explained to the child, is to use certain parts of his/her brain to increase the effectiveness of his/her own natural pain control system. In this way, both the child and parents can understand the potential impact of hypnotherapeutic intervention on circuitry in the brain that relates to pain perception.

Hypnotherapy is a psychological intervention that helps the child to have a narrowed and channeled focus of attention, so that the child can be open to possibilities of altered sensations, emotions, and beliefs. Muscle relaxation is often an accompaniment of a hypnotic state but is not necessary for hypnotherapy to occur. The primary focused goals of hypnotherapy are: (1) to capture attention; (2) to reduce distress; (3) to reframe the pain experience; and (4) to help the child to dissociate from the pain. This process typically involves three stages: (1) "induction" (help the child to dissociate from the environment); (2) "deepening" (enhance the dissociation); and (3) suggesting that the child find a "favorite place" (that is safe, fun, interesting, and in which the child feels in control). Images can be suggested to enhance imaginative involvement and the child can be asked to notice the sights, smells, texture of clothes, sounds, etc. around him/her. Helping the child to use his/her sensory system often helps to enhance involvement of the child in his/her favorite place.

For acute pain experiences such as medical procedures, exciting and challenging events can happen within this imaginative involvement. For example, a child might see himself or herself playing basketball and making the winning basket for the team and "saving the team," or the child might be playing soccer and noticing the goal ahead and the ball in front of his/her feet, while the rest of the team is right behind him/her. Sometimes the use of focal hypnoanesthesia can be helpful to reduce pain during a medical procedure. For example, a "magic glove" can be "placed" on a hand that is to have an intravenous line placed. Recall of past anesthetic experiences (e.g., a foot or hand numbed when placed in snow) can also be used.

For children with chronic pain, a "central sensory control station" can be suggested as being located in the part of the brain that "thinks with pictures." This can be described as the center for control of sensory signals coming from the body. Various suggestions for what this might "look like" can be provided (e.g., colored lights, knobs, and switches, such as what a pilot might see in a plane cockpit). The child can be asked to signal with a finger when he/she "finds" the central control station, and to signal again when he/she finds the "switch or lever" that controls the feelings coming from the affected body part (e.g., foot, stomach). At that point, it can be suggested that the switch is like a rheostat (dimmer switch) rather than an on/off switch and that the child can slowly turn the switch until he/she has "just as much feeling (in that body part) as he/she wants to have." It might be suggested that if he/she turned the switch "all the way off," that body part might become numb, and so he/she should turn it "just enough." It can also be suggested that, as these changes begin to take place, as evidence of a change in the whole system, the child might notice new sensations, such as tingling, in his/her hands or feet (children typically will notice this before they notice decreased sensation in the part that hurts). It can be suggested that the brain is now beginning to learn what "it" needs to do to quiet the pain signals to help that part of the body feel better. Analogies can be given, such as learning to ride a bicycle. "In the beginning, it took work and concentration. But, after a while, the brain learned what it needed to do and then you could ride without thinking about it." Post-hypnotic suggestions could then be provided for the beginning of change and ease of entering this special state of mind whenever the child needed to, or perhaps at bedtime.

Ultimately, hypnotherapy can be an effective tool for changing the mind/body dualism to a new paradigm in which all systems are connected. This treatment can facilitate feelings of control and the belief that physical changes are possible. This paradigm shift heralds the beginning of reduction of pain and enhancement of functioning. Hypnotherapy can play a major role metaphorically in increasing feelings of control, competence, and hope.

Conclusion

Popular interest in and use of complementary and alternative therapies clearly have outpaced scientific evaluation of these modalities. At present, significant gaps in the available scientific knowledge base limit the ability of health professionals to guide parents and pediatric patients with regard to complementary and alternative approaches to treatment of cancer or the side effects of cancer treatment. Most CAM approaches, especially in pediatric samples, remain relatively or completely unstudied from the standpoint of controlled clinical trials research. Increased resources are currently being allotted to their evaluation in adult samples at the local, national, and international levels, and several clinical trials are currently underway. The popularity of CAM interventions for children with cancer renders the scientific evaluation of their safety, efficacy, and effectiveness for children key research objectives.

Acknowledgments

This study was supported in part by NCCAM grant K01AT005093 (PI: S Evans).

References

1. National Center for Complementary and Alternative Medicine *What is Complementary and Alternative Medicine*? 2010 http://nccam.nih.gov/health/whatiscam/ (accessed March 8 2011).
2. Barnes PM, Bloom B, Nahin RL. Complementary and alternative medicine use among adults and children: United States, 2007. *National Health Statistics Reports* **12**:1–23.
3. Post-White J. Complementary and alternative medicine in pediatric oncology. *Journal of Pediatric Oncology Nursing* 2006;**23**:244.
4. Burgio GR, Locatelli F. Alternative therapies and the Di Bella affair in pediatrics. a questionnaire submitted to Italian pediatric oncologists and hematologists. *Haematologica* 2000;**85**:189–194.
5. Bishop FL, Prescott P, Chan YK, Saville J, von Elm E, Lewith GT. Prevalence of complementary medicine use in pediatric cancer: a systematic review. *Pediatrics* 2010;**125**:768–776.
6. Post-White J, Fitzgerald M, Hageness S, Sencer SF. Complementary and alternative medicine use in children with cancer and general and specialty pediatrics. *Journal of Pediatric Oncology Nursing* 2009a;**26**:7.
7. Kelly KM. Bringing evidence to complementary and alternative medicine in children with cancer: focus on nutrition-related therapies. *Pediatric Blood & Cancer* 2008;**50**:490–493.
8. Nathanson I, Sandler E, Ramírez-Garcia G, Wiltrout SA. Factors influencing complementary and alternative medicine use in a multisite pediatric oncology practice. *Journal of Pediatric Hematology Oncology* 2007;**29**: 705–708.
9. Tomlinson D, Hesser T, Ethier M, Sung L. Complementary and alternative medicine use in pediatric cancer

reported during palliative phase of disease. *Support Care Cancer* 2011;**19**:1857–1863.

10. Hamidah A, Rustam ZA, Tamil AM, Zarina LA, Zulkifli ZS, Jamal R. Prevalence and parental perceptions of complementary and alternative medicine use by children with cancer in a multi-ethnic Southeast Asian population. *Pediatric Blood & Cancer* 2009;**52**:70–74.

11. Naja F, Alameddine M, Abboud M, Bustami D, Halaby RA. Complementary and alternative medicine use among pediatric patients with leukemia: the case of Lebanon. *Integrative Cancer Therapies* 2010;**10**:38–46.

12. Längler A, Spix C, Edelhäuser F, Kameda G, Kaatsch P, Seifert G. Use of homeopathy in pediatric oncology in Germany. *Evidence-Based Complementary and Alternative Medicine.* 2011;**2011**:867151.

13. Clerici CA, Veneroni L, Giacon B, Mariani L, Fossati-Bellani F. Complementary and alternative medical therapies used by children with cancer treated at an Italian pediatric oncology unit. *Pediatric Blood & Cancer* 2009;**53**:599–604.

14. Genc RE, Senol S, Turgay AS, Kantar M. Complementary and alternative medicine used by pediatric patients with cancer in Western Turkey. *Oncology Nursing Forum* 2009;**36**:E159–E164.

15. Roth M, Lin J, Kim M, Moody K. Pediatric oncologists' views toward the use of complementary and alternative medicine in children with cancer. *Journal of Pediatric Hematology Oncology* 2009;**31**:177–182.

16. Pillai AK, Sharma KK, Gupta YK, Bakhshi S. Anti-emetic effect of ginger powder versus placebo as an add-on therapy in children and young adults receiving high emetogenic chemotherapy. *Pediatric Blood & Cancer* 2011;**56**:234–238.

17. Ladas EJ, Kroll DJ, Oberlies NH, *et al.* A randomized, controlled, double-blind, pilot study of milk thistle for the treatment of hepatotoxicity in childhood acute lymphoblastic leukemia (ALL). *Cancer* 2010;**116**:506–513.

18. Thygeson MV, Hooke MC, Clapsaddle J, Robbins A, Moquist K. Peaceful play yoga: serenity and balance for children with cancer and their parents. *Journal of Pediatric Oncology Nursing* 2010;**27**:276–284.

19. Gottschling S, Reindl TK, Meyer S, *et al.* Acupuncture to alleviate chemotherapy-induced nausea and vomiting in pediatric oncology: a randomized multicenter crossover pilot trial. *Klinische Pädiatrie* 2008;**220**:365–370.

20. Liossi C, White P, Hatira P. Randomized clinical trial of local anesthetic versus a combination of local anesthetic with self-hypnosis in the management of pediatric procedure-related pain. *Health Psychology* 2006;**25**:307–315.

21. Phipps S, Barrera M, Vannatta K, *et al.* Complementary therapies for children undergoing stem cell transplantation: report of a multisite trial. *Cancer* 2010;**116**: 3924–3933.

22. Post-White J, Fitzgerald M, Savik K, *et al.* Massage therapy for children with cancer. *Journal of Pediatric Oncology Nursing* 2009b;**26**:16–28.

13

Fantasy, Art Therapies, and Other Expressive and Creative Psychosocial Interventions

Shulamith Kreitler, Daniel Oppenheim, Elsa Segev-Shoham

Introduction

Increased awareness on the part of health practitioners of the psychological difficulties attending children with cancer and undergoing treatment has led to the development and application of various psychosocial means designed to help the children live through the ordeal and mitigate their suffering.

The present chapter describes various forms of expressive and creative interventions, including different modalities of art therapy practiced in wards of pediatric cancer around the world, each presented by expert practitioners. Each type of intervention is characterized by a particular methodology and is targeted to attain specific goals. Yet, in practice each of the interventions is often used for attaining different goals, similar to those targeted by other interventions. Moreover, often several types are applied together, either at the discretion of the practitioner, tailored to the needs and possibilities of a particular patient, or in prestructured multimodal comprehensive packages [1, 2].

In general, in this broad domain there are many detailed case reports, for example, [4, 5], descriptions of particular projects and techniques and relatively few well-designed studies with a sufficient number of participants focused on any one of the described therapy modalities or on comparing the effects of two or more therapies. This is due partly to the tendency to apply various techniques together, and partly to the necessity of maintaining flexibility in adapting the therapies to a great variety of children in difficult medical situations [5]. This makes it difficult to provide evidence-based support in the strict sense of the term for the particular effects of any of the therapies.

The most frequently cited objectives of the different therapies are the following: distraction of attention, blocking or inhibiting of distress reactions, mitigating side effects of medical procedures or treatments (e.g., pain, nausea, fatigue), reducing fear of the unknown, reducing negative emotions, promoting positive emotions, providing means for self-expression, increasing self-esteem, strengthening sense of control, extending coping skills, and facilitating cooperation with the medical procedures [6, 7].

Fantasy Involvement

The sedative and possibly healing power of imagery has been recognized in many cultures since ancient times [8]. In recent years there has been growing use of images as a therapeutic modality in medical contexts, with children and adults [9]. Fantasy could be considered as a process that plays a role in all the expressive and affective interventions. The National Cancer Institute [10] has also recommended guided imagery as a major means of alleviating the child's discomfort and fear before and during cancer procedures. It is often coupled with hypnosis, which provides the relaxation or concentration part and uses imagery to present suggestions in the course of hypnosis and post-hypnotically. Also, without hypnosis, it is often applied in the context of art therapy and only rarely as a single modality [11].

When used alone, it represents a therapy that focuses on engaging the child in some imaginary activity. The child is asked to imagine some kind of experience, object, event or situation. All the child's senses may be involved, namely, not only visual sensations

Pediatric Psycho-oncology: Psychosocial Aspects and Clinical Interventions, Second Edition.
Edited by Shulamith Kreitler, Myriam Weyl Ben-Arush and Andrés Martin.
© 2012 John Wiley & Sons, Ltd. Published 2012 by John Wiley & Sons, Ltd.

which are most common, but also sounds, tastes, smells, or a combination of these. When the focus is on visual imagery, the child may be asked to imagine being in a favorite room or place, in a flower garden, watching some kind of sport activity, or animals, TV or movies; when the focus is on auditory imagery, the fantasy may involve hearing conversations with significant others, favorite songs, environmental sounds (waves, etc.), playing a musical instrument, or listening to music; when the focus is on movement imagery, the child is asked to imagine flying, swimming, skating, or any other pleasurable activity [12]. When applied in regard to pain, the focus is either on providing distraction, in which case any pleasant absorbing fantasy will do [13], or on combating pain by changing the perception of the pain, for example, imagine that you blow the pain away or make it fade out [14–16]. The process of imagining may range from free unstructured suggestions to imagining anything one desires, to providing step-by-step instructions about how to proceed. Precise instructions would include steps, such as the following:

We are going to make a journey to a nice place which you will greatly enjoy; please sit comfortably and close your eyes; breathe slowly. Now choose a place where you want to be. Now that you have reached it, observe carefully who is there in that place; then focus on the objects in that place; try to see the colors and the forms; try to hear the sounds. Are there any smells, etc.? You may now come back from that place.

Not only the process of imagining but also the image itself may be subjected to different degrees of guidance or shaping by the therapist. For example, in order to initiate the procedure of imagining, the therapist may show the child a TV cartoon and introduce the child to a particular character or location. Also the theme of the image may be suggested to the child, for example, a road, a wheel, or a circus. In other contexts, the therapist would wait for the child to offer an image and would shape it by suggestions so that it exerts its optimal therapeutic impact or at least does not develop into an anxiety-laden negative image, as can sometimes happen. The goals of guided imagery are reduction of anxiety, promoting positive feelings and sometimes "fighting cancer" (i.e., promoting healing). Studies showed that guided imagery has significant effects in reducing distress in children undergoing diagnostic procedures [17] or chemotherapy [18, 19]. One session of imaginative involvement with children 3–10 years old reduced more distress than standard care in bone marrow aspirations [20]. Another study with 25 pediatric oncology patients, found that 21 agreed to use the exercises of guided imagery and 19 showed substantial reductions in pain and nausea associated with their practice, especially if they begin the exercises at the time of their initial diagnosis [21]. There is evidence that children project their disease concerns and anxieties onto the images they produce [22]. Studies demonstrating the effect of guided imagery on immune function in adults [23] have yet to be replicated in children. Also, there is a need for research focused on the processes accounting for the beneficial effects of imagery.

Guided Imagery Combined with Computerized Art Therapy

Computerized animation is a special variety of guided imagery which was developed in order to help pediatric oncology and hematology patients to meet the challenges of serious illness regardless of distance from the hospital, language, time and religion [24]. The goal of providing the children a safe environment in which to express their feelings in a nonverbal way was attained by constructing a graphic program, adapted for use of children from the age of 4 years onward, which allows the child creative exploration and discovery. It was created by using a digital camera, video-phone and scanner, with hand-painted drawings and graphics, computerized video animation, computer CD games and audiocassettes with music, sounds from nature and voices. One such program, called "The Bridge," is based on nonverbal communication, which aids in projecting unconscious imagery. It stimulates the five senses and awakens the child's imagination. The computerized program is introduced to the child in the hospital under the supervision of an art therapist. Each child receives an art therapy menu, adapted to his/her emotional, psychological and medical condition. The program allows freedom of choice of colors, forms and even medium, and encourages the child to produce images by using the different expressive options. The scanned images are transferred to the home computers. Patients are requested to print and/or store the images on disk-on-keys or CDs. Siblings and parents are invited to participate, so that family interactions and communication are promoted. The program may be activated by the child at home so that it assists the medical staff with home medical management.

Visual Arts

Art therapy based on the visual arts is probably the most widely applied modality of art therapy. It uses painting, drawing, sculpture, photography, ceramics, and the fabric arts in order to enable the children to express their conscious and unconscious concerns about the disease and to externalize their anxieties, as well as to promote self-awareness and self-confidence and to try out new solutions to their problems in a safe environment. A variety of materials are used (e.g., clay, wood, beads, buttons, cloth, paper), in a variety of forms (e.g., finger painting, drawing, using computer graphic programs), with a variety of produced outputs (e.g., paintings, sculpted objects, drawn images, embroidery, photographs).

The three poles of this therapeutic modality are the therapist, the patient, and the image, whereby the art therapist is often called upon to act in the triple role of artist, teacher and therapist. The emphasis is on creativity and expressiveness, often coupled with spontaneity and improvising. This therapeutic modality is characterized by three major dimensions: (1) the expressive–creative dimension, based on the relation between the patient and the image, wherein the therapist is the facilitator in the image production process; (2) the cognitive–symbolic dimension, based on the relationship between the therapist and the patient through and about the produced image, wherein the therapist helps the patient to understand the image; and (3) the interactive–analytic dimension, based on direct communication between the therapist and the patient, where the therapist uses the image and its meanings in order to help the patient understand himself or herself [6].

Art therapy may take place in the hospital, in the child's home or in the therapist's clinic; it may consist of individual sessions or group sessions; it may or may not be accompanied or followed by analysis of the art work and discussion in the group setting or between the therapist and the child. During each session the therapist may offer techniques, subject-matter, media and/or free choices in line with the changing needs of the patient and the therapeutic goals. The child may decide consciously what to convey through the art work, or simply start in a random fashion to produce something.

A common form of art therapy is letting the children participate in a kind of fine art workshop encouraging them to express themselves freely while producing works of art, designed even for public display, with their consent (as conducted by Gericot in the Gustave Roussy Cancer Institute, Villejuif, France, 2005–2011). The themes that are often found in the children's works of art manifest projections of their distress (e.g., drawings of castles where they can "hide," disfigured bodies), their anger, as well as attempts to overcome the distress (e.g., drawings of doctors healing a child).

Varieties of Art Therapy

Special kinds of art therapy have been developed. For example, structured art therapy consists of asking the children to draw specific themes, once or even more than once in consecutive sessions. Standard themes would be the "mandala" (color–feeling wheel), the "change-in-family" drawing and the "scariest" drawing. The structured aspect of these drawings allows the therapist to ask highly focused questions and interpret the drawings within the context of the individual's reality [25].

Another interesting kind of art therapy focuses on mask making. Jones [26] described its application with pediatric oncology patients, in a public hospital. The masks were produced from papier-mâché, over a period of 5–8 weeks. The project included a video recording of each patient's mask-making process, photographs of each mask, and a closing semi-structured interview. Analysis showed that the project promoted creativity, individual expression, symbolization, objectification of feeling, expression of disease-related concerns, while supporting adaptive denial, self-representation, expression of wishes, fantasy development, and production of a transitional object. It also enabled the children to gain control of some aspect of their time in the hospital. The oncologists reported that the mask making decreased the children's anticipatory anxiety, possibly by providing distraction, but did not increase the children's social interaction.

Computer-assisted art therapy (CAAT) is another fairly common kind of art therapy [27–29]. It uses computer technology to create and share images. Concerning *production*, CAAT provides the following possibilities: performing computer drawing by applying different graphic software; using image banks to select images, constructing new images out of given graphic elements or improving on self-produced images; creating animated graphics; combining drawings and photos; adding to the images multi-media components, such as music and motion. Note that the use of computers obviates the need to rely on materials (e.g., colors, cloth) which may jeopardize pediatric oncology patients whose immune systems are compromised. Concerning *storing* of the products, CAAT enables easy storage of the products, in multiple locations, and with easy access to the products stored on disk or CDs. Possibly the most innovative developments occur in regard to *communication*. CAAT enables the products to be shared with sick and healthy children in other countries. It also presents the possibility for electronic exhibitions, open to any interested spectator around the globe. Most importantly, it promotes online interactive communication between the art producers and the art therapist, in real time. This enables not only computer support for art therapy at a distance, but also bridges the gap between producing static images and dynamic performance.

Bibliotherapy

Bibliotherapy is a therapy that uses literary products (i.e., books) as a therapeutic means for providing relief, enhanced self-understanding, promotion of coping skills and personal growth. It is an interactive process with three essential components: the client or patient, the trained facilitator or therapist, and literary products (e.g., stories, poetry, plays, folktales). In the context of pediatric oncology, different kinds of books are used for a variety of goals, for example, for distraction during medical procedures; for providing health-relevant information about the procedures; for fun (e.g., humor, adventure books); for relaxation and reduction of anxiety; and for psychotherapeutically relevant goals, such as enhancing the child's self-esteem and self-identity. The most salient and interesting is the psychotherapeutic use. The underlying philosophy is that "the world is made up of stories, not facts" [31]. The patient is exposed to a structured selection of literary themes designed to encourage self-exploration, self-expression. The theoretical rationale for this type of psychotherapy is the assumption that life is a narrative and that psychotherapy is the production, improvement and understanding of this narrative. The characteristic processes applied in bibliotherapy are the following: transcending the patient's enclosure within the confines of his or her own narrow set of problems; coping within an imaginary protected setting; attaining a timeout period that enables release from one's own problems by identifying with the problems of the literary figures; promoting self-awareness by encouraging the child to talk freely about one's problems and feelings while discussing those of the literary figure that may resemble one's own; providing emotional relief by identifying emotionally with problems and solutions of the depicted figures; coping with taboo issues, such as death, loss, abandonment that embody the child's innermost fears by presenting the themes symbolically and sometimes by providing in fantasy wish fulfillment of taboo desires through the explicit or implicit narrative. Even a short-term application of bibliotherapy is expected to facilitate integration of the traumatic event or situation and to help identify sources of strength, thus promoting self-esteem, the experience of a continuity of life events, social functioning and increased life satisfaction [32].

The basic technique used in bibliotherapy consists of the therapist telling the child a story in his/her own language or reading the child a story. There are, however, many possible variations of the basic technique. The story may sometimes but not always be accompanied by showing relevant pictures. The reading is often followed by a discussion of the themes by the therapist and the child. Sometimes the story is told or read to a group of children and is followed by group discussion. Another variation includes the following three phases: first, the therapist tells or reads a story to the child, then the child tells it back to the therapist, and, finally, they both discuss it. Sometimes the reading of the story is amended or amplified by fantasy, for example, the child is asked to suggest additions or changes in the story, or the child and therapist exchange presents between themselves in the form of stories [33, 34].

The story told or read by the therapist may refer directly to cancer (there are books about children with cancer, for example, Cothern [35] and Noonan [36]), but may also deal with other themes, selected by the therapist as pertinent to the child's current needs.

There are specializations within bibliotherapy—poetry therapy [37, 38], folktale or mythology therapy, according to the preferences and needs of the patients. Each type of literature contributes something unique, for example, poetry provides special images, rhymes and rhythms; folktales provide metaphors and generally applicable "lessons"; stories provide absorbing plots with figures with whom one may identify. Books of humor constitute a special subcategory that is conceptualized as "humor therapy" (see pp. 152–3).

There is empirical evidence that telling the child a story featuring their favorite hero, who helps the child cope with the situations which are gradually increasing in difficulty, reduces the children's distress during treatments [2; see also Chapter 10 of this book]. Storytelling incorporated within a multimodal treatment package was shown to reduce distress as well as nausea, vomiting and other side effects [1]. In a study with patients with leukemia, 6–19 years old, undergoing bone marrow transplantation, even after one intervention of storytelling there was already less self-reported pain and anxiety [39]. The therapeutic effect of books and stories may be exercised simply by reading the material, but the effect is usually enhanced when the material has been also discussed.

Writing

Writing is a form of therapy that consists of the patients writing poetry, stories, personal memoirs, testimonials, or diaries (also called journaling). Writing may be considered the creative part of bibliotherapy. Patients often feel the need to write. Some patients tend to write either because they are basically verbal types or because they feel that nonverbal means of expression are too infantile for them or not common in their culture. Some patients start writing on their own initiative, whereas others need to be encouraged. Again, some do it on their own, others dictate it to others, still others need the help of someone else who acts as a therapist. According to the Lahad method [44], the child is asked to write a story on the basis of memory or fantasy, in line with six basic guiding questions, which are assumed to provide the child a steady framework enhancing his/her sense of security to express his/her thoughts. The written products sometimes assume the form of metaphorical stories (e.g., fighting a cruel ruler who kills most of his citizens, because he acts under an ancient curse that he can only be evil), at other times they are outright documentary material (e.g., a girl, 11 years old, diagnosed with an advanced brain tumor, wrote an almost day-by-day account, starting with the day of her diagnosis and ending a week prior to her death). Often patients write poems of a classical or modern type [40]. Some patients produce a written product only once, or only during a certain period of time; others write sporadically, and still others keep on writing all through their illness.

Part of the effect of writing is due to the emotional relief it provides. Another factor may be the sense of control and freedom it gives to the writer who is constrained in a situation where he/she may feel overwhelmed, helpless and dominated by external factors (e.g., the disease, the treatments, hospital regulations). Studies of the effects of writing in people in general showed that those who were asked to write about consequential events felt in the short term worse than those who were asked to write about trivial events, but in the long run they had fewer health problems and better immunological functioning. Findings of this kind were explained as due to two factors. The first is expression, which reduces the need for inhibition and the stress it involves. The second factor is the use of language, which enables distancing from the event and assimilating it while processing it and organizing the material [41–43].

Play

Play is being used to alleviate distress, pain and various side effects of chemotherapy. One study showed that even adding to the medical procedure an expandable whistle-like toy ("party blower") makes the child's crying less likely and enables relaxation by paced breathing [46]. Another study examined the effects of playing video games on children (9–20 years old, with various cancer diagnoses) in the course of chemotherapy. Most (69%) of the children in the experimental group who played the games reported a sizable reduction in nausea as compared with 23% in the control group who

had no video games. Further, in the second part of the study, the introduction and withdrawal of the opportunity to play video games were followed by reduction and exacerbation of nausea, respectively. Notably, playing video games was associated with an increase in systolic blood pressure, indicating an increase in arousal [47]. Another study with three participants, 11–17 years old, suffering from acute lymphocytic leukemia, showed that playing video games in the course of chemotherapy was associated with self-reported reductions in anticipatory symptoms (e.g., insomnia, nail-biting 24 hours prior to treatment) and state anxiety, observer-rated distress due to side effects (e.g., dizziness, nausea), and self-reported as well as observer-rated post-chemotherapy side effects. The mentioned distress signs were exacerbated when the games were withdrawn; the signs were reduced again when the video games were reintroduced [48]. A study with children undergoing bone marrow transplantation for acute lymphocytic leukemia showed that non-directed play was as effective as hypnosis (including the use of imagery, muscle relaxation, and suggestions of mastery) in reducing the children's self-rated pain and fear [49]. Playing games forms part of several intervention packages in pediatric oncology that have reported overall positive effects on the well-being of the treated children or adolescents [1, 17, 50–52]. It is likely that computer games will be increasingly used, complementing the common video games. The beneficial effect that playing has on children in treatment for cancer is mostly attributed to the distraction of the children's attention from the painful procedures they are undergoing [1, 48]. However, it seems likely that further processes may play a role, such as gaining a sense of control, and overcoming distress by fantasy. The possible involvement of fantasy indicates a likely blurring of boundaries between proper play and play therapy.

Play Therapy

Play therapy is a therapeutic medium that uses playing with dolls and other toys in order to provide support to children in distress and help them resolve problems [53]. Play therapy is designed to assist the child to cope with stressful situations, enhance the child's sense of mastery, help the child establish an atmosphere of normality under conditions that deviate from normality, and reduce helplessness and anxiety. The goal of play therapy is often to help the child adapt the reality to the self and the self to reality.

Play therapy may be conducted in the form of individual sessions or group sessions with several sick children, whereby mutual support and the possibility for creating social ties are provided [54, 55]. Significant others may act as observers, watching the child's play. They may gain thereby a better understanding of the child's means of coping, as well as feelings and perceptions of the situation and even of themselves.

Play therapy may be carried out in different forms. Toys and dolls can be given to the child who is left alone with them, to play as he or she wishes. This non-directive procedure can be amended by suggesting a general playing theme to the child, such as "this is a hospital ward" or "they are all going on a trip." Play therapy may be enacted also in a directive–interactive manner, whereby the therapist lets the child start out with the play, offers an interpretation or suggestion for the next step, and so on, closing with a discussion between the therapist and the child. The number of sessions also varies in line with the needs of the child and the particular play therapy technique used by the therapist.

EXAMPLE

Here are some examples of play therapy sessions in the context of the hospital ward. A 4-year-old girl, diagnosed with Hodgkin's disease, used to play for hours with a set of dolls presented to her by the therapist. The play changed from one session to the other but one element kept recurring: she used to hide one doll somewhere in her bed and would start crying because she "lost" it. When this happened, the therapist asked what was the matter, whereby the girl would urge her to help her in finding the missing doll. When the doll was found, which was invariably the case, the girl would cry with joy and make a big party for the dolls. In one of the follow-up visits to the hospital she volunteered of her own accord the meaning of the game: "even when you die, they will look for you and find you." The theme of coping with one's own pending death recurs in accounts of play therapy with pediatric oncology patients [e.g., 56–58].

Examples of further themes that recur in play therapy with pediatric oncology patients are misunderstanding of the child as to why he or she was in the hospital [58], family relations under the threat of death [57], and loneliness due to difficulty of interpersonal relations

with friends [59]. Most examples use projection and symbolization by the children in their endeavors to find a solution to a problem by means of therapist-guided play therapy.

Drama Therapy and Psychodrama

Drama therapy is a mode of therapy which uses theatrical forms of expression as a therapeutic medium [60]. The best known form of drama therapy is psycho-drama, originally developed by Jacob L. Moreno [61]. It employs guided dramatic action, supplemented by action methods and role playing, in order to facilitate insight into the patient's problems, promote the patients' awareness and understanding of themselves and reality, and enable the learning of new skills and the enhancement of emotional well-being. Like some other forms of art therapy (e.g., bibliotherapy), psychodrama enables the patients to approach real-life problems and emotionally-laden themes through the safe distance of fictionalized situations and characters. In addition, the dramatic medium and the largely non-verbal form of expression combine to lower the patients' control, so that they may reveal more about themselves than they would otherwise do. The special characteristic components of psychodrama are acting out and fantasy. The patient is encouraged to act out in a protected setup, and give free rein to his/her fantasy in a spontaneous, creative manner. The product is a creative expression of imagination which assumes a concrete form in reality through action. Thus, the restricting structures are released, coupled with the production of new structures which often spell out new solutions to both old and new problems.

Accordingly, psychodrama provides a safe, supportive environment to practice new and more effective roles and behaviors, rehearse new roles, try out solutions, and explore new options. In general, it offers the opportunity to see reality from different points of view. Finally, since it relies on action, it is often more empowering than traditional verbal therapies. The overall procedure includes the steps that lead the patient from reality to fiction to a better reality.

The basic components of psychodrama are the protagonist, the auxiliary egos (i.e., others who play significant others or inner forces within the person), the audience, the director (i.e., therapist), and the stage (physical space). The three major structural components involved in psychodrama are warm-up, action, and sharing (e.g., through discussion) [62].

Drama therapy may be enacted according to a script previously discussed or produced spontaneously. It can follow a script produced by the child spontaneously, or by the therapist, or by both, sometimes even following a script out of a book or play. The drama may be enacted by the child or children and sometimes with puppets (dolls or marionettes). The boundary between theater and drama therapy becomes blurred sometimes, so that psychodramatic elements are embedded within the context of theater, presenting therapeutically relevant themes, thus combining entertainment, catharsis, and therapy. One example is the STOP GAP drama therapy workshops of California that visit hospitals performing theater and psychodrama.

Drama therapy can be applied in any space, small or large, closed or open, in the presence of others (adults, children) or without them [63]. However, essentially the presence of spectators, either an active or passive audience, is conceptualized as an integral component of drama therapy. Others may often be called upon to fulfill various roles in the unfolding drama.

EXAMPLE

In one session with a 12-year-old child suffering from leukemia, psychodrama was enacted in the sick room in the hospital, with two other patients. The child assumed the role of "the sick child," whereas the two patients played in turn the roles of "two doctors" discussing the case of "the sick child" and concluding that he would recover, then the roles of "the fear" and "the hope" dwelling within "the sick child," fighting it out between themselves until "the hope" won the upper hand. This psychodramatic enactment served the goal of confronting the child's fears and strengthening his hope. In a series of psychodramatic sessions with a group of survivors of childhood cancer, the enacted themes were problems of being accepted again in the group of children, the sense of having missed out because of the long time spent in the hospital, the feeling of being different from other children, not being understood by others, and means of making others understand.

Drama therapy is often used to prepare the child for medical procedures, undertaken for diagnostic or treatment purposes. This use of drama therapy, sometimes called behavioral rehearsal, consists in going with the child through the different steps of the procedure he or she is to undergo, whereby the child may assume in turn the roles of patient, nurse, and doctor. Puppets may sometimes be used. The dramatic enactment, which may be repeated more than once, familiarizes the child with the situation, reducing fear of the unknown, and strengthening the sense of control [64]. This kind of application of drama therapy has been reported to have highly beneficial effects on the mood and cooperation of the child [65].

Dramatic Play Therapy in the Hospital Setting

Dramatic play therapy represents a special variety of drama therapy. It combines the therapeutic advantages of drama and of play to form a unique tool to address the sick child's special needs. Its enactment requires the patient, a drama therapist, one or more other individuals (adults or children), dolls or puppets and often other toys and objects. The drama unfolds in line with a script that has been prepared in advance or is being improvised on the spot. Change of roles often takes place. Dramatic play therapy is of special importance in the context of hospitalization. Hospitalization could be traumatic for children because the hospital is an unfamiliar environment, with little privacy, reduced control over the situation, in which frightening and painful procedures occur.

There are several clear-cut advantages of dramatic play therapy in the hospital setting. It enables children: (1) to re-enact familiar activities and thus reduce the strangeness and threat of the unknown environment; (2) to reorganize their life and thus gain a better understanding of what is happening to them; (3) to assume in the play an active role and thus regain the sense of control that has been impaired by the disease and the hospitalization; (4) to express aggression under controlled conditions and thus attain relief for the sustained frustration; and (5) to express their dreams, needs and feelings, by projecting them onto the dolls.

Dramatic play therapy is often used to help prepare children for diagnostic or therapeutic medical procedures (even surgery) both by providing them information about what is going to take place and by reducing fear and tension through the enactment of the events. In this context, the actual use of real accessories, such as gloves or syringes, is of great help in preparing a child for a medical procedure.

EXAMPLE

The patient was a 6-year-old girl diagnosed with histiocytosis at the age of 2.3 years. She has undergone many medical tests pre-and post-diagnosis, mostly under general anesthesia. The recurrent painful tests made her highly anxious. Her anxiety was further exacerbated through the anxiety of her parents, who felt that the girl had terminal disease. The goal of the play therapy was to prepare the girl for an MRI test without anesthetic. The play therapy was based on using two glove puppets representing mother and father, a small doll representing a baby, and a plastic tube representing the MRI machine. The major protagonists of the play were Mother, Father, and Baby. The Doctor joined in later. The patient and the drama therapist were present all through. In the first session the patient was a spectator. In the beginning, the Father and Mother decided not to tell Baby that they were going for an MRI but instead to deceive her by telling her that they were going on a trip. At this point the patient interfered and the first session ended with her admitting to the drama therapist that she knew the show was about her. In the second session, the patient chose for herself the role of the mother and for the drama therapist the role of the baby. Baby started to question Mother about where they were going. When she was told about the MRI test, she wanted to know why and how it would be done. Mother showed her by simulation with the plastic tube how the MRI test would be performed. At this point Baby raised concerns about frightening sounds in the course of the medical test (made sounds) and asked to be hugged. The Doctor joined the play and explained that the patient would be put to sleep so that she does not move in the course of the test. Baby resisted this suggestion because she was afraid that she would not wake up. The Doctor suggested that when she gets to the clinic for the MRI, she could ask not to be put under anesthetic. The session ended with Mother holding Baby. Following the suggestion of the drama therapist, the patient and her mother took the dolls home for the weekend in order to play with them. The therapy was highly successful: the girl underwent MRI without anesthetic. She lay completely still for 45 minutes, with her mother holding her hand. The girl and her mother were strengthened by the success, learned to cope with different procedures and even helped other parents.

Cinema and Video Therapy

Focus on Viewing

Cinema therapy is the use of cinema in order to diagnose and help individuals in distress. Conservative cinema therapy consists in showing the patient a film selected by the therapist especially for the patient with the intent of illustrating some particular problem relevant for the patient. For example, the film *Life is Beautiful* (by Robert Begnini) portrays a father who turned the stay in a concentration camp into a kind of game for the child and thus helped him survive the horror with a minimum anxiety and without paying too high a price in mental health. Other examples include *The Miracle Maker* about Helen Keller (by Arthur Penn), Charlie Chaplin's *The Kid*, and *Patch Adams*, demonstrating humor therapy. Films involve powerful sensory experiences, appealing to various senses and portraying situations that often resemble those in actual daily life. Hence they may be used profitably in order to transmit to patients, also children, various therapeutically important messages, such as "you're not the only one to suffer this problem," "others in your situation have survived it," and "every cloud has a silver lining." The transmission of the messages is enhanced by the experiential impact of film, and the indirect way in which it is communicated. The film may be watched by the child alone or in the company of an adult (e.g., parent, sibling, other patients), at home or in the hospital, once or several times, and with a variety of screening devices. Further, viewing the film may be preceded by some kind of focusing by the therapist and may be followed by discussion. Conservative cinema therapy may be considered a film-based variety of bibliotherapy.

Focus on Producing

Another variety of cinema or video therapy consists in actually producing a film. The underlying assumption is that the film-making process offers various artistic and organizational activities that resemble those used by therapists and which may provide useful and challenging psychological exercises. This variety of cinema therapy requires a film-making expert, a therapist and a patient. Working together, this team produces a film primarily for the benefit of one single viewer: the patient.

Video therapy consists of helping a child to produce a video film. Snapshot and video cameras, tape, CD and computers are used, along with traditional art therapy tools, such as storytelling, music, and painting. The focus is on producing video animation, but further means such as sculpting, modeling and drawing are also used in these projects. The children are encouraged to invent the plot, write the script, draw and sculpt the background scenario, design and decide where, when and how the video takes place, and then film and edit the film. In this kind of video art therapy the child assumes alternately the roles of director, actor, author and producer of his or her own movie. Five major stages are involved in the process: (1) text-writing (scenery preparation), in which the child learns how to prepare a 'story board'; (2) directing, in which the child directs others, maybe children or patients, parents, siblings, members of the medical staff; (3) filming, in which the child chooses whether to film, photograph or act in front of the camera; (4) editing, in which the child introduces into the film the changes he or she considers appropriate to shape a product with a specific purpose, for example, a movie that can be used as a therapeutic tool in the future; and (5) screening, in which the child assumes control of when, where and to whom the movie will be screened.

When the video film is completed, the child is encouraged to take it home as his or her own work. However, it can also be used for discussion in individual sessions or group sessions, in order to improve the children's or the caretakers' insight.

Video art therapy can make unique contributions to the child's well-being. First, it provides distraction, which helps to alleviate pain and anxiety. This is achieved by involving the child in an interesting and totally engrossing activity, satisfying insofar as it appeals to the child's narcissistic needs, and with enough variety to hold the child's attention for longer periods of time. Second, it provides catharsis by enabling the child to express his or her innermost fears and problems by means of unconscious projection and symbolic representations in the video plot and images. Third, it contributes significantly to improving the child's mood and quality of life by providing satisfaction, fun and entertainment. Fourth, it promotes interaction between the child and his or her family by involving the whole family in the video production, which the family keeps as a document commemorating happy moments in this difficult period. Fifth, it boosts the child's ego by providing activities and encouraging creativity that may reveal new strengths and discover new talents. Ego-strengthening is particularly important both because the circumstances increase the child's sense of helplessness, and because through the newly acquired strength the child finds new ways of coping. Sixth, it contributes to improving the child's body image by involving the child in bodily activities.

Clowning

We present the major elements of the clown's intervention in the Department of Pediatric Oncology, Gustave Roussy Cancer Institute. Twice a week, two clowns come to the ward [66], as others do in many pediatric departments in France (e.g., the 'Rire Médecin'), and elsewhere (e.g. the Clown Care Unit of The Big Apple Circus, active in several pediatric hospitals in the US). The clowns work in the corridors and the waiting hall area as well as in the rooms, with children and adolescents, even with the terminally ill, individually or collectively in a group, but also with the parents and the caregivers. Each clown has his or her own style, personality, and particular skill: they play music, perform magic tricks, dance, speak too fast, stutter, or mime, etc. They come in different varieties—big or small, fat or lean, with long hair or bald heads, skilful or clumsy, but all wear red noses. Their names are Dr Giraffe, Dr Basket, Dr Cauliflower, Dr Lulu Leek. They perform brief and improvised shows in the corridors by themselves or by drawing into the dance, the game or the little scene a child, or anyone else who happens to be in the vicinity. The children become spectators or actors, and eventually receive a red nose. The clowns wear a decorated white coat, carry props in their doctor's bags, some of which are made out of medical or nursing devices (e.g., balloons made of gloves, whistles or telephones made of syringes or stethoscopes).

The Clowns' Work

The clowns offer joy and laughter, but do much more than simply amuse the children. Children know about their illness and the complex and precise treatments they need. They usually accept these constraints, which are nonetheless hard to endure. This is why they enjoy, by way of revenge, the anarchy, nonsense and fantasy introduced by the clowns through their clothes, the way they walk or dance, the way they talk or shout, telling fake and horror stories, disturbing the parents and nurses. Playful and musical noises are heard, instead of silence or aggressive noises (pagers, pump alarms, cries, etc.). The clowns are fully aware of the fact that the children may sometimes feel frustration because they have to endure painful treatments and operations. Therefore they readily provide the children an outlet to engage in aggressive behavior: the children can bite and be bitten, they can tear off Giraffe's Velcroed tail, they can push a clown, and so on. The clowns also transform the function of a place from its intended use: the nurse's room turns into a dance hall, a child's room becomes a ring or a circus, and the whole ward turns into a playground, in addition to its original function to provide medical care services.

The clowns help the children regain possession of and pride in their bodies by showing that they are proud of their own strange and distorted bodies, when they demonstrate how to put a handicap to good use, when they grimace together with the child, when they transform a child's neck brace into a royal necklace. They express openly the emotions the children may feel (fear, terror, love, anger, etc.) and show how these can be understood and integrated in a play and in a story. Thus, the children know that even their most intense or violent emotions have a place in the ward and that they can also do something positive with them.

Illness plays a key role in the clowns' games. Illness is the implicit theme in the background when ropes are cut and magically restored, when a ball disappears in the nose and reappears in the mouth, when a child removes Giraffe's horn and puts it on his own nose, or on the nurse's head. Pranks of this kind may illustrate the child's etiopathological theories, for example, "Where does my illness come from? Somebody has put it inside me. If I could give it to someone else, or if only it could disappear magically." The games enacted by clowns allow the children to express their illness theories, without fully believing in them or feeling bound to explain them, and to maintain them, without conflicting with the medical theories which they know and accept. When the clowns parody the caregivers, they allow the children to revolt under safe conditions. This may give the children not only an emotional outlet, but may also help to avoid non-compliance.

The clowns participate in the care of the child, working in close collaboration and harmony with the medical staff, fully aware of the risk that both the children and the nurses may contrast the "good doctors" (the clowns) with the "bad and naughty ones" (the pediatricians and nurses). They have to determine the specific role they intend to play in the midst of all the other professionals (psycho-oncologists, teachers, art therapists, etc.). They must be experienced professional clowns, trained for this specific setting, functioning in line with a strict code of ethics. They have regular meetings with a psycho-oncologist who can help to shed light on some of the complexities of the situation in pediatric oncology and to deal with their own emotional reactions.

Humor Therapy

The potentially beneficial effects of laughter and humor on health have long been known: "The arrival of a good clown exercises a more beneficial effect upon the health of a town than 20 asses laden with pills" (Sir Thomas Sydenham) or "If it were not for laughs, we would be sicker than we are" (William Frey, both professor of medicine and researcher of humor).

A growing body of research is beginning to provide empirical evidence supporting the contribution of humor and laughter to strengthening the immune system, moderating the effects of stress, and serving as an efficient coping and defense mechanism [67–69]. The popular screenplay *Patch Adams* highlighted the healing aspects of laughter in the medical context, whereas the show *Andre Vincent is Unwell* (in the Edinburgh Festival, 2002), which showed the suffering of a cancer patient in the form of stand-up comedy, has contributed to shattering the notion that cancer is a taboo subject in comedy. Some notable initiatives to bring humor therapy into the oncology wards include The Hamptons Comedy Festival (2002), and the East Coast's premier comedy organization dedicated to using comedy to fight cancer, which launched in 2002 the Comedy Fights Cancer/Laughter Promotes Healing initiative, and brings comics to cancer patients in hospitals in the form of large shows or bedside performances. At Loma Linda University Cancer Institute, humor-based treatment complements chemotherapy so that during the treatments the patients are encouraged to watch videos or read literature from the Laughter Library, with the SMILE (Subjective Multidimensional Interactive Laughter Evaluation) software guiding their choices of material. "Humor carts" (conceived by humor therapist Judy Goldblum-Carleton) exist in over 40 hospitals in the USA, bringing to pediatric oncology wards humor therapists who have learned how to create fun and laughter in the sick children. The largest and most ambitious project is Rx Laughter (created by Dunay Hilber and led by Margaret Stuber and Lonnie Zeltzer, and conducted by the Johnson Cancer Center, the Mattel Children's Hospital at UCLA and the UCLA Neuropsychiatric Institute and Hospital) which applies for therapeutic entertainment carefully selected cartoons and TV classic films in order to study how best to use humor for pain reduction and prevention or treatment of diseases in children and adolescents.

Research shows that children (5–10 years) with cancer do not differ in humor from healthy children and that they more often rated a cartoon as funny even without understanding the joke, which indicates they had a tendency for humor [70]. A study with 43 school-aged children with cancer showed that children scoring high on the Multidimensional Sense of Humor Scale had better psychological adjustment than those scoring low, regardless of the amount of cancer stressors, insofar as coping humor moderated the daily hassles of living with cancer. Moreover, the high scorers had a lower incidence of infections when the number of reported cancer stressors increased, and better immunological functioning (as assessed by salivary IgA levels and absolute neutrophil counts [71]). Major mechanisms involved are partly physiological (e.g., muscular relaxation) and partly psychological (e.g., better coping) [72]. Both types of effects appear to be mediated by the cognitive changes brought about by humor [73, 74]. Humor consists of shifts in the meanings assigned to the situation and the major protagonists. The shifts express awareness both of the problem inherent in the situation and of its insolubility, at least for the time being. Hence, humor makes it easier to accept reality, even if it is neither humorous nor "a laughing matter."

Music Therapy

Music therapy is a general name for different ways of using music to help the patient cope, or more specifically, for providing a feeling of satisfaction and harmony [75], facilitating relaxation, moderating physical symptoms, such as pain and nausea and reducing anxieties, loneliness and stress [76]. Music is particularly adapted to goals of this kind because of its harmonious structure, its use of components that are not found in their pure form in external reality (e.g., tones, melody) and its structural properties, manifested especially in its rhythm [77]. The major processes involved in music therapy are promoting nonverbal interaction, expressing repressed emotions, enabling diversion, providing fun and entertainment and indirectly facilitating the acceptance of the new reality. There are a great variety of ways to exercise music therapy [78]. The major means include the following: exploring and stating one's musical preferences; listening to the desired music usually in the company of the therapist, nurses or other patients; listening to live music played or sung by an individual present (e.g., the therapist); engaging in relaxation exercises or anxiety-relieving fantasies with background music [79]; using musical instruments or playing rhythm instruments, including improvisational drumming; learning to play instruments, such as the guitar, omnichord, shakers, bells and drums; composing original songs or melodies; drawing under the inspiration of musical pieces; playing music on the inspiration of a drawing (the child's own, another child's or a printed painting); listening to special musical tones or chords (e.g., electronic music, Indian gongs, or even vibrations produced by tones) [80]. The sessions may last from 15 minutes to one hour, and may be conducted in individual sessions, even at the patient's bedside, or in groups, which may be open also to family members and other visitors.

Music therapy was shown to be of great help in reducing the distress of children undergoing painful medical procedures [81, 82]. A study with 65 pediatric hematology/oncology patients whose mean age was 7 years (range: birth to 17) showed significant improvement in the children's ratings of their mood in terms of the "faces pain scale" (a pictorial scale of faces depicting various degrees of pain, including numbers, colors and definitions) from pre-to post-music therapy, whereas the parents perceived an improved play performance after music therapy in preschoolers and adolescents. Notably, 49% of the parents in this study said that the music therapy brought them comfort and reduced their own anxiety [83]. In children with myeloid leukemia, music therapy was observed to promote the child's behavior from being "just a patient" into playing temporarily a more active social role [84]. Playing music for children in isolation (in the course of bone marrow transplantation) is of particular help because it decreases their loneliness and sense of detachment from the world [85–87]. It may even help reduce anxieties in terminally sick children [88, 89]. Music therapy was also observed to promote more engaging behaviors in the children than other activities, such as unstructured play or reading taped storybooks with the therapist [90].

EXAMPLE

K., a 13-year-old girl diagnosed with lymphoma, suffered badly from the disease and the treatments. She became so distressed by the changes in her appearance caused by the treatments that she refused to have any contacts with others. One purpose of music was to provide the girl with diversion and relaxation in the course of chemotherapy. While listening to the music she loved (ballet music with clear rhythm and musical patterns), she was encouraged to make a fantasy voyage by using imagery. The voyage led her to distant worlds that opened a window to dreams and space. Another function of music in this case was to enable K. to meet with her friends at school. She agreed to meet them when they were all listening to their preferred music.

Singing and Chorus

Songs and singing as therapeutic means share a few elements with music therapy but also differ from it in basic respects. First, the elements of singing are more intrinsically human than musical components. Second, producing singing sounds involves activation of a bodily organ, unlike musical sounds whose production does not necessarily depend on the body. Due to the origin of singing in the human body, listening to singing sounds activates the listener's body in a way different from listening to musical sounds. Since singing is a product of the human voice, it may be expected to be related most intimately to the expression of emotions. Thus, it is natural for human beings to express their joy, suffering, pain, even despair through sounds, which are often not words but rather vowels or combinations of sounds mimicking the emotion (e.g., Aah, Ooh, Oiy, Rrrr). When combined and sounded in a kind of protracted melody (e.g., undulating sound, repetitive sounds in staccato), these moans and other sound combinations form the elements of singing. This affinity of sounds to emotions may constitute the understructure which promotes the therapeutic use of singing [91, 92]. Further, since singing and composing songs do not require accessories or even training (at least not at the basic level), singing provides a ready means for creative expression [93]. A highly specific property of singing that enhances its therapeutic potential is the fact that it uses the human voice in two capacities—expressive and communicative. Notably, the two functions may use nonverbal or verbal means or both, so that reactivity and interaction can be both verbal and nonverbal [94]. Thus, when singing, the patient may use words or, for that matter, sounds or nonsense syllables at his or her discretion—all the time, part of the time or not at all.

Singing may be used with individual patients or with groups, in which case it assumes the form of a chorus. Singing in groups strongly enhances the community feeling of the sick children on the ward and greatly reduces the sense of loneliness. Family members, other patients, and friends may be invited to join the session. A child may be induced to listen to recorded singing or to singing by the therapist or an actual singer, and may be encouraged to join the singing to the extent that he or she wishes or is able to. Often children prefer to sing on their own. Of course, the quality of the singing plays no role at all. The singing may take place anywhere on the ward or outside it and often does not need any accessories [95, 96].

Dance and Movement Therapy

The American Dance Therapy Association defines dance or movement therapy as "the psychotherapeutic use of movement as a process which furthers the emotional, cognitive and physical integration of the individual." In recent years more specific goals were developed in regard to helping patients, including oncology patients and children [97]. Dance therapy relies almost exclusively on nonverbal expression, and uses for therapy mainly muscular and kinesthetic responses. The special focus of dance therapy is bodily movements. This is of particular importance in the case of pediatric oncology patients whose body image may be impaired following surgery and oncological treatments. Therapeutic use of movements may restore the children's contact with the body and lead them to accept their body despite the changes it has undergone temporarily or permanently [98].

Dance therapy may be conducted for single patients or groups. When children dance in groups, there may or may not be coordination between them. When each child in a group dances for himself or herself without coordination in the movements of the children in the group, the outcome resembles "a collective monologue" in the sphere of language [99]. The extent of the movements may also vary greatly. Dance therapy may be enacted in space, with the child moving in space as much as the body enables or as minimally as the child is able and willing to move. Dance therapy may not involve changing location in space but be focused only on bodily movements. Thus, dancing may involve the whole body or parts of it, so that sometimes only the fingers or eyelids dance. The dance may even be enacted only in fantasy, when the child is unable or unwilling to move, or simply too exhausted to move. Hence, dance therapy may be performed in the child's bed.

Dance therapy may use music as background or not. The dance may be performed according to the child's own rhythm and patterns or according to externally presented rhythm, with or without musical tones. When the melodious aspect of music is distracting for the child, rhythm alone may be used. Some children find it beneficial to move in time with rhythm that is familiar to them or precisely unfamiliar, even bizarre.

Dance therapy may be expressive to varying degrees. It is completely expressive when the movements are free, improvised by the child as he or she goes along, and do not conform to any code or style of motion taught to the child or agreed upon prior to the dance. Often at least some elements of diverse motional codes or styles are incorporated into the child's dance. Some therapies focus primarily on the performance of prescribed movements, which may follow distinct dance styles (e.g., Latin American or Indian or local folk dancing) or specific movement codes reflecting a conceptual or symbolic tradition (e.g., yoga), a particular theory or a physiological conception (e.g., Alexander, Aikido, Feldenkrais,

Hanna Somatic, Chi Kung and Tai Chi Chuan) [94, 98, 100, 101]. Movement therapies of this kind offer the patient primarily renewed contact and awareness of one's body and an enhanced sense of bodily control.

Movement therapy may also include the special practices of swimming or splashing in water, taking hot or cold baths, and massage (insofar as it is medically approved) which resembles passive movement. These motional practices may be enjoyable for the child and contribute to restoring his or her acceptance of the body and mastery over one's body following the changes in body image in the course of treatments.

Animal-Assisted and Pet-Facilitated Therapies

The ancient Greeks had already recognized the psychological effects of contact with animals, but the earliest documented reports of the use of animals in therapy date from the late eighteenth century in the UK and beginnings of the twentieth century in the USA. The rapidly accumulating evidence shows the beneficial impact of contact with animals on patients with different diagnoses, regardless of where the patients stay. Animal-assisted therapy has been reported to be particularly effective with children and adolescents [102].

There are various forms of practicing animal-assisted therapy. For example, the child may own a pet or actually help to take care of an animal, alone or as part of a team of children, usually under the guidance or active participation of an adult, who may be the therapist. The child may interact with the animal, touching it or talking to it, in the presence of the therapist. The child may simply watch the animal and learn about it and its behavior, for example, fish in an aquarium. A pet may be adopted by the ward as "our animal" without the active participation of the children in taking care of it. The adopted pet will not be allowed on the ward, but may stay somewhere else on the hospital grounds or at home with the child or children going to visit it.

The major observed effects of animal-assisted therapy were increase in trust, social contacts, cooperation and readiness to communicate; reduction of anxiety, depression, distress, loneliness, stress and the sense of threat; increase in relaxation; enhanced responsiveness to the sensory environment; increased physical activity; promotion of responsibility; and improvement in confidence, self-image and self-esteem [103, 104].

Up to now there has been a relatively limited use of animal-assisted therapy in oncology, mainly because of fear of infection in patients with suppressed immune system function. However, even though the experience is limited, the results showed that contact with animals markedly decreased depression and distress in oncology patients in regular hospital units [105, 106] and hospices [107, 108]. There is an increasing number of anecdotal reports about the introduction of animals into pediatric oncology units while observing adequate precautions to prevent infections, for example, restricting contact with the animals merely to observing them, communicating with them without touching them, and in general avoiding any physical contact with the animals.

Animal-assisted therapy may be expected to be particularly effective in the context of pediatric oncology because it focuses on social interaction in its basic and simplest form. It offers the chance for forming and maintaining a simple companionship, a bond based on give and take without the damaging intervention of prior conceptions, biases, and emotions, such as shame, guilt and sense of inferiority. The contact with the animal is mostly nonverbal and consists in interaction for its own sake. One gives as much or as little as one can give and is appreciated for this. Hence, this kind of therapy provides the child the chance for feeling accepted despite limitations, such as fatigue, sadness, sense of restricted ability to give, and changed body image. The contact with the animal gives the children the feeling that they are needed and appreciated for what they are. The animal may become a friend indeed because it is a friend in need.

Further contributions of animal-assisted therapy are that through the animal the ward or the sick room gains an element of normality and everyday-life atmosphere, which may be important for children hospitalized for longer periods of time or whose daily routine has been ruptured in other ways. Last but not least, animals and pets may give the sick child something to think about, possibly fantasize about, outside the range of the disease and the treatments. Being preoccupied with the animal even for limited periods of time enables dissociation from the painful and anxiety-evoking treatment.

Parties and Outdoor Entertainment

It has become traditional in pediatric oncology wards to organize parties, shows, picnics, outings, and other forms of entertainment, for the children, considering their state of health. Children who are confined to the bed or ward are entertained in the spot where they have to stay, whereas others who may be freer to move are taken outside the hospital into the community, on trips and even to other countries. These entertainments are always planned in cooperation with and under the guidance of the medical staff. Moreover, members of the medical staff participate in these events mainly for medical reasons in order to make sure that the health of the children is not compromised in any way and to take care of any unusual medical occurrence.

Since such entertainment events are so common, it is likely that they contribute in some form to the well-being of the children. The reasons seem clear. First, the explicit goal of such events is to provide fun and entertainment, at least in partial compensation to the children for the suffering they have been undergoing. Second, elements of different forms of art therapy are often incorporated into these events, such as play, humor, clowns, jesters, magicians, music, dance, singing and storytelling. These art therapeutic components exert their beneficial effect also in this setting. Third, since some of the restrictions and rules that govern the children's behavior are lifted on these occasions (e.g., one may scream, laugh loudly, throw things around, be impertinent), the children may enjoy a cathartic effect to counterbalance their frustrations and anger. Fourth, on these occasions the children get the opportunity to interact with the medical staff on a more day-to-day level, not necessarily with less distance, but often without the role-bound limitations of "doctor" and "patient." This experience may help the children accept the need for compliance in the regular hospital routine. And last but not least, the entertainment occasions sound loud and clear the encouraging message that "life goes on" and soon the child may perhaps be able to rejoin it.

Conclusion

This chapter has presented a variegated colorful panorama of a great number of therapeutic modes and media, most of which go under the name of "art therapy." Though each of the therapies is unique, they share a number of characteristics. The shared elements concern the goals, the therapeutic processes, and the manner of application or practicing.

A variety of goals are listed by the different therapies, including mostly palliation of physical symptoms, improvement of mood, boosting of body image and increasing self-esteem. Despite differences in formulation, it is evident that all the goals boil down to improving the child's quality of life, and do not refer to survival or improving the recovery chances of the child.

The therapeutic processes involved in art therapeutic media were summarized aptly by Luzzatto and Gabriel [6] as 'the six "C"s': Catharsis by creating conditions for externalizing pent-up emotions; Creativity by promoting self-expression through artistic media; Communication by expressing for others what one feels and how one perceives reality; Containment by providing legitimacy to attitudes and emotions difficult to acknowledge as part of oneself; Connections by enabling integration between different forces within oneself and outside oneself; and Changing the image by facilitating transformations in meanings.

Finally, there are many similarities in the manner in which art therapies are practiced. First, the approach is mostly multidisciplinary and consists in applying several art therapeutic media jointly in the same session or in a sequence with the same child or group of children. It seems to be the rare case when art therapy is focused on one medium exclusively. This seems to be rooted in the orientation of art therapies towards the person as a whole, including his or her emotional, cognitive, physiological, emotional and behavioral needs [109]. The holistic orientation may create the desire to address as many of the child's needs as possible. Second, the application of art therapeutic means is more often tailored to the specific needs and problems of the patient as conceptualized in the "here and now" rather than adhering to a strict structured protocol. There seems to be a great sensitivity in art therapists to changing situations, needs, interests and problems of the patient. Hence the tendency to use a variety of art therapeutic means for attaining basically the same goals. Third, the art therapies use artistic means to attain goals other than art, without pretending to teach the arts for their own sake or to turn the children into artists at present or in the future. Fourth, in many of the art therapies there is an interplay between the more passive and more active forms of application, for example, between viewing films and producing films, between reading stories and inventing stories, between listening to songs and singing. This interplay introduces an element of tension into the practice of art therapy but widens immensely the potential of the medium to appeal to the child and awaken his or her response. Fifth, art therapies focus on the use of nonverbal means, which are appropriate for children and promote their expressiveness. And last but not least, art therapies seem to be open to incorporating new media and widening the scope of the applied therapies. At present we are witnessing the expansion of art therapy into the domains of computerized art and video art. In future, we may witness the incorporation of virtual reality media, electronic music, or installation art. However, in art therapy the message is not the medium. Rather, the message underlying and inspiring the diverse present and future forms of art therapy is that even though the child is sick, he or she is still a child, and we have to do all in our power to keep it that way.

Acknowledgments

The authors would like to thank all those who have contributed to this chapter: Tlalit Asna, Ofra Levanoni, AnaLia Magen, Michal M. Kreitler, Lorna Saint Ange, Elsa Segev-Shoham, Herzel Gavriel, Yoseph Horowitz, Dina Soberano, Jennifer Zellas, Drs Yoseph Horovitz and Herzel Gavriel, and Michal Gressel.

References

1. Hilgard JR, LeBaron S. *Hypnotherapy of Pain in Children with Cancer*. Los Altos, CA: William Kaufmann, 1984.
2. Jay SM, Elliott CH, Woody PD, *et al*. An investigation of cognitive-behavior therapy combined with oral valium for children undergoing painful medical procedures. *Health Psychology* 1991;**10**:317–322.
3. Montanaro RL.Creative art therapy programs for pediatric oncology patients: a comparative case study. Master's thesis, the arts and administration program of the University of Oregon, 2007.
4. Rudloff LM. An illustrated study of a young man with cancer. *American Journal of Art Therapy* 1985;**24**:49–62.
5. Prager A. Pediatric art therapy; strategies and applications. *Art Therapy* 1995;**12**:32–38.
6. Luzzatto P, Gabriel B. Art psychotherapy. In: Holland JC (ed.) *Psycho-oncology*. New York: Oxford University Press, 1998; pp. 743–757.
7. Malchiodi C. *Expressive Therapies*. New York: The Guilford Press, 2005.
8. Kunzendorf RG. *Mental Imagery*. New York: Plenum Publishing, 1991.
9. Klein NC. *Healing Images for Children: Teaching Relaxation and Guided Imagery to Children Facing Cancer and Other Serious Illnesses*. Watertown, WI: Inner Coaching, 1999.
10. National Cancer Institute. *Young People with Cancer: A Handbook for Parents*. U.S. Department of Health and Human Services, 2001. Available from: http://www.nci.nih.gov/cancertopics/youngpeople (accessed September 2006).
11. Hockenberry MH. Guided imagery as a coping measure for children with cancer. *Journal of the Association of Pediatric Oncology Nurses* 1989;**6**:29.
12. Hockenberry-Eaton M, Barrera P, Brown M, *et al*. Pain management in children with cancer. Texas Cancer Council, 1999. Available at: www.childcancerpain.org.
13. Kleiber C, Harper DC. Effects of distraction on children's pain and distress during medical procedures: a meta-analysis. *Nursing Research* 1999;**48**:41–49.
14. Liossi C, White P, Hatira P. A randomized clinical trial of a brief hypnosis intervention to control venepuncture-related pain of pediatric cancer patients. *Pain* 2009;**142**:255–263.
15. Liossi C. *Procedure Related Cancer Pain in Children*. Oxford: Radcliffe, 2002.
16. French GM, Painter EC, Coury DL. Blowing away shot pain: a technique for pain management during immunization. *Pediatrics* 1994;**93**:384–388.
17. Zeltzer L, LeBaron S. Hypnosis and nonhypnotic techniques for reduction of pain and anxiety during painful procedures in children and adolescents with cancer. *Journal of Pediatrics* 1982;**101**:1032–1035.
18. Cotanch P, Hockenberry M, Herman S. Self-hypnosis, antiemetic therapy in children receiving chemotherapy. *Oncological Nursing Forum* 1985;**12**:41–46.
19. Genuis ML. The use of hypnosis in helping cancer patients control anxiety, pain and emesis: a review of recent empirical studies. *American Journal of Clinical Hypnosis* 1995;**37**:316–325.
20. Kuttner L, Bowman M, Teasdale M. Psychological treatment of distress, pain and anxiety for young children with cancer. *Journal of Developmental & Behavioral Pediatrics* 1988;**9**:374–382.
21. Olness K. Imagery (self-hypnosis) as adjunct therapy in childhood cancer: clinical experience with 25 patients. *American Journal of Pediatric Hematology/Oncology* 1981;**3**:313–321.
22. Achtenberg J, Lawlis GF. *Imagery and Disease*. Champaign, IL: Institute for Personality and Ability Testing, 1984.
23. Schneider J, Smith CS, Whitcher S. *The Relationship of Mental Imagery to White Blood Cell (Neutrophil) Function: Experimental Studies of Normal Subjects*. Memo. East Lansing, MI: Michigan State University, 1983.
24. Magen A, Ben Arush M. Computerized art therapy and guided imagery for pediatric oncology and hematology. *Medical and Pediatric Oncology* 1999;**23**:151.
25. Sourkes BM. Truth to life: art therapy with pediatric oncology patients and their siblings. *Journal of Psychosocial Oncology* 1991;**9**:81–96.
26. Jones VM. Mask making as art therapy with pediatric oncology patients. *Dissertation Abstracts International: Section B: The Sciences and Engineering* 1997;**57**:5330.
27. Collie K. Computer support for distance art therapy. Paper presented at Human Factors in Computing '98. CHI98, Los Angeles, CA, USA, April 18–24, 1998.
28. Collie K. Internet art therapy. Paper presented at Discipline and Deviance: Genders, Technologies, Machines. Duke University, Durham, NC, USA, October 2–4, 1998.
29. Malchiodi CA. *Art Therapy and Computer Technology: A Virtual Studio of Possibilities*. London: Jessica Kingsley, 2000.
30. Gericot C, Perrignon J. *La Porte Bleue: Autoportraits d'enfants atteints de Cancer*. Paris: Institut Gustave Roussy/Les Arènes, 2000.
31. Remen RN. *Kitchen Table Wisdom: Stories that Heal*. New York: Putnam, 1996.
32. Borden W. Narrative perspectives in psychosocial intervention following adverse life events. *Social Work* 1992;**37**:135–141.
33. Gardner AR. *Therapeutic Communication with Children: The Mutual Storytelling Technique*. Northvale, NC: Jason Aronson, 1986.
34. Mair M. Kelly, Bannister and a story-telling psychology. *International Journal of Personal Construct Therapy* 1989;**2**:1–14.
35. Cothern N. Healing with books: literature for children dealing with health issues. *Ohio Reading Teacher* 1994;**28**:8–15.

36. Noonan W. Healing tales: the metaphors of folktales help cancer patients in their therapy. *Creation Spirituality* 1992;**4**:28–30.

37. Leedy JJ. *Poetry as Healer: Mending the Troubled Mind.* New York: Vanguard Press, 1985.

38. Lerner A. *Poetry in the Therapeutic Experience*, 2nd edn. St. Louis: MMB Music, 1994.

39. Hilgard JR, LeBaron S. Relief of anxiety and pain in children and adolescents with cancer: Quantitative measures and clinical observation. *International Journal of Clinical and Experimental Hypnosis* 1982;**4**:417–442.

40. Gorelick K. Poetry therapy. In: Malchiodi C (ed.) *Expressive Therapies*. New York: The Guilford Press, 2005; pp. 117–140.

41. Pennebaker JW, Kiecolt-Glaser J, Glaser R. Disclosure of traumas and immune function: health implications for psychotherapy. *Journal of Consulting and Clinical Psychology* 1988;**56**:239–245.

42. Booth RJ, Petrie KJ, Pennebaker JW. Changes in circulating lymphocyte numbers following emotional disclosure: evidence of buffering? *Stress Medicine* 1997;**13**: 23–29.

43. Esterling BA, LaAbate L, Murray E, *et al.* Empirical foundations for writing in prevention and psychotherapy: mental and physical health outcome. *Clinical Psychology Review* 1999;**19**:79–96.

44. Lahad M. *All Life Stretches before You*. Haifa, Israel: Nord, 1992 (in Hebrew).

45. Oppenheim D, Pittolo V, Gericot C, *et al.* A writing workshop for children with cancer. *Archives of Disease in Childhood* 2008;**93**:708–709.

46. Manne S, Bakeman R, Jacobsen P, *et al.* An analysis of an intervention to reduce children's distress during venipuncture. *Health Psychology* 1994;**13**:556–566.

47. Redd WH, Jacobsen PB, Die-Trill M, *et al.* Cognitive-attentional distraction in the control of conditioned nausea in pediatric cancer patients receiving chemotherapy. *Journal of Consulting and Clinical Psychology* 1987;**55**: 391–395.

48. Kolko DJ, Rickard-Figueroa JL. Effects of video games on the adverse corollaries of chemotherapy in pediatric oncology patients: a single-case analysis. *Journal of Consulting and Clinical Psychology* 1985;**53**:223–228.

49. Katz ER, Kellerman J, Ellenberg L. Hypnosis in the reduction of acute pain and distress in children with cancer. *Journal of Pediatric Psychology* 1987;**12**:379–394.

50. LeBaron S, Zeltzer LK. Behavioral intervention for reducing chemotherapy-related nausea and vomiting in adolescents with cancer. *Journal of Adolescent Health Care* 1984;**5**:178–182.

51. McGrath PA, de Veber LL. The management of acute pain evoked by medical procedures in children with cancer. *Journal of Pain and Symptom Management* 1986;**1**:145–150.

52. Wall VJ, Womack W. Hypnotic versus active cognitive strategies for alleviation of procedural distress in pediatric oncology patients. *American Journal of Clinical Hypnosis* 1989;**31**:181–190.

53. Walker C. Use of art and play therapy in pediatric oncology. *Journal of Pediatric Oncology Nursing* 1989;**6**:121–126.

54. Cooper SE, Blitz JT. A therapeutic play group for hospitalized children with cancer. *Journal of Psychosocial Oncology* 1985;**3**:23–37.

55. Lingnell L, Dunn L. Group play: wholeness and healing for the hospitalized child. In: Sweeney DS, Horneyer LE (eds) *The Handbook of Group Play Therapy: How to Do it, How it Works, Whom it's Best For.* San Francisco, CA: Jossey-Bass/Pfeiffer, 1999; pp. 359–374.

56. Manheimer L. Harry: A 10-year-old's last summer. In: Oremland EK, Oremland JD (eds) *Protecting the Emotional Development of the Ill Child: The Essence of the Child Life Profession.* Madison, CT: Psychosocial Press, 2000; pp. 59–71.

57. McCall J. Dana: A 7-year-old girl with leukemia. In: Oremland EK, Oremland JD (eds) *Protecting the Emotional Development of the Ill Child: The Essence of the Child Life Profession.* Madison, CT: Psychosocial Press, 2000; pp. 73–84.

58. Tacata J. Brief encounters. In: EK Oremland, JD Oremland (eds) *Protecting the Emotional Development of the Ill Child: The Essence of the Child Life Profession.* Madison, CT: Psychosocial Press, 2000; pp. 85–91.

59. Goodman RF. Childhood cancer and the family: Case of Tim, age 6, and follow-up at age 15 In: Webb NB (ed.) *Play Therapy with Children in Crisis: Individual, Group, and Family Treatment*, 2nd edn. New York: Guilford Press, 1999; pp. 380–404.

60. Clayton GM. *Living Pictures of the Self: Applications of Role Theory in Professional Practice and Daily Living.* Victoria, Australia: ICA Press, 1993.

61. Moreno JL. *Psychodrama*, Vols 1–3, 4th edn. McLean, VA: ASGPP, 1994.

62. Dunne PB. *The Narrative Therapist and the Arts: Expanding Possibilities Through Drama, Movements, Puppets, Masks and Drawings.* Los Angeles, CA: Drama Therapy Institute of Los Angeles, 1992.

63. Landy R. Drama therapy and psychodrama. In: Malchiodi C. (ed.) *Expressive Therapies*. New York: The Guilford Press, 2005; pp. 90–116.

64. DuHamel KN, Johnson Vickberg SM, Redd WH. Behavioral interventions in pediatric oncology. In: Holland JC (ed.) *Psycho-oncology*. New York: Oxford University Press, 1998; pp. 962–977.

65. Ancelin-Schuetzenberger A. The drama of the seriously ill patient: fifteen years' experience of psychodrama and cancer. In: Holmes P, Karp M. (eds.), *Psychodrama: Inspiration and Technique.* New York: Tavistock/Routledge, 1991; pp. 203–224.

66. Henderson SW, Rosario K. But seriously: clowning in children's mental health. *Journal of American Academy of Child and Adolescent Psychiatry* 2008;**47**:983–986.

67. Lefcourt RM. *Humor: The Psychology of Living Buoyantly*. New York: Kluwer Academic/Plenum Publishers, 2001.

68. Martin RA. Humor, laughter and physical health: methodological issues and research findings. *Psychological Bulletin* 2001;**127**:504–519.

69. Vaillant GE. Adaptive mental mechanisms: their role in a positive psychology. *American Psychologist* 2001;**55**:89–98.

70. LaRue E, Zigler E. Psychological adjustment of seriously ill children. *Journal of the American Academy of Child Psychiatry* 1986;**25**:708–712.

71. Dowling JS. Sense of humor, childhood cancer stressors, and outcomes of psychosocial adjustment, immune function, and infection. *Dissertation Abstracts International, Section B: The Sciences and Engineering* 2001;**61**:3506.

72. Buckman ES. *Handbook of Humor: Clinical Applications in Psychotherapy*. Melbourne, FL: Krieger, 1994.
73. Kreitler S, Drechsler I, Kreitler H. How to kill jokes cognitively? The meaning structure of jokes. *Semiotica* 1988;**68**:297–319.
74. Kreitler H, Kreitler S. Dependence of laughter on cognitive strategies. *Merrill-Palmer Quarterly of Behavior and Development* 1970;**16**:163–177.
75. Bruscia KE. *Case Studies in Music Therapy*. Barcelona, Spa in: Barcelona Publishers, 1991.
76. Bunt L. *Music Therapy: An Art Beyond Words*. London: Routledge, 1998.
77. Kreitler H, Kreitler S. *Psychology of the Arts*. Durham, NC: Duke University Press, 1972.
78. Forinash M. Music therapy. In: Malchiodi C. (ed.) *Expressive Therapies*. New York: The Guilford Press, 2005, pp. 46–67.
79. Bonny H, Savary L. *Music and Your Mind: Listening with a New Consciousness*. New York: Harper & Row, 1973 (reprint 1990).
80. Lane D. Music therapy interventions with pediatric oncology patient. In: Froehlich MA (ed.) *Music Therapy with Hospitalized Children: Creative Arts Child Life Approach*. Cherry Hill, NJ: Jeffrey Books, 1996.
81. Hockenberry MJ, Bologna-Voughan S. Preparation for intrusive procedures using noninvasive techniques in children with cancer: state of the art vs new trends. *Cancer Nursing* 1985;**8**:97–102.
82. Malone A. The effects of live music on the distress of pediatric patients receiving intravenous starts, venipunctures, injections, and heel sticks. *Journal of Music Therapy* 1996;**23**:19–33.
83. Barrera ME, Rykov MH, Doyle SL. The effects of interactive music therapy on hospitalized children with cancer: a pilot study. *Psycho-Oncology* 2000;**11**:379–388.
84. Aasgaard T. An ecology of love: aspects of music therapy in the pediatric oncology environment. *Journal of Palliative Care* 2001;**17**:177–181.
85. Brodsky W. Music as an intervention for children with cancer in isolation rooms. *Music Therapy* 1989;**8**:17–34.
86. Kuttner L. *A Child in Pain: How to Help, What to Do*. Point Roberts, WA: Hartley & Marks, 1996.
87. Pfaff V, Smith, KE, Gowan D. The effects of music assisted relaxation on the distress of pediatric cancer patients undergoing bone marrow aspirations. *Children's Health Care* 1989;**18**:232–236.
88. Fagan TS. Music therapy in the treatment of anxiety and fear in terminal pediatric patients. *Music Therapy* 1982;**2**:1.
89. Garrison WT, McQuiston S. *Chronic Illness during Childhood and Adolescence: Psychological Aspects*. Newbury Park, CA: Sage, 1989.
90. Robb SL. The effect of therapeutic music interventions on the behavior of hospitalized children in isolation: developing a contextual support model of music therapy. *Journal of Music Therapy* 2000;**37**:118–146.
91. Bailey L. The use of songs in music therapy with cancer patients and their families. *Music Therapy* 1984;**4**:5–17.
92. Dileo C. Songs for living: the use of songs in the treatment of oncology patients. In: Dileo C. (ed.) *Music Therapy and Medicine: Theoretical and Clinical Applications*. Silver Spring, MD: AMTA, 1999; pp. 151–166.
93. Turry A, Turry AE. Creative song improvisations with children and adults with cancer. In: Dileo C. (ed.) *Music Therapy and Medicine: Theoretical and Clinical Applications*. Silver Spring, MD: AMTA, 1999; pp. 85–91.
94. Newham P. *Using Voice and Movement in Therapy: The Practical Application of Voice Movement Therapy*. London: Jessica Kingsley, 1999.
95. Logis M, Turry A. Singing my way through it: facing the cancer pain and fear. In: Hibben J. (ed.) *Inside Music Therapy: Client Experiences*. Phoenixville, PA: Barcelona, 1999; pp. 97–117.
96. O'Callaghan C. Pain, music creativity and music therapy in palliative care. *The American Journal of Hospice and Palliative Care* 1996;**13**:43–49.
97. Loman S. Dance/movement therapy. In: Malchiodi C (ed.) *Expressive Therapies*. New York: The Guilford Press, 2005; pp. 68–89.
98. Levy FJ, Fried JP, Leventhal F. *Dance and Other Expressive Art Therapies: When Words Are Not Enough*. London: Routledge, 1995.
99. Piaget J. *The Language and Thought of the Child* (Trans. Marjorie and Ruth Gabain). New York: Humanities Press, 1959.
100. Behar-Horenstein LS, Ganet-Sigel J. *The Art and Practice of Dance/Movement Therapy*. Boston, MA: Pearson Custom Publishing, 1999.
101. Halprin A. *Dance as a Healing Art: Returning to Health Through Movement and Imagery*. Mendocino, CA: Life-Rhythm, 2000.
102. Kale M. Kids and animals: a comforting hospital combination. *Interactions* 1992;**10**:17–21.
103. Carpenter S. Therapeutic roles of animals. *Journal of the American Veterinary Medical Association* 1997;**211**: 154–155.
104. Willis DA. Animal therapy. *Rehabilitation Nursing* 1997;**2**:78–81.
105. Muschel IJ. Pet therapy with terminal cancer patients. *Social Casework* 1984;**65**:451–458.
106. Raveis VH, Mesagno F, Karus D, *et al.* Pet ownership as a protective factor supporting the emotional well-being of cancer patients and their family members. Memorial Sloan–Kettering Cancer Center, Department of Social Work Research Unit (mimeograph), 1993.
107. Chinner TL, Dalziel FR. An exploratory study on the viability and efficacy of pet-facilitated therapy project within a hospice. *Journal of Palliative Care* 1991;**7**:3–20.
108. Slavin P. A sense for who needs them. *Hospice* 1996;**7**: 21–26.
109. Kreitler H, Kreitler S. Art therapy: Quo vadis? *Art Psychotherapy* 1978;**5**:199–209.

14

Palliative Care for Children with Advanced Cancer

Stefan J. Friedrichsdorf, Lonnie Zeltzer

Introduction

More than 12,000 children and adolescents 0–19 years of age are diagnosed with cancer each year in the US [1, 2]. The large majority of them are fortunately cured of their malignancy with more than 80% of children with cancer alive five years after diagnosis, compared with about 62% in the mid-1970s [3]. However, an overwhelming number of children experience considerable suffering during their cancer treatment and unfortunately not all survive; cancer remains the leading cause of death for children with life-limiting conditions in the United States [4]. A total of 34,500 childhood cancer deaths were reported in the USA during 1990–2004. In 2004 alone (last available data), 2,223 children and adolescents died due to a malignancy. Among these, leukemias were the most common diagnoses (25.5%), followed by brain and other nervous system neoplasms (25.0%) [4].

Comprehensive palliative care is the expected standard of care for patients with advanced illness [5, 6], however, access to, and availability of palliative care expertise for the majority of children with life-threatening conditions, are still lacking compared with adult services. In the US, the vast majority of infants, children, and teenagers with advanced illnesses who are near the end of life do not have access to interdisciplinary pediatric palliative care (PPC) services either in their community or at the nearest children's hospital.

Definition of Palliative Care

This chapter will present a philosophy of cancer care that promotes communication between providers, patients (regardless of age), and parents throughout the illness with the goal of achieving the best possible quality of life for the child and family. PPC provides solace for infants, children and teenagers suffering from a life-threatening or a life-limiting condition regardless of whether curative treatments succeed or fail, many of which continue for years.

According to the Association for Children's Palliative Care (ACT) and the British Royal College of Pediatrics and Child Health [7]:

[PPC is] an active and total approach to care, embracing physical, emotional, social and spiritual elements. It focuses on enhancement of quality of life (QOL) for the child and support for the family and includes management of distressing symptoms, provision of respite and care through [disease], death and bereavement.

In the words of an ill child: "Palliative care no longer means helping children die well, it means helping children and their families to live well, and then, when the time is certain, to help them die gently" (Mattie Stepanek, 1990–2007) [8].

Our emphasis will be on including communication as a primary tenet of palliative care, and on integrating palliative care along the entire disease trajectory, whether the anticipated outcome is cure, chronic disease or death. Pediatric Palliative Care usually starts at the diagnosis of a life-threatening conditions, in conjunction with curative therapies supporting the primary care team, and follows the entire trajectory of the disease.

History of Palliative Care

Palliative Care was first describe by Homer in *The Iliad* around 800 BC, performed by the army physicians Podaleirios and Machaon, for Erypylos, who had

Pediatric Psycho-oncology: Psychosocial Aspects and Clinical Interventions, Second Edition.
Edited by Shulamith Kreitler, Myriam Weyl Ben-Arush and Andrés Martin.
© 2012 John Wiley & Sons, Ltd. Published 2012 by John Wiley & Sons, Ltd.

received a lethal injury during a fight (Homer: *Iliad*, XI. Book, 809–848) [9].

During the Roman Empire, a building was erected in Epidauros in Greece especially for the care of dying people in 50 AD.

Some accounts associate the name of the early Umayyad caliph Al-Walid I (668–715), who ruled from 705 to 715, with the founding of a hospice, possibly a leprosarium, in Damascus, Syria (Alia A. K. Al-Ghunaim, personal communication, 2008) [10].

In medieval Europe, hospices (often inside monasteries) provided care to people on pilgrim routes. The Latin word *hospes* initially meant "stranger," but with time evolved to *hospitium*, which at first described the warmth between guest and host, and later the building where this was experienced [11].

The modern era of hospice and palliative care stems from the dedication and enthusiasm of an English physician, Dame Cicely Saunders. She had previously trained as a nurse, and before entering medical school, worked as a voluntary nurse at St Luke's Home for the Dying Poor in London. After qualifying from medical school, Saunders worked at St Joseph's Hospital in Hackney, London, where she explored the use of opioids to achieve pain control in dying patients. She discovered that regular doses of opioids in higher doses than were then standard practice could relieve patients' pain and allow them to talk openly about their illness. Saunders wrote and taught about her experiences, and by 1967 had persuaded the National Health Service to support the building of St Christopher's Hospice in Sydenham, England.

In North America, nurses and physicians became interested in the ethos of palliative care at St Christopher's. In 1974, funded by the National Cancer Institute, the Connecticut Hospice began offering home-based care. The same year, in New York, a team of specialists in care of the dying started a consulting service at St Luke's Hospital. In 1975, Mount established the Palliative Care Service at The Royal Victoria Hospital, Montreal. Hospice and palliative care were thus demonstrated to be concepts that could be practiced in very varied settings [11].

Sister Francis Domenica founded in 1982 the first stationary free-standing children's hospice, "Helen House," in Oxford, UK, which then prompted development of numerous care models for children with life-limiting and terminal conditions worldwide. Free-standing Children's Hospices (usually inpatient facilities with 8–12 beds) now exist in many countries, including Australia, Canada, Costa Rica, Germany, Great Britain, Poland, and the

USA. Palliative home care services were introduced in the late 1970s, 1980s and 1990s in Costa Rica, Poland, Ukraine, the United Kingdom, the USA and other countries.

The first inpatient pediatric palliative care unit in the USA was opened at St Mary's Hospital for Children in Bayside, New York in 1985 [12]. Initially the majority of admissions were children with chronic disorders, but as AIDS became common among inner city children, the program started to care for affected families, as well as children with cancer and other forms of terminal illness.

In 2011, in the USA and Canada there are now more than 35 advanced hospital-based PPC services available, four of them offering PPC fellowships (Akron, OH, Boston, MA, Minneapolis, MN, and Philadelphia, PA). Free standing-respite homes ("Children's Hospice") are found in San Francisco, Phoenix, Vancouver, Montreal (with more being at different stages of realization) and there are various services providing pediatric palliative home care.

Extent of Need for Pediatric Palliative Care for Children with Cancer

Although the prognosis for children with cancer has improved considerably over the past four decades, the disease remains the leading cause of non-accidental death in childhood. Sadly, advances in the control of symptoms in children dying of cancer have not kept pace with treatment directed at curing the underlying disease. In two retrospective studies of bereaved parents of 221 pediatric cancer patients conducted by Wolfe *et al.*, the majority of distressing symptoms (such as pain, dyspnea and nausea/vomiting) were not treated, and when treated, therapy was commonly ineffective [5, 13].

Barriers to the Provision of Pediatric Palliative Care

There are assumptions and barriers which may hinder the implementation of PPC into the care of a child with cancer. Here are some of the main assumptions.

Assumption #1: Pediatric Palliative Care Starts When Curative Treatments Stop

Pediatric palliative care may erroneously be considered to commence only when curative treatment stops and/or when a child is close to dying.

The traditional model of palliative care has represented the relief of symptoms to be the major goal of treatment only when aggressive therapy directed at a cure has been unsuccessful. The overall improvement in prognosis in childhood cancer, and the enormous emotional issues involved in trying to save a child's life can prevent both caregivers and parents from abandoning cancer-directed therapy. Pursuit of intensive cancer-directed therapy can overshadow attention to quality of life and symptom control, which can result in substantial suffering during the last phase of a child's life.

However, it is often not possible for parents and/ or the child to forgo further cancer-directed therapy, and this should not be required in order to achieve optimal palliative care. The need to ensure that everything possible has been done may be the only way that some parents can live and cope with their child's death [14].

The World Health Organization (WHO) [15] defines Palliative Care as follows:

Palliative care is an approach that improves the quality of life of patients and their families facing the problem associated with life-threatening illness, through the prevention and relief of suffering by means of early identification and impeccable assessment and treatment of pain and other problems, physical, psychosocial and spiritual.

Palliative care:

- Provides relief from pain and other distressing symptoms.
- Affirms life and regards dying as a normal process.
- Intends neither to hasten nor postpone death.
- Integrates the psychological and spiritual aspects of patient care.
- Offers a support system to help patients live as actively as possible until death.
- Offers a support system to help the family cope during the patients illness and in their own bereavement.
- Uses a team approach to address the needs of patients and their families, including bereavement counseling, if indicated.
- Will enhance quality of life, and may also positively influence the course of illness.
- Is applicable early in the course of illness, in conjunction with other therapies that are intended to prolong life, such as chemotherapy or radiation therapy, and includes those investigations needed to better understand and manage distressing clinical complications.

The WHO Definition of Palliative Care for Children, adapted, adds the following to the above [15].

Active total care of the child's body, mind and spirit, and also involves giving support to the family. Such care:

- Begins when illness is diagnosed, and continues regardless of whether or not a child receives treatment directed at the disease.
- Demands that health providers evaluate and alleviate a child's physical, psychological, and social distress.
- Requires a broad interdisciplinary approach.

- Includes the family and makes use of available community resources; it can be successfully implemented even if resources are limited.
- Can be provided in tertiary care facilities, in community health and hospice centers, and in children's homes.
- Should be developmentally appropriate and in accordance with family values.

Earlier recognition by both physicians and parents that the child had no realistic chance of cure led to a stronger emphasis on treatment to lessen suffering and integrate PPC in pediatric cancer patients [7]. PPC therefore starts at diagnosis of a life-threatening disease or life-limiting condition, continues through the trajectory of the illness, and does not equal end-of-life care (but certainly includes it). PPC extends beyond the child's death to the family during bereavement.

Assumption #2: Parents Have to Choose between "Fighting for a Cure" Or "Giving Up"

Parents and pediatric patients will often opt for continued treatment of the underlying cancer even when there is no realistic hope for cure [13, 16]. This is often motivated either by hope for a miracle, a desire to extend life, or a desire to palliate symptoms related to progressive disease. In discussions of treatment options with families, Wolfe *et al.* suggest the following statement, "The very nature of miracles is that they are rare. However, we have seen miracles, and they have occurred both on and off treatment" [17]. In other words, a child does not have to continue on cancer-directed therapy in order to preserve hope, especially when the therapy significantly impacts the child's remaining quality of life. Regardless, decisions regarding continued cancer-directed therapy need to be carefully considered, weighing the potential for life extension and impact on quality of life.

Caring for a dying child is emotionally very difficult. It may be particularly challenging for physicians and other caregivers to consider the integration of palliative care because this may be perceived as "giving up." More importantly, parental loss of a child is certainly considered to be the most difficult type of loss [18, 19]. As a result, the emotional cost of recognizing that a child may die impedes planning for optimal care and support.

Hope for cure and pediatric palliative care include each other. PPC translates into aggressive management to maintain or improve quality of life and children can graduate from palliative care. Despite the prevailing myth to the contrary, life-saving care and excellent symptom relief can be provided simultaneously.

Assumption #3: Pediatric Palliative Care Means "Giving Up Hope"

PPC explicitly does not mean giving up hope. In fact, in order to explore the family's goals of care a question such as "Tell me, what are you hoping for?" may be asked by the PPC clinician. Not infrequently families may respond with "Cure from cancer" or "A miracle." The clinician may respond "I hope this too—I'm with you. What else are you hoping for?" By following the avenue of hope further, families may wish for very aggressive pain and symptom management, the possibility to go outside or home, to hold their child more often, to have more family to visit, or many other things. Even when the underlying condition cannot be cured, PPC will not give up hope.

Assumption #4: Pediatric Palliative Care Means "Doing Nothing"

A clinician trained in PPC will never say, "There is nothing else we can do." In fact, he or she will say, "There is always a lot we can do." Even when the underlying condition cannot be cured, sophisticated medical technology will be used to control symptoms and improve a child quality of life. PPC translates into aggressive pain and symptom management and providing the best possible quality of life and is therefore a very active and aggressive approach to symptom management and family support.

A recent groundbreaking randomized controlled trial (RCT) in 151 adults with advanced lung cancer demonstrates that an early palliative care intervention (at the point of diagnosis) providing appropriate and beneficial treatments, actually increased quality of life, decreased depression, and led to a prolonged life (11.6 months vs. 8.9 months, $p = 0.02$) [20]. These results underscore the need for palliative care early in a serious illness and refute the notion that palliative care means giving up. Patients received palliative care alongside their curative treatment. Although this is only one study, it is an exciting one and results are not surprising: PC clinicians regularly see these outcomes in practice—especially in pediatric patients.

Assumption #5: Pediatric Palliative Cancer Care Should Only Occur in a Children's Hospital

Some have suggested that a home death may promote better family adjustment and healing [21, 22]. This may be related to fewer feelings of helplessness and greater opportunity for family intimacy offered by being at home. Others have found family relationships to be better when the child died in the hospital [23]. While many have suggested that most children prefer to die at home, this too has not been systematically evaluated.

Dr. Ann Goldman from the Department of Hematology/Oncology at Great Ormond Street in London, UK, implemented a "Symptom Care Team," a team of nurses who were introduced at cancer diagnosis to the child and family. All children received home visits after their first discharge. Children with high-risk cancer or relapses then already knew the "Symptom Care Team," which provides a 24/7 service, from the time of diagnosis. From 1978 to 1981, before the implementation of the "Symptom Care Team," only 19% of patients with cancer died at home. In 1989–1990, after implementation of the team, 77% of the children dying from malignancies did so at home [24].

Parents of terminally ill children often wish for home care [14, 25] and there is a not surprisingly positive correlation between availability of palliative home care and the number of children dying at home [13, 26–28]. Most families regard caring for their dying child as a positive experience [29].

The number of children with complex chronic conditions who die at home internationally range from Washington State 20%, Poland 23%, Germany 40%, to England and Wales 52% [30–33].

It is critically important to discuss preferences regarding the primary location of care as early as possible. A parental decision to care for their terminally ill child at home involves consideration of medical, psychological, social and cultural factors together with such practical considerations as the availability of respite care, physician access, and financial resources [34]. Whatever the decision is regarding the primary location of care, families should be reassured that they can change from one option to another and that the primary team will remain closely involved [29].

The WHO states that PPC can be provided in tertiary care facilities, in community health and hospice centers, and in children's homes and over the last decade it has become clear that clinically advanced palliative cancer care for children can indeed be provided at home, in free-standing children's hospices as well as in Pediatric hematology/oncology units [15].

Assumption #6: Increasing the Dose of Opioids Causes Respiratory Depression and Quickens Death

An enduring misconception is the belief that in the management of pain and dyspnea, opioids will hasten death and should only be administered as a last resort. This was contradicted in the adult literature [34] and our PPC teams commonly observe that administering opioids and/or benzodiazepines, together with comfort care to relieve dyspnea and pain, not only prolongs life but also improves the child's quality of life [35].

A retrospective cohort study (n = 223 adult oncologic patients) reviewing the mean survival in relation to opioid use and found less than a two-fold increase in their initial opioid dose resulted in 9 days survival, and more than a two-fold increase in their initial opioid dose resulted in 22 days survival [36].

Assumption #7: Pediatric Palliative Care Takes Patients Away from Primary Pediatric Cancer Specialists

PPC is complementary and does not aim to get care completely transferred from the pediatric hematologist/oncologist. In fact, the PPC philosophy at most programs will strongly support maintaining the primary relationship between the child, family and cancer specialist and rather add aspects of advanced PPC not included into the care yet. This may involve second opinion regarding decision-making, symptom management, coordination of care, and/or implementation of palliative home care.

Financial Barriers to PPC

Numerous financial barriers may impede early integration of palliative care. The communication required on the part of physicians, nurses, social workers, child life workers, and others, is very time-consuming as we guide families from diagnosis to death. Lack of reimbursement for communication time, typical of pediatrics in the USA, is a much larger problem in this setting. More significantly, many US state Medicaid hospice programs are based on the federal Medicare model, which was designed for adult patients with cancer. Admission is restricted to patients with a life expectancy of six months or less. This stipulation makes it difficult to provide hospice services to many pediatric patients, whose providers and parents may find it difficult to recognize when a child meets this criterion.

Furthermore, US hospice benefits may not cover treatments intended to improve the quality of a child's remaining life, such as transfusions, ventilator support for neuromuscular disorders, or palliative surgery. The total daily reimbursement for hospice services in 2011 is $147. At present only a fraction of dying children are receiving hospice care in the US [37, 38].

Communication and Decision-Making

Optimal palliation requires the establishment of open and ongoing communication between all care team members, the child and the family. Wolfe and colleagues [17] have shown that parents first recognize that the child has no realistic chance for cure more than three months after the primary oncologist realizes this likelihood [7]. Involvement of a child psychologist or social worker was associated with parents and physicians coming to understand the child's terminal prognosis closer together in time. The study also showed that earlier recognition by the physician and parent that the child had no realistic chance for cure was associated with better integration of palliative care. Thus, early and ongoing interdisciplinary discussions aimed at informing parents of the possibility of a child's death might be critical to easing suffering during the end of a child's life.

Introducing Palliative Care

Many have suggested strategies for "breaking bad news" [39–41], however, it remains less clear how to discuss palliative care with families. Billings [42] suggests the following introduction of palliative care to families: "Palliative care is a special service, a team approach to providing comfort and support for persons living with life-threatening illness and for their families," leaving out reference to the terminal prognosis. Often the most effective communication begins with open-ended questions such as, "What concerns you most about you/your child's illness?", "How is treatment going for you/your child and your family?," "As you think about your/your child's illness, what is the best and worst that might happen?," "What are your/your child's hopes (expectations, fears) for the future?" [43]. These open-ended questions provide a means to explore the possibility of a child's dying.

Discussing Palliative Care with Children

Very little is known regarding communication about palliative care with children with advanced cancer; however, knowledge of the developmental understanding of death should help guide this generally unexplored area (Table 14.1). Most children learn to recognize when something is "dead" before they reach 3 years of age, but at this early age death, separation, and sleep are almost synonymous in the child's mind. As children become preschool age, they can recognize that a dead person cannot function, but may believe that death is temporary. Their egocentric reasoning can lead them to believe they can cause death with their thoughts or actions.

School-age children begin to have logical thought and during these years they normally acquire a much more complete understanding of death. By the age of 7,

Table 14.1 Overview of children's concepts of death.

Age range, years	Concept
Birth to 2	Death is perceived as separation or abandonment
	Protest and despair from disruption in caretaking
	No cognitive understanding of death
2 to 6	Death is reversible or temporary
	Death is personified and often seen as punishment
	Magical thinking that wishes can come true
6 to 11	Gradual awareness of irreversibility and finality
	Specific death of self or loved one difficult to understand
	Concrete reasoning with ability to see cause-and-effect relationships
Older than 11	Death is irreversible, universal, and inevitable
	All people and self must die, although latter is far off
	Abstract and philosophical reasoning

Source: [107]. Reproduced with permission from *Pediatrics*, Vol. 105, pages 445–447, Table 1, Copyright 2000.

most children understand that death is irreversible, universal, that the dead do not function, and that people die from both internal and external causes. They can be interested in the specific details of death, and in the latter part of this phase they are able to envision their own deaths. As children become adolescents, their thinking about death is usually consistent with reality. They can begin to also appreciate the effect death has on other people and on society as a whole. However, their future orientation makes it difficult for them to recognize their own deaths as a present possibility, although they can conceive this occurring at some point in the future.

Children with chronic, advanced illness appear to have a precocious understanding of the concepts of death and their personal mortality [44–47]. Yet, for each individual child, prior experience, social and cultural factors will impact greatly on their understanding of death. Importantly, studies have indicated that children with cancer want to know about their prognosis.

In a survey of 50 children with cancer, ages 8–17, 95% of patients wanted to be told if they were dying [48]. Although most of the children felt that treatment decisions were up to the physicians, 63% of the adolescents and 28% of the younger children wanted to make their own decisions about palliative therapy. Nitschke *et al.* [49] reported on their experience of including children between 6 and 20 years in a "final stage conference" in which progression of disease, minimal chance of cure, imminence of death, and therapeutic options were discussed. These children appeared capable of making rational decisions about further therapy. Others have suggested that children under 11 years of age may not be able to grasp these concepts [50, 51]. The approach should be tailored to the individual child and family.

In order to preserve a relationship that is built on trust and caring, the caregiver should always be honest with the child. Children will often know when they are dying and may feel tremendous isolation if they are not given permission to talk openly about their illness and impending death [52]. Furthermore, it is now generally accepted that children give their assent in medical decision-making [53]. When talking to children, it is important to stay open and receptive when the child initiates a conversation. "Teachable moments" may be fleeting, and an immediate response is necessary to capitalize on them. Alternatively, many children communicate best through nonverbal means such as artwork or music. For example, they may be more willing to "talk things over" with puppets or stuffed animals rather than real people. Finally, euphemistic expressions about death can be very confusing or even frightening for children (for instance, equating death with sleep may result in the child being afraid of going to bed), and should always be avoided.

Resuscitation Status

It can be very difficult to initiate discussions about the appropriateness of cardiopulmonary resuscitation efforts for children with advanced cancer [54]. As a result, medical caregivers may avoid these conversations until respiratory or cardiac collapse appears imminent or may not initiate them at all [55]. This may account for why 45% of children with advanced cancer who die in hospital die in the intensive care unit [7]. Clearly, parents would be better able to consider this decision if they were not in the midst of a crisis. Thus advanced discussion about resuscitation status may be very beneficial to the child and family.

Wolfe and Grier [17] suggest approaching this sensitive topic by framing it as "in the worst case scenario, we would like you to consider whether your child should undergo cardiopulmonary resuscitation (CPR) efforts if we believe he or she has an irreversible problem." This approach, along with reassurance that a life-threatening event is not imminent, may allow parents to maintain hope while facing this decision. It may also be helpful to reassure parents that should the child's condition improve, this status would be reconsidered. At the same time, if parents are unable to make a decision about resuscitation status, caregivers should not labor the point, and recognize that for some parents this is an impossible decision to make. Ideally, optimal palliative care should be delivered wherever the child is residing, even in the intensive care unit.

Careful thought should be placed on the exact words used during a discussion about resuscitation status. Parents often think that agreeing to "do not resuscitate" (DNR) status is choosing death over life for their children. It is helpful to explain that it is the uncontrolled cancer that would be the cause of death. More concretely, using the phrase "do not resuscitate" may imply that, when attempted, resuscitation is always successful. However, among children with far-advanced cancer, the likelihood of being extubated once on a ventilator and surviving is extremely low. Thus, when approaching families about this issue, it is recommended to use the phrase: "do not attempt resuscitation" (DNAR) [56].

A recent study by Baker and colleagues [57] demonstrated that placing a "Do not resuscitate" (DNR) order did clearly not result in reduction of the level, quality and priority of children's medical cancer care.

Cancer-Directed Therapy

Chemotherapy

Chemotherapy can both prolong life and lessen pain and suffering. However, administration of treatments may also lead to increased numbers of physician–patient interactions, visits to clinic, admissions to the hospital and most importantly treatment-related complications requiring increased supportive care. Among adult patients, a number of studies show improved quality of life in patients receiving chemotherapy compared to those who were not [58–62]. Possible reasons for this include placebo effect, provision of hope, and/or increased medical attention associated with being on treatment.

The impact of chemotherapy in children with advanced cancer has not been studied and may depend on the developmental stage of the child and awareness of disease state. For example, increased interactions with medical personnel may outweigh any improvements in quality of life for the child. Parents may also have differing views on the role of continued cancer-directed therapy. Wolfe and colleagues [7] found that only 13% of parents reported that the primary goal of cancer-directed therapy for their child during the end-of-life care period was to lessen suffering. The majority of parents maintained a primary goal of extending life. Communication around this issue must be very clear and tailored to the individual family. The decision about whether or not to continue cancer-directed therapy must carefully balance considerations of efficacy, potential treatment-related complications and psychological impact.

Phase I Trials

The goal of phase I research is to determine the toxicities and maximum-tolerated dose of an investigational drug or drugs. However, only one-third of adults enrolled in a phase I trial were able to state the purpose of the trial [63]. Most cancer patients who participate in phase I trials are strongly motivated by the hope of therapeutic benefit and not altruistic feelings. Yet overall, the chance of tumor response in phase I trials is low, ranging from 4–6% [63, 64]. In children, the response rate is similar [65]. At the same time the chance of fatal toxicity is also low, at approximately 0.5% [64, 65]. Physicians also tend to assume more positive potential benefit from experimental chemotherapy than statistics would warrant [63]. Although these biases are not presented to the family with any intention of doing harm, they may make the informed consent process exceedingly difficult and potentially raise serious ethical questions [66].

Similar to discussions around chemotherapy, it is critical to ensure effective communication when discussing phase I therapy for children with advanced cancer. Furthermore, it is strongly recommended that children give their assent to participation in clinical trials [67].

Radiation Therapy

Approximately half of all courses of radiation therapy are delivered with palliative intent with the goal of relieving symptoms, and complete elimination of the tumor is not necessary [68]. Larger fraction sizes over shorter timeframes can be used in most cases, as late-arising complications are not of major concern [69]. Munro and Sebag-Montefiore [70] have devised the concept of "opportunity cost," that is, what the time spent on the treatment of a dying patient costs in terms of lost opportunities in his or her remaining lifespan. Common indications for palliative radiation [68] include:

- pain relief from bone metastases or pulmonary metastases, and tumors causing nerve root and soft tissue infiltration;
- control of bleeding;
- control of fungation and ulceration;
- relief of impeding or actual obstruction, for example, of the large airways;
- shrinkage of tumor masses causing symptoms, such as brain metastases, skin lesions, and other sites;
- oncological emergencies, such as spinal cord compression, superior vena-caval obstruction.

In the absence of symptoms to palliate, there is probably little value in giving treatment unless it is apparent that significant problems are incipient.

Complementary and Alternative Medicine (CAM)

Complementary therapies are categorized by the National Centers for Complementary and Alternative Medicine (NCCAM) as therapies that are outside the realm of traditional therapy. As such, what is considered "outside traditional medicine" becomes a moving target over time. Roughly 40–50% of parents use CAM for their child with cancer, with an increase in use when relapse occurs or the child does not respond to front-line therapy [71–75]. The most commonly used CAM therapies are herbal remedies, nutritional supplements and diet, and faith healing. Parents' religiosity is a significant predictor of CAM use for their children [76]. In the majority of cases, parents do not tell their child's physicians that these CAM therapies are being used.

Randomized controlled trials (RCT) of CAM therapies are limited for children with cancer, especially those in palliative care, or have methodological limitations. This problem has led to mixed findings. For example, in a RTC of massage, music, and other therapies for patients undergoing stem cell transplantation, Phipps et al. [77] found no added benefit with CAM therapies. In a study by Wu et al. [78], a history of prior manipulation therapy was associated with a significantly poorer prognosis for children with osteogenic sarcoma. However, most prospective smaller studies show promising results with various types of CAM, including play and music therapy [79, 80]. There are more studies about CAM, especially hypnosis, for procedure-related pain than for use in palliative care. Clinically, more programs are including art, music, and play therapies, hypnotherapy, and yoga in pediatric palliative care.

Pain and Symptom Management

In two retrospective studies of bereaved parents of 221 pediatric cancer patients conducted by Wolfe et al.

[5, 13], the majority of distressing symptoms (such as pain, dyspnea and nausea/vomiting) were not treated, and when treated, therapy was commonly ineffective. A dying child is often highly symptomatic, and providing symptom relief is one of the most compelling imperatives of Pediatric Palliative Care (PPC). Importantly, Wolfe et al. [7] also found that earlier recognition by both physicians and parents that the child had no realistic chance of cure led to a stronger emphasis on treatment to lessen suffering and integrate PPC in pediatric cancer patients. Consequently, proponents in the field urge that PPC be provided as an option early on—ideally at the point of diagnosis or early in treatment.

In children with advanced cancer, any distress should be considered a medical emergency requiring direct evaluation of the patient and immediate implementation of interventions. The constellation of symptoms that a child dying of cancer may experience is determined by the site of the tumor and any metastatic disease, and the side effects or complications of treatment. In children, many tumors spread widely and aggressively, so that the terminal stage of illness may be short when compared to an adult with cancer [81].

Pain management forms a major part of the care of a child dying of cancer, but other symptoms may also need to be addressed. The extent to which the precise underlying cause of a symptom needs to be established should be tempered by the child's ability to tolerate investigations; it may be more appropriate to just try to alleviate the suffering.

The primary and/or PPC team addressing pain or other distressing symptoms must provide prompt and effective management. Managing pain in children with advanced cancer or at end-of-life will usually require the integration of pharmacology with non-pharmacological, integrative therapies. Not uncommonly, children may require the addition of adjuvant analgesia or invasive approaches. Needless to say, any underlying pathology causing pain needs to be addressed concurrently, if appropriate and feasible in the specific clinical scenario.

Pain Management

A principle of pharmacokinetics teaches us that unless the drug reaches the site of action, it cannot be expected to exert its dynamic effect.

With morphine the situation is that when the drug dose not reach the patient, what hope is there for pain relief? [82]

More than 80% of children with advanced cancer experience pain, regardless of the underlying diagnosis and this symptom is often inadequately controlled [13, 83]. Under-treatment of pain may be related to several critical barriers to effective pain management. These include a general deficit in knowledge and experience [84, 85], the unsubstantiated fear of inducing addiction [86–89], the symbolic implication that beginning a morphine infusion is equivalent to "giving up on a patient" [90], and importantly the inappropriate fear of hastening death through respiratory depression, excess sedation, or both [91]. Open communication regarding these issues among medical caregivers and the family may be an important means to overcoming these barriers.

In the twenty-first century, pediatric hematology/oncology patients and their families should expect nothing less than state-of-the-art analgesia, that is, a combination of the following approaches, so-called "Broad-band Analgesia" [92]:

(1) Administration of non-opioid analgesics (e.g., acetaminophen/paracetamol plus ibuprofen or celecoxib, if appropriate in the clinical setting).

(2) Administration of opioids (e.g., morphine, fentanyl, hydromorphone, oxycodone, or methadone) by various routes.

(3) Applying the four World Health Organization (WHO) principles of pain management [93]:

"By the Clock": Regular scheduling of analgesia ensures a steady blood level, reducing the peaks and troughs of PRN (pro re nata = "as needed") dosing. PRN dosing may take several hours and higher opioid doses to relieve pain and results in cycle of under-medication and pain, alternating with periods of overmedication and drug toxicity [94]. Commonly used opioid drug regimes include immediate release oral morphine every four hours or controlled-release morphine twice daily plus (for both strategies) 1/10–1/6 of the 24-hours morphine requirement as an hourly immediate-release breakthrough pain medication as needed. Patient-controlled analgesia (PCA) pumps provide a continuous intravenous or subcutaneous infusion, with extra doses by demand (a single PCA bolus dose usually equals the total hourly dose).

"By the Appropriate Route": The least invasive route of administration, decided by the child, has to be chosen, making painful intramuscular of pain medication unnecessary and obsolete (e.g., oral, sublingual, buccal, intranasal, transdermal, intravenous, subcutaneous, rectal). Novel routes of administration usually make use of high liphophilicity of certain opioids to cross skin or mucosa.

"With the Child": The analgesic treatment should be individualized according to the child's pain, response to treatment, frequently reassessed and modified as required. Some children may require extremely high doses of opioids (sometimes more than 100 times the standard dose) to control severe pain.

"By the Analgesic Ladder": The choice of analgesic drugs should be based on the WHO analgesic ladder, i.e., severe pain requires strong pain medication, namely opioids.

(4) Importantly, state-of-the-art pain and symptom management requires combining pharmacological approaches with rehabilitative, supportive, and integrative therapies (e.g., cuddle/hug by parent, massage, music, imagery, diaphragmatic breathing, hypnosis, biofeedback or aromatherapy). Utilizing these modalities effectively stimulates efferent inhibiting pathways descending from the periaqueductal gray, decreases nociception, and provides effective self-coping skills to the child and his or her family. More on integrating complementary, physical, and psychological approaches to cancer pain management can be found in [95, 96].

(5) If the combination of the above four basic analgesic strategies are inadequate to manage pain successfully, the use of adjuvants or co-analgesics may be appropriate (e.g., anticonvulsants/gabapentinoids, tricyclic antidepressants, benzodiazepines, N-methyl-D-aspertate receptor [NMDA] antagonists, bisphosphonates, antispasmodics, low-dose general anesthetics).

(6) Anesthetic or neurosurgical options may also be required (e.g., epidural/intrathecal infusions or neurolytic blocks). Successful approaches in adult palliative care also include intraventricular opioids or percutaneous cervical cordotomy.

Only if all the above approaches have been exhausted concurrently, and not earlier, would it be necessary to consider sedation to unconsciousness, hence making the latter a very rarely needed intervention (estimated less than once per year in large pediatric cancer programs).

Medications, which *cannot* be recommended in pediatric analgesia include:

• *Codeine*: A large percentage of children, estimated as 36%, show remarkably inefficient hepatic conversion of codeine to morphine and achieve no analgesia [97]. The prevalence of nausea and vomiting is higher than with any other opioid. Up to 5% of Caucasians are ultra-rapid CYP 2D6 metabolizers, producing dangerously high morphine doses with reported deaths in children [98].

- *Meperidine/pethidine* (e.g., Demerol^{TM}), and *propoxyphene* (e.g., Darvocet^{TM}) due to their neurotoxic metabolites.
- *Fixed combination analgesia*, usually acetaminophen plus an opioid such as hydrocodone (e.g., Vicodine^{TM}), oxycodone (e.g., Percocet^{TM}), or codeine (e.g., Tylenol No 3^{TM}). The fixed ratio of acetaminophen to the opioid leaves dangerous choices: Either using suboptimal opioid doses or, when using adequate opioid doses administering a liver-toxic dose of acetaminophen. Also it is unclear, if a child takes a scheduled fixed-combination formulation, what to choose for a rescue dose—also, can we be certain that caregivers will not administer additional doses of the drug, if their child remains in pain (and thereby grossly increasing the risk of an acetaminophen overdose)? It also remains unclear how to increase/titrate the opioid to effect. State-of-the-art pediatric analgesia therefore suggests the individual titration of stand-alone acetaminophen with a single opioid, the latter titrated to effect.

Symptom Management

Children with advanced cancer exhibit a high prevalence of distressing symptoms, including nausea/vomiting, anxiety, constipation, cachexia, diarrhea, dyspnea, and fatigue. However, unlike pain, these symptoms are usually not regularly assessed on pediatric oncology units in daily practice, thereby impeding the aggressive management of those symptoms.

Management of distressing symptoms usually follows the following steps:

Step 1: Regular symptom assessment (e.g., using the MSAS tool [99, 100]).
Step 2: Clinical examination and history taking.
Step 3: Treating underlying pathologies (if feasible and appropriate in the individual case).
Step 4: Implementing supportive and integrative (non-pharmacological) therapies.
Step 5: Pharmacological treatment.

A treatment strategy going straight from Step 1 (e.g., "nausea") to step 5 (e.g., "administer ondansetrone") omitting steps 2, 3 and 4 often may fail in our experience.

The detailed management of distressing symptoms would be beyond the scope of this chapter and we would like to refer to recent textbooks including Wolfe *et al. Textbook of Interdisciplinary Pediatric Palliative Care* [101] and Goldman *et al. Oxford Textbook of Palliative Care for Children* [102].

Meaningfulness and Quality of Life at the End of Life

Adequate pain and symptom management, strengthening relationships with loved ones, and avoiding inappropriate prolongation of dying are among a set of priorities elicited from adult patients with terminal illness [103]. Similar research has not been conducted in children or their parents. However, experience teaches us that these are critical considerations.

Religion, spirituality or life philosophy plays an important role in the lives of most parents whose children receive palliative cancer care [104].

The families' sense of spirituality or engagement in a religious community may provide a structure for positive coping strategies for both parent and child [105]. "The goal is to add life to the child's years, not simply years to the child's life" [106]. Facilitating memory building during this period can be the greatest gift to the child and family.

For many children, the social context of school and friendship is most important. The care team should encourage the child's continued participation in a school setting, even if attendance is limited by the child's physical deterioration to "social" visits. Whether the child is based at home or in an institution, regular social contact with other children and adults should be strongly encouraged. This may involve a shift of attitude in families that have been very protective about visitors for fear of introducing infection to the child on chemotherapy.

Intense support of siblings during the final phase of a child's life is critical to ensuring healing. Siblings of a dying child often hold misconceptions and misunderstandings about the child's illness. Specific, concrete information about the dying child's illness as well as the siblings' own health, may do much to allay fears [107]. Many children's books on dying, death, and bereavement are available for families to use in helping siblings mourn (Table 14.2).

Conclusion

High-quality care for children with advanced cancer is now the expected standard [37, 106]. However, there remain significant barriers to achieving optimal care related to lack of formal education, reimbursement issues and the emotional impact of caring for a dying child. Whenever possible, treatment should focus on continued efforts to control the underlying illness. At

Table 14.2 Lifecycle stories for children.

Book	Notes
Al-Chokhachy, E. *The Angel with the Golden Glow.* Marblehead, MA: The Penny Bear Co., 1998	A story about a special little boy and his family and how they savored every moment they shared.
Branderburg, A. *The Two of Them.* New York: Mulberry Books, 1979	The story of the special relationship between a girl and her grandfather.
Breebart, J. and Breebart, P. *When I Die, Will I Get Better?* Belgium: Peter Bedrick Books, 1993	A story about rabbit brothers written by a 6-year-old boy as he tries to come to terms with the death of his younger brother.
Brown, L. and Brown, M. *When Dinosaurs Die.* Boston: Little, Brown & Co., 1996	A guide for understanding death, using dinosaurs as the characters.
Buscaglia, L. *The Fall of Freddie the Leaf: A Story of Life for All Ages.* Thorofare, NJ: Slack, Inc., 1982	Freddie and his companion leaves change with the passing seasons, finally falling to the ground with winter's snow.
Carlstrom, N. *Blow Me a Kiss, Miss Lilly.* New York: HarperCollins, 1990	The relationship between a young girl and her elderly neighbor during her illness.
Coerr, E. and Young, E. *Sadako and the Thousand Paper Cranes.* New York: G.P. Putnam & Sons, 1993	Sadako's journey through illness and death, illustrating her courage and strength.
Coleman, W. *When Someone You Love Dies.* Minneapolis, MN: Augsburg, 1994	Advice and support for children ages 8–12 and their parents on fears and questions they have when someone they love dies.
Fahy, M. *The Tree that Survived the Winter.* New York: Paulist Press, 1989.	For survivors who find joy and compassion on the other side of suffering.
Gootman, M. *When a Friend Dies: A Book for Teens about Grieving and Healing.* Minneapolis, MN: Free Spirit Publishing Inc., 1994	A book of wisdom and compassion for grieving teens, their parents and educators.
Grollman, E. *Straight Talk about Death for Teenagers.* Boston: Beacon Press, 1993	For teenagers who have lost a friend or relative to death. Includes a journal section to record memories, feelings, and hopes.
Holden, D. *Gran-Gran's Best Trick: A Story for Children Who Have Lost Someone They Love.* Washington, DC: Magination Press, 1989	A young girl whose beloved grandfather battles cancer learns that those we love never leave our hearts and that this is "love's best trick."
Johnson, J. and Johnson, M. *Where's Jess?* Omaha, NE: Centering Corp., 1982.	When a brother or sister dies, a child may have these questions and feelings.
Levy, J. *The Spirit of Tío Fernando: A Day of the Dead Story.* Morton Grove, IL: Albert Whitman & Company, 1995	This bilingual story describes a young boy's understanding of death through the Mexican Day of the Dead celebration.
London, J. and Long, S. *Liplap's Wish.* San Francisco: Chronicle Books, 1994	Little bunny Liplap wrestles with his grandmother's death and finds solace in his mother's tale about the First Rabbits becoming "stars in the sky."
Mills, J.C. *Gentle Willow.* New York: Magination Press, 1993	How friends help a willow tree face a terminal illness.
Mundy, M. *Sad Isn't Bad.* St. Meinrad, IN: Abbey Press, 1998	A good grief guidebook for children dealing with loss.
Romain, T. *What on Earth Do You Do When Someone Dies?* Minneapolis, MN: Free Spirit Publishing, 1999	Children's questions about death. Isaiah goes on a search for heaven after his grandfather dies and finds it where he least expects it.

Table 14.2 (*Continued*).

Book	Notes
Sasso, S. E. *For Heaven's Sake, What is Heaven? Where Do We find It?* Woodstock, VT: Jewish Lights Publishing, 1999	A beautiful life cycle story.
Stickney, D. *Water Bugs and Dragonflies.* Cleveland, OH: The Pilgrim Press, 1982	
Varley, S. *Badger's Parting Gifts.* New York: A Mulberry Paperback Book, 1984	An aging badger prepares for his death.
Viorst, J. *The Tenth Good Thing about Barney.* New York: Atheneum Books, 1971	Plans for a funeral for pet cat Barney.
Wigand, M. *Heavenly Ways to Heal from Grief and Loss.* St. Meinrad, IN: Abbey Press, 1998	Let the angel in you lend strength and comfort as you journey from grief to grace.
Wild, M. *Old Pig.* New York: Penguin Books, 1995	Old Pig and her grand-daughter say "good-bye" in the best way they know.

the same time, children and their families should have access to interdisciplinary care aimed at promoting optimal physical, psychological and spiritual well-being. Open and compassionate communication can best facilitate meeting the goals of these children and families. Future research efforts should focus on ways to enhance communication, symptom management and quality of life for children with advanced cancer and their families. Being present with children with advanced cancer and their families is at the same time a great gift and intensely rewarding on a personal level.

Persistent myths and misconceptions have led to inadequate symptom control in children with advanced cancer. Pediatric Palliative Care advocates the provision of comfort care, pain, and symptom management concurrently with cancer-directed treatments. Families no longer have to opt for one or the other. They can pursue both, and include integrative care to maximize the child's quality of life.

Acknowledgments

Thanks to Joanne Wolfe (Boston, MA) and Anne Tournay (Irvine, CA) who authored and co-authored this chapter in the first edition of this book and who allowed us to edit and integrate into the current chapter.

References

1. Ries LAG SM, Gurney JG, Linet M, Tamra T, Young JL, Bunin GR (eds.) *Cancer Incidence and Survival among Children and Adolescents: United States SEER Program 1975–1995*, National Cancer Institute, SEER Program. Bethesda, MD: NIH, 1999.
2. Li J , Thompson TD , Miller JW , Pollack LA , Stewart SL. Cancer incidence among children and adolescents in the United States, 2001–2003. *Pediatrics.* 2008;**121**: e1470–1477.
3. Ries LAG, Krapcho M, Stinchcomb DG, *et al.* (eds.) *SEER Cancer Statistics Review, 1975–2005.* Bethesda, MD: National Cancer Institute, 2008.
4. Linet MS , Ries LA , Smith MA , Tarone RE , Devesa SS. Cancer surveillance series: recent trends in childhood cancer incidence and mortality in the United States. *Journal of National Cancer Institute* 1999;**91**:1051–1058.
5. Wolfe J , Hammel JF , Edwards KE , *et al.* Easing of suffering in children with cancer at the end of life: is care changing? *Journal of Clinical Oncology* 2008;**26**:1717–1723.
6. Wolfe J , Hinds PS , Sourkes B. The language of pediatric palliative care. In: Wolfe J, Hinds PS, Sourkes B (eds.) *Textbook of Interdisciplinary Pediatric Palliative Care*: Oxford: Elsevier; 2011; pp. 3–6.
7. Wolfe J , Klar N , Grier HE , Duncan J , Salem-Schatz S , Emanuel EJ , *et al.* Understanding of prognosis among parents of children who died of cancer: impact on treatment goals and integration of palliative care. *JAMA.* 2000;**284**:2469–2475.
8. Mattie Stepanek (patient).
9. Homer. *The Iliad*, XI. Book, 809–848.
10. Alia AK Al-Ghunaim, personal communication, 2008.
11. Saunders C. Foreword: The early hospices. In: Doyle D, Hanks G, MacDonald N (eds.) *Oxford Textbook of Palliative Medicine.* Oxford: Oxford University Press, 1993; pp. v–ix.
12. Armstrong-Dailey A , Zarbock S. Introduction. In: Armstrong-Dailey A, Zarbock S (eds.) *Hospice Care for Children.* Oxford: Oxford University Press, 2001.
13. Wolfe J , Grier HE , Klar N , *et al.* Symptoms and suffering at the end of life in children with cancer. *New England Journal of Medicine* 2000;**342**:326–333.
14. Vickers JL , Carlisle C. Choices and control: parental experiences in pediatric terminal home care. *Journal of Pediatric Oncology Nursing* 2000;**17**:12–21.

15. WHO website http://www.who.int/cancer/palliative/definition/en.

16. Goldman A , Heller KS. Integrating palliative and curative approaches in the care of children with life-threatening illnesses. *Journal of Palliative Medicine* 2000;**3**:353–359.

17. Pizzo PA, Poplack DG (eds.) *Principles and Practice of Pediatric Oncology*, 4th edn. Philadelphia, PA: Lippincott Williams & Wilkins, 2002.

18. Saunders CM. A comparison of adult bereavement in the death of a spouse, child, and parent. *Omega* 1979–1980;**10**:302–322.

19. Whittam, E.H. Terminal care of the dying child: psychosocial implications of care. *Cancer* 1993;**71**:3450–3462.

20. Temel JS , Greer JA , Muzikansky A , Gallagher ER , Admane S , Jackson VA , *et al.* Early palliative care for patients with metastatic non-small-cell lung cancer. *New England Journal of Medicine* 2010;**363**:733–742.

21. Lauer ME , *et al.* A comparison study of parental adaptation following a child's death at home or in the hospital. *Pediatrics* 1983;**71**:107–112.

22. Lauer ME , *et al.* Long-term follow-up of parental adjustment following a child's death at home or hospital. *Cancer* 1989;**63**:988–994.

23. Birenbaum LK , Robinson MA. Family relationships in two types of terminal care. *Social Science & Medicine* 1991;**32**:95–102.

24. Goldman A , Beardsmore S , Hunt J. Palliative care for children with cancer: home, hospital, or hospice? *Archives of Disease in Childhood* 1990;**65**:641–643.

25. Chambers EJ , Oakhill A. Models of care for children dying of malignant disease. *Palliative Medicine* 1995;**9**:181–185.

26. Sirkia K , Saarinen UM , Ahlgren B , Hovi L. Terminal care of the child with cancer at home. *Acta Paediatrica* 1997;**86**:1125–1130.

27. Goldman A. Home care of the dying child. *Journal of Palliative Care* 1996;**12**:16–19.

28. Friedrichsdorf S BS , Menke A , Wamsler C , Zernikow B. Pediatric palliative care provided by nurse-led home care services in Germany. *European Journal of Palliative Care* 2005;**12**:79–83.

29. Collins JJ , Stevens MM , Cousens P. Home care for the dying child: a parent's perception. *Australian Family Physician* 1998;**27**:610–614.

30. Feudtner C , Silveira MJ , Christakis DA. Where do children with complex chronic conditions die? Patterns in Washington State, 1980–1998. *Pediatrics*. [Research Support, U.S. Gov't, P.H.S.]. 2002;**109**:656–660.

31. Friedrichsdorf SJ , Brun S , Zernikow B , Dangel T. Palliative care in Poland: The Warsaw Hospice for Children. *European Journal of Palliative Care* 2006;**13**:35–38.

32. Friedrichsdorf SJ , Menke A , Brun S , Wamsler C , Zernikow B. Status quo of palliative care in pediatric oncology: a nationwide survey in Germany. *Journal of Pain Symptom and Management* 2005;**29**:156–164.

33. Higginson IJ , Thompson M. Children and young people who die from cancer: epidemiology and place of death in England (1995–9). *BMJ*. [Research Support, Non-U.S. Gov't]. 2003;**327**:478–479.

34. Thorns A , Sykes N. Opioid use in last week of life and implications for end-of-life decision-making. *Lancet.* 2000;**356**:398–399.

35. Friedrichsdorf SJ. Pain management in children with advanced cancer and during end-of-life care. *Pediatric Hematology-Oncoogyl* 2010;**27**:257–261.

36. Bengoechea I , Gutierrez SG , Vrotsou K , Onaindia MJ , Lopez JM. Opioid use at the end of life and survival in a Hospital at Home unit. *Journal of Palliative Medicine* 2010;**13**:1079–1083.

37. Field MJ , Behrman RE (eds.) *When Children Die: Improving Palliative and End-Of-Life Care for Children and Their Families. Institute of Medicine of the National Academies Report 2003*. Washington, DC: The National Academy Press, 2003.

38. Friebert, S. *National Hospice and Palliative Care Organization Facts and Figures: Pediatric Palliative and Hospice Care in America, 2009*. Retrieved Oct 2009 from http//www.nhpco.org.

39. Buckman R. *How to Break Bad News*. Baltimore, MD: Johns Hopkins University Press, 1992.

40. Suchman AL , *et al.* A model of empathic communication in the medical interview. *JAMA* 1997;**277**:678–682.

41. Girgis A , Sanson-Fisher RW. Breaking bad news: consensus guidelines for medical practitioners. *Journal of Clinical Oncology* 1995;**13**:2449–2456.

42. Billings JA. What is palliative care? *Journal of Palliative Medicine* 1998;**1**:73–82.

43. Lo B , Quill T , Tulsky J. Discussing palliative care with patients. ACP-ASIM End-of-Life Care Consensus Panel. American College of Physicians—American Society of Internal Medicine. *Annals of International Medicine* 1999;**130**:744–749.

44. Schonfeld DJ. Talking with children about death. *Journal of Pediatric Health Care* 1993;**7**:269–274.

45. Spinetta J , Rigler D , Karon M. Anxiety in the dying child. *Pediatrics* 1973;**52**:841–845.

46. Spinetta J The dying child's awareness of death: a review. *Psychological Bulletin* 1974;**81**:256–260.

47. Greenham DE , Lohmann RA. Children facing death: recurring patterns of adaptation. *Health and Social Work* 1982;**7**:89–94.

48. Ellis R , Leventhal B. Information needs and decision-making preferences of children with cancer. *Psycho-Oncology* 1993;**2**:277–284.

49. Nitschke R , *et al.* Therapeutic choices made by patients with end-stage cancer. *Journal of Pediatrics* 1982;**101**:471–476.

50. Leikin SL , Connell K. Theraputic choices by children with cancer. *Pediatrics* 1983;**103**:167.

51. Shumway CN , Grossman LS , Sarles RM. Theraputic choices by children with cancer. *Pediatrics* 1983;**103**:168.

52. Hilden JM , Watterson J , Chrastek J. Tell the children. *Journal of Clinical Oncology* 2000;**18**:3193–3195.

53. Bartholome WG. Informed consent, parental permission, and assent in pediatric practice. *Pediatrics* 1995;**96**:981–982.

54. Goold SD , Williams B , Arnold RM. Conflicts regarding decisions to limit treatment: a differential diagnosis. *JAMA*, 2000;**283**:909–914.

55. SUPPORT (1995): a controlled trial to improve care for seriously ill hospitalized patients. The study to understand prognoses and preferences for outcomes and risks of treatments (SUPPORT). The SUPPORT Principal Investigators. *JAMA* 1996;**275**:1232; and *JAMA* **274**:1591–1598.

56. Foex BA. The do-not-attempt resuscitation ("DNAR") order. *Anaesthesia* 2000;**55**:292.

57. Baker JN , Kane JR , Rai S , Howard SC , Hinds PS. Changes in medical care at a pediatric oncology referral center after placement of a do-not-resuscitate order. *Journal of Palliative Medicine* 2010;**13**:1349–1352.

58. Cassileth BR , *et al.* Survival and quality of life among patients receiving unproven as compared with conventional cancer therapy. *New England Journal of Medicine* 1991;**324**:1180–1185.

59. Coates A , *et al.* Improving the quality of life during chemotherapy for advanced breast cancer; a comparison of intermittent and continuous treatment strategies. *New England Journal of Medicine* 1987;**317**:1490–1495.

60. Ellis PA , *et al.* Symptom relief with MVP (mitomycin C, vinblastine and cisplatin) chemotherapy in advanced non-small-cell lung cancer. *British Journal of Cancer* 1995;**71**:366–370.

61. Poon MA , *et al.* Biochemical modulation of fluorouracil: evidence of significant improvement of survival and quality of life in patients with advanced colorectal carcinoma. *Journal of Clinical Oncology* 1989;**7**:1407–1418.

62. Geels P , *et al.* Palliative effect of chemotherapy: objective tumor response is associated with symptom improvement in patients with metastatic breast cancer. *Journal of Clinical Oncology* 2000;**18**:2395–2405.

63. Daugherty C , *et al.* Perceptions of cancer patients and their physicians involved in phase I trials. *Journal of Clinical Oncology* 1995;**13**:1062–1072.

64. Decoster G , Stein G , Holdener EE. Responses and toxic deaths in phase I clinical trials. *Annals of Oncology* 1990;**1**:175–181.

65. Shah S , *et al.* Phase I therapy trials in children with cancer. *Journal of Pediatric Hematology Oncology* 1998;**20**:431–438.

66. Emanuel EJ. A phase I trial on the ethics of phase I trials. *Journal of Clinical Oncology* 1995;**13**:1049–1051.

67. American Academy of Pediatrics Informed consent, parental permission, and assent in pediatric practice. Committee on Bioethics, American Academy of Pediatrics. *Pediatrics* 1995;**95**:314–317.

68. Kirkbride P. The role of radiation therapy in palliative care. *Journal of Palliative Care* 1995;**11**:19–26.

69. Gaze MN , *et al.* Pain relief and quality of life following radiotherapy for bone metastases: a randomised trial of two fractionation schedules. *Radiotherapy & Oncology* 1997;**45**:109–116.

70. Munro AJ , Sebag-Montefiore D. Opportunity cost: a neglected aspect of cancer treatment. *British Journal of Cancer* 1992;**65**:309–310.

71. Bishop FL , Prescott P , Chan YK , *et al.* Prevalence of complementary medicine use in pediatric cancer: a systematic review. *Pediatrics.* 2010;**125**:768–776.

72. McLean TW , Kemper KJ. Complementary and alternative medicine therapies in pediatric oncology patients. *Journal of the Society for Integrative Oncology* 2006;**4**:40–45.

73. Paisley MA , Kang TI , Insogna IG , Rheingold Sr. , Complementary and alternative therapy use in pediatric oncology patients with failure of frontline chemotherapy. *Pediatric Blood & Cancer.* 2011;**56**:1088–1091.

74. Meyers CD , Stuber ML , Zeltzer LK. Spirituality, complementary, and alternative medicine. In: Brown RT (ed.) *Comprehensive Handbook of Childhood Cancer and Sickle Cell Disease: A Biopsychosocial Approach.* Oxford: Oxford University Press, 2006; pp. 189–204.

75. Tomlinson D , Hesser T , Ethier MC , Sung L. Complementary and alternative medicine use in pediatric cancer reported during palliative phase of disease. *Support Care Cancer* 2010 Oct. 24. E-pub ahead of print.

76. McCurdy EA , Spangler JG , Wofford MM , *et al.* Religiosity is associated with the use of complementary medical therapies by pediatric oncology patients. *Journal of Pediatric Hematology-Oncology* 2003;**25**:125–129.

77. Phipps S , Barrera M , Vannatta K , *et al.* Complementary therapies for children undergoing stem cell transplantation: report of a multisite trial. *Cancer.* 2010;**116**:3924–3933.

78. Wu PK , Chen WM , Lee OK , *et al.* The prognosis for patients with osteosarcoma who have received prior manipulative therapy. *Journal of Bone and Joint Surgery, British* 2010;**92**:1580–1585.

79. van Breemen C. Using play therapy in paediatric palliative care: listening to the story and caring for the body. *International Journal of Palliative Nursing* 2009;**15**:510–514.

80. Barry P , O'Callaghan C , Wheeler G , Grocke D. Music therapy CD creation for initial pediatric radiation therapy: a mixed methods analysis. *Journal of Music Therapy* 2010;**47**:233–263.

81. Goldman A. Life threatening illnesses and symptom control. In: Doyle D, Hanks G, MacDonald N (eds) *Oxford Textbook of Palliative Medicine.* Oxford: Oxford University Press, 1998.

82. Ghooi RB , Ghooi SR. A mother in pain. *Lancet.* 1998;**352**:1625.

83. Sirkia K , *et al.* Pain medication during terminal care of children with cancer. *Journal of Pain Symptom and Management* 1998;**15**:220–226.

84. Ingham JM , Foley KM. Pain and the barriers to its relief at the end of life: a lesson for improving end of life health care. *Hospital Journal* 1998;**13**:89–100.

85. Buchan ML , Tolle SW. Pain relief for dying persons: dealing with physicians' fears and concerns. *Journal of Clinical Ethics* 1995;**6**:53–61.

86. Porter & Hick (1980).

87. Levin DN , Cleeland CS , Dar R. Public attitudes toward cancer pain. *Cancer* 1985;**56**:2337–2339.

88. Fife BL , Irick N , Painter JD. A comparative study of the attitudes of physicians and nurses toward the management of cancer pain. *Journal of Pain Symptom and Management* 1993;**8**:132–139.

89. Elliott TE , *et al.* Physician knowledge and attitudes about cancer pain management: a survey from the Minnesota cancer pain project. *Journal of Pain Symptom Management* 1995;**10**:494–504.

90. Field MJ , Cassel CK , Institute of Medicine (U.S.) Committee on Care at the End of Life. *Approaching Death: Improving Care at the End of Life.* Washington, DC: National Academy Press, 1997; pp. xvii, 437.

91. Solomon MZ , *et al.* Decisions near the end of life: professional views on life-sustaining treatments. *American Journal of Public Health* 1993;**83**:14–23.

92. Friedrichsdorf SJ , Kang TI. The management of pain in children with life-limiting illnesses. *Pediatric Clinics of North America* 2007;**54**:645–672, x.

93. WHO. *Cancer Pain Relief and Palliative Care in Children.* Geneva: World Health Organization, 1998.

94. APS. *Principles of Analgesic Use in the Treatment of Acute Pain and Cancer Pain.* Washington, DC: American Pain Society, 2008.

95. Casillas J and Zeltzer LK. Cancer pain in children. In: Ballantyne JC, Fishman SM, Rathmell JP (eds.) *Bonica's Management of Pain*, 4th edn. Hagerstown, MD: Lippincott Williams & Wilkins, 2009, pp. 669–680.

96. Krane EJ , Casillas J , Zeltzer LK. Pain and symptom management. In: Pizzo PA, Poplack DG (eds.) *Principles and Practice of Pediatric Oncology*, 6th edn. Philadelphia: Lippincott Williams & Wilkins, 2010, pp. 1256–1287.

97. Williams DG , Patel A , Howard RF. Pharmacogenetics of codeine metabolism in an urban population of children and its implications for analgesic reliability. *British Journal of Anaesthesia* 2002;**89**:839–845.

98. Koren K. Codeine, ultrarapid-metabolism genotype, and postoperative death. *New England Journal of Medicine* 2009;**8**:827–828.

99. Collins JJ , Byrnes ME , Dunkel IJ , Lapin J , Nadel T , Thaler HT , *et al.* The measurement of symptoms in children with cancer. *Journal of Pain Symptom and Management* 2000;**19**:363–377.

100. Collins JJ , Devine TD , Dick GS , *et al.* The measurement of symptoms in young children with cancer: the validation of the Memorial Symptom Assessment Scale in children aged 7–12. *Journal of Pain Symptom and Management* 2002;**23**:10–16.

101. Wolfe J, Hinds PS, Sourkes BM (eds.) *Textbook of Interdisciplinary Pediatric Palliative Care.* Oxford: Elsevier, 2011.

102. Goldman A, Hain R, Liben S (eds.) *Oxford Textbook of Palliative Care for Children.* Oxford: Oxford University Press.

103. Singer PA , Martin DK , Kelner M. Quality end-of-life care: patients' perspectives. *JAMA* 1999;**281**:163–168.

104. Hexem KR , Mollen CJ , Carroll K , Lanctot DA , Feudtner C. How parents of children receiving pediatric palliative care use religion, spirituality, or life philosophy in tough times. *Journal of Palliative Medicine.* 2011;**14**:39–44.

105. Barnes LJ , *et al.* Spirituality, religion, and pediatrics: Intersecting worlds of healing. *Pediatrics* 2000;**104**: 899–908.

106. American Academy of Pediatrics Committee on Bioethics and Committee on Hospital Care. Palliative care for children. *Pediatrics* 2000a;**106**:351–357.

107. American Academy of Pediatrics. Committee on Psychosocial Aspects of Child and Family Health. The pediatrician and childhood bereavement. *Pediatrics* 2000b;**105**:445–447.

Part B
Survivorship

15

Neuropsychological Sequelae of Childhood Cancer

Matthew C. Hocking, Melissa A. Alderfer

Introduction

Almost 11,000 children under the age of 14 are diagnosed with a form of childhood cancer annually [1]. Leukemias and brain or central nervous system (CNS) tumors are the two most common childhood cancer diagnoses, representing 33% and 20% of the total diagnoses respectively [2]. While a childhood cancer diagnosis in 1975 carried with it only a 58% chance of survival, advances in cancer treatments have significantly improved the overall survival rates across all cancers to 82.5% over the period between 2001 and 2007 [2]. Notably, survival rates for the most common form of childhood leukemia, acute lymphoblastic leukemia (ALL), improved from 57.5% to 90.5% over the past 30 years. Similarly, CNS tumor survival has improved from 57% to 75% [2].

Survivors of childhood cancer, however, often experience costs associated with survival, typically referred to as "late effects," that are persistent and can be degenerative in nature. Over 62% of adult survivors of childhood cancer experience at least one significant health problem secondary to their cancer treatment [3]. Neurocognitive late effects in survivors of ALL [4] and CNS tumors [5] also are common and negatively affect survivor quality of life [6]. Given the dramatic improvements in survival rates and the increased recognition of treatment-related late effects, oncologists have shifted their perspective regarding the desired outcome of treatment from survival only to survival plus good quality of life.

Treatment protocols for ALL and CNS tumors typically involve multiple therapy modalities directed at the CNS. Indeed, much of the success in improvements in survival for these disease groups has been attributed to therapeutic regimens that proactively prevent the spread of further CNS disease (e.g., CNS prophylaxis for ALL). Such CNS prophylaxis approaches, including using intrathecal (IT) methotrexate (MTX) during the maintenance phase of treatment for ALL, however, affect the developing brains of children and contribute to neurocognitive late effects [7].

This chapter will provide an overview of the neurocognitive sequelae experienced by survivors of childhood cancer, focusing primarily on survivors of ALL and CNS tumors. This chapter will: (1) briefly describe the treatment regimens for these two diseases, highlighting how they affect the CNS and lead to neurocognitive late effects; (2) review the literature on neurocognitive outcomes in pediatric ALL and CNS tumor survivors focusing on known risk factors for poorer outcomes; (3) outline standards of clinical care for this group of survivors; (4) provide an overview of the current intervention efforts to reduce neurocognitive late effects; and, (5) present future directions for research and clinical care.

Treatment Regimens for ALL and CNS Tumors and Their Effect on the Central Nervous System

Treatment of childhood ALL generally lasts two to three years and consists of three distinct phases: induction, consolidation/intensification, and maintenance. Because leukemia cells infiltrate the CNS, and systemic chemotherapies cannot cross the blood–brain barrier, throughout each phase of ALL therapy, children receive treatments that target the CNS. Such treatments, termed CNS prophylaxis, include intrathecal chemotherapy (chemotherapy injected into the spinal fluid) and/or cranial radiation (in high risk or relapsed ALL). Cranial radiation used to be a standard component of treatment protocols for ALL but was removed

Pediatric Psycho-oncology: Psychosocial Aspects and Clinical Interventions, Second Edition.
Edited by Shulamith Kreitler, Myriam Weyl Ben-Arush and Andrés Martin.
© 2012 John Wiley & Sons, Ltd. Published 2012 by John Wiley & Sons, Ltd.

over the last 25 years from most protocols in favor of multi-agent systemic and intrathecal chemotherapy regimens in order to reduce the risk of CNS toxicity given equivalent survival outcomes, for example, [8].

Compared to childhood ALL, childhood CNS tumors and their treatments are much more varied due to the multiple tumor types and locations. Tumor-directed treatment regimens generally include multiple modalities and consist of some combination of surgical resection, chemotherapy, and cranial or craniospinal radiation. Treatment regimens for CNS tumors generally are shorter in duration than for ALL, but often are more invasive and damaging to a child's developing brain due to the higher doses of cranial or craniospinal radiation than typically used in ALL and the potential complications associated with surgical resection (e.g., hydrocephalus, cerebellar mutism). Surgical resection of the brain tumor itself may impact areas of the brain that are responsible for a variety of important functions, including coordination, language, memory and other higher order cognitive skills (e.g., attention, executive function) and contribute to diminished neurocognitive functioning [9]. The multiple modalities of treatment used in pediatric brain tumors likely interact with one another and contribute to neurocognitive late effects that are generally more severe than what is seen in ALL. Indeed, even children with cerebellar tumors treated with surgery alone demonstrate deficits in attention, processing speed and memory [10].

Despite differences in treatment for ALL and CNS tumors, the various modalities used in these protocols are known to affect the development of children's brains. Myelination and white matter proliferation, the physiological processes allowing for rapid communication between neurons and eventually higher order cognitive skills, begin during the third or fourth month of gestation and continues through early adulthood [11]. It is these physiological processes that are most vulnerable to the effects of cancer treatments directed at the CNS. Both cranial radiation and intrathecal chemotherapy are associated with white matter injury, demyelination, and leukoencephalopathy [12]. The effects of treatment on the development of white matter in particular are considered to be the greatest contributor to neurocognitive late effects [13]; abnormalities in white matter are associated with deficits in attention, memory, and processing speed [14]. Several studies have shown that children treated with cranial radiation, particularly those treated at a younger age with less time for myelination, demonstrate reduced white matter volumes as survivors [13, 15, 16]. Reduced white matter volume, in turn, has been associated with problems with attentional functioning [17], working memory [18], IQ, verbal and nonverbal reasoning [13].

Neurocognitive Sequelae in Survivors of Childhood Acute Lymphoblastic Leukemia

The first effective CNS prophylactic treatments for ALL included cranial radiation administered at 2400cGY and five doses of intrathecal methotrexate [19]. While the first investigators studying intelligence among ALL survivors receiving this therapy [20] found no significant impact of this treatment, subsequent studies [21] revealed significant reductions in intelligence (IQ) scores over time for the majority of children receiving this therapy. As data accumulated, an early narrative and quantitative meta-analysis of 31 published reports demonstrated a preponderance of evidence supporting significant declines in IQ over time with an average decrement across studies for survivors of ALL compared to controls of about 10 IQ points [22]. Evidence of deficits in academic achievement, memory, processing speed, attention and concentration [23, 24] were also documented.

Based in part on reports of the negative neuropsychological and physiological effects of cranial radiation [24], experimental prophylactic regimens reducing the total amount of cranial radiation or eliminating it completely were soon introduced. Comparisons of the neurocognitive functioning of children randomly assigned to these various treatment protocols quickly followed. Again, the earliest of these studies had somewhat conflicting findings. Rowland and colleagues demonstrated that children receiving 2400 cGY of cranial radiation as part of their treatment exhibited significantly lower full scale IQ scores and poorer academic achievement than those receiving IT methotrexate alone or IT methotrexate plus intravenous intermediate dose methotrexate. However, Mulhern and colleagues [25, 26] comparing children receiving IT methotrexate alone, IT methotrexate plus 1800 cGY cranial radiation and IT methotrexate plus 2400 cGY cranial radiation found no significant differences between the three groups; over time, all three groups showed significant declines in IQ and arithmetic academic achievement. A relatively recent meta-analysis of 28 empirical studies published between 1980 and 2004 [4] concluded that children with ALL receiving IT methotrexate plus cranial radiation performed significantly more poorly on measures of overall intellectual functioning when compared to those receiving methotrexate alone. Some evidence suggests that differences between those receiving cranial radiation plus IT methotrexate and IT methotrexate alone become more obvious with longer-term follow up (e.g., 20 years post-diagnosis) [27]. Individual studies also suggest that impairments in concentration, attention, and memory are greater for children receiving cranial radiation compared to those receiving intrathecal chemotherapies alone [28, 29].

With the elimination of cranial radiation from most CNS prophylaxis treatment regimens, attention turned to the impact of IT chemotherapy alone on neurocognitive functioning. A narrative review of 33 studies published between 1981 and 1997 [30] summarized that the majority of studies comparing children with ALL who received IT methotrexate to controls found declines in at least one area of cognitive functioning as measured by intelligence tests. Additionally, data were accumulating to suggest that CNS prophylaxis with IT methotrexate was related to poorer academic achievement and neuropsychological deficits in attention and nonverbal memory. A more recent narrative review of 21 studies published between 1997 and 2008 [31] indicated that 8 of 10 studies reporting on overall IQ and 4 of 8 studies examining academic achievement found no declines for ALL survivors treated with chemotherapy only compared to controls; however, subtle neuropsychological deficits were evident in the areas of attention, processing speed, visuospatial skills and memory. A meta-analysis providing a statistical synthesis of 13 studies published between 1992 and 2004 comparing children with ALL receiving IT chemotherapy only to control groups (11 of which overlapped with the review of Buizer and colleagues) revealed that ALL survivors exhibited significant impairment in multiple domains of intellectual functioning, including perceptual reasoning skills, working memory, and processing speed [32]. Additionally, academic achievement in both math and reading were poorer among the ALL survivors compared to controls and there was some evidence of executive functioning and verbal memory deficits. As data continue to accrue [18, 27, 33, 34], findings continue to be somewhat inconsistent; however, deficits in visual processing, attention, concentration, and working memory continue to be found [35]. The inconsistencies across these studies may be attributable to the fact that only a subset of survivors who receive IT chemotherapy alone experience impairment—about 30% [36]. Given the size of this subset, differences between groups may not be apparent statistically when average levels of functioning are compared unless large samples are available.

Across the various treatment regimens for CNS prophylaxis there seems to be a core set of factors identified as predictors of poorer neurocognitive outcomes.

For example, females seem more vulnerable to neurocognitive deficits following CNS-directed therapies [37]. It has been hypothesized that these gender-linked differences in neurocognitive outcomes may relate to varied sexual dimorphism in male and female brains. Boys have a higher percentage of white matter within their brains than do girls, making girls potentially more sensitive to agents that disrupt white matter development and functioning [38]. Young age during treatment is also related to poorer neurocognitive outcomes, and in this case is believed to be a proxy for underlying neurodevelopmental maturity [39]. Regardless of age, patients undergoing CNS prophylactic treatment have been found to lose white matter volume at a similar rate [16]. Because younger age is associated with less fully developed white matter, they tend to lose a greater overall percentage of their white matter which has been linked with greater intellectual deficits [39]. Time since treatment is a third variable that relates to the degree of neurocognitive impairment with greater deficits seen with longer-term follow-up. Deficits can begin to appear within 1 to 2 years of treatment, however, some studies have found that effects can be delayed for up to 10 years after treatment [40] and some suggest that the subtler deficits associated with IT chemotherapy only regimens may take even longer to materialize [27]. Generally it has been accepted that the effects of CNS-directed therapies do not cause declines in cognitive abilities, but rather cognitive growth is slowed in comparison to same age peers and eventually may plateau. Of course, with standardized tests that use age-based norms, this manifests as declining scores over time [9].

Neurocognitive Sequelae in Survivors of Childhood CNS Tumors

Childhood CNS tumor survivors often experience a number of medical late effects across multiple areas, including deficiencies in hormones, hearing impairments, and neurological difficulties [41]. The totality of these late effects contributes to pediatric CNS tumor survivors having the poorest health-related quality of life among childhood cancer survivors [42]. The often pervasive neurocognitive late effects, however, are the most debilitating for these survivors and largely responsible for their poor quality of life.

Although conducting "clean" research on the neurocognitive late effects of CNS tumor survivors with adequate sample sizes is difficult due to the heterogeneity of tumor types and treatment regimens, there is strong evidence documenting the significant deficits in overall intellectual functioning (IQ) [43]. A recent meta-analysis on neurocognitive outcomes in survivors of childhood CNS tumors that incorporated data from 39 studies concluded that this group of survivors experiences clinically significant deficits in across multiple domains of neurocognitive functioning compared to normative data [5]. The meta-analysis indicated medium-to-large effect sizes for deficits in overall IQ, verbal IQ and non-verbal IQ [5].

A notable series of longitudinal studies demonstrated that children with medulloblastoma treated with surgical resection and craniospinal radiation evidence significant and continued declines in IQ over time [44, 45]. One study found that these declines occur at an average rate of approximately 2.5 IQ points per year [45]. Children who were younger at the time of radiation treatment displayed more immediate declines in IQ (i.e., within the first year after radiation) that continued over time, while older children did not demonstrate declines in IQ until approximately two years after the conclusion of treatment [44]. Although the sample demonstrated increases in raw scores on the subtests comprising the IQ measure, these increases occurred at a slower rate than expected when compared to norms for same-age peers, resulting in decreases in IQ scores over time [45]. This suggests that children treated with craniospinal radiation do not lose previously acquired skills or information but have difficulty acquiring new skills and knowledge at the expected rate [45].

Given these findings, researchers have focused on the core neurocognitive processes of these survivors that likely account for these difficulties with knowledge acquisition [45]. The processes of attention, working memory and processing speed have received the most consideration since normal, developmental improvements in these areas generally account for a large proportion of the variance in measures of general intelligence in healthy children [46] and ALL survivors [47]. Indeed, survivors of childhood CNS tumors experience deficits across a wide array of core areas [43] including working memory [48], executive functioning [49], processing speed [50], verbal memory [51], and attention [52–54]. Furthermore, the recent meta-analysis found large effect sizes for deficits in verbal memory, language, visual-spatial skills, and attention [5].

Research has illustrated that survivors of CNS tumors experience difficulties across multiple domains of attention. A study that serially administered a widely used measure of sustained attention to children with primary brain tumors throughout the course of radiation therapy and up to five years off treatment showed significant increases in survivor inattentiveness in the years following radiation [52]. Another study

found that children with posterior fossa tumors treated with or without cranial radiation demonstrate deficits in selective attention abilities, although those who received cranial radiation had the most significant deficits [53]. Such difficulties likely make it challenging for survivors to efficiently and quickly focus on important stimuli while resisting distraction and could contribute to their problems with acquiring new information at expected rates. Evidence suggesting that reductions in white matter volumes following radiation have indirect effects on IQ through declines in attentional functioning support this hypothesis [55].

Several factors influence the nature and severity of the neurocognitive sequelae experienced by survivors. The type and location of the tumor, the specific tumor-directed treatments used [41], the presence of post-surgical complications [56, 57], and the age of the child during treatment [13, 58] have all been related to neurocognitive outcomes. Receiving cranial radiation and, even more so, receiving cranial radiation at a young age (typically younger than age 8) are considered the most significant risk factors for developing neurocognitive late effects due to the effects of radiation on white matter development in younger children [13, 17]. Through a series of studies using magnetic resonance imaging to examine white matter volume, Mulhern and colleagues highlighted the associations between age at time of radiation, white matter volume, and IQ and indices of attentional functioning, with younger children during treatment showing reduced white matter volume and more neurocognitive deficits [13, 17].

Additionally, post-surgical complications warrant further consideration for their role in the development of neurocognitive late effects. One study comparing the neurocognitive outcomes in pediatric medulloblastoma survivors with and without ventriculoperitoneal-shunts for hydrocephalus following tumor resection, revealed that those with shunts had significantly lower IQs, nonverbal reasoning skills, and academic skills than those survivors without shunts [56]. Another study demonstrated that, compared to matched medulloblastoma survivor controls, medulloblastoma survivors who developed cerebellar mutism syndrome following surgical resection had significantly worse performances on measures of attention, processing speed, working memory, executive function, and academic skills 12 months following the diagnosis of cerebellar mutism syndrome [57]. These studies highlight the many complexities in terms of conducting research on neurocognitive outcomes in pediatric CNS tumor survivors and delivering clinical care to these at-risk groups.

Standards of Clinical Care for Survivors of Childhood ALL and CNS Tumors

Given that 40–60% of childhood cancer survivors are at risk for neurocognitive impairment [39, 59], the Long-term Follow-up Guidelines of the Children's Oncology Group (COG; www.survivorshipguidelines. org) includes recommendations for neurocognitive screening and intervention for survivors of childhood cancer. These guidelines are evidence-based, developed and updated periodically after review of the available literature, and informed by the collective clinical experiences of a multidisciplinary panel of experts in late effects of pediatric cancer treatment. Version 3.0 of these guidelines was completed in October 2008 after a review of the literature spanning through 2007.

These guidelines recommend formal neuropsychological evaluation around the time that medical treatment ends for children whose therapy has included antimetabolites (i.e., Methotrexate, high dose IV Cytarabine), cranial or total body irradiation, and/or neurosurgery. This evaluation is recommended even in the absence of overt clinical manifestations of CNS injury to serve as a baseline against which future functioning can be compared. After that, follow-up evaluation is recommended as clinically indicated. For example, as soon as the child begins to have difficulties in school, or perceived changes in their cognitive functioning, testing should be repeated. In the absence of noted changes, repeat testing is also recommended based upon the child's specific medical and developmental risk factors and the anticipated trajectory of the emergence of late cognitive effects [60]. For example, repeat testing should be considered when the child transitions to a new level of schooling (i.e., junior high to high school; high school to college).

Given the pattern of potential deficits as outlined above, formal neurocognitive evaluation is recommended to include measures of intelligence, processing speed, academic achievement, memory, attention, visual motor integration, comprehension of verbal instructions, verbal fluency, executive function and planning. Finally, it is recommended that patients with identified neurocognitive deficits be provided with intervention in the form of specialized educational plans and that emerging interventions, such as psychotropic medications (e.g., stimulants) or evidence-based cognitive rehabilitation training, be considered [60].

Intervention Efforts

Given the clear evidence of the neurocognitive sequelae in survivors of childhood ALL and CNS tumors, interventions are needed that address the pattern of deficits seen in these survivors in order to improve outcomes and enhance quality of life. However, the research on interventions for these concerns is in its early stages and needing additional empirical investigations. Although there are multiple innovative, ongoing studies currently examining the benefits of a variety of approaches (e.g., computer programs), only two intervention approaches have been tested in separate multisite randomized, clinical trials: stimulant medication [61] and cognitive remediation [62].

Stimulant medication is a common and effective treatment approach to address symptoms associated with ADHD. Methylphenidate, in particular, is the most common stimulant used to treat ADHD and works by increasing the availability of dopamine in the prefrontal cortex [63]. The benefits of methylphenidate in children with ADHD have been well documented, particularly on measures of attention and behavior [64], Given the similarities in the types of attentional deficits between survivors of childhood cancer and children with ADHD, several trials have examined the efficacy of methylphenidate in survivors of ALL and CNS tumors with mixed findings. Using randomized, double-blind, placebo-controlled designs, a series of studies have found significant methylphenidate-related improvements on teacher and parent ratings of attention and teacher ratings of social skills after 3 weeks [65, 66] and 12 months [66]. Another study using a similar design found acute benefits of methylphenidate when compared to placebo on measures of processing speed but not attention after 3 weeks of methylphenidate use [67]. However, benefits of methylphenidate use were found at 12-month follow-up on indices of sustained attention, processing speed, and parent and teacher reports of functioning [61].

Despite these generally promising findings, it is unclear whether methylphenidate is an appropriate treatment approach for childhood cancer survivors. One study examining the benefits of a moderate dose of methylphenidate after three weeks of use found that only 45% of the sample could be classified as responders to the medication trial [68]. This response rate is much lower than the 75% rate seen in children with ADHD [68]. In general, those with more teacher and parent-identified problems with attention prior to the trial of methylphenidate were more likely to have a positive response [68]. Additionally, female survivors and those with lower baseline IQ are more likely to report more severe medication-related side effects [69]. Additional research is needed in order to identify those survivors who are most likely to benefit from a trial of stimulant medication.

A second line of intervention research has focused on the application of cognitive rehabilitation or remediation in survivors of childhood cancer. Cognitive remediation is well established in the fields of adult and pediatric brain injury rehabilitation with most studies finding small-to-moderate, yet clinically relevant, improvements in functioning across multiple domains [70, 71]. Through a series of studies involving single-case [72] and pilot designs [73], Butler and colleagues adapted and refined a cognitive remediation program (CRP) that was subsequently evaluated in a multisite, randomized controlled trial with 161 survivors of childhood cancer who had documented difficulties with attention [62]. The intervention evaluated in this trial consisted of 20 2-hour sessions and contained instruction on meta-cognitive and academic strategies, components of cognitive-behavioral interventions, and progressive massed practice of all exercises and strategies. The intervention was compared to a wait-list control group. Participants in the intervention group underwent assessments of academic achievement, attentional functioning, working memory, and memory at baseline and 6 months after the conclusion of treatment while those in the control group were evaluated at baseline and again 6 months later. Compared to the control group, those receiving the CRP exhibited significant improvements in academic performance, parent-rated attention, and use of metacognitive strategies [62]. The CRP, however, failed to produce significant improvements in the measured neurocognitive outcomes, such as attention and working memory. Completion of all 20 sessions was an issue for this intervention, particularly for older survivors and African-American survivors [62]. While the findings are promising, refinements to this intervention approach are needed in order to enhance the benefits of the intervention while increasing the acceptability and feasibility of the intervention by reducing the demand on survivors and families.

Future Directions

This review has highlighted the significant progress that has been made in understanding the neurocognitive sequelae in survivors of childhood cancer. However, there are many directions for future research that require careful study in order to further the field and promote the best outcomes possible for this group of survivors. An ongoing challenge of research on the neurocognitive late effects of childhood cancer survivors relates to the rapid developments and improvements in cancer treatments. Protocols for treating childhood cancer change so quickly that it is often

difficult for research on the neurocognitive late effects to keep up with these changes in treatments over time. Additionally, after a new treatment's effects on neurocognitive functioning become understood through several years of research, a new treatment breakthrough is likely to occur that will require further study on its associated neurocognitive sequelae. Proton radiation, for example, is a potential treatment for cancers affecting the CNS that may reduce the severity of neurocognitive sequelae in children due to its potential in reducing the amount of exposure of healthy brain tissue to radiation [74, 75]. As technology advances and more children are treated with risk-adapted protocols [76], it is important for psychologists and neuropsychologists to be involved in the development of cooperative research protocols (e.g., Children's Oncology Group) that incorporate regular neuropsychological assessments in order to better understand the neurocognitive sequelae of these new treatment approaches.

From research and clinical perspectives, brief screening approaches are needed to effectively and efficiently identify those survivors demonstrating neurocognitive difficulties who are in need of additional evaluations and resources. Such screeners should be incorporated into treatment protocols and routine clinical care throughout the course of treatment and into survivorship. Routine, serial, brief assessment batteries that include elements of standardized neurocognitive tests and self- and informant-reports of functioning could be regularly implemented across pediatric cancer centers in order to compile substantial data on neurocognitive outcomes in survivors and address a largely unmet need in clinical care [77]. The Childhood Cancer Survivor Study Neurocognitive Questionnaire [78] is a self-report measure of neurocognitive functioning for childhood survivors that holds promise as a tool that could be widely used to screen survivors for the need for further neurocognitive testing and deserves additional research given its potential clinical utility.

An unexplored area of research is the role of other systems (e.g., family, school, peers) on the development and expression of neurocognitive late effects in childhood cancer survivors. A comprehensive model of childhood cancer survivorship suggests that several child and family factors, including family adaptation and functioning, and school factors influence the course of neurocognitive late effects in survivors [79]. Such factors deserve empirical investigations in order to establish their relevance as risk and protective factors and potential intervention targets or mechanisms. Assessments of the family system, in particular, should be included in future research on neurocognitive sequelae in survivors given the family's potential to influence survivor outcomes [80].

The field is ripe for innovations in clinical interventions that address survivors' neurocognitive late effects. The previously discussed randomized controlled clinical trial of an intensive cognitive remediation program [62] holds promise as an intervention program for survivors. However, improvements to this treatment are needed to make it more feasible for families and cost-effective (e.g., fewer session, delivered in the home) and to help the benefits of the intervention generalize, such as incorporating elements that address family systems factors [62]. Ongoing trials involving computer-based interventions (e.g., Cogmed RM^{TM}) offer potential as effective and cost-efficient approaches that target important areas of neurocognitive functioning for survivors of childhood cancer, such as working memory [81] and executive function [82]. In the future, it will be important to investigate whether such cognitive training may be effective to preserve functioning in children with cancer at greatest risk for long-term neurocognitive sequelae.

Finally, scientific and technological advances have made it possible to study the underlying neurobiological and genetic mechanisms of the neurocognitive sequelae in childhood cancer survivors. Earlier research using quantitative magnetic resonance imaging (MRI) techniques [83] and diffusion tensor imaging [84], which can examine the integrity of white matter in survivors, has highlighted the importance of better understanding how alterations in various brain structures secondary to disease and treatment influence the development of neurocognitive late effects in survivors. In one study, for example, MRI scans showing temporary changes in white matter in children under the age of 5 undergoing chemotherapy for ALL were associated with declines in neurocognitive functioning [85]. A recent study using diffusion tensor imaging to examine white matter fractional anisotropy found impairments in white matter tracts that correlated with decreased processing speed [86]. Another study that screened survivors using EEG found that changes in event-related potential mismatch negativity were associated with declines in neurocognitive functioning [87]. Genetic polymorphisms also have been identified as possible contributing risk factors to the development of neurocognitive late effects in children treated for ALL [88]. These imaging, scanning, and genetic screening approaches should be incorporated into research protocols in order to better understand the neuropathology of these neurocognitive late effects and identify those at greatest risk for developing neurocognitive late effects.

Understanding who is more likely to experience long-term neurocognitive declines at the time of cancer therapy based on genetic or structural markers (e.g., changes in white matter during active chemotherapy) could lead to greater implementation of risk-adapted treatment protocols that aim to spare neurocognitive functioning by reducing or eliminating unnecessary therapy directed at the CNS. Furthermore, cognitive remediation programs could be implemented preventively to those at greatest risk in the early stages of cancer treatment in an effort to prevent and ameliorate these neurocognitive sequelae [9].

References

1. American Cancer Society. *Cancer Facts and Figures*. Atlanta, GA: American Cancer Society, 2009.
2. Howlader N, *et al.* (eds.) *SEER Cancer Statistics Review, 1975–2008*. Bethesda, MD: National Cancer Institute, 2011.
3. Oeffinger KC, *et al.* Chronic health conditions in adult survivors of childhood cancer. *New England Journal of Medicine* 2006;**355**:1572–1582.
4. Campbell LK, *et al.* A meta-analysis of the neuro-cognitive sequelae of treatment for childhood acute lymphocytic leukemia. *Pediatric Blood & Cancer* 2007;**49**:65–73.
5. Robinson KE, *et al.* A quantitative meta-analysis of neurocognitive sequelae in survivors of pediatric brain tumors. *Pediatric Blood & Cancer* 2010;**55**:525–531.
6. Ellenberg L, *et al.* Neurocognitive status in long-term survivors of childhood CNS malignancies: a report from the Childhood Cancer Survivor Study. *Neuropsychology* 2009;**23**:705–717.
7. Gaynon PS, *et al.* Children's Cancer Group trials in childhood acute lymphoblastic leukemia, 1983–1995. *Leukemia* 2000;**14**:2223–2233.
8. Tubergen DG, *et al.* Prevention of CNS disease in intermediate-risk acute lymphoblastic leukemia: comparison of cranial radiation and intrathecal methotrexate and the importance of systemic therapy: a Childrens Cancer Group Report. *Journal of Clinical Oncology* 1993;**11**:520–526.
9. Askins MA, Moore IIIBD. Preventing neurocognitive late effects in childhood cancer survivors. *Journal of Child Neurology* 2008;**23**:1160–1171.
10. Steinlin M, *et al.* Neuropsychological long-term sequelae after posterior fossa tumor resection during childhood. *Brain* 2003;**126**:1998–2008.
11. Casey BJ, Giedd JN, Thomas KM. Structural and functional brain development and its relation to cognitive development. *Biological Psychology* 2000;**54**:241–257.
12. Mulhern RK, Butler RW. Neurocognitive sequelae of childhood cancers and their treatment. *Pediatric Rehabilitation* 2004;**7**:1–14.
13. Mulhern RK, *et al.* Risks of young age for selected neurocognitive deficits in medulloblastoma are associated with white matter loss. *Journal of Clinical Oncology* 2001;**19**:472–479.
14. Gunning-Dixon FM, Raz N. The cognitive correlates of white matter abnormalities in normal aging: a quantitative review. *Neuropsychology* 2000;**14**:224–232.

15. Reddick WE, *et al.* A typical white matter volume development in children following craniospinal irradiation. *Neuro-Oncology* 2005;**7**:12–19.

16. Reddick WE, *et al.* Subtle white matter volume differences in children treated for medulloblastoma with conventional or reduced dose craniospinal irradiation. *Magnetic Resonance Imaging* 2000;**18**:787–793.

17. Mulhern RK, *et al.* Attentional functioning and white matter integrity among survivors of malignant brain tumors of childhood. *Journal of the International Neuropsychological Society* 2004;**10**:180–189.

18. Ashford J, *et al.* Attention and working memory abilities in children treated for acute lymphoblastic leukemia. *Cancer* 2010;**116**:4638–4645.

19. Simone J, *et al.* "Total therapy" studies of acute lymphocytic leukemia in children. current results and prospects for cure. *Cancer* 1972;**30**:2123–2134.

20. Soni SS, *et al.* Effects of central-nervous-system irradiation on neuropsychologic functioning of children with acute lymphocytic leukemia. *New England Journal of Medicine* 1975;**293**:113–118.

21. Meadows, AT, *et al.* Declines in IQ scores and cognitive dysfunction in children with acute lymphocytic leukemia treated with cranial irradiation. *Lancet* 1981;**2**:1015–1018.

22. Cousens P, *et al.* Cognitive effects of cranial irradiation in leukemia: a survey and meta-analysis. *Journal of Child Psychology and Psychiatry and Allied Disciplines* 1988;**29**: 839–852.

23. Cousens P, *et al.* Cognitive effects of childhood leukemia therapy: a case for four specific deficits. *Journal of Pediatric Psychology* 1991;**16**:475–488.

24. Rowland JH, *et al.* Effects of different forms of central nervous system prophylaxis on neuropsychologic function in childhood leukemia. *Journal of Clinical Oncology* 1984;**2**:1327–1335.

25. Mulhern RK, Fairclough D, Ochs J. A prospective comparison of neuropsychologic performance of children surviving leukemia who received 18-Gy, 24-Gy, or no cranial irradiation. *Journal of Clinical Oncology* 1991;**9**: 1348–1356.

26. Ochs J, *et al.* Comparison of neuropsychologic functioning and clinical indicators of neurotoxicity in long-term survivors of childhood leukemia given cranial radiation or parenteral methotrexate: a prospective study. *Journal of Clinical Oncology* 1991;**9**:145–151.

27. Harila MJ, *et al.* Progressive neurocognitive impairment in young adult survivors of childhood acute lymphoblastic leukemia. *Pediatric Blood & Cancer* 2009;**53**: 156–161.

28. Langer T, *et al.* CNS late effects after ALL therapy in childhood, Part III: neuropsychological performance in long-term survivors of childhood ALL: impairments of concentration, attention and memory. *Medical and Pediatric Oncology* 2002;**38**:320–328.

29. Spiegler B, *et al.* Comparison of long-term neurocognitive outcomes in young children with acute lymphoblastic leukemia treated with cranial radiation or high-dose or very high-dose intravenous methotrexate. *Journal of Clinical Oncology* 2006;**20**:3858–3864.

30. Moleski M. Neuropsychological, neuroanatomical, and neurophysiological consequences of CNS chemotherapy for acute lymphoblastic leukemia. *Archives of Clinical Neuropsychology* 2000;**15**:603–630.

31. Buizer AI, de Sonneville LM, Veerman AJ. Effects of chemotherapy on neurocognitive function in children with acute lymphoblastic leukemia: a critical review of the literature. *Pediatric Blood & Cancer* 2009;**52**:447–454.

32. Peterson CC, *et al.* A meta-analysis of the neuropsychological sequelae of chemotherapy-only treatment for pediatric acute lymphoblastic leukemia. *Pediatric Blood & Cancer* 2008;**51**:99–104.

33. Jansen NC, *et al.* Neuropsychological outcome in chemotherapy-only treated children with acute lymphoblastic leukemia. *Journal of Clinical Oncology* 2008;**20**: 3025–3030.

34. Lofstad, GE, *et al.* Cognitive outcome in children and adolescents treated for acute lymphoblastic leukemia with chemotherapy only. *Acta Paediatrica,* 2009;**98**: 180–186.

35. Winick N. Neurocognitive outcome in survivors of pediatric cancer. *Current Opinion in Pediatrics,* 2011;**23**: 27–33.

36. Mulhern RK, Butler RW. Neuropsychological late effects. In: Brown RT (ed.) *Comprehensive Handbook of Childhood Cancer and Sickle Cell Disease: A Biopsychosocial Approach.* New York: Oxford University Press, 2006; pp. 262–278.

37. Moore IIIBD. Neurocognitive outcomes in survivors of childhood cancer. *Journal of Pediatric Psychology* 2005; **30**:51–63.

38. Jain N, *et al.* Sex-specific attention problems in long-term survivors of pediatric acute lymphoblastic leukemia. *Cancer* 2009;**115**:4238–4245.

39. Mulhern RK, Palmer SL. Neurocognitive late effects in pediatric cancer. *Current Problems in Cancer* 2003;**27**: 177–197.

40. Kato M, *et al.* Ten-year survey of the intellectual deficits in children with acute lymphoblastic leukemia receiving chemoimmunotherapy. *Medical and Pediatric Oncology* 2003;**21**:435–440.

41. Turner CD, *et al.* Late effects of therapy for pediatric brain tumor survivors. *Journal of Child Neurology* 2009;**24**:1455–1463.

42. Zeltzer L, *et al.* Psychological status in childhood cancer survivors: a report from the Childhood Cancer Survivor Study. *Journal of Clinical Oncology* 2009;**27**:2396–2404.

43. Mulhern RK, *et al.* Late neurocognitive sequelae in survivors of brain tumors in childhood. *Lancet Oncology* 2004;**5**:399–408.

44. Palmer SL, *et al.* Predicting intellectual outcome among children treated with 35–40 Gy craniospinal irradiation for medulloblastoma. *Neuropsychology* 2003; **17**:548–555.

45. Palmer SL, *et al.* Patterns of intellectual development among survivors of pediatric medulloblastoma: A longitudinal analysis. *Journal of Clinical Oncology* 2001;**19**: 2302–2308.

46. Fry AF, Hale S. Relationships among processing speed, working memory, and fluid intelligence in children. *Biological Psychology* 2000;**54**:1–34.

47. Schatz J, *et al.* Processing speed, working memory, and IQ: a developmental model of cognitive deficits following cranial radiation therapy. *Neuropsychology* 2000;**14**: 189–200.

48. Callu D, *et al.* Cognitive and academic outcome after benign or malignant cerebellar tumor in children. *Cognitive and Behavioral Neurology* 2009;**22**:270–278.

49. Spiegler B, et al. Change in neurocognitive functioning after treatment with cranial radiation in childhood. Journal of Clinical Oncology 2004;**22**:706–713.

50. Mabbott DJ, et al. Core neurocognitive functions in children treated for posterior fossa tumors. Neuropsychology 2008;**22**:159–168.

51. Nagel BJ, et al. Early patterns of verbal memory impairment in children treated for medulloblastoma. Neuropsychology, 2006;**20**:105–112.

52. Kiehna EN, et al. Changes in attentional performance of children and young adults with localized primary brain tumors after conformal radiation therapy. Journal of Clinical Oncology 2006;**24**:5283–5290.

53. Mabbott DJ, et al. The effects of treatment for posterior fossa brain tumors on selective attention. Journal of the International Neuropsychological Society 2009;**15**:205–216.

54. Reeves C, et al. Attention and memory functioning among pediatric patients with medulloblastoma. Journal of Pediatric Psychology 2006;**31**:272–280.

55. Reddick WE, et al. Developmental model relating white matter volume to neurocognitive deficits in pediatric brain tumor survivors. Cancer 2003;**97**:2512–2519.

56. Hardy KK, et al. Hydrocephalus as a possible additional contributor to cognitive outcome in survivors of pediatric medulloblastoma. Psycho-Oncology 2008;**17**:1157–1161.

57. Palmer SL, et al. Neurocognitive outcome 12 months following cerebellar mutism syndrome in pediatric patients with medulloblastoma. Neuro-Oncology 2010;**12**:1311–1317.

58. Sands SA, et al. Long-term quality of life and neuropsychologic functioning for patients with CNS germ-cell tumors: from the First International Germ-Cell Tumor Study. Neuro-Oncology 2001;**3**:175–183.

59. Hewitt M, SL. Weiner P, Simone JV (eds.) Childhood Cancer Survivorship: Improving Care and Quality of Life. Washington, DC: National Academies Press, 2003.

60. Nathan PC, et al. Guidelines for identification of, advocacy for, and intervention in neurocognitive problems in survivors of childhood cancer: a report from the Children's Oncology Group. Archives of Pediatrics and Adolescent Medicine 2007;**161**:798–806.

61. Conklin HM, et al. Long-term efficacy of methylphenidate in enhancing attention regulation, social skills, and academic abilities of childhood cancer survivors. Journal of Clinical Oncology 2010;**28**:4465–4472.

62. Butler RW, et al. A multicenter, randomized clinical trial of a cognitive remediation program for childhood survivors of a pediatric malignancy. Journal of Consulting and Clinical Psychology 2008;**76**:367–378.

63. Nelson JC. Sympathomimetics. In: Kaplan HI, Saddock BJC (eds.) Comprehensive Textbook of Psychiatry. Baltimore, MD: Williams & Wilkins, 1995.

64. Brown RT, et al. Treatment of attention-deficit/hyperactivity disorder: overview of the evidence. Pediatrics 2005;**115**:749–757.

65. Mulhern RK, et al. Short-term efficacy of methylphenidate: arandomized, double-blind, placebo-controlled trial among survivors of childhood cancer. Journal of Clinical Oncology 2004;**22**:4795–4803.

66. Netson KL, et al. Parent and teacher ratings of attention during a year-long methylphenidate trial in children treated for cancer. Journal of Pediatric Psychology 2011;**36**:438–450.

67. Conklin HM, et al. Acute neurocognitive response to methylphenidate among survivors of childhood cancer: a randomized, double-blind, cross-over trial. Journal of Pediatric Psychology 2007;**32**:1127–1139.

68. Conklin HM, et al. Predicting methylphenidate response in long-term survivors of childhood cancer: a randomized, double-blind, placebo-controlled, crossover trial. Journal of Pediatric Psychology 2010;**35**:144–155.

69. Conklin HM, et al. Side effects of methylphenidate in survivors of childhood cancer: a randomized, double-blind, placebo-controlled trial. Pediatrics 2009;**124**:226–233.

70. Anderson V, Catroppa C. Advances in postacute rehabilitation after childhood-acquired brain injury: a focus on cognitive, behavioral, and social domains. American Journal of Physical Medicine and Rehabilitation 2006;**85**:767–778.

71. Cicerone KD, et al. Evidence-based cognitive rehabilitation: updated review of the literature from 2003–2008. Archives of Physical Medicine and Rehabilitation 2011;**92**:519–530.

72. Butler RW. Attentional processes and their remediation in childhood cancer. Medical and Pediatric Oncology 1998;**30**:75–78.

73. Butler RW, Copeland DR. Attentional processes and their remediation in children treated for cancer: a literature review and the development of a therapeutic approach. Journal of the International Neuropsychological Society 2002;**8**:115–124.

74. Merchant TE, et al. Proton versus photon radiotherapy for common pediatric brain tumors: comparison of models of dose characteristics and their relationship to cognitive function. Pediatric Blood & Cancer 2008;**51**:110–117.

75. Semenova J. Proton beam radiation therapy in the treatment of pediatric central nervous system malignancies: a review of the literature. Journal of Pediatric Oncology Nursing 2009;**26**:142–149.

76. Mulhern RK, et al. Neurocognitive consequences of risk-adapted therapy for childhood medulloblastoma. Journal of Clinical Oncology 2005;**23**:5511–5519.

77. Krull KR, et al. Screening for neurocognitive impairment in pediatric cancer long-term survivors. Journal of Clinical Oncology 2008;**25**:4138–4143.

78. Krull KR, et al. Reliability and validity of the Childhood Cancer Survivor Study Neurocognitive Questionnaire. Cancer 2008;**113**:2188–2197.

79. Peterson CC, Drotar D. Family impact of neurodevelopmental late effects in survivors of pediatric cancer: review of research, clinical evidence, and future directions. Clinical Child Psychology and Psychiatry 2006;**11**:349–366.

80. Hocking MC, et al. Neurocognitive and family functioning and quality of life among young adult survivors of childhood brain tumors. The Clinical Neuropsychologist. In press.

81. Hardy KK, Willard VW, Bonner M. Computerized cognitive training in survivors of childhood cancer: a pilot study. Journal of Pediatric Oncology Nursing 2011;**28**:27–33.

82. Kesler SR, Lacayo NJ, Jo B. A pilot study of an online cognitive rehabilitation program for executive function skills in children with cancer-related brain injury. Brain Injury 2011;**25**:101–112.

83. Mulhern RK, et al. Neurocognitive deficits in medulloblastoma survivors and white matter loss. Annals of Neurology 1999;**46**:834–841.

84. Khong P-L, *et al.* White matter anisotropy in post-treatment childhood cancer survivors: preliminary evidence of association with neurocognitive function. *Journal of Clinical Oncology* 2006;**24**:884–890.

85. Wilson DA, *et al.* Transient white matter changes on MR images in children undergoing chemotherapy for acute lymphocytic leukemia: correlation with neuropsychologic deficiencies. *Radiology* 1991;**180**:205–209.

86. Aukema EJ, *et al.* White matter fractional anisotropy correlates with speed of processing and motor speed in young childhood cancer survivors. *International Journal of Radiation Oncology Biology and Physics* 2009;**74**:837–843.

87. Jarvela LS, *et al.* Auditory event related potentials as tools to reveal cognitive late effects in childhood cancer patients. *Clinical Neurophysiology* 2011;**122**:62–72.

88. Krakinovic M, *et al.* Polymorphisms of genes controlling homocysteine levels and IQ score following the treatment for childhood ALL. *Pharmacogenomics* 2005; **6**:293–302.

16

Survivorship in Childhood Cancer

Elena Krivoy, Meriel E.M. Jenney, Amita Mahajan, Monique Peretz Nahum[1]

Introduction

In treating and controlling cancer, the most dramatic evidence of progress is that seen in childhood cancer. Formerly almost uniformly fatal, pediatric cancer has become a commonly curable illness in the past 30 years. For children diagnosed with cancer, the current five years cancer-free survival rate is 80% and the ten years survival rate is approaching 75% [1].

In 2010, it is estimated that 1 in 250 adolescents and young adults aged 15–40 in the USA, and 1 in 715 people in United Kingdom is a survivor of a childhood malignancy [2]. This population is at an increased risk for late health problems, with a relative risk (RR) of 16 compared to siblings, according to the last Childhood Cancer Survivor Study (CCSS) report [3]. Late effects such as delayed growth and other endocrinological problems, musculo-skeletal sequelae, neurocognitive impairment, reduced fertility, cardiotoxicity, and second malignancies have been extensively reported in many publications [4, 5]. In Nordic countries, childhood cancer survivors constitute 0.1% of the national population, and they have a persistent overall RR of 5.9 for a second malignant neoplasm [6].

Over half of all childhood cancer survivors may experience at least one chronic medical problem [7]. Late effects depend on cancer type and site, treatment, gender, and age at diagnosis. Teenagers and female cancer patients have a higher risk for specific late effects, such as fertility or sexual function and for psychosocial difficulties than other survivors [8].

The fact that so many children with cancer live long enough to become young, even aging adults, is one explanation why pediatric oncology clinicians, and researchers are among the leaders in identifying the chronic and late effects of cancer and their treatment. Curing a child is not enough; it is an obligation to consider that the quality of children's lives is as important as their duration [9]. Does this population also have a higher incidence of disturbances in psychosocial adjustment, given their frequency of chronic medical complications, their "at-risk" status of disease recurrence, and the psychological trauma of their earlier illness experiences?

The dramatic improvement in survival rates has led to a shift in research toward the concerns of long-term survivors, into areas not traditionally considered as part of pediatric psychology. It is now appropriate to address the problems that survivors are having with issues such as employment, marriage, and parenthood.

A review of the literature on the psychosocial outcomes of childhood cancer survivors shows varied and sometimes contradictory results. This inconsistency in outcomes is likely caused by small sample sizes, varied outcomes measures used across studies, differences in the populations studied (e.g., the inclusion of brain tumor survivors with significant neurocognitive problems, or not), and differences in the selection of population norms for the comparison group [10].

Following Completion of Treatment

The Transition

At first sight, completion of therapy would appear to be a positive experience for families. However, it is frequently a time of distress, anxiety, and uncertainty. The significance of this transition phase for families can be under-estimated by their carers. Patients and families are often ambivalent about terminating the use of chemotherapeutic agents known to be responsible for cancer remission [11]. Consequently, they often report heightened anxiety, fears, and feeling of vulnerability as active treatment ends [12] The protocols and

Pediatric Psycho-oncology: Psychosocial Aspects and Clinical Interventions, Second Edition.
Edited by Shulamith Kreitler, Myriam Weyl Ben-Arush and Andrés Martin.
© 2012 John Wiley & Sons, Ltd. Published 2012 by John Wiley & Sons, Ltd.

treatment modalities, which have provided structure and reassurance, are replaced by a "wait and see" period recurrence is still a possibility.

A formal conference at the end of treatment is appropriate to address these issues and prepare the family for the future. This provides a sense of closure to the active treatment. It also provides an opportunity to move from active treatment to a focus on a healthy lifestyle and a perspective that reflects an understanding of the disease, and of potential late-effects.

Physical Sequelae of Successful Therapy

Successful therapy can be associated with a number of potential long-term physical sequelae. The functional status of individual patients in adolescence and adulthood largely depends on the severity of these effects and how effectively they develop coping strategies. The presence or absence of long-term physical toxicity may be one of the major determinants of psychological well-being in adulthood. The physical sequelae of successful treatment have been extensively reported elsewhere [13–15]. They include physical disfigurement (e.g. radiotherapy to face, keloid scar, chronic hair loss or amputation) or limitation of function, e.g. following limb salvage procedures for bone tumors, neurological deficit, chronic bladder and bowel dysfunction. Growth impairment, abnormalities of puberty, obesity and other endocrine abnormalities are reported in a number of survivors, particularly following cranial radiotherapy or bone marrow transplantation (BMT). Radiation therapy has been associated with risk of severe age-related and dose-related physical late effects [16].

The central nervous system (CNS) late effects include a range of neuropsychological disorders varying from subtle learning difficulties to overt neurological deterioration depending on the modality of treatment given. Common problems include deficiencies in mental processing speed, verbal and non-verbal memory, freedom from distractibility, attention and arithmetic.

Studies of mortality of long-term survivors suggest that there is an increased risk of early death of 7% at 30 years [16]. The patients at most risk of increased late mortality are those who survived relapse of their primary tumor and those with a second malignant neoplasm (SMN).

In the latest Children Cancer Survivor Study report [17], the cumulative incidence of SMN was 11% among 14,359 patients, within 30 years of diagnosis. The presence or absence of these late-effects may have a significant influence on the subsequent psychological adjustment of the survivors.

Psychological Adjustment of Child and Adolescent Cancer Survivors and Impact on Social Skills

Overview

The psychological impact of having had childhood cancer can continue long after treatment ends for survivors and their families. However, reassuringly most survivors appear to have a reasonable level of psychosocial adjustment. This adjustment in the years after completion of therapy depends on a number of variables. The age at diagnosis, level of academic functioning and family cohesiveness are major determinants in childhood and adolescence. In adulthood, the presence or absence of physical sequelae and economic status (specifically successful employment) are important factors influencing adequate psychosocial adjustment.

The diagnosis of cancer and subsequent treatment may challenge the child's normal development by limiting opportunities, restricting play and other activities, delaying the attainment of autonomy and potentially compromising family and peer relationships. These effects may differ specifically as a function of the child's age. For infants, cancer is most likely to affect parent–child relationships, restrict mobility, or limit opportunities to socialize with peers. For older children, the impact of cancer can lead to reduced schooling, compromised peer relationships, more time with adults, concern about body image and awareness of vulnerability and possible death. Cancer in adolescence may extend the period of dependency on parents and may reduce opportunities to establish close interpersonal relationships, for example, with the opposite sex. We will explore these issues for children with cancer at different ages and stages of maturity.

Psychological Adjustment in Childhood in the First Few Years Following Completion of Therapy

A number of issues are of particular importance for the intellectual and psychological well-being of the prepubertal child. These include freedom from symptoms, growth, spontaneous progression through puberty and normal physical development. Adjusting to normal family life rather than being the center of attention may also be challenging for some. A number of studies have investigated peer relationships, interactions and perceptions during the critical period of reintegration into school during the late-treatment phase and immediately following completion of therapy. For example, in a study evaluating teacher ratings of children who were either on treatment or had terminated therapy within the past year [18], 24 patients (ages 8–18 years) were compared with matched classroom controls.

A wide variety of malignancies were represented, although children with brain tumors were not included. The teachers completed a modified version of "Revised Class Play."

This instrument was modified to obtain teachers' impressions of three fundamental dimensions of interpersonal style: "sociability–leadership,", "aggressive–disruptive," "sensitive–isolated." When compared to matched controls, children with cancer were perceived by teachers as being: (1) less sociable and prone towards leadership; and (2) more socially isolated and withdrawn. The same cohort was also evaluated for peer and self-perceptions of sociability, social isolation, overall popularity, mutual friendships and feelings of loneliness. The reports from peers suggested that children with cancer were perceived as being more socially isolated. However, no significant differences were found in their popularity, number of friends or self-worth [19]. In contrast, Spirito et al. [20] examined the social adjustment of 56 children aged 5–12 years who had been off-treatment for at least 6 months. In comparison with their healthy peers, teachers rated the survivors as being better adjusted socially. Specifically, the children were rated as being teased less and arguing less frequently with classmates. The survivors themselves, however, reported fewer friends of the same age and greater loneliness and isolation.

In other settings, the impact of chronic illness itself has been shown to affect psychological adjustment but the influence is variable. Spirito et al. [20] noted that chronic illness frequently disrupts peer interactions because of observed physical limitations and differences. Other reported studies specifically examining the social competency of children with chronic illnesses, however, show generally good adjustment. The degree of psychosocial adjustment and social competence among survivors of childhood cancer appears to be most closely associated with the functional status of the child, parental education, and family functioning [21]. Newby et al.[22] reported that social skills, as rated by both parents and teachers, are best predicted by academic functioning. They demonstrated a significant association between fewer school-related difficulties and better psychological adjustment.

Adequacy of family support and adaptability are strongly associated with good psychological adjustment. The family represents the primary system that influences adjustment. Following completion of therapy, the interactions of child and family assume an important role. Kupst et al. [23] reported that coping and perceived adjustment in survivors were positively associated with mothers' coping and adjustment, particularly in the younger age group (those less than 7 years at diagnosis). Although several investigators have examined psychosocial functioning of survivors and their families, comparatively few studies concentrate exclusively on parents. Investigators have observed high rates of posttraumatic stress symptoms (PTSS) in parents. Parents also report persistent feelings of loss, uncertainty, and anxiety about the recurrence of the disease or the emergence of late effects in their child. These findings may help to explain why some parents of adult patients continue to accompany their children to follow-up appointments [24].

Psychological Adjustment during Adolescence

Adolescence is a time of change and normal psychological progression through adolescence is well described in a number of models [25]. Newman and Newman [26] have identified five tasks related to adolescence: (1) relationship with peers; (2) emotional independence; (3) preparation for career; (4) sense of morality; and (5) development of sex-role identity. The adolescent survivor from cancer has to cope also with fear of relapse, insecurity about the future, damage to self-esteem, loss of autonomy, and, for some, distorted appearance and body image. It is therefore not surprising that in a number of individuals, normal progression through adolescence may be compromised. Despite this, most research suggests that the majority of adolescent survivors show positive psychosocial functioning.

A study among adolescent and adult survivors of childhood and adolescent cancer from all 10 Canadian provinces, the majority of whom had been diagnosed and treated more than 10 years previously, showed that survivors in general reported more specific physical health problems than a population control with no cancer history. However, quality of life differences were very small and not clinically important. For the majority of survivors, reported quality of life, self-esteem, optimism and life satisfaction were comparable with those of their peers [27]. Few studies have specifically explored the psychosocial consequences of diagnosis and treatment of cancer on issues related to the career-development process. In one study, Stern and Norman [28] prospectively examined whether adolescents with a history of cancer differ from healthy adolescents in their responses to career development tasks. Adolescent patients showed a greater tendency to prematurely foreclose on a career choice and were well ahead of healthy adolescents on career maturity progress. Meadows et al. [29] compared a cohort of 95 long-term survivors to their healthy siblings, finding no significant difference in social competence, frequency of adverse behaviors, or school achievement compared to siblings. In another study, Noll *et al.* [30] found that adolescent survivors were rated by peers as being more socially isolated, although friendships and popularity were not affected. Again, most studies highlight that the most important determinants of the level of psychological adjustment are the survivors' functional status (degree of physical/cognitive impairment) and adaptability.

A number of studies emphasize the importance of family functioning in predicting overall adjustment during this period. One surprising finding is that the survivors from families who report significant cohesiveness exhibit poorer adjustment [22]. Specifically, a higher frequency of behavioral problems in the survivors, as reported by the teachers, was associated with reports of greater cohesiveness within families. Family cohesiveness, which is generally considered to be a positive attribute of family life for healthy children, appears to be associated with more adjustment difficulties in young people who have survived cancer [31]. A possible explanation for this is that adolescents who have survived cancer have a greater need for autonomy than their healthy peers.

Finally, length of time following completion of treatment also appears to significantly affect overall psychological adjustment; children and adolescents who had completed therapy longer ago were rated by parents and teachers as being better adjusted than those who had only recently completed therapy [22].

Adolescents appear to experience significant initial anxiety and emotional turbulence following cessation of therapy, perhaps because of fear of possible recurrence. It appears that the psychological adjustment improves with the passage of time since therapy.

Psychosocial Adjustment during Adulthood

The ability to establish identity and functional independence and the ability to form intimate relationships are hallmarks of a successful transition from adolescence to adulthood. A number of studies have attempted to look at adult psychosocial functioning after childhood cancer. Again, variability in methods used and deficits in design have contributed to conflicting findings.

Discrepancies have arisen due to small sample sizes, the inclusion of largely chronic attendees where follow-up is not universal (a self-selected cohort), and the use of siblings as controls despite the documented emotional and behavioral difficulties among siblings of survivors [32]. Most studies of adult psychosocial outcomes have relied on questionnaires that assess current function but are therefore dependent on the respondent's understanding of the issues explored.

Irrespective of the incidence of psychological problems reported in the various studies, once again the key determinants appear to be functional status, specifically freedom from symptoms, and the individuals' or the families' resilience and adaptability. Even if there are no long-term medical or psychological problems, there is still the issue of the continuing stigma of having had cancer earlier in life, which may restrict employment and career choices. In a study assessing the eligibility for compulsory military service of childhood cancer survivors, it was reported that childhood cancer survivors were less likely to meet the requirements set for military service. Furthermore, 30% were rejected just on the basis of a former diagnosis of cancer [33].

In a large study exploring psychosocial adjustment of long-term survivors, Koocher and O'Malley [34] utilized both patient and parent self-reports as well as interview data from 117 survivors. They reported that, although most long-term survivors were able to lead relatively normal lives in terms of academic, vocational and social functioning, nearly half showed some evidence of significant psychological problems, primarily in the form of anxiety and difficulties in interpersonal relationships. A similar study limited to survivors of childhood Hodgkin's disease [35], utilizing interview data and study staff ratings, documented maladjustment defined by social incompetence and poor interpersonal relationships in nearly a third of their sample. A more recent study of 102 adult survivors of childhood acute leukemia and Wilms' tumor did not find increased incidence of psychiatric disorder in this population or a significant difference in current social functioning, but did report significant long-term problems with interpersonal functioning and day to-day coping [36]. A number of other studies found generally low levels of psychological distress with an absence of significant psychopathology [20, 37]. Only three factors were identified that were associated with an increased risk of maladjustment: (1) older patient age at follow-up; (2) greater number of relapses; and (3) presence of severe functional impairment.

In general, it appears that those studies relying primarily on self-report demonstrate a better outcome [38–40], compared to those utilizing parent, teacher or staff reports, which seem to show higher levels of maladjustment [34, 35]. It may well be that self-reports are biased towards minimization of affective distress and a propensity to present oneself in a more favorable light, or it may simply reflect successful coping mechanisms [41–43]. These studies have demonstrated a high incidence of a repressive adaptive style in cancer survivors, which may account for their lower scores of affective distress using self-report measures.

Individuals identified as repressors have lower scores on measures of anxiety, depression and anger expression, i.e. are better functioning. It has been hypothesized that repressive defenses may decrease the self-report of negative psychological outcomes for this population. This highlights the difficulties in the interpretation of self-reporting. Whether patients repress symptoms or demonstrate self-denial, the identification of a lack of adjustment is difficult and requires careful assessment. These may be the patients at greatest risk for later problems and interventions may be particularly important for this cohort.

Successful relationships in survivors depend both on achieving a biological cure and a positive psychological adaptation as well as the successful negotiation of adolescent developmental milestones. Marriage can be viewed as a surrogate marker of positive psychological functioning among adult survivors.

In the Children's Cancer Survivor Study, a study looking at self-reported data from 10,425 cancer survivors in North America [44], 32% reported being married or living in a stable, committed relationship, 6% being divorced or separated and 62% having never been married. Survivors of central nervous system (CNS) tumors were even less likely to be married. These figures are significantly lower than those in the general population.

A recent study [45] on a cohort of 6044 cancer children from Italy reported that 77% had not married, and that sexual functioning and romantic relationship skills may be disturbed in survivors. Zebrack [46], in a review of 599 survivors aged 18–39 years old, found that 52% of females and 32% of males reported problems in sexual functioning that were significantly associated with health-related quality of life, and that males were more distressed by sexual difficulties. Van Dijk et al. [47] who reviewed 60 survivors with a mean age of 24 years, found that 28% had no sexual experience, 44% were unable to feel sexually attractive because of poor body image, low emotional expression, scars, or risk of infertility. Survivors treated in adolescence had a delay in achieving psychosexual milestones when compared with those treated in childhood.

In summary, it would appear that while severe psychopathology is relatively rare, mild to moderate adjustment difficulties may be present in a significant proportion of adult survivors. The majority of individuals seem to overcome these difficulties reasonably well and appear to have adequate social functioning. The available evidence also suggests that repressive adaptation is a stable personality trait that might be expected to endure after completion of therapy. However, a significant proportion of survivors continue to have problems with interpersonal relationships.

Survivors of Brain Tumors during Childhood

Survivors of brain tumors during childhood have additional problems that warrant further discussion. It is in this group of patients that the physical and psychological sequelae of successful therapy are the most profound. Brain tumors are the second commonest malignancy in childhood, after acute lymphocytic leukemia, and account for nearly 20% of all malignancies in childhood. This subgroup represents a major cause of acquired neurological disability. A number of studies attest to the physical, cognitive, linguistic and behavioral problems experienced by children with primary brain tumors [48].

Psychological testing reveals that between 40% and 100% of long-term survivors of CNS tumors have some form of cognitive dysfunction [49], the variation being attributable to the type of tumor and use of radiotherapy. Impaired intelligence as evidenced by a reduction in full-scale IQ is seen in the majority of patients with medulloblastoma treated conventionally with localized radiotherapy [50].

There is also increasing evidence that cognitive and academic abilities may deteriorate progressively over time [51]. Two neuropsychological processes contribute to this progressive decline. Children may lose previously acquired information and skills, but more importantly the acquisition of new skills and information happens at a much slower rate than in healthy age-related peers [52, 53]. The dose of radiotherapy and the age at which it was administered correlate significantly with the neurocognitive outcome (the higher the dose and the younger the age, the greater the impairment).

In addition to the reduction in full-scale IQ, children with intracranial tumors show evidence of impairment across a range of cognitive functions, including visual attention and memory, verbal fluency, perceptual abilities, freedom from distraction and social problem solving [54–56].

Such cognitive impairments can create serious problems in a classroom setting. It is important to establish whether early intervention can limit this progressive decline and this is currently under investigation. A recent study looking at various aspects of cognitive impairment demonstrated that nonverbal and information processing skills continued to decline progressively while other deficits remained relatively stable over time. Literacy skills, however, increased with time, and progress was achieved with educational intervention, emphasizing the gains that can occur with remediation [51, 57].

Post-Traumatic Stress Disorder

A cluster of anxiety and avoidance symptoms has been identified in some pediatric cancer survivors and their parents. These symptoms are consistent with a trauma response and have led researchers to propose that the long-term psychosocial impact of cancer may best be understood by using the framework of post-traumatic stress disorder (PTSD) [58, 59].

There are many aspects of cancer diagnosis and treatment that evoke intense fear and helplessness. Treatment can be visualized as a chronic process of traumatic stress, including painful invasive procedures, repeated hospitalizations, separation from family members, and painful complications following treatment. In addition, late-effects of treatment, such as infertility and growth problems, physical changes, such as amputation and cardiac and pulmonary dysfunction; and cognitive changes can serve as lifelong reminders. For individuals who are treated during childhood, these long-term effects are understood and recognized in new ways at each level of development and provide lifelong opportunities for re-traumatization. However, despite research documenting psychological symptoms in children that are consistent with PTSD in the months and years following cancer treatment, recent work has found that pediatric cancer survivors actually report fewer PTSD symptoms than do their parents [58] and on formal measures tend to respond in a manner similar to children who have never been ill. Kazak et al. [60], described rates and concordance of PTSD and PTSS in adolescent childhood cancer survivors and their mothers and fathers. Rates of PTSD and PTSS tend to be higher in parents of adolescent cancer survivors than in the survivors themselves. Fathers, who are sometimes seen more peripherally involved in the care of the child, were similar to mothers in current PTSS, showing that the experience has long-lasting effects for them. Additionally, the potentially traumatic effect of childhood cancer is seen in adolescent siblings [61].

The finding that PTSS tend to be reported by only one member of a given family is new. This suggests the importance of evaluating all family members for PTSS. Reckitis et al. [62] tried to evaluate risk of suicide ideation (SI) after childhood cancer, in comparison with a sibling comparison group. In accordance with this study, adult survivors are at increased risk for SI. Risk of SI is related to cancer diagnosis and post-treatment mental and physical health, even many years after completion of therapy. The association of suicidal symptoms with physical health problems is important because these may be treatable conditions for which

survivors can seek follow-up care, underscoring the need for a multidisciplinary approach to survivor care.

Current Strategies to Minimize Long-Term Medical and Cognitive Problems

It is important to recognize that to minimize the incidence of psychological maladjustment in the long term, constant efforts must be made to reduce the incidence of medical and cognitive problems. For a number of childhood cancers, the survival rates have improved to a level where the intensity and duration of therapy, particularly radiotherapy and mutilating surgery, can be reduced. Effective systemic chemotherapy has allowed the use of lower doses and volumes of radiotherapy with a profound improvement in quality of life for the survivors and with no reduction in the survival rates [63, 64].

Additionally, modifications in the delivery of radiation, for example, the use of conformal radiotherapy and more accurate imaging with field reduction, have also diminished the musculoskeletal and other complications associated with the use of this modality of treatment [65]. Treatment planning and modern radiation equipment, in particular Intensity Modulated Radiation Therapy can reduce the dose to the surrounding tissues and decrease the incidence of SMN. It is now well known that cranial radiation used to treat children with ALL has significant long-term sequelae in terms of poorer academic achievement and psychosocial functioning [48]. The most important clinical intervention in recent years has been to abandon the routine use of this modality in the treatment of childhood acute lymphoblastic leukemia, preserving its use only in those with disease in the CNS or undergoing total body irradiation as part of conditioning for BMT (at a significantly lower dose). Infertility following cancer therapy is a major issue that affects about 15% of cancer childhood survivors [66]. Gonadal damage after cancer treatment results from either gonadotoxicity of systemic chemotherapy (alkylating agents), radiation to spinal or pelvic area, cranial radiation which disrupts the hypothalamic-pituitary axis, or total body radiation.

However, recent advances in the field of reproductive medicine have potentially opened opportunities for the preservation of the reproductive potential of young cancer patients with good long-term prognosis for survival. According to the Committee on Bioethics for Fertility Preservation in Children and Adolescents [67], fertility preservation should be considered for children with cancer before treatment: For males, post-pubertal sperm cryopreservation should be offered. For prepubertal boys, strategies such as cryopreservation of testicular tissue or germ cells are still experimental, and delay in cancer treatment should be avoided as this increases the risk of DNA damage and malformations. For girls, oophoropexy should be done before pelvic irradiation, post-pubertal girls may have gonadal suppression by gonadotrophic hormone (GnRH) analogs or cryopreservation of oocytes; but again, it is important to avoid delays in cancer treatment.

The management of bone tumors involving the extremities requires surgical resection, historically by amputation. Limb-salvage surgery, with endoprosthetic replacement, is being increasingly performed when feasible. In 2009, the Children Cancer Survivors Study [68] reported good global function and social integration in 629 patients with lower-extremity bone tumors.

Strategies to Cope with Long-Term Sequelae

The majority of pediatric oncology centers have evolved a mechanism to follow up survivors of childhood cancer well into adult life. "Long-term follow-up" or "after completion of therapy" (ACT) clinics have been set up in most centers to counsel patients and their parents about late effects and to detect subtle late effects as early as possible. These clinics are usually multidisciplinary and involve input from a number of specialists, such as endocrinologists, neurologists and cardiologists. Most units would have access to the services of a clinical psychologist and family therapy unit. If there is a perceived need for intervention, particularly psychological support or counseling, this should be provided.

It has been suggested that continued monitoring of cancer survivors in specialty clinics might increase anxiety and potentially stigmatize a group who is without disease and only at minimal risk of new complications. One way to minimize this would be to formulate individualized follow-up plans that are based on an individual's risk. A growing literature base is becoming available to guide decisions about the clinical follow-up of long-term survivors largely based on retrospective cohort studies, and prospective evaluation of new treatments is now needed. Information to guide the follow-up of survivors will come from national population-based cohort studies, large multicenter clinical studies, and randomized clinical trials designed to evaluate both survival and long-term toxicities associated with different strategies. As this information accumulates, the level of clinical surveillance can be developed to match the clinical need. An evidence base is clearly required [69]. Some centers have tried novel approaches to reduce symptoms of distress and improve family functioning and development. Intervention programs combining cognitive-behavioral and family therapy are well received and appear to be effective in reducing the symptoms of post-traumatic stress and anxiety [54]. Other programs have been directed more specifically at helping the child with cancer acquire the social skills to cope with school life. Clearly, return to school can be a difficult time for children with cancer but there are early indications [70] that this can be eased with intervention [71]. Whether or not these interventions have an impact on later functioning remains to be established.

Conclusion

It appears that most children have an impressive ability to come to terms with their cancer experience and develop adequate psychosocial adjustment in later life. At the same time, it is important to recognize that a proportion of survivors experience genuine difficulties in adjustment, which may be aggravated by physical sequelae or adverse social or family circumstances.

As future studies of survivorship issues are undertaken, attempts to understand physical and psychological effects of childhood cancer must be made in parallel. It is only by adopting equal emphasis in both mental and physical health that young adults will have the best chance to attain their full potential.

In 2008, the SIOP Working Committee on Psychosocial Issues in Pediatric Oncology issued a position paper on resilience in survivors of childhood cancer, with the conclusion:

The long-term goal of the cure and care of the child with cancer is that he/she become a resilient, fully functioning, autonomous adult with an optimal health- related quality of life, accepted in society at the same level of his/her age peers.

Survivors can and do learn positive coping strategies from their cancer experience. The goal is to encourage parents and health care professionals from the point of diagnosis through long-term follow up, to engage in those age-appropriate behaviors that will promote resilience in long-term survivors.

Note

1. This chapter is based and updated from Dr. Amita Mahajan's text in the first edition.

References

1. Rowland JH, Mariotto A, Aziz NA, *et al.* Cancer survivorship, United States, 1971–2001. *Morbidity and Mortality Weekly Report.* 2004;**53**:526–530.
2. Hamish W, Wallace B, Anderson Richard A, *et al.* Fertility preservation for young patients with cancer: who

is at risk and what can be offered? *Lancet Oncology* 2005;**6**:209–218.

3. Vrooman M, Najita J, Goodman P, *et al.* Long-term outcome after cancer in infancy: a report from the Childhood Cancer Survivor Study (CCSS). Paper presented at 11th International Conference in Long-Term Complications of Treatment of Children and Adolescents with Cancer, Williamsburg, Virginia, USA, 2010.

4. Fryer C. Late effects in childhood cancer survivors: a review with a framing effect bias? *Pediatric Blood & Cancer* 2011;**10**:/1002/pbc.22975.

5. Green D, Lange JM, Peabody EM, *et al.* Pregnancy outcome after treatment for Wlims tumor: a report from the National Wilms Tumor Long Term Follow-up Study. *Journal of Clinical Oncology* 2010;**28**:2824–2829.

6. *Journal of National Cancer Institute* 2009;**101**:806–813.

7. Hudson MM, Mertens AC, Yasui Y, *et al.* Health status of adult long term survivors of childhood cancer. *JAMA* 2003;**290**:1583–1592.

8. Woodward E, Jessop M, Glaser A, *et al.* Late effects in survivors of teenage and young adult cancer: does age matter? *Annals of Oncology* Mar 22. [E-pub ahead of print, 2011.]

9. Rowland J. Looking beyond cure: pediatric cancer as a model. *Journal of Pediatric Psychology* 2005;**30**:1–3.

10. Zeltzer L, Recklitis C, Buchbinder D, *et al.* Psychological status in childhood cancer survivors: a report from the Childhood Cancer Survivor Study. *Journal of Clinical Oncology* 2009;**27**:2396–2404.

11. Lewis S, La Barbera JD. Terminating chemotherapy: another stage in coping with childhood leukemia. *American Journal of Pediatric Hematology Oncology* 1983;**5**:33–37.

12. Haase JE, Rostad M. Experiences of completing cancer therapy: children's perspectives. *Oncology Nursing Forum* 1994;**21**:1483–1492.

13. Oeffinger KC, Mertens AC, Sklar CA. Chronic health conditions in adult survivors of childhood cancer. *New England Journal of Medicine* 2006;**355**:1572–1582.

14. Geenen MM, Cardous-Ubbink MC, Kremer LC, *et al.* Medical assessment of adverse health outcomes in long-term survivors of childhood cancer. *JAMA* 2007;**297**:2705–2715.

15. Reulen RC, Winter DL, Lancashire EL, *et al.* Health-status of adult survivors of childhood cancer: a large-scale population-based study from the British Childhood Cancer Survivor Study. *International Journal of Cancer* 2007;**121**:633–640.

16. Armstrong GT Stovall M, Robinson LL. Long-term of radiation exposure among adult survivors of childhood cancer: a result from the Childhood Cancer Survivor Study. *Radiation Research* 2010;**174**:840–850.

17. Friedman DL, Whitton J, Leisenring W, *et al.* Subsequent neoplasms in 5-year survivors of childhood cancer, the Childhood Cancer Survivor Study. *Journal of National Cancer Institute* 2010;**102**:1083–1095.

18. Noll R, Bukowski W, LeRoy S, *et al.* Social interaction between children and their peers: teacher ratings. *Journal of Pediatric Psychology* 1990;**7**:75–84.

19. Noll R, LeRoy S, Bukowski W, *et al.* Peer relationships and adjustment in children with cancer. *Journal of Pediatric Psychology* 1991;**6**:307–326.

20. Spirito A, Starck L, Cobiella C, *et al.* Social adjustment of children successfully treated for cancer. *Journal of Pediatric Psychology* 1990;**15**:359–371.

21. Wallander J, Varni J, Babani H, *et al.* Family resources as resistance factors for psychologically ill and handicapped children. *Journal of Pediatric Psychology* 1989;**14**:157–174.

22. Newby WL, Brown RT, Pawletko TM, *et al.* Social skills and psychosocial adjustment of child and adolescent cancer survivors. *Psycho-oncology* 2000;**9**:113–126.

23. Kupst MJ, Natta MB, Richardson CC, *et al.* Family coping with pediatric leukemia: ten years after treatment. *Journal of Pediatric Hematology Oncology* 1995;**5**:33–37.

24. Hardy K, Bonner M, Masi R, *et al.* Psychosocial functioning in parents of adults survivors of childhood cancer. *Journal of Pediatric Hematology Oncology* 2008;**30**:153–159.

25. Havinghurst R. *Developmental Tasks and Education.* New York: David McKay, 1992.

26. Newman B, Newman P. *Development Through Life: A Psychosocial Approach.* Chicago: The Dorsey Press, 1987.

27. Maunsell E, Pogany L, Barrera M, *et al.* Quality of life among long-term adolescent and adult survivors of childhood cancer. *Journal of Clinical Oncology* 2006;**24**:2527–2535.

28. Stern M, Norman SL. Career development of adolescent cancer patients: a comparative analysis. *Journal of Counseling Psychology* 1991;**38**:431–439.

29. Meadows AT, McKee K, Kazak AE. Psychosocial status of young adult survivors of childhood cancer: a survey. *Medical and Pediatric Oncology* 1989;**17**:466–470.

30. Noll RB, Bukowski WM, Davies WH, *et al.* Adjustment in the peer system of adolescents with cancer: a two year study. *Journal of Pediatric Psychology* 1993;**18**:351–364.

31. Kazak A. Implications of survival: pediatric oncology patients and their families. In: Bearison DJ, Mulhern RK (eds.) *Pediatric Psycho-Oncology Psychological Perspectives on Children with Cancer.* New York: Oxford University Press, 1994; pp. 171–192.

32. Sahler OJZ, Mulhern R, Dolgin MJ, *et al.* Sibling adaptation to childhood cancer collaborative study: prevalence of sibling distress and definition of adoptions levels. *Journal of Developmental & Behavioral Pediatrics* 1994;**15**:353–366.

33. Paivi ML, Heikki AS, Toivo TS, *et al.* Military service of male survivors of childhood malignancies. *Cancer* 1999;**85**:732–740.

34. Koocher G, O'Malley J. *The Damocles Syndrome.* New York: McGraw-Hill, 1981.

35. Cella D, Tan C, Sullivan M, *et al.* Identifying survivors of pediatric Hodgkin's disease who need psychologic interventions. *Journal of Psychosocial Oncology* 1988;**5**:83–96.

36. Mackie E, Hill J, Kondryn H, *et al.* Adult psychosocial outcomes in long-term survivors of acute lymphoblastic leukemia and Wilms' tumor: a controlled study. *Lancet* 2000;**355**:1310–1314.

37. Elkin TD, Phipps S, Mulhern RD, *et al.* Psychological functioning of adolescent and young adult survivors of pediatric malignancy. *Medical and Pediatric Oncology* 1997;**29**:582–588.

38. Fritz GK, Williams JR. Issues of adolescent development for survivors of childhood cancer. *Journal of the American Academy of Child and Adolescent Psychiatry* 1988;**58**:712–715.

39. Fritz GK, Williams JR, Amylon M. After treatment ends: psychosocial sequelae in pediatric cancer survivors. *American Journal of Orthopsychiatry* 1988;**58**:552–561.

40. Greenberg HS, Kazak AE, Meadows AT. Psychological functioning in 8–16-year-old cancer survivors and their parents. *Journal of Pediatrics* 1989;**114**:4889–4893.
41. Worchel FF. Denial of depression: adaptive coping in pediatric cancer patients? *Newsletter of Society of Pediatrics* 1989;**13**:8–11.
42. Canning EH, Canning RD, Boyce TB. Depressive symptoms and adaptive style in children with cancer. *Journal of American Academy of Child and Adolescent Psychiatry* 1992;**31**:1120–1124.
43. Phipps S, Srivastava DK. The repressor personality in children with cancer. *Health Psychology* 1997;**16**:521–528.
44. Rauck A, Green DM, Yasui Y, *et al.* Marriage in survivors of childhood cancer: a preliminary description from the Childhood Cancer Survivor Study. *Medical and Pediatric Oncology* 1999;**33**:60–63.
45. Pivetta E, Maule MM, Pisani P, *et al.* Marriage and parenthood among childhood cancer survivors: a report from the Italian AEIOP Off-Therapy Registry. *Haematologica* 2011;**96**:744–751.
46. Zebrack BJ, Foley S, Wittmann D, *et al.* Sexual functioning in young adult survivors of childhood cancer. *Psychooncology* 2010;**19**:814–822.
47. Van Dijk EM, Van Dulmen-den Broeder E, Kaspers GJ, *et al.* Psychosexual functioning of childhood cancer survivors. *Psychooncology* 2008;**17**:506–511.
48. Ellenberg L, Liu Q, Gioia G, *et al.* Neurocognitive status in long term survivors of childhood CNS malignancies: a report from the Childhood Cancer Survivor Study. *Neuropsychology* 2009;**23**:705–717.
49. Glauser TA, Packer RJ. Cognitive deficits in long-term survivors of childhood brain tumors. *Child's Nervous System* 1991;**7**:2–12.
50. Dennis M, Spiegler BJ, Hethrington CR, *et al.* Neuropsychological sequelae of the treatment of children with medulloblastoma. *Journal of Neurooncology* 1996;**29**:91–101.
51. Anderson VA, Godber T, Smibert E, *et al.* Cognitive and academic outcome following cranial irradiation and chemotherapy in children: a longitudinal study. *British Journal of Cancer* 2000;**82**:255–262.
52. Hopewell JW. Radiation injury to the central nervous system. *Medical and Pediatric Oncology Supplement* 1998;**1**:1–9.
53. Twaddle V, Britton PG, Kernahan J, *et al.* Intellect after malignancy. *Archives of Disease in Childhood* 1986;**61**:700–702.
54. Kazak AE, Simms S, Barahat P, *et al.* Surviving cancer completely intervention program (SSCIP): a cognitive-behavioral and family therapy intervention for adolescent survivors of childhood cancer and their families. *Family Process* 1999;**38**:175–191.
55. Garcia-Perez A, Sierrasesumaga L, Narbona-Garcia J, *et al.* Neuropsychological evaluation of children with intracranial tumors: impact of treatment modalities. *Medical and Pediatric Oncology* 1994;**23**:116–123.
56. Butler RW, Hill JM, Steinherz PG, *et al.* Neuropsychologic effects of cranial irradiation, intrathecal methotrexate and systemic methotrexate in childhood cancer. *Journal of Clinical Oncology* 1994;**12**:2621–2629.
57. Kreitler S, Ben Arush M, Krivoy E, *et al.* Psychosocial aspects of radiotherapy for the child and family with cancer. In: Halperin EC, Constine LS, Tarbell NJ, Kun LE (eds.) *Pediatric Radiation Oncology*, Philadelphia: Lippincott, Williams and Wilkins, 2011; pp. 447–455.
58. Buttler R, Rizzi L, Handwergwe B. The assessment of posttraumatic stress disorder in pediatric cancer patients and survivors. *Journal of Pediatric Psychology* 1996;**21**:499–504.
59. Kazak AE, Barakat LP, Meeske E, *et al.* Posttraumatic stress, family functioning and social support in survivors of childhood leukemia and their mothers and fathers. *Journal of Consulting and Clinical Psychology* 1997;**65**:120–129.
60. Kazak AE, Alderfer M, Rourke MT, *et al.* Posttraumatic stress disorder (PTSD) and posttraumatic stress symptoms (PTSS) in families of adolescent childhood cancer survivors. *Journal of Pediatric Psychology* 2004;**29**:211–219.
61. Alderfer M, Labay L, Kazak A. Brief report: does posttraumatic stress apply to siblings of childhood cancer survivors? *Journal of Pediatric Psychology* 2003;**28**:281–286.
62. Reckitis C, Diller L, Xiaochun L, *et al.* Suicide ideation in adult survivors of childhood cancer: a report from the Childhood Cancer Survivor Study. *Journal of Clinical Oncology* 2010;**28**:655–661.
63. D'Angio G, Breslow N, Beckwith B, *et al.* Treatment of Wilms' tumor: results of the Third National Wilms' Tumor Study. *Cancer* 1989;**64**:349.
64. Donaldson S, Link M. Combined modality treatment with low-dose radiation and MOPP chemotherapy for children with Hodgkin's disease. *Journal of Clinical Oncologyl* 1987;**5**:742.
65. Donaldson S, Kaplan H. Complications of treatment of Hodgkin's disease in children. *Cancer Treatment Report* 1982;**66**:977.
66. Byrne J, Mulvihill JJ, Myers MH, *et al.* Effects of treatment on fertility in long-term survivors of childhood or adolescent cancer. *New England Journal of Medicine* 1987;**317**:1315–1321.
67. Fallat ME, Hutter J, the Committee on Bioethics. Section on hemato/oncology and section on surgery. *Pediatrics* 2008;**121**:461–469.
68. Nagarajan J, Mogil R, Neglia JP, *et al.* Self-reported global function among adult survivors of childhood lower-extremity bone tumors: a report from the Childhood Cancer Survivor Study (CCSS). *Journal of Cancer Survivors* 2009;**3**:59–65.
69. Wallace H, Blacklay A, Eiser C, *et al.* Developing strategies for long term follow up of survivors of childhood cancer. *British Medical Journal* 2001;**232**:271–274.
70. Haase J, Rostad M. Experiences of completing cancer therapy: children's perspectives. *Oncology Nursing Forum* 1994;**21**:1483–1492.
71. Annett RD, Erickson SJ. *European Journal of Cancer Care* 2009;**18**:421–428.

Part C
Death and Bereavement

17

Care of a Child Dying of Cancer

Sergey Postovsky, Myriam Weyl Ben-Arush

Introduction

In the case of a dying child, the goal of therapy is to maintain the child's comfort and provide support to the child and the family [1–3]. It is the responsibility of the health care team to provide the child in the last phase of his or her life adequate control of pain as well as of all other bothersome symptoms.

Despite the significant success that has been achieved in the past two decades in the treatment of children with cancer, it is estimated that long-term survival may be achieved only in about 75–80% of patients [4]. This implies that at least every fourth child suffering from cancer will eventually die.

The life of a child lasts to its last second. Loss of a child's life is a tragic and illogical event for all those involved and especially for the child's parents who have come to believe, as so many people do, that it is the children who should witness their parents' death and not vice versa.

The last days, hours and minutes of a child's life will most probably remain engraved forever in the parents' mind. Moreover, the way their child dies may play a critical role in the future life of parents and possibly of the other siblings too. Therefore, it is difficult to overestimate the importance of a competent, comprehensive and sensitive management during the terminal phase of a child's life.

Burden of Physical and Psychosocial Distress at the End of Life

Knowing the most probable scenario of approaching death may potentially facilitate better preparation to the optimal management of a child's end-of-life period [5]. Based on our knowledge of prevailing signs and symptoms that should be addressed by a treating palliative team during the final period of a patient's life, it is possible and desirable to create a therapeutic plan before this period becomes actually evident. Knowledge informing such treatment plans has been obtained from surveys that have usually been performed retrospectively, asking the parents of deceased pediatric cancer patients some time after their deaths.

Several groups of investigators have performed and published results of such surveys [6–9]. Physical fatigue was the most common symptom reported by parents of children who had died of cancer, according to one survey performed in Sweden [6]. Other frequent symptoms reported in this study were reduced mobility, pain, poor appetite and nausea. These symptoms were mentioned as frequently as above 60% of all reported cases by 449 parents of 368 deceased children. The frequency of symptoms varied according to diagnosis. Thus, for instance, patients with sarcomas and neuroblastoma more frequently complained of physical fatigue, pain, poor appetite and weight loss than children with brain tumors or leukemia. Otherwise, patients with brain tumors more frequently suffered from difficulties in swallowing, impaired speech, and paralysis. This difference in frequency of reported symptoms may be explained by several factors. First, most patients with brain tumors die from the local effects of the tumor itself, which rarely metastasize beyond the CNS. The majority of such patients are treated with steroids as part of their palliative therapy. Steroids may facilitate better appetite and weight gain, which is certainly not the case among patients with other types of cancer. In the dying patient with a brain tumor, the most prominent symptoms are connected to the specific location of the tumor, more that to the degree of systemic spread of the disease. In contrast, in many patients with extraneural malignant tumors, as well as in patients with leukemia/lymphoma, there is frequently progressive and widespread disease involving many organs and systems such as the skeletal system. Such a pattern of involvement causes the almost universal

Pediatric Psycho-oncology: Psychosocial Aspects and Clinical Interventions, Second Edition.
Edited by Shulamith Kreitler, Myriam Weyl Ben-Arush and Andrés Martin.

occurrence of symptoms like pain, decreased appetite, and weight loss.

The age of a patient may also influence the frequency of reported complaints. Parents of children dying between the ages of 9 to 15 years reported a higher number of symptoms than other parents. This may be explained by the relatively more mature descriptive abilities of older children, who are generally able to describe and discern the various symptoms they are suffering from.

In another study performed by Dutch specialists [8], it was shown that although most physical symptoms (82%) were recognized by the treating team, only 18% of them were addressed completely, with 26% more resolved to a partial degree. The five most frequent symptoms reported by parents were pain, poor appetite, fatigue, lack of mobility, and vomiting. The psychological burden at the end of life is not less significant. The management of psychological symptoms is even more difficult. The recognition of these symptoms is not efficient enough, and their successful management often can be more the exception than the rule. Thus, according to the results of this study, only 43% of psychological symptoms reported by parents were addressed by the medical professionals and, of these, only 9% were resolved completely, and 25% more were resolved partially. It should be stressed that not all symptoms at the end of life are amenable to correction. For instance, immobility or other physical movement limitations caused by irreversible neurological damage (e.g., pre-existing spinal cord compression) could remain unresolved. Thus, not all the persistent burden of physical and/or psychological suffering is a sign of failure on the part of the treating team.

The main flaw in such surveys is their retrospective nature. It is not always possible for parents to recall in detail all the signs and symptoms which were present during the final period of their child's life. In addition, the emotional stress under which parents usually find themselves may potentially interfere with the validity of their recollections. But the most serious obstacle for the objectivity of findings of such surveys is that that signs and symptoms described are those that are no longer present but are reported and interpreted by their parents, who actually give information that has not been experienced by they personally but rather is transformed by their very personal and not objective experience.

Another means of obtaining data on the frequency and prevalence of symptoms at the end of life is by retrieving pertinent data from medical records. There are several potential drawbacks hampering obtaining objective results in this way. First, these data are

retrieved retrospectively, so some information may be not recorded or not recorded in the correct way. Second, parents spend usually significantly more time with their dying child than treating personnel. This may result in that most of the relevant data not being recorded in the medical files. This is true for patients who spend most of the time in hospital and even more when children remain at home and receive palliative care by providers who are not closely connected to the treating hospital.

DNR and DNAR Orders

Parents are frequently reluctant to discuss the "Do Not Resuscitate" (DNR) order regarding their children because they tend to equate such a decision with the abandonment of hope and capitulation in the face of impending death. Parents may sometimes consider a decision of this kind as outright betrayal of their child. Such fears actually do not correspond to reality and are not justified. Thus, for instance, Baker et al. [10] analyzed the possible influence of DNR orders on subsequent changes in the medical care of two hundred cancer patients and found that, despite written DNR orders, the medical interventions that the children were receiving at the time of this order, with the exception of chemotherapy, were continued in 66.7% to 99.3% cases. Other studies have shown that a DNR order itself does not shorten the patient's remaining life. For example, of 22 patients reported by Postovsky et al. [11], the mean time from the last day of anticancer treatment until death was 63 days in the group with DNR orders and 56.5 days in the group without DNR orders ($p = $ NS).

The responsibility of the palliative team is to help parents make a correct decision in the best interests of their child. It may be prudent to initiate conversations with parents about this topic long before a child suffering from progressive cancer approaches imminent death. This approach conforms also to the modern concept that promotes incorporating palliative care into the standard care of a child sick with cancer from the very initial stages of the child's disease [12].

It is important to note that resuscitative measures may be successful in the "technical" sense of the word, allowing the treating team to sustain the continued performance of the vital functions, but at the same time rendering the child unconscious and leaving him/her without any ability to communicate with parents and other loved ones. Given the progressive nature of the child's cancer, and the mostly irreversible nature of the symptoms causing the present distress, the net result of resuscitation may often exert a devastating effect on both the sick child and his/her relatives. Hence, it is of vital importance to introduce parents to the concept of "Do Not *Attempt* to Resuscitate" (DNAR) [13]. In certain instances, avoiding unnecessary interventions may be more appropriate than to "go ahead to the end" and thus to prolong suffering.

Whatever the situation may be, it is advisable to discuss all issues regarding possible interventions in the end of the child's life before the critical moment approaches, and to put on the patient's medical chart written notification to forgo or to initiate (and to what extent) resuscitation efforts. Planned discussion of the DNAR order long before the patient's final deterioration, which may be rapid and not always anticipated, allows parents to ponder upon the possibility of their child's final phase of life without the enormous psychological and emotional strain that usually accompanies witnessing the dying process of their beloved child. Furthermore, it is likely to enable the parents to take a more considered and reasoned decision in the best interests of their child. In view of the above considerations, discussion of the DNAR order appears to be of paramount importance. It is very useful to clarify with parents all aspects of this order, for example, not to initiate intubation and indirect cardiac massage, without concurrently forgoing drug therapy such as anti-seizures drugs and oxygen supply.

When discussing various aspects of the treatment of a child during his/her last days and hours, it is always useful to remember that the parents are those who are the primary decision-makers for the child. This is true not only because of the legal aspects of this situation, but primarily because no one else knows better what their child would have preferred if he/she had been able to decide for themselves in a given situation. Hence, in most circumstances parents should be encouraged to clearly express their intention to initiate or forgo resuscitation during the terminal phase of their child's cancer.

Unfortunately, all too often in clinical practice, a DNR order is only written near the time of the child's death. McCallum, Byrne and Bruera [14] noted that the median time intervening between DNR and death was less than 24 hours in the case of 77 pediatric patients with cancer and other life-threatening diseases; and in 8% of the cases, the DNR order was not given at all. Only in 13 cases did death occur in the pediatric or oncology ward or at home, while the majority of deaths were registered in the intensive care unit. Postovsky et al. [11] showed that DNR orders were written on 61% of the charts of patients suffering from progressive cancer and, in several cases, DNR orders were given close to death (within the last 24 hours of the child's remaining life). Ordering DNR during the last 24 hours of the patient's life is not timely, as this brief time span does not provide parents and other relatives with a sufficient amount of time to fully and optimally prepare for their child's death. In addition, the medical staff, including psychologists and social workers, may not be informed long enough before and will not be able to provide all the needed support to the grieving family members. Therefore, prescribing a DNR order in close proximity to the patient's death should be regarded as suboptimal and should be considered only as the default decision in the very rare situations when the child's death was unanticipated [14].

Wolfe *et al.* [9] noted that there is a significant discrepancy in the understanding of the ultimate prognosis between physicians and the parents of pediatric cancer patients. In general, physicians realized that there was no realistic chance of cure significantly earlier than the parents of children with progressive cancer (mean 106 versus 206 days before child's death, $p = 0.01$).

Earlier recognition of the incurability of a child's cancer and earlier initiation of discussion of all aspects of management of the terminal phase will enable both the treating physician and the child's parents to come to terms with instituting the DNR order long before the approach of the final phase.

A well-documented phenomenon is when adult cancer patients unrealistically estimate their chances of a cure. Such unrealistic expectations may play an important positive role when struggling with a potentially life-threatening disease, allowing patients to maintain hope and encourage them to adhere to treatment plans. On the other hand, such high expectations may adversely affect decisions made by patients, which would not match the unfavorable course of the patient's disease.

In the practice of pediatric oncology the situation is even more complicated. In the majority of cases, parents serve as legal guardians for their children and they are morally and legally obligated to take the decisions in the best interests of their children during all stages of disease, including end of life. In a study performed by Mack *et al.* [15], the authors reported that frequently there was a discrepancy between the parents' and the physicians' estimation regarding the chances of a cure for children during the first year of treatment after establishing the cancer diagnosis. Most parents (61%) were more optimistic than the treating physicians about the chances for a cure for their child. It is interesting that parents were frequently unaware of the opinions of their child's doctors. Thus, most parents (70%) believed that their child's oncologist held the same view as they did, regarding the prospect of a cure. Only 4% of parents reported that they were more optimistic than their physicians. This difference in attitude between the parents and their child's doctors regarding the estimation of their child's chances of survival was statistically significant ($p < 0.0001$). The reason for such overly unrealistic parental optimism lies, at least partly, in the far from ideal communication process frequently found between the treating physician and the child's parents. When a pediatric oncologist who is discussing a child's present status with parents leaves room for interpretation of data and conclusions made during such sessions, the parents tend to fill in the gaps with their own conclusions and may return home after such sessions in an overly positive mood and with optimistic expectations for their child's survival. According to Mack et al. [15], lack of confidence by the doctor in imparting information to parents and lack of sufficient time dedicated to such kinds of conversations are two important factors which may hamper the efficacy of discussion, thus suggesting that physicians play an important role in parents' unrealistic optimism.

Maintaining the life of a child is an inherent instinct of every parent, so it is not surprising that no one wants to hear about his/her child's approaching demise. That may be why if there is some space left for interpretation of data delivered to parents by pediatric oncologists, it can be filled with thoughts, feelings and actions that are overall too optimistic for the bleak reality.

Possible problems may arise when clearly clarified written permission from the parents has not been procured in time when the child in the terminal phase of cancer is rapidly deteriorating and develops cardiopulmonary arrest. In a situation of this kind, it may be advisable to initiate resuscitation using indirect cardiac massage and artificial ventilation with an Ambu bag. Concurrently, an emergency session with the parents may be organized, sometimes at the patient's bedside. It should be conducted in a sensitive and empathic manner, preferably by the treating pediatric oncologist who has been in close contact with the family all through the child's disease. The session could be decisive regarding continuation or withdrawal of resuscitative measures. But if the parents do not give their permission to abandon life-supporting therapy, these measures should be continued in full.

It is to be emphasized that, even if parents choose to proceed with resuscitation, despite the apparent futility of this mode of action, they neither should be nor can be blamed for this. Under no circumstances is it the parents' fault but is rather a failure of the palliative team to come to terms with the parents when the possibility of withdrawing resuscitative measures was contemplated.

Despite the apparent "finality" of a DNAR order, in clinical reality it sometimes is not the case. It is not inconceivable that even a child with widespread multiform glioblastoma of the brain, resistant to treatment, who has lost consciousness and has deteriorated hemodynamically, may sometimes regain cognitive status and resume cardio-respiratory functioning, provided all the necessary supportive measures have been properly instituted. Given the current status of medical knowledge, we are not always able to assess a clinical situation accurately. Thus, even a child with widespread brain tumor may deteriorate because of seizures or transient elevation of intracranial pressure, namely, causes that are potentially treatable but may go unrecognized in a child with cancer, who might be referred to as "terminal." If such a child is treated promptly and correctly with anti-seizure drugs and Mannitol, he/she may be stabilized and even discharged home for quite a long period of time. The correct decision in this kind of situation is a matter of the art of medicine and clinical experience.

Palliative Sedation in Pediatric Cancer Patients

Most children with progressive cancer in the terminal phase of their life suffer from various symptoms, where pain is the most common [2, 12, 16–19]. With modern treatment modalities, effective control of pain, vomiting and other symptoms of physical distress is attainable in more than 90% of pediatric cancer patients [18, 19].

Difficult symptoms are identified as those symptoms which, despite their severity, may be alleviated by standard, sometimes rather rigorous, therapy, without causing unbearable side effects. This therapy does not cause sedation and excessive side effects that outweigh the positive effects of the therapy itself. This therapy should be effective within an acceptable timeframe when it is applied to a dying patient [20].

Symptoms of suffering would be designated as refractory symptoms [20], when all our interventions: (1) are incapable of providing adequate relief; (2) or are associated with excessive and intolerable side effects; (3) or are unable to provide relief to the dying child within the relevant period of time.

When all the interventions directed at alleviating the suffering of a child in the terminal phase of his cancer have proven to be ineffective, conducting therapy that is accompanied by sedation may be the only and last mode of action we have in use. This therapy is frequently designated terminal sedation.

The definition of terminal sedation is rather elusive. First, we do not always actually know if the child has entered the terminal phase of the disease because our ability to predict survival in patients with advanced cancer is sometimes limited. Second, there is an often-stated belief that terminal sedation is aimed at terminating the patient's suffering by hastening death. According to this belief, terminal sedation is a form of slow euthanasia [19–21]. Morita *et al.* [22] showed that palliative sedation does not affect survival of adult cancer patients. Actually, this therapy may even prolong life, since alleviating suffering decreases the severe physiologic stress that may exhaust the patient and accelerate death.

It is to be emphasized that alleviating pain in dying children enhances the child's quality of life and eases the distress of their grieving parents. There is a major difference between palliative sedation and euthanasia. Palliative sedation is intended to alleviate the existing symptoms of physical and existential suffering, while euthanasia is primarily a course of action initiated by the physician and intended to hasten death [23–25]. The aim of palliative sedation is not to shorten the duration of the remaining life but to alleviate pain and other symptoms, although some risk of facilitating death exists [20, 23]. In order to minimize this risk, palliative sedation should be applied only by personnel who have special expertise and training in palliative care and with thorough monitoring with regular reassessment of the child's status.

As a result, several other terms for this mode of action have been proposed, such as:

(1) palliative sedation [26];
(2) sedation for intractable distress of a dying patient [23, 27];
(3) sedation in the imminently dying [28];
(4) heavy sedation [27].

We prefer the term "palliative sedation" in order to avoid the possible negative connotations of termination of life.

Regardless of the term, it is sedation for intractable problems near the end of life. Therefore, it is justified to raise the question: what problems may be encountered that could serve as indications of initiation of palliative sedation?

The following are the most frequent ones:

(1) severe uncontrollable pain;
(2) refractory dyspnea;
(3) refractory seizures;
(4) various psychiatric disturbances, such as confusion, agitation, or restlessness;
(5) existential suffering [29–31].

Palliative sedation is directed solely at alleviating otherwise uncontrollable suffering. This is the main and only aim that we pursue when initiating this treatment.

There is no intent to shorten the life of a suffering patient.

Nevertheless, under certain circumstances, when we apply palliative sedation to a dying child, we cannot exclude the potential for accelerating death. In order to provide a moral justification for applying palliative sedation, a certain moral code has been devised. It is called the principle of double effect [20, 25, 32, 33].

Palliative sedation in terms of the principle of double effect means that:

(1) Our primary and only aim is to help the patient.
(2) Palliative sedation is undertaken with the intention to achieve the possible alleviation of suffering without intending to shorten life even though this may be foreseen.
(3) We do not want to end suffering by termination of life.
(4) Palliative sedation is undertaken in a dying child when all other interventions have been unsuccessful.

There exist various methods of palliative sedation. Usually it is a combination of administering an opioid drug with some other drug that has sedative properties [18–20, 34, 35]. Because many dying children with cancer have severe pain, we advocate the use of an opioid as part of sedation in most cases.

Ideally, a decision regarding conducting palliative sedation is a multistep process. First, a palliative team should perform a thorough clinical and laboratory re-evaluation of the patient and, if needed, restaging of the disease in a given child. The primary goal of this re-evaluation is to be reassured that we are dealing with refractory symptoms in a child with terminal cancer. Second, a revision of all therapies, including psychological intervention, directed toward the alleviation of suffering is performed. Further, with the consensus of all involved medical and psychosocial staff, including the treating senior physician, nurses, the psychologist and the social worker, the possibility of presenting the proposal of palliative sedation to the child's parents is discussed. If such a decision is made, the next step is the discussion of the issue with the patient's parents.

Not all parents are ready immediately to accept a proposal of this kind at this stage, because of the immense emotional significance carried by such a decision. Hence, sometimes the performance of other additional medical tests, usually some kind of imaging scan, may be useful in order to help parents understand the real state of affairs and to accept the reality of the situation. After their agreement, palliative sedation is commenced.

Because the majority of cancer patients at the end of life suffer from pain, one of the components of palliative sedation is usually morphine, administered intravenously or subcutaneously. Usually the patient gets some opioid medication at the start of palliative sedation. Hence, all that is often necessary is merely to adjust the dose of the opioid drug to the extent that pain becomes absent or minimal and to switch to the parenteral route of administration, if this has not been done before.

If the patient has not been placed on opioids earlier and is in pain, at the beginning of palliative sedation, one usually applies a loading dose of morphine in order to switch off the child's consciousness, while maintaining a subsequent continuous intravenous drip of morphine with the aim of keeping the patient unconscious without, however, causing respiratory depression. This is usually achieved with doses of morphine between 0.5 and 5 mg/hour with upward titration when needed. Sometimes significantly higher doses are used to achieve the desirable effect. Use of morphine is especially convenient when the patient suffers from cancer with lung metastases causing respiratory distress and the feeling of air hunger [18].

Use of Meperidine in the practice of clinical pediatric oncology is limited mainly to the treatment of chills, as a side effect resulting from transfusion of various blood products or infusion of Amphotericin B. In these situations Meperidine may be a rapidly effective drug. When Meperidine is administered in repeated doses or as a continuous infusion, its toxic metabolite, normeperidine, may accumulate in the plasma and exert its excitatory effect, potentially leading to convulsions. Therefore, it is recommended to avoid the use of Meperidine as an opioiate in the context of palliative sedation [36, 37].

In addition to its known sedative effects, Midazolam also has prominent anticonvulsive properties. Therefore, it is especially useful for patients with seizures at present or in the past and for those who have intracranial metastases or brain tumor as a primary cancer [18, 38]. After the loading dose of 0.2–0.3 mg/kg of Midazolam, it should be continued by intravenous drip.

It is to be emphasized that initiating palliative sedation is not always dictated by unbearable and uncontrolled pain. Therefore, morphine or some other opioid is not always administered and hence must not necessarily be viewed as an integral component of this kind of treatment. For example, if palliative sedation is initiated in a child with a brain tumor because of intractable seizures, sedation only with Midazolam or other sedative agents may suffice.

It is important to try to avoid any temporal association between initiation or performance of palliative sedation and the occurrence of death because such an association, even if it is merely coincidental, may be of great negative symbolic significance in the minds of parents. It is still customary in clinical practice to conduct palliative sedation with the combination of morphine, chlorpromazine and Phenergan. Chlorpromazine has cholinergic properties and tends to decrease the level of arterial pressure. Hence, it may precipitate a cardiovascular collapse in a patient, and should not be used in the context of palliative sedation. Because of the possibility of ensuing death as a result of administering chlorpromazine, it is preferable to avoid using this drug as much as possible. For the same reason, increments in drug doses should be made gradually rather than by push.

Role of Nutrition and Hydration During the Terminal Phase

Providing a sick person with fluids and food is a basic requirement of human and compassionate care [39–41]. Timely and correct nutritional support may significantly improve outcome in patients with cancer. More specifically, they have been shown to facilitate successful recovery after surgical interventions [42] and recovery after high-dose chemotherapy with stem cell support [43]. Nutritional support represents a highly emotion-laden theme with serious ethical considerations in the practice of pediatric palliative care. It is widely assumed that forgoing nutrition and fluids to a terminally ill child contradicts the very essence of compassionate care. This point of view is frequently supported by parents and other lay persons who tend to think that withholding fluids and food may lead to the patient's accelerated demise. Given the fact that most pediatric cancer patients have a central line in place during their last phase of life, it might seem tempting to use it as a vehicle for providing nutrition and hydration to the dying child. Nevertheless, one has to keep in mind all the possible and unfortunately not rare drawbacks of total parenteral nutrition (TPN), which may occur with even higher frequency in debilitated cancer patients [44]. Since in most instances the projected life expectancy is very short, and TPN may be potentially useful when it is given for sufficiently long periods of time (say, weeks to months), TPN cannot play a central role in the context of palliative medicine.

Exceptions to this conclusion would be those rare instances when the terminal phase of cancer is expected to be prolonged in a child who cannot be fed in any other way (for example, cases in which a surgically uncorrectable intestinal obstruction or severe respiratory distress develop in a child with pulmonary metastases after insertion of a nasogastric tube).

It has been shown that most patients with progressive cancer do not feel hunger and thirst. McCann, Hall and Groth-Juncker [45], in their study of 32 adult patients with a life expectancy of 3 months or less (31 patients suffered from cancer), found that 63% of patients never experienced any hunger and 34% additional patients complained about being hungry only during the initial phase of starvation. Similarly, 62% of patients either experienced no thirst or experienced thirst only initially during their terminal illness. In those patients who had some complaints about either hunger or thirst, it was possible to achieve alleviation by very simple measures, such as providing small amounts of food, or water and by moistening of lips. In another study, Torelli, Campos and Meguid [46] tried to determine whether providing TPN may actually improve the quality of life and alter the ultimate outcome of terminally ill adult cancer patients. The authors evaluated the possible influence of TPN provided either as an adjunct to in-hospital intensive therapy for cancer or for in-hospital supportive treatment, and found that in both settings providing TPN was of no value either for quality of life or for the ultimate outcome of these patients. Unfortunately, no similar studies have been performed with terminally ill pediatric cancer patients. But common sense and clinical experience suggest that the same holds true for pediatric oncology as well.

A lot has been written about the ethical aspects of forgoing nutritional support to terminally sick patients [39, 41, 47, 48]. A current concept prevailing in medicine is that nutrition and hydration are medical interventions as much as any other treatment modalities and, therefore, their administration should be subsumed under the same moral and ethical principles [31, 49]. It is ethically justified to withhold or even withdraw some medical interventions in patients suffering from progressive cancer in the terminal phase, in order to prevent unnecessary suffering by providing futile treatments [41]. According to this postulate, providing nutrition and hydration should be ruled only by medical indications. However, in the reality of pediatric palliative oncology, this apparently clear decision to forgo provision of nutrition to the child dying of cancer is not so easily accepted.

Very often, parents, and sometimes even the treating medical personnel, find it emotionally too difficult to agree not to give food or fluids to a dying child. In certain instances, when there is no consensus between the parents of a dying child and the treating physician, it may be prudent to provide the child with hydration through either a nasogastric tube [50] or a central/peripheral line while forgoing nutritional support.

Explaining to the parents that the fluids contain a certain amount of glucose necessary for providing energy may facilitate parental agreement to accept the physician's proposal.

Place of Death

It is generally assumed that most people would prefer to die at home surrounded by close family members and friends. It is logically easy to assume that children do not constitute an exception to this general rule [51, 52]. As McCallum, Byrne and Bruera [14] put it: "death in hospital is the default situation when support for death in the home is inadequate." Unfortunately, it is only rarely that the child's death occurs at home. There are several possible reasons for this. First, the progressive nature of cancer itself is often accompanied by multiple symptoms, sometimes difficult to control, which necessitate hospitalization of a dying child. Second, the intense psychological impact that the imminent death of the child poses for other family members may preclude the child's staying at home in the last phase of sickness. Third, there are sometimes certain human, financial and other difficulties that limit or even completely preclude the possibility of managing the terminal phase of cancer in an ill child at home. This becomes all too evident when we consider that, in order to enable successful terminal care of the child with cancer at home, it is necessary to create a palliative care team specifically dedicated to the management of such children [53]. Optimally, this multidisciplinary team should consist of a pediatric oncologist, a pediatric oncology nurse, a psychologist and a social worker. The presence of a chaplain may be very helpful as well.

If death at home is not an option, the dying child spends the last days in the hospital. But even in a hospital ward the medical personnel should make everything possible in order to create a sense of "home" for the dying child and the relatives. It is insensitive and therefore unacceptable to ask parents to leave the room where their child is dying, even using the excuse that it is too stressful for parents to witness the last agony of their loved one. These last minutes spent together may be very precious for those who continue to live, indeed they are too precious to be ignored or slighted. It is likely that they may even help the parents undergo a normal bereavement process during this difficult time.

It is the responsibility of the palliative team to do everything possible in order to mask signs of agony by properly performed medical assistance to a dying child (by optimal dosing of opioids and sedatives). It may sometimes be very useful to explain tactfully to parents about the physiologic changes their child is undergoing during the process of dying as soon as they occur, while constantly reassuring parents that all possible sources of suffering during this period have been properly addressed and controlled. Only very rarely in the clinical practice of pediatric oncology does it happen that parents do not want to be present at the bed of their dying child. In that case the parents' wishes should be respected and a quiet place should be provided for them to stay or wait not far from the child's ward. In these cases it is very helpful if a psychologist or another person familiar to the parents stays near the grieving parents.

One possible solution, when death at home or in hospital seems to be not suitable, albeit presumably a costly one, is the creation of a palliative care unit capable of providing comprehensive palliative treatment both to patients with curable diseases and to those whose lives can no longer be saved. Experience with the establishment of such a unit has been reported by Golan *et al.* [54], who showed that palliative care units may lead to a decrease in the number of deaths occurring both in the hospital and at home. Dedicated primarily and mainly to provide palliative care for patients with incurable cancer, such a unit can also admit children with good prognosis as well for supportive or chemotherapy treatments, according to overall bed availability. Since for many parents and children themselves (especially adolescents), terminology such as palliative care and hospice are frequently synonyms of imminent death, thus, early introduction to this unit, when there is no immediate prospect of death, may facilitate a smoother transition to this unit if required at a later stage. The palliative care unit existing in Israel is geographically located outside but in near proximity to the department of pediatric oncology of one of the largest medical centers in the country. Such a location allows the medical and psychosocial personnel of the department of pediatric oncology to maintain close contact with the dying child and his/her parents, and thus this avoids the feeling of abandonment and separation by the patients and families which may otherwise occur when death takes place either in a hospice or at home. Death at home may be too distressing for those who spend the last moments by their dying child (siblings, grandparents and other close relatives); sometimes it is just impossible to leave the dying child at home due to prominent suffering. Alternatively, transfer of such a patient to a hospital or the department of pediatric oncology may be inappropriate because of the nature of care he or she needs at this stage of life. In such a situation,

hospitalization of terminally ill pediatric cancer patient in a palliative care unit seems most appropriate for the dying child and the family.

Conclusion

For a parent, witnessing the death of their child is a tragic event, one that cannot be compared in its severity and intensity to anything else. The physician is often unable to prevent this death but is responsible for making it as peaceful and free of suffering as possible. The ultimate gratification of the physician in his work as a palliative care specialist is rendering it possible for the bereaved parents to find meaning and solace in the death of their child. This is achieved by vigorous control of all physical symptoms in a dying child and by close attention to all existential, emotional and social demands of both the child and his or her relatives.

References

1. Masera J, Spinetta JJ, Jankovic M, *et al.* Guidelines for assistance to terminally ill children with cancer: a report of the SIOP Working Committee on psychosocial issues in pediatric oncology. *Medical and Pediatric Oncology* 1999;**32**:44–48.
2. McGrath P. Development of the World Health Organization guidelines on cancer pain relief and palliative care in children. *Journal of Pain & Symptom Management* 1996; **12**:87–92.
3. Wolfe J. Suffering in children at the end of life: recognizing an ethical duty to palliate. *Journal of Clinical Ethics* 2000;**11**:157–163.
4. Gatta G, Capocaccia R, Coleman MP, *et al.* Childhood cancer survival in Europe and the United States. *Cancer* 2002;**95**:1767–1772.
5. Bradshaw G, Hinds PS, Flensing BS, Gattuso JS, Razzouk BI. Cancer-related deaths in children and adolescents. *Journal of Palliative Medicine* 2005;**8**:86–95.
6. Jalmsell L, Kreicbergs U, Onelöv E, Steineck G, Henter J-I. Symptoms affecting children with malignancies during the last month of life: a nationwide follow-up. *Pediatrics* 2006;**117**:1314–1320.
7. Pritchard M, Burghen E, Srivastava DK, *et al.* Cancer-related symptoms most concerning to parents during the last week and last day of their child's life. *Pediatrics* 2008;**121**:e1301–1309.
8. Theunissen JMJ, Hoogerbrugge PM, van Achterberg T, *et al.* Symptoms in the palliative phase of children with cancer. *Pediatric Blood & Cancer* 2007;**49**:160–165.
9. Wolfe J, Grier HE, Klar N, *et al.* Symptoms and suffering at the end of life in children with cancer. *New England Journal of Medicine* 2000;**342**:326–333.
10. Baker JN, Kane JR, Rai S, *et al.* Changes in medical care at a pediatric oncology referral center after placement of a Do-Not-Resuscitate order. *Journal of Palliative Medicine* 2010;**13**:1349–1352.
11. Postovsky S, Levenzon A, Ofir R, Weyl Ben Arush M. "Do not resuscitate" orders among children with solid

tumors at the end of life. *Pediatric Hematology-Oncology;* 2004;**21**:661–668.

12. American Academy of Pediatrics Committee on Bioethics and Committee on Hospital Care. Palliative care for children. *Pediatrics* 2000;**106**:351–357.

13. Foex BA. Do-not-attempt resuscitation ("DNAR") order. *Anaesthesia* 2000;**55**:92.

14. McCallum DE, Byrne P, Bruera E. How children die in hospital. *Journal of Pain & Symptom Management* 2000; **20**:417–423.

15. Mack JW, Cook EF, Wolfe J, Grier HE, *et al.* Understanding of prognosis among parents of children with cancer: parental optimism and the parent–physician interaction. *Journal of Clinical Oncology* 2007;**25**:1357–1362.

16. Wolfe J, Klar N, Grier HE, *et al.* Understanding of prognosis among parents of children who died of cancer: impact on treatment goals and integration of palliative care. *JAMA* 2000;**284**:2469–2475.

17. Stevens MM, Dalla-Pozza L, Cavalletto B, *et al.* Pain and symptom control in paediatric palliative care. *Cancer Survivors* 1994;**21**:211–231.

18. Collins JJ, Grier HE, Kinney HC, Berde CB. Control of severe pain in children with terminal malignancy. *Journal of Pediatrics* 1995;**126**:653–657.

19. Galloway KS, Yaster M. Pain and symptom control in terminally ill children. *Pediatric Clinics of North America* 2000;**47**:711–746.

20. Cherny NI, Portenoy RK. Sedation in the management of refractory symptoms: guidelines for evaluation and treatment. *Journal of Palliative Care* 1994;**10**:31–38.

21. Meisel A. Legal myths about terminating life support. *Archives of Internal Medicine* 1991;**151**:1497–1501.

22. Morita T, Tsunoda J, Inoue S, Chihara S. Effects of high dose opioids and sedatives on survival in terminally ill cancer patients. *Journal of Pain & Symptom Management* 2001;**21**:282–289.

23. Chater S, Viola R, Paterson J, Jarvis V. Sedation for intractable distress in the dying: a survey of experts. *Palliative Medicine* 1998;**12**:255–269.

24. Quill TE, Lo B, Brock DW. Palliative options of last resort: a comparison of voluntary stopping eating and drinking, terminal sedation, physician-assisted suicide, and voluntary active euthanasia. *JAMA* 1997;**278**:2099–2104.

25. Rushton CH. Ethical decision making at the end of life. In: Armstrong-Dailey A, Zarbock S (eds.) *Hospice Care for Children*, 2nd edn. Oxford: Oxford University Press, 2001; pp. 323–352.

26. Yanov ML. Responding to intractable terminal suffering; letter. *Annals of Internal Medicine* 2000;**133**:560.

27. Krakauer EL, Penson RT, Truog RD, *et al.* Sedation for intractable distress of a dying patient: acute palliative care and the principle of double effect. *Oncologist* 2000;**5**: 53–62.

28. Sulmasy DP, Ury WA, Ahronheim JC, *et al.* Responding to intractable terminal suffering; letter. *Annals of Internal Medicine* 2000;**133**:560–561.

29. Morita T, Tsunoda J, Inoue S, Chihara S. Terminal sedation for existential distress. *American Journal of Hospital Palliative Care* 2000;**17**:189–195.

30. Rousseau P. Existential suffering and palliative sedation: a brief commentary with a proposal for clinical guidelines. *American Journal of Hospital Palliative Care* 2001; **18**:151–153.

31. Cherny NI. Sedation in response to refractory existential distress: walking the fine line. *Journal of Pain & Symptom Management* 1998;**16**:404–406.

32. Quill TE, Dresser R, Brock DW. The rule of double effect: a critique of its role in end-of-life decision making. *New England Journal of Medicine* 1997;**337**:1768–1771.

33. Sulmasy DP, Pellegrino ED. The rule of double effect: clearing up the double talk. *Archives of Internal Medicine* 1999;**159**:545–550.

34. Kenny NP, Frager G. Refractory symptoms and terminal sedation of children: ethical issues and practical management. *Journal of Palliative Care* 1996;**12**:40–45.

35. Fainsinger RL, Waller A, Bercovoci M, *et al.* A multicentre international study of sedation for uncontrolled symptoms in terminally ill patients. *Palliative Medicine* 2000;**14**:257–265.

36. Kaiko RF, Foley KM, Grabinski PY, Heindrich G, Rogers AG, Inturrisi CE, *et al.* Central nervous system excitatory effects of Meperidine in cancer patients. *Annals of Neurology* 1983;**13**:180–185.

37. Marinella MA. Meperidine-induced generalized seizures with normal renal function. *Southern Medical Journal* 1997;**90**:556–558.

38. Postovsky S, Moaed B, Krivoy E, *et al.* Practice of palliative sedation among children with brain tumors and sarcomas at the end of life. *Pediatric Hematology-Oncology* 2007;**24**:409–415.

39. MacFie J. Ethics and nutritional support. *Nutrition* 1995;**11**:213–216.

40. Morita T, Tsunoda J, Inoue S, Chihara S. Perceptions and decision-making on rehydration of terminally ill cancer patients and family members. *American Journal of Hospital Palliative Care* 1999;**16**:509–516.

41. Nelson LJ, Rushton CH, Cranford RE, Nelson RM, Glover JJ. Forgoing medically provided nutrition and hydration in pediatric patients. *Journal of Law & Medical Ethics* 1995;**23**:33–46.

42. Bozzetti F, Gavazzi C, Miceli R, *et al.* Perioperative total parenteral nutrition in malnourished, gastrointestinal cancer patients: a randomized, clinical trial. *Journal of Parenteral and Enteral Nutrition* 2000;**24**:7–14.

43. Weisdorf SA, Lysne J, Wind D, *et al.* Positive effect of prophylactic total parenteral nutrition on long-term outcome of bone marrow transplantation. *Transplantation* 1987;**43**:833–838.

44. Wesley Jr., Efficacy and safety of total parental nutrition in pediatric patients. *Mayo Clinic Proceedings* 1992;**67**: 672–675.

45. McCann RM, Hall WJ, Groth-Juncker A. Comfort care for terminally ill patients: the appropriate use of nutrition and hydration. *JAMA* 1994;**272**:1263–1266.

46. Torelli GF, Campos AC, Meguid MM. Use of TPN in terminally ill cancer patients. *Nutrition* 1999;**15**:665–667.

47. Sullivan RJ. Jr., Accepting death without artificial nutrition or hydration. *Journal of General Internal Medicine* 1993;**8**:220–224.

48. Barber, M.D., Fearon, K.C.H., Delmore, G., Loprinzi, C.L. Should cancer patients with incurable disease receive parenteral or enteral nutritional support? *European Journal of Cancer* 1998;**34**:279–285.

49. Bozzetti F, Amadori D, Bruera E, *et al.* Guidelines on artificial nutrition versus hydration in terminal cancer patients. *European Association for Palliative Care: Nutrition* 1996;**12**:163–167.

50. Boyd KJ, Beeken L. Tube feeding in palliative care: benefits and problems. *Palliative Medicine* 1994;**8**:156–158.
51. Lauer ME, Camitta BM. Home care for dying children: a nursing model. *J. Pediatrics* 1980;**97**:1032–1035.
52. Mulhern RK, Lauer ME, Hoffmann RG. Death of a child at home or in the hospital: subsequent psychological adjustment of the family. *Pediatrics* 1983;**71**:743–747.
53. Sirkia K, Saarinen UM, Ahlgren B, Hovi L. Terminal care of the child with cancer at home. *Acta Paediatrica* 1997;**86**:1125–1130.
54. Golan H, Bielorai B, Greber D, *et al.* Integration of a palliative and terminal care center into comprehensive pediatric oncology department. *Pediatric Blood & Cancer* 2008;**50**:949–955.

18

Psychological Intervention with the Dying Child

Shulamith Kreitler, Elena Krivoy

Introduction: Psychological Intervention as a Component of Palliative Care

In recent years there has been increased attention to the suffering of pediatric cancer patients at the end of life, which has led to enhanced efforts to respond adequately to the psychological needs of children and adolescents confronting death [1, 2]. These efforts have been facilitated by the increasing conviction that palliative care needs to be integrated firmly into the curative program of pediatric cancer [3]. There is evidence of special efforts that are made in different pediatric departments to provide psychological care for the young patients facing death [4–6]. However, psychological care of the dying child has not yet become a standard element in the treatment of the child with cancer. In our view, psychological interventions targeted at dealing with the emotional needs of the children and their families need to be considered as indispensable components within this broadened system of medical care. This would be consistent with the consideration of the rights of young patients no less than of those of adults, and would manifest respect for the young patient as a whole person deserving the best quality of life and of death that we can provide.

Death Awareness in Children

It is only in recent years that it has become evident that the suffering of children in the terminal stage may be due not only to physical symptoms but may also reflect their awareness of imminent death, no less than it may be the case in adults [7]. This awareness may be more or less logical, conscious and verbally expressible depending on the child's level of development and previous experiences, although the seriousness of the disease may itself accelerate the development of the child's cognitive insights [8]. Information about children's conceptions of death is important for any attempt to help children confronting death. Awareness of death in children has been studied from two complementary perspectives: the cognitive one, focusing on children's conceptions of death in general, and the experiential one, focusing on children's construction of their state.

Children's Conceptions of Death

Studies of the development of death conceptions in children adopt either the "comprehensive stages" approach or follow the developmental sequence of specific themes that make up the conception of death.

The comprehensive stages approach is based on the assumption that the child's conception of death is some kind of an integrated conceptualization that depends primarily on the child's cognitive abilities and changes in an orderly sequence, although the rate of moving from one stage to another may differ across children. The developmental sequence has been described as following closely the Piagetian model [9]. The empirical data has been collected in different countries and by means of different research tools [e.g., 10–11]. In the sensorimotor stage of infancy (0–2 years), babies below 6 months of age have no understanding of death because it requires a grasp of the constancy and identity of objects which are still missing. Hence, they react to death only as the absence of familiar persons (i.e., separation, loss), demonstrated sometimes by stranger anxiety. Toddlers identify objects but are limited by their inability to assume a frame of reference other than their own, which is being alive. In the preoperational stage (2–7 years) of early childhood, there is no real understanding of the universality and

Pediatric Psycho-oncology: Psychosocial Aspects and Clinical Interventions, Second Edition.
Edited by Shulamith Kreitler, Myriam Weyl Ben-Arush and Andrés Martin.
© 2012 John Wiley & Sons, Ltd. Published 2012 by John Wiley & Sons, Ltd.

irreversibility of death. Death is conceived as a state similar to sleep, characterized by the activities of the living, e.g., eating, going fishing. At the stage of concrete operations (7–11/12 years) of middle childhood, children will personify death, often in evil images (e.g., devil, bogeyman) and will tend to regard death as punishment for evil deeds. By the age of 9 or 10 years, most children have an adult conception of death as universal and irreversible, further influenced by the religious conceptions of their culture. In the stage of formal operations (over 12 years), the adolescents have a good understanding of death. Hence, the possibility of non-being poses for them a great anxiety-provoking threat, which religious beliefs may mitigate to some extent.

The stages view led to the conclusion that, up to the age of 10, terminally ill children are not concerned with their possible death and this supported the recommendation not to discuss this theme with them [12, 13]. Both the conclusion and the recommendation seem inadequate. One fault of this approach is that it is concerned mainly with verbal expression of concepts by the children and hence captures only partial, possibly distorted aspects of the phenomenon. Moreover, it expects consistency across children, where there may be none. It is, however, important insofar as it reveals the situation when one focuses on verbal expression, which may be the preferred mode of communication by specific psychotherapists or children.

The 'specific themes' approach follows the development of particular aspects of the death conception, mainly non-functionality (i.e., death ends all life-sustaining functions), irreversibility, universality, causality and personal mortality. Kenyon's [14] excellent review shows that each of the five themes develops differently and separately. For example, the causes of death shift from non-natural ones (e.g., violence, accident) in 5–6-year-olds to natural ones (e.g., illness) in 8-year-olds, to spiritual ones (e.g., invocation by God) in 11-year-olds. Awareness of personal mortality follows more closely the binary developmental track: from denial in 3–4-year-olds to confirmation in 8- and 11-year-olds. This suggests that there are no stages defined by a bundle of features but different developmental trajectories following individual tracks. Further, each of the themes of the death concept is affected differently by major factors, such as age, gender, cognitive ability, and culture.

Most important is the effect of experience on the development of death concepts. Studies of children 5–12 years old showed that having lost a loved one through death was related to less accurate death scores, especially in regard to causality and universality [15], or was not correlated with death concept scores at all

[e.g., 16]. Yet, children with cancer differed from matched healthy children in their concepts about personal mortality and death-as-justice [17]. They more often acknowledged personal mortality and less often viewed death as a punishment. Moreover, within the oncology group, those who had experienced the death of a close friend or relative had a deeper understanding of personal mortality, universality and irreversibility of death, irrespective of age. Similarly, children with leukemia (4–9 years old) did not differ from healthy children in their overall death scores, but had better understanding of the irreversibility and non-functionality of death [18]. Yet, independently of disease, anxiety was found to lower scores of understanding different death aspects, notably universality, irreversibility, non-functionality and personal mortality [19, 20]. These findings suggest that personal experience with death in the form of a life-threatening disease like cancer may override the effects of death anxiety observed in healthy children, which may cause distortions or denial.

Children's Awareness of Dying

The research findings about children's conceptions of death need to be complemented by findings about the awareness of death in dying children. The issue was studied from the early 1950s, relying first on clinical observations and semi-structured interviews with children and their parents [e.g., 21], then on the accounts of parents and hospital staff [22] and later on examining directly the terminally ill children, for example, by means of projective techniques [23]. All studies showed unequivocally that children were aware of the seriousness of their condition and their impending death. This conclusion is further supported by rich documentary material of stories, poems, drawings and dreams of dying children [24–27].

Some children actually express their awareness in words (e.g., J., a 4-year-old, said one week prior to his death of leukemia: "Mommy, I don't want you to cry when I die, I want to see your smile"), while others do it in a symbolic form, using images, drawings, toys and other objects. Thus, G., an 8-year-old with retinoblastoma, had an imaginary rabbit whom she treated for weeks until one day she declared that it was going to die on Wednesday "because when rabbits get that sick they cannot live much longer." The form of expression may depend on the level of the child's conscious awareness [24], the child's conformity with the social rules of "mutual pretense" in regard to impending death [26] or the child's habitual form of thinking [28].

In one of the most widely known descriptions of the development of awareness of death in sick children, five stages were defined [25]:

Stage 1, defined as "seriously ill," reflects the children's experiences of admission to the hospital for diagnostic tests, the ensuing medical treatments and the changed caring attitude assumed toward them by the adults. Most of their fears at this stage are of the unknown rather than of the prognosis.

The children pass into stage 2, defined as "seriously ill and will get better" after they have experienced a remission and a few rapid recoveries of disease-related symptoms, such as nosebleeds. After having received drugs which make them feel better and noticing that most people treat them in a normal way again, they conclude that eventually they will get better.

Stage 3, defined as "always ill and will get better," sets in after they have been through the relapse-remission cycle and have noticed the uneasy avoidance response of the adults around them. The fears focus on recurrence but there is still the belief that despite it one can still recover.

Stage 4, defined as "always ill and will never get better," sets in after more relapses, pain and drug complications. At this stage the children become aware that they are getting weaker, that they can plan only for very short terms and they start grieving about all those things of the future that they will most probably not do. They get used to the sickness staying always with them.

Children move onto stage 5, defined as "dying," following an event such as the death of another child on the ward. The similarity in disease and treatments between themselves and the deceased child may spur the sick children to integrate all their knowledge about the disease and treatments and get to the startling, disastrous conclusion that they themselves are dying. The pace at which they reach this conclusion varies from one child to another, but eventually they all reach that awareness. It is then that they begin expressing their awareness of impending death, verbally and symbolically. The awareness may be accompanied by decreased communication with adults, from whom the dying children tend to hide their new awareness, and by lowered cooperation with different medical procedures that have not helped in the past. Slowly their world starts narrowing down in terms of themes, activities and interests: they play less, they move around less, and they are concerned more with death. Gradually death comes to permeate their minds and thinking.

The above description demonstrates that the awareness of one's death is a slowly developing process, fed, on the one hand, by the child's personal experiences of disease and treatments, and, on the other hand, by information obtained from the adults, mostly indirectly through eavesdropping and observing their behaviors toward oneself or among themselves (e.g., special caring, crying surreptitiously).

In parallel, another process occurs—gradual dying in a psychological sense. As noted, the children lose interest in many things, give up plans for the future, do not look forward to holidays, refer to the shortness of time they have, prepare less for the future ("you don't have to work hard to become a ghost," said a 5-year-old two weeks prior to his death).

The findings concerning awareness of one's own death seem to differ in various respects from those concerning death conceptions discussed earlier. The disparities are due partly to differences in research tools (drawings, stories, semi-structured interviews and observations in the studies of death awareness versus verbal expressions and questionnaires in the studies of conceptions). Additionally, the disparities may arise out of the basic difference there may be between dealing with death in general or the death of others and confronting one's own death. According to Kastenbaum [30, p. 88], the simple proposition "I will die" presupposes a wealth of cognitions, such as awareness of being a person with a life of one's own, of belonging to a class of mortal beings, of awaiting the certain occurrence of death at an uncertain timing, of accepting the finality of death as the ultimate separation of oneself from the world, and the necessity of preparing for an event about which one knows absolutely nothing. All these considerations, further compounded by the emotional component of sadness about not being any more, underscore the conclusion that "relying solely on the terminally ill child's overt expressions of anxiety yields incomplete or misleading information" [31, p. 176]. In providing palliative psychological care to a dying child, one is well advised to use all available channels of communication—verbal and nonverbal—keeping in mind what children may be expected to know or understand of death, without losing sight of the important distinction between death in general and one's own death.

Pediatric Psychological Palliative Care (PPPC)

The pediatric cancer patient in the terminal stage is a very special kind of patient who may require a special type of psychological palliative care. Not only are the patients young but they may be suffering from various physical symptoms and may be confronting death; they may have special needs (emotional, existential, spiritual and cognitive); and there may be explicit or more often implicit restrictions on communication with them for they are guarded and cared for by their parents, who may have the final say in regard to the treatment and information provided to the patients. Due to these and other characteristics of the patients, their state, concerns and the setup, we suggest calling the kind of psychological intervention designed for the patient at the end-of-life Pediatric Psychological Palliative Care (PPPC) to distinguish it from psychological intervention practiced in other stages of pediatric oncology.

The concept of PPPC has several implications. A major implication concerns the goals. PPPC is not designed to cure any psychological ailment or disorder but to improve the child's state, overall or any particular aspect, and sometimes prevent, moderate or delay any adverse effects of physical or psychological state. Further, the palliative aspect indicates that we should regard the child's welfare in a holistic manner, be attentive to multiple domains and help wherever we can, but stay within the boundaries of palliative care, that is to say, let ourselves be guided primarily by concerns of the here-and-now rather than promoting the emergence or resolution of problems that may be significant mainly for the future.

An important assumption of the PPPC is that the pediatric patient needs to be approached as a "whole person," namely, as a person with different and varied needs, including the emotional, social, cognitive, existential, and spiritual, all of which have to be addressed if and when mentioned by the patient.

A major characteristic of PPPC is that it enables and encourages the child to express himself or herself in whatever form he or she prefers by creating a safe atmosphere and offering an empathic and maximally permissive listening. No prescriptions, criticism or instructions accompany the listening. The psychologist is equally receptive to an adolescent who spends the sessions discussing Buber's I–Thou conception, another who may prefer to sit silently, and still another who may fill up pages with colored lines.

As a component of palliative care, PPPC is primarily a client-centered responsive kind of intervention. This indicates that it is initiated and functions mainly in response to the needs and possibilities of the child at a given time and place and adapts its tools in line with these needs and possibilities, rather than in accordance with some preconceived scheme or theory about the needs of a dying child. For example, it is not advisable to approach the dying child with the preconception that a dying individual should resolve previously unresolved issues ("close up circles," so to speak). Some children may express the wish or need to do so, whereas others may shy away from it or not be at all aware of such issues. Whereas there may be a justification for promoting the resolution of unresolved issues within the framework of some psychotherapeutic conceptions, within the framework of palliative care it is justified only if the patient herself or himself is aware of the need to do so.

In line with the general approach of palliative care which deals primarily with symptoms, PPPC too is focused on specific issues, in an attempt to resolve particular problems or conflicts so as to reduce distress as much as possible. For example, when a patient is anxious or depressed, PPPC is geared to identify the particular source of the anxiety or depression in the here-and-now and resolve or moderate it, without necessarily attempting to provide the patient with tools to deal with anxiety and depression in general and without expecting that the problem that has caused the anxiety or depression will not recur.

As noted, PPPC advocates the adaptation of tools to the needs and possibilities of the child. A whole variety of tools stands at the disposal of the PPPC practitioner. Rather than starting, for example, with the common assumption that play or drawing are the major vehicles of communication with children in therapy, PPPC advocates the use of whatever tool is adequate at a given time for a particular child handling a specific issue. In the framework of PPPC it is legitimate to use drawing at the beginning of a therapeutic session with the child, then switch over to verbal discussion, and perhaps even finish with dance-like movements enacted by both therapist and child.

Similarly, in regard to other rules and routines concerning therapy. It is usual in psychological interventions to set fixed times and even locations for the therapy. PPPC does not necessarily abide by these conventions. It does not make sense to strictly limit the psychological intervention sessions to the routine of a fixed number of times per week or to conduct the therapy only in the therapist's room. Rather, if necessary, PPPC may take place twice a day on some days and at the child's bedside when the child so prefers or is unable to move.

The same goes for the convention of treating the child alone, without the presence of others. This convention too may be set aside in favor of treating the child with other close persons (e.g., a parent, a sibling), if the child expresses the need or the wish to do so.

Further, PPPC considers the child within the framework of the whole family system, including whoever is actively involved in or affected by the child's disease, namely, the parents in the first place, but also grand-parents and siblings and in exceptional cases also other relatives. Their involvement may range all the way from active participants to observers.

In general, pediatric palliative care is essentially based on team work [7], which is multidisciplinary [32]. Hence, PPPC should be viewed as part of the total palliative care of the patient, and its practice is to be coordinated with the other palliative care measures administered to the sick child. Beyond coordination, PPPC requires cooperation with the rest of the palliative team. Implementing the cooperation may vary with the specific patient. Sometimes it entails mainly getting information from the other team members and providing them information about the patient's psychological state; in the case of other patients, it may entail mobilizing the whole team for the attainment of a goal that has come up in the framework of the PPPC, such as making up with a sibling, or fulfilling the child's wish for a leave-taking party; in still other cases it may imply providing the child opportunities to raise the bothering issues with any member of the team preferred by the child.

Finally, since PPPC is designed for children in advanced disease stages, it is to be initiated only when the child enters the terminal phase. However, the child and the parents may be dismayed and scared if they are suddenly exposed to PPPC. Therefore, it may be advisable to let the child and family meet the person or team of PPPC earlier, in an informal manner, maybe as part of getting acquainted with the ward and hospital services. If the child and family have at least had a chance of meeting the person or team of the PPPC before it is launched as a full-fledged intervention, they may be better able to respond to it and benefit from it without being threatened or embarrassed.

Concerns of the Dying Child and How to Deal with Them Psychologically

In this section we will deal with different issues and problems that often come up in the treatment of children in the terminal phase and what to do about them in the framework of PPPC. However, it is necessary to emphasize that these issues do not always come up, nor are they the only ones. The basic principle of PPPC is to be attentive to the child's needs without enforcing the discussion of any theme according to a preordained scheme.

Fear of Abandonment and Separation

Some of the more characteristic fears of children and adolescents in the terminal phase are fears of abandonment, of being left alone, or simply of loneliness. Some are even scared of falling asleep for fear that precisely

then they will be left alone. The physical presence of others, especially family members, reassures them that nothing evil will happen to them. Some children may even need recurrent physical contact in order to feel reassured. In some cases, this fear is manifested as fear of the dark, because in the darkness one is less certain of the presence of others. In other cases, the fear of abandonment or of loneliness is explicitly expressed as fear of being separated from one's family. For example, Rachel, a 7-year-old girl with leukemia, is quoted as saying: "I am so worried because . . . I think I may die and I don't want to leave my family . . . Promise me that if I die before you and Daddy that you and Daddy will be buried beside me" [33, p. 30].

This cluster of fears may be an expression of the child's fear of separation, of leaving her family and friends, of being lost [34]. Hence, it is possible that this fear expresses fear of death. Indeed, fear of annihilation, fear of separation, and fear of vanishing are identified components of death anxiety [35]. However, it could also express the child's sense of helplessness and weakness as compared with the tasks of confronting forces partly known to be strong and evil (e.g., pain) and partly not yet experienced. It is only natural for the child to feel the need of support, reinforcement through the presence of others who may be a great help when things get tough. Some children deal with the fear of loneliness and separation by invoking the presence of imaginary figures, as for example, Rachel [33] who could feel the presence of her guardian angel, but only when she was alone. PPPC would not try to allay the fears or tell the child "there is nothing to fear"; on the contrary, it would encourage the child to ask for the presence of others and encourage others to stay with the child. Indeed, it would even praise the child for asking for help and for preparing in this way to face the hardships in store.

The described complex of fears seems to be related to anticipatory reactions to impending separation from mother, family, or friends that have been widely documented in children [36]. The response to separation is typically biphasic, including a first phase of agitation with increased behavioral and physiological activation, reflecting active coping, followed by a second phase of depression, apathy and withdrawal, reflecting passive coping. The manifestations may be observed in play behavior, activity level, sleep and eating patterns, heart rate, body temperature and immune functions [37].

Fears of Leaving the Familiar and of Confronting the Unfamiliar

Leaving the familiar means primarily leaving parents, siblings, family at large and friends. But additionally it may mean leaving one's clothes, familiar objects, one's bed and desk, one's home, in short, all those things one has learned over the years to love, to use, to call "my own." Indeed, it may mean leaving behind, being disconnected from everything on which one's sense of pride, security and even identity had been based.

Confronting the unfamiliar represents a different experiential complex. It may indicate being in a strange, bizarre environment, completely different from anything one has known before, possibly experiencing things one has never experienced or been told before, acting in a setting of which one knows nothing and for which no one has ever prepared the child in any way. Whereas leaving the familiar may evoke in the child fear, anger and sorrow, confronting the unfamiliar may evoke plain terror, regardless of how self-confident the child may be. Children deal with these in different ways. Studying examples of children's coping may help the PPPC practitioner devise means of helping other children.

Here are some examples concerning leaving the familiar. Naama, a 6-year-old, dying of a brain tumor, organized a set of rituals for taking leave of her things, each in turn, for example, kissing it, whispering to it, touching it. Joseph, a 9-year-old with leukemia, started to wrap up his beloved things as presents, and stuck on each a note indicating to whom he wanted the object to be given. He had to stop because this procedure evoked great anxiety in his mother. She blamed him for "robbing" her of his things, which she wanted to keep. In the framework of PPPC the mother was led to understand that Joseph wanted to make sure his things would not grieve for him but be happily used by other children. Older children may assume the attitude of "I have outgrown these things, like an old pair of pants; they are of no use to me any more."

The examples for confronting the unfamiliar are different. Moshe, a 12-year-old, with Ewing's sarcoma, "populated" the hereafter with many different individuals whom he expected to help him. He started out with saying that he knew his grandfather, who had recently died, would wait for him. A few days later he wondered about whether his grandpa would look in the hereafter for his pals who had previously died. Then he said he thought this is the thing his grandpa would do "and this is a good thing 'cause they would all be like my friends." Some children try to construct an imaginary world based on movies they have seen and stories they had read. Preparing for the unknown may be one reason why children in this state were reported to be eager to read books about death [e.g., 27].

Fear of Punishment

Another class of fears focuses on being punished. Sometimes children talk of being attacked, hit, molested, beaten or incarcerated by other people or forces, familiar or unfamiliar, which may appear to the children in the form of monsters, "bad people," witches, ghosts, skeletons or other symbolic figures. Personifications of death, which assume these forms, were found to be common in children in the middle years of childhood, 6–8 years [38, pp. 61–62]. This fear may reflect the child's fear of the unknown that lies ahead. It may also arise out of the child's feeling that there may be tasks to handle in the future which he may not be able to master. PPPC would lead us to strengthen the child by reminding him or her of all the tasks in the past which they were afraid they could not handle but eventually handled successfully. Memories of past successful coping are designed to lead to the conclusion that there is no reason to assume the child would not be able to do in the future as well as it had done in the past. Also, there is no reason to assume at all that there would be tests, hardships and bad things to experience. The monsters and other symbolic evil figures may be overcome by means of guided imagery which may be taught to the child or performed with her.

However, fear of punishment may also have to do with the children's past—with the sense of guilt or remorse about "bad" things the children think they have done in the past or "good" things they have failed to do. For example, some children and adolescents are guilt-ridden because they have not been good to their parents, have not treated their siblings well, have lied, taken things that do not belong to them, have evaded their duties, had forbidden thoughts, and so on. The therapeutic attitude of PPPC would stress that such and similar things may be bad, but doing bad things is part of being human, all children do things of this kind, and adults know that children do them. The bad that human beings do is offset by the good things that one does. PPPC would urge the child to recall as many good things that it had done in the past, recount them and dwell on them. Some children and adolescents may express the tendency to re-evaluate conceptions of good and evil. It would be advisable to help them along this route. But if the child shows no such tendency, it would not be advisable at this stage to plunge into a process of checking one's values, which might contribute to undermining the child's sense of security.

Fear of punishment and the sense of guilt may be related to the child's religious beliefs and concern with the afterlife [39]. The child's conception of life after death may focus on punishments meted out to the evil human beings by superior powers, on suffering and hell. PPPC would focus on humanizing the scene in the afterlife, complementing the conception by elaborating on the concepts of paradise and good angels, mitigating the child's sense of guilt and self-blame, dwelling on the good deeds the child had done, and reminding the child of the suffering it had already suffered through the illness and the treatments which may obviate the need for further suffering.

Fear of Pain and Suffering

Some children and adolescents may have fears of pain and suffering. It would be natural for them to have those fears both because of what they have already undergone themselves and because of what they may have observed in other children on the ward or in the clinic. Sometimes the fears refer to specific symptoms, such as being immobilized, suffocating, losing control over bowel movements, losing a limb, or not being able to see. Fears of this kind may reflect the child's fear of the unknown lying ahead, focused on one's body rather than on the external environment (as in fear of the unfamiliar). But they may also reflect distrust of the physicians and nurses taking care of them. Some children develop with time a growing distrust when they become aware of the fact that although the physicians do for them the utmost, there are limits to what they can do. Nevertheless, it is of utmost importance that the child stay convinced that the doctors really do the utmost for him or her, and even when they cannot heal, they can alleviate pain and suffering. Maybe a good way to put it is that the child patient has to make the shift from curative to palliative medicine, just as the doctors had done. In this context, PPPC often consists of helping the child express his or her fears, communicate them to the doctor and be courageous enough to insist on getting all the help medicine can offer. A fair number of children still need to be convinced that they are not to blame for feeling pain, that they do not have to feel ashamed for confessing they feel pain, and that it is not a sign of weakness not to want to feel pain. Some are not even sure that pain can be controlled to a large if not full extent.

Fear of Death

Sometimes children in the terminal phase will refer directly to their fear of death. In the literature there are three major approaches to death anxiety: "the displacement theory," "the existential theory," and "the pragmatic theory." The first maintains that there is no true death anxiety because consciously we have never experienced death and unconsciously it is inconceivable because the unconscious knows no negation [40]. Thus, that which appears to be death anxiety is in fact anxiety displaced from other unresolved conflicts and problems. The second approach views death anxiety as rooted in the awareness of our mortality and as an inalienable aspect of our existence, mostly handled through repression [41]. The third approach maintains that we are actually not afraid of death itself but of a variety of things that have come to be associated with death, such as pain, suffering, separation, loneliness, or punishment [42], which are often based on mistakes and misinformation.

All three approaches may contribute to handling death anxiety in the framework of PPPC. The displacement theory would advocate resolving conflicts the child may have; the existential theory would advocate legitimizing death anxiety (e.g., "it is natural"); the pragmatic approach would advocate easing the process of dying as much as possible and allaying the fears that relate to the different real or imagined connotations of death, as discussed earlier. In each case, PPPC would advocate applying the methods which best respond to the issues raised directly or indirectly by the child.

Being Told the Truth

For children in the terminal phase, being told the truth reduces to being told about impending death. As noted above, many of the young patients are aware of this eventuality on a certain level of consciousness. Some children and adolescents do not raise the issue at all with the doctors or parents. The reason may be denial, desire to deal with this issue on one's own terms or safeguarding one's parents.

Denial is not an all-or-nothing phenomenon but may be partial and subject to fluctuations [42]. In the framework of PPPC, awareness is not considered as an asset in its own right. Hence, as long as the child cooperates with the basic medical requirements, PPPC respects the child's right to denial.

Some children and adolescents in the terminal phase may feel more comfortable discussing death and dying with individuals other than their doctors and parents. PPPC respects the right of children to choose the person with whom they want or do not want to discuss their own death. Respecting their right may entail helping the adults understand, tolerate and accept this behavior, which may not always be easy, particularly not for parents.

Sometimes more complex situations occur. Nir, a 17-year-old adolescent suffered from a recurrence of ALL (leukemia) after 13 years. He knew very soon that he was dying, but his father, who assumed complete and exclusive control of Nir's treatment, was not ready to accept the fact and refused to talk about it. Nir pressured him to discuss it but to no avail. The psychologist had a few sessions with the father. When finally the father was able to tell his son that he knew he was dying, Nir calmed down and died peacefully 48 hours later.

This example demonstrates that discussing death with the parents may sometimes be important for the children for reasons, such as getting confirmation that the parent respects them sufficiently to be able to accept them as mature partners, or being reassured that the parent is not angry with them for dying, that the parent knows they have done everything in order to stay alive but may not succeed in this venture.

On several occasions dying children who knew of their impending death explained to the psychologist that they wanted nevertheless to be "told the truth" as a sign that they are sufficiently respected to be considered as worthy and able to get the right information.

Protecting One's Parents

Concern over one's parents is an issue that may bother quite a number of children in the terminal phase. They are concerned about the suffering and pain of their parents and try to hide from them how much they suffer. Dalia was a 10-year-old girl with sarcoma who stayed on the ward for five months, almost continuously. When she went home, mostly over the weekend, she developed high fever and other complications (e.g., neutropenia, low magnesium level) which necessitated her return to the hospital. Her mother stayed with her most of the time, despite the fact that there was another 3-year-old boy at home. Dalia felt that her mother suffered because she had to neglect the small brother. Dalia started gently communicating to her mother that she felt better, had no pain, was in good mood and could take care of herself. She even said "I am not a 3-year-old baby that you have to look after all the time." Notably, the mother was persuaded to go home and leave Dalia alone for periods that grew longer until the psychologist succeeded in improving communication between the mother and daughter so that Dalia could tell her mother what she had been doing.

Protecting one's parents may take diverse forms. Sometimes the child would simply hide from the parent his or her pain, or choose to deceive the parent by enacting a happy play or appearing to be immersed in some trivial task, or insist on staying in the hospital because she or he believes that care at home would be too difficult for the parents. Dan, an 11-year-old boy

with sarcoma, told the psychologist "My mother need not suffer for me; it does not help me but it harms her, she will live after I die." However, Zehava, who was only 8 years old, disclosed another surprising insight: "Mummy and daddy when they come here don't cry, they cry when they are not in the room, but outside, in the corridor; it is better to cry alone, I also cry alone when they don't see, I don't want them to cry because of me." Thus, it is possible that a child may imitate the parent in hiding one's grief.

PPPC indicates the need for improving communication between parents and children so that, if they wish, they can openly discuss the issue of whether to share one's pain and suffering with each other. It is through communication that they may find out, for example, as Itay the 8-year-old did, that when his parents spoke of being strong they did not mean not complaining about pain, or, as Tami the 5-year-old did, that her parents suspected she was dissimulating and it pained them that she did not trust them enough to share her pain with them. In both cases the improved communication led to increased sharing on the part of the children. Increased communication can also lead initially to decreased sharing as, for example, in the case of Avi, who found out that his disease reminded his mother of the Holocaust. Following several common sessions with the psychologist, Avi and his mother understood how misleading it was to equate their predicament with the Holocaust.

Guilt in Regard to One's Parents

A dying child may feel guilty for letting down his or her parents by dying before the child could realize their wishes and expectations of him or her. "My father wanted me to be an officer in the army, now I will only be a dead child," said Gil, a 7-year-old with sarcoma. A girl on the ward wrote a note to her parents asking them for forgiveness "because all you put into me is going down the drain." This girl felt guilty because she could not give her parents back what she thought they deserved in return for everything they had given her.

There are several ways to deal with this issue in the framework of PPPC. One way is to let the child see that its parents did not bring it into the world in order to fulfill their expectations; they created life for life's sake. Another way is to let the child perceive that the future is only one aspect of life, complementing the present and the past but not replacing them and not outweighing them in importance. Still another way is to let the child perceive all the happiness she had given its parents and let the parents tell the child how happy she had made them all through. Which one or more of these different ways is adequate for any specific child depends on the child.

Loss of Respect for Authorities

Children and adolescents in the last phases of terminal disease sometimes suffer from a crumbling respect for authorities. It may have its roots in the gradually emerging awareness that the doctors are unable to provide the means for full recovery, do not always know what the next step in the disease would be, sometimes cannot even help in fully controlling pain. This awareness is all the more disconcerting because it has come to replace the complete trust that the child and his family had in the medical institution. In addition, there is the growing recognition on the part of the child that even the all-powerful parents, who have always shielded the child from all evil and have satisfied all his needs, are unable to prevent impending death in the future and all of the suffering at present. These are very difficult and painful insights because parents and doctors are mainstays of one's sense of security and confidence in the benevolence of life and reality. Instead of the shielded security of childhood and teenage years, the patient stays with "a tattered cloak" of make-beliefs, half-truths, and uncertainties. The 13-year-old boy with sarcoma who used this metaphor added "this cloak gives you no warmth."

It is difficult to evaluate for whom these insights are harder: for the smaller child who up to the occurrence of the disease has lived in a state of complete trust in one's parents, or for the adolescent who has already started his or her exploration of reality and has had a chance "to see through the veil of certainty," to use another metaphor of a sick teenager. For the younger children the collapse of trust may be more extensive, but for the adolescents it is no less vital because it is precisely the trust in their parents that gives them the courage to explore.

The insights about the inability of doctors and parents to avoid the evil bring in their wake disappointment, frustration, enhanced sense of helplessness, and weakness. As far as the parents are concerned, various feelings may be evoked, starting with anger for their having misled the child, through guilt about feeling that way, to pity which generates the desire to protect the parents since "they are not stronger than I am."

PPPC tries to help the patient recognize that having limits on one's capacity does not mean the absence of all ability and effectiveness. The extreme all-or-nothing approach is to be complemented by the realistic approach which takes into account abilities, knowledge and goodwill, coupled with the recognition of limitations to what one can achieve. From one child we have learned "that sometimes my math teacher gives me a good grade because I tried hard even though I did not have the solution." In other words, it is justified to respect people for what they are trying to achieve and for the effort they put into it even if they fail. Also, not all failures are identical. Some failures are closer to success than others.

Loss of Control

Loss of control at present and in the future bothers some of the children and teenagers in the terminal phase. Due to their experiences in previous stages of the disease and treatments, the patients have noticed the gradual loss of control over their body, appearance, actions, feelings and behaviors. Since control is tightly bound with the sense of identity, diminished control indicates a threat to one's self-identity and comfort of being in the world.

PPPC concentrates in these cases on constructing the sense of control, both from bottom up and from top to bottom. Examples of the bottom-up approach include insisting on the child deciding about small or concrete things, such as where to put objects in his or her room, what to wear, where to sit, who would visit and when. Examples of the top-down approach include discussing with the child the issue of control in general, the limitations on control, the illusion of having control even when one has little or no control, and "respect for reality" which has not been constructed so as to enable each and everyone to have control over most things. Helping the child remember events and situations when it felt it had control or no control provides examples that help the child gain insight about how control functions and its limitations.

Sadness and Sorrow

The terminal phase of illness is often the period when the child or adolescent starts the process of grieving and mourning over oneself. PPPC enables the children to express their sadness. One child said, "Look at me, so young and such a pretty body, what a pity." Dying children and adolescents may become poignantly aware of all the things in the present and especially in the future which they would miss by being no more. They may think of careers, of getting married and having kids, of traveling in the world, of participating in parties, of having fun, of loving and being loved. The more they know of the world and of life the deeper the potential sorrow. In the framework of PPPC there are a variety of ways to deal with this important issue. One way consists in elaborating on moments of joy and happiness from the child's past. This serves not only to raise the mood at present but also communicates the message that "life has been wonderful and has had its exquisite moments even if they belong to the past" or "no one can take from me wonderful moments I have experienced." Another way we have learned from one of our patients. Silvia was an 11-year-old girl when it became evident that she would die from Wilms' disease. Her physical suffering was intense. She expressed a wish to have a party. A party was organized for her on the ward and many of her friends participated. Silvia enjoyed the party enormously and a few days later she asked for another party. "I know we had a party but that was long ago, like 'last year'." A series of six parties was organized for Silvia, which she experienced as if they stretched over a time period of years. In the last party she asked to be dressed in a white dress "like a bride," and insisted on video photos to be taken of her all in white, to show everyone "next year." What Silvia attempted to do was to compress the future as much as possible, reduce it to fun and parties and live as many of its delightful moments as she could. Silvia acted out in reality or quasi-reality what many others do in fantasy and daydreams. A similar insight was expressed by Avi, a 15-year-old, who drew "a bird's song," consisting only of different colored dots and lines. He explained that life was the dots and lines, which in the case of some people were strewn around over a larger space and in the case of some over a much smaller space.

Anger

Anger often appears in the process of coping with the awareness of death, although not necessarily as a specific stage in a sequence, as claimed by Kübler-Ross [25]. It may appear in varied forms. Sometimes it takes the form of envy of others in general or of specific others (e.g., a sibling or a schoolmate) who are not sick and stay alive. In others it may appear as rebellion or refusal to cooperate with the medical treatment ("anyway it does not help at all"). It often accompanies the complaint of injustice ("Why me?" or "It is not fair that I should die, I have done so little . . . "). It may also take the form of a desire to destroy, to vent out the anger ("I want to see everyone dead when I am dead," said one 4-year-old). A 15-year-old girl dying of leukemia was full of rage to such an extent that she could not tolerate anything living in her vicinity, no animal, no flower, no picture of an animal, not even anything that moves of its own accord. Indeed, she put herself into a world of total death, as a kind of protest against her fate.

PPPC provides a framework for expressing the anger. It enables the child or adolescent to externalize the anger by using the variety of expressive means suggested by the psychologist (e.g., words, enacted movements, drawings, fantasy). The mere expression may already be helpful. Once released, the emotion may be more manageable. PPPC turns the anger into a legitimate emotion and thus frees the patient of the need to hide it or fight it, and encourages him or her to devote these energies instead to confronting the situation that had produced the anger. Some of the patients get into a fierce dialogue with life, fate or God in their efforts to overcome the anger. Some find within themselves an answer that brings with it some comfort; others find in themselves the courage to face the silence. In the context of this confrontation not a few seek solace in faith and religion.

Wish Fulfillments

Some children use wish-fulfillments in order to solve problems they have when facing death. Fulfilling wishes, which is possible to fulfill at this stage, is a most important and potent means of PPPC. For many children it is an exhilarating experience to find out that their wishes may not only be fulfilled, but often without delay and without compromising. The fulfillment of some of these wishes may get to be reported in the media, as for example, the visit of a famous artist or entertainer in the children's ward because a sick child wanted to meet him or her. Some wishes are touchingly modest, as to own some object, see a certain picture, wear a certain piece of jewelry, listen to a particular music and so on. One 10-year-old girl on the ward had a wish to kiss her mother's breasts (in a kind of regression to early infancy); another boy (a 12-year-old dying of a brain tumor) wanted to have in his room in the hospital many different colored balloons; another older boy (a 14-year-old) wanted to have privacy because "I am not a public ground where everyone can come and go when they want."

Some wish-fulfillments require special effort on the part of the parents, such as the wish of one dying girl to see her recently divorced parents staying together at least in her room, or the wish of another girl to spend the last weeks of her life at home rather than in the hospital. PPPC tries to create an atmosphere in which the children can express wishes and makes a point of promoting the fulfillment of the patients' wishes as promptly as possible. Fulfilling the patients' wishes may require a close cooperation between the parents, the medical staff and the psychologist.

Hope and Self-comforting

Dying children and adolescents often seek hope, comfort, or consolation openly. Some may beg for it ("tell me something that will give me hope"), others may tell of their success in finding it ("I saw an angel and he was smiling at me" or "I dreamt I went to heaven and then came back and was all healthy; I know this can happen to you"). In their effort to get hope they often turn to faith and religion, even if their upbringing has not been strictly orthodox and even if they do not know too much about religion. Contact with higher powers (e.g., God, angels), high-ranking individuals (e.g., the prime minister) or close people who had died before (e.g., the child's grandmother) may be very comforting to some children. To the question that is sometimes asked "Will they help me?," the psychologist can only answer, "I hope so." No doubt, the belief itself is helpful.

Search for Meaning

Although children and adolescents are generally not expected to deal with abstract issues of this kind, some nevertheless do and raise questions, such as "Who am I?," "What is the meaning of my life?," "What was my role in life and did I fulfill it?," "Why was I born?," and "Why do I die?" PPPC considers it as its function to help young patients confronting death to explore these issues and chart for themselves some kind of answer. Help in this domain does not mean indoctrination, persuasion, or providing answers; rather it means encouraging the child to look for himself or herself, explore optional answers, provide information when the child asks for it, sometimes rephrasing clearly what the child has been trying to say or conceptualize. The major characteristic feature of the approach of PPPC is that meaning resides in the act of assigning meaning. Hence, meaningfulness is the product of the meaning or meanings the human being assigns to the facts, rather than of the facts or events as such. Assigning meaning may be a laborious process that may lead to unexpected results. Sometimes it reveals that events that seemed in the past highly meaningful lose some of their meanings, whereas others which had been hardly noticed assume great significance. Some young people draw a lot of comfort from the discovery that by relating events to one another and by exploring interactions among components one may discover meanings that had not been evident in considering other relations or partial sections of the past. Other children find comfort in realizing that "no one can finish the whole job, and others will go on with the job in the future," for example, "my younger sister will make nice drawings for my

mother because she loves them" and "my older brother said that he will not go to the army and help my father because I cannot help him." The search may end with the conclusion "I don't know" or "I will find out only after I die." It may, however, also end with the realization that there is no sense in anything. The psychologist may then help in avoiding the subsequent emergence of despair.

Sometimes the search for meaning focuses on concern with self-identity. This issue may be of enhanced importance in adolescence, the period when a child is focused on developing his or her identity and individuality. With a curtailed life expectancy that greatly limits the options for actions and experiences, the youngster may feel that he or she has missed out on developing their self-identity. PPPC would promote the child's enhanced sense of uniqueness and individuality by encouraging the child to dwell at length on behaviors, experiences, daydreams, friendships that demonstrate how special he or she is, how different from anyone else they know. Further, PPPC would encourage the child to express his or her individuality also in the context of the terminal phase in the hospital in a variety of ways, such as through clothing, choice of objects to be placed around, and so on. It is of special importance, particularly in the case of adolescents, to promote cultivation of their external appearance, insofar as attractiveness may be one of the earmarks of individuality.

General Issues in Providing PPPC

As noted earlier, two major principles of PPPC are considering the child patient within the context of the whole family system and considering PPPC within the total context of palliative care provided to the sick child.

The Dying Child and the Family

Providing PPPC to a sick child in the terminal phase means treating the child and his or her family, that is to say, together with the family, within the family, sometimes through the family. The family consists naturally first and foremost of the parents, but includes also grandparents and siblings insofar as they are involved with the treatment of the sick child. In practice this entails, for example, dealing with the anxieties of the parents that may transfer to the child; helping the parents and the child talk openly, especially about their emotions; and promoting mutual communication of needs and desires [44].

Often taking care of the family may require improving communication also within the family, for example, between the two parents who may not be communicating openly concerning their sick child or in general, as well as between the parents or the sick child and a sibling who may suffer from anger, envy or guilt in regard to the dying child. Tension-laden situations of this kind call for the attention of the psychologist because they may project on the sick child and even interfere with satisfying the child's needs. PPPC advocates adopting a flexible approach and treating the family as a whole, or in pairs or each member individually, as required for a speedy resolution of the problems.

The parents are not only the primary care-takers of the child in the hospital no less than at home; they are also the prime decision-makers in regard to anything that concerns the child. While this in no way restricts the responsibility of the medical treatment and palliation team in the hospital, it increases the child's sense of security, belongingness and identity.

However, treating the child in the context of the family does not mean that the psychologist is free to communicate to the parents everything that has taken place in the therapeutic session with the child. The child's right to privacy has to be defended no less than the parents' rights. It is also important that the therapeutic session provides a safe haven for the child to express thoughts and feelings that he or she finds difficult to express elsewhere. However, the psychologist may ask the child's permission to share with the parents any theme that came up in therapy and which may be important to communicate to the parents so as to improve the child's state or quality of life. Involving the parents is important all along, but in particular in regard to themes that have any operational implications. Asking the child for permission is one way to empower the child and help him or her resume control of their life. More importantly, the psychologist will encourage, enable and help the child and the parents to discuss among themselves themes that were discussed in therapy as well as others. Further, with the consent of both parties, in some or all PPPC sessions, both child and parents may participate.

PPPC and the Treatment Team

Workers in the field have noted how difficult it may be to produce cooperation between the treatment team, the family and the child, coordinating their sometimes different needs [7]. Communication and cooperation between the nursing staff and the family may sometimes require psychological intervention [45]. When PPPC has become a part of the palliative therapy in a specific ward or clinic, the treating teams are trained in

the specific techniques and issues of PPPC and may only need adjustment or focused intervention for particular cases.

PPPC advocates treatment of the therapeutic staff both in general and in regard to cases of specific patients. The purpose is double—both to help in providing PPPC to the dying child and to keep burnout of the staff as low as possible. Treatment of the staff includes providing understanding of the psychological setup of the child and his or her family, analyzing and—if necessary—improving communication and cooperation with the child's family, working through one's reactions and difficulties in the course of treating the child, and resolving the pain and shock after the child's demise.

The involvement of the staff in PPPC may sometimes require imparting information about the child's psychological needs and state. In view of the child's right to privacy and in order to enhance the child's sense of security, it is advisable that, if at all possible in view of the child's state and age, no information be imparted without prior discussion with the child and his or her fully informed consent.

Issues of Time and Place

There are two difficult operational issues loaded with heavy emotional connotations with which PPPC may be concerned and which involve the child, the parents and the staff. These have to do with the decision about palliative sedation and with the location in which the child will stay in the last period of his or her life. The decision of palliative sedation is all the more difficult because it is a decision for another human being who is one's own child and it relinquishes the last vestige of hope for the child's survival. One of the hard tasks of PPPC is to help the parents confront their inner attitudes and decide or express the decision they have already undertaken [46].

Determining the location for the child to spend the terminal period requires a decision of a different order. The desire of the parents to protect their child and provide the warmest and most comfortable environment is of prime importance, but it is necessary to consider also the child's desire and needs as well as the logistics of treatment at home that may be difficult [1]. The home is also for many children the most favorable environment, but not for all. It is of paramount importance to find out what the child's desires in this respect really are. For example, some children, perhaps the youngest, would prefer home at all costs, but others may feel safer and more protected medically in the hospital. Again, some children would like to take leave of their beloved objects at home or perform symbolically important acts like bathing in their own bathtub or extend as much as possible the illusion of normal daily routine at home. Other children, however, may prefer to forgo the pain of leave-taking of places and objects or may be at a stage where these symbolic acts have already become meaningless. PPPC means that special means and care are applied for helping in clarifying or identifying the child's desires in this as in other respects and encouraging their expression so that they may be implemented with all possible promptness, care, devotion and love.

References

1. Wolfe J, Hammel JF, Edwards KE, *et al.* Easing of suffering in children with cancer at the end of life: is care changing? *Journal of Clinical Oncology* 2008;**26**:1717–1723.
2. Friedrichsdorf SJ, Menke A, Brun S, *et al.* Status quo of palliative care in pediatric oncology: a nationwide survey in Germany. *Journal of Pain & Symptom Management* 2005;**29**:156–164.
3. American Academy of Hospice and Palliative Medicine, Center to Advance Palliative Care: National Consensus Project for Quality Palliative Care: Clinical practice guidelines for quality palliative care: executive summary. *Journal of Palliative Medicine* 2004;**7**:611–627.
4. Ben-Arush MW. Current status of palliative care in Israel: a pediatric oncologist's perspective. *Journal of Pediatric Hematology Oncology* 2011;**33**:S56–S59.
5. O'Mahony S, Blank AE, Zallman L, *et al.* The benefits of a hospital-based inpatient palliative care consultation service: preliminary outcome data. *Journal of Palliative Medicine* 2005;**8**:1033–1039.
6. Duncan J, Spengler E, Wolfe J. Providing pediatric palliative care: PACT in action. *American Journal of Maternal/Child Nursing* 2007;**32**:1–9.
7. Glazer JP, Hilden JM, Poltorak DY. *Pediatric palliative medicine Child and Adolescent Psychiatric Clinics of North America* 2006;**15**:xvii–xx.
8. Spinetta J, Rigler D, Karon M. Anxiety in the dying child. *Pediatrics* 1973;**52**:841–845.
9. Poltorak DY, Glazer JP. The development of children's understanding of death: cognitive and psychodynamic considerations. *Child and Adolescent Psychiatric Clinics of North America* 2006;**15**:567–573.
10. Nagy M. The child's view of death. In: Feifel H (ed.) *The Meaning of Death*. New York: McGraw-Hill, 1959; pp. 95–96.
11. Speece MW, Brent SB. The development of children's understanding of death. In: Corr CA, Corr DM (eds.) *Handbook of Childhood Death and Bereavement*. New York: Springer Publishing Company, 1996; pp. 29–50.
12. Rando T. (1984) *Grief, Dying and Death: Clinical Interventions for Caregivers.* Champaign, IL: Research Press.
13. Spinetta JJ. The dying child's awareness of death. *Psychological Bulletin* 1974;**4**:256–260.
14. Kenyon BL. Current research in children's conceptions of death: a critical review. *Omega: Journal of Death and Dying* 2001;**43**:63–91.
15. Cotton CR, Range LM. Children's death concepts: relationship to cognitive functioning, age, experience with death, fear of death, and hopelessness. *Journal of Clinical Child Psychology* 1990;**19**:123–127.
16. Mahon M. Children's concept of death and sibling death of trauma. *Journal of Pediatric Nursing* 1993;**8**:335–344.
17. Jay SM, Green V, Jonson S, Caldwell S, Nitschke R. Differences in death concepts between children with cancer and physically healthy children. *Journal of Clinical Child Psychology* 1987;**16**:301–306.
18. Clunies-Ross C, Lansdown R. Concepts of death, illness and isolation found in children with leukemia. *Child Care, Health, and Development* 1988;**14**:373–386.
19. Cobbs, B. Psychological impact of long-term illness and death of a child on the family circle. *Journal of Pediatrics* 1956;**49**:746–751.
20. Orbach I, Gross Y, Glaubman H, Berman D. Children's perceptions of various determinants of the death concept as a function of intelligence, age and anxiety. *Journal of Clinical Child Psychology* 1986;**15**:120–126.
21. Candy-Gibbs SE, Sharp KC, Petrun CJ. The effects of age, object and cultural/religious background on children's concepts of death. *Omega: Journal of Death and Dying* 1984- 5;**15**: 329–346.
22. Solnit AJ, Green M. Psychologic considerations in the management of death on pediatric hospital services. *Pediatrics* 1959;**24**:106–112.
23. Morrissey Jr., Children's adaptations to fatal illness. *Social Work* 1963;**8**:81–88.
24. Waechter EH. Children's reactions to fatal illness. In: Krulik T, Holaday B, Martinson IM (eds.) *The Child and Family Facing Life-threatening Illness*. Philadelphia, PA: Lippincott, 1987; pp. 108–119.
25. Kübler-Ross E. *On Children and Death*. New York: Macmillan, 1983.
26. Bertoia J, Allen J. Counselling seriously ill children: use of spontaneous drawings. *Elementary School Guidance and Counselling* 1988;**22**:206–221.
27. Bluebond-Langner M. *The Private Worlds of Dying Children*. Princeton, NJ: Princeton University Press, 1978.
28. Jampolsky GG. Taylor, P. *There is a Rainbow behind Every Dark Cloud*. Tiburon, CA: Celestial Arts, 1978.
29. Kreitler S. *Symbolschöpfung und Symbolerfassung: Eine experimentalpsychologische Studie Studie. [Symbol Creation and Symbol Perception: An Experimental Psychological Study]*. Munich: Reinhardt, 1965.
30. Kastenbaum R. *The Psychology of Death*, 2nd edn. New York: Springer, 1992.
31. Lonetto R. *Children's Conceptions of Death*. New York: Springer, 1980.
32. Freyer DR, Kuperberg A, Sterken DJ, Pastyrnak SL, Hudson D, Richards T. Multidisciplinary care of the dying adolescent. *Child Adolesc Psychiatric Clin N Am* 2006;**15**:693–715.
33. Bertoia J. *Drawings from a Dying Child: Insights into Death from a Jungian Perspective*. London: Routledge, 1993.
34. Rochlin G. How younger children view death and themselves. In: Grollman EA (ed.) *Explaining Death to Children*. Boston: Beacon Press, 1967; pp. 51–85.
35. Lifton RJ. *The Broken Connection*. New York: Simon & Schuster, 1979.
36. Field F Coping with separation stress by infants and young children. In: Field TM, McCabe PM,

Schneiderman N (eds) *Stress and Coping*. Hillsdale, NJ: Erlbaum, 1985; pp. 197–219.

37. Reite M, Short R, Kaufman IC, Stynes AJ, Pauley JD. Heart rate and body temperature in separated monkey infants. *Biological Psychiatry* 1978;**13**:91–105.

38. Lonetto, R, Templer DI. *Death Anxiety*. New York: Hemisphere, 1986.

39. Kavanaugh RE. *Facing Death*. New York: Penguin Books, 1977.

40. Freud, S. *Thoughts for the Times for War and Death*. In: Collected Works of Sigmund Freud,Vol. **4** London: Hogarth Press, 1953/1913; pp. 288–317.

41. Becker, E. *The Denial of Death*. New York: The Free Press, 1973.

42. Hinton, J. *Dying. Harmondsworth*, UK: Penguin Books, 1967.

43. Kreitler, S. Denial in cancer patients. *Cancer Investigation* 1999;**17**:514–534.

44. Sourkes, B.M. Psychotherapy with the dying child. In: Chochinov HM, Breitbart W (eds.) *Handbook of Psychiatry in Palliative Medicine*. New York: Oxford University Press, 2000; pp. 265–272.

45. Lipton H. The dying child and the family: the skills of the social worker. In: Sahler OJZ (ed.) *The Child and Death*. St. Louis: Mosby, 1978; pp. 52–71.

46. Kaplinsky C. Quality of death: the death of sick children. *In: Kreitler S. Confronting Dying and Death*. New York: Nova Science (in press).

19

Providing Support for Families Experiencing the Death of a Child

David J. Schonfeld

Introduction

Although bereavement is a normative experience and not a "disorder," it is often a profound experience that can be, at least temporarily, disabling. It is common to hear people say "it's not like someone died" when trying to compare and contrast other stressors in life. Indeed, there are fortunately few, *if any*, experiences that are worse than witnessing the physical suffering, increasing debility and ultimate death of one's own child. Attempts to alleviate or minimize the suffering of grieving family members should therefore be a high priority in programs that aim to meet the needs of families of children with potentially life-limiting conditions.

Anticipatory Grieving

While the focus of this chapter is on supporting families after the death of a child (see Chapter 17 for discussion of providing support to children who are dying and their families), the process of grieving for family members begins well before the death occurs, often as early as the time the diagnosis is first confirmed or even suspected. Such anticipatory grieving allows family members and others with connections to the child to allow themselves to experience graduated feelings of loss while the child is still alive. In this way, they can "practice" grieving in a somewhat safer context; when they begin to feel overwhelmed by feelings of loss, they can quickly comfort themselves by the realization that the individual is, in fact, still alive and can hope and anticipate that further treatment or other interventions can prevent the death. In this way, anticipatory grieving allows people the opportunity to start some of the work of grieving before the death has occurred. There

are, though, several common challenges that this poses that should be understood by clinicians carrying for children with potentially life-limiting conditions.

As with bereavement in general, the course and timeframe of anticipatory grieving for individuals are neither consistent nor predictable. Individuals do not follow a steady and linear course. They may seem to be accepting of the inevitability of the child's death and be taking actions, such as planning the funeral or discussing what the family will do to adjust to the loss, and then become overwhelmed by the associated feelings and re-engage only moments later in discussions of the need to pursue more aggressive treatments. This can be confusing to health care providers who oversee the child's medical treatment and cause tension between the providers and the family.

What makes this all the more challenging is that the course and timing of anticipatory grieving for individual members of the family are often quite different. Conflicts can result from the lack of synchrony. For example, one parent may reach some degree of resignation and acceptance of the impending death and begin to disengage from the child, stating, for example, the need to return to work or to provide needed attention to the siblings as the reason for less frequent visits to the hospital or increased emotional distance. If the spouse is at a different point in the process, this may lead to perceptions of abandonment (of both the child and the spouse) and the spouse may attempt to compensate by becoming even more involved with the child or less accepting of the eventuality of death. The health care providers then find themselves dealing with parents who present conflicting preferences on the course of medical treatment and who are less able to provide support to each other.

Pediatric Psycho-oncology: Psychosocial Aspects and Clinical Interventions, Second Edition.
Edited by Shulamith Kreitler, Myriam Weyl Ben-Arush and Andrés Martin.
© 2012 John Wiley & Sons, Ltd. Published 2012 by John Wiley & Sons, Ltd.

Members of the health care team also experience anticipatory grieving. Conflicts arise when members of the health care team have different levels of acceptance of the eventuality of the child's death or when there are conflicts between the views of the health care team and the family. For example, the physician may have accepted that further treatment is unlikely to be curative, while a nurse caring more directly with the child may be questioning unexplored options; conversely, the physician who has spent less time providing direct support to a child who is struggling with the side effects of aggressive treatment may be more inclined to suggest additional aggressive treatment while the nurse may be more in favor of palliative care and the withdrawal of curative interventions.

Anticipating the death of a child is painful, so family members understandably may wish for resolution of their anticipatory grieving. In the absence of a wholly unanticipated cure, the only likely means of ending the process of anticipatory grieving is the child's death. Parents and other family members may therefore find themselves at times wishing the child would die soon. The parent may then become overly involved (e.g., unable to leave the bedside even to shower or meet other basic needs) in part to compensate for extreme guilt that may result from a realization of this wish. Understanding that this is a common thought, even among parents who care deeply for their children, may help to alleviate some of the feelings of guilt.

Open communication, among family members and with the health care team, can help to minimize some of the conflicts that result from anticipatory grieving. If individuals are aware that others care about the child, but may be experiencing grief and coping in different ways, they may be less judgmental of different behaviors or may feel less abandoned. There may be more opportunities for family members to express, and have met, their unique needs for support. Meetings of health care teams involving all disciplines can be used to explore and resolve misperceptions and growing conflicts among team members. The current health care environment that increasingly relies on technology as a means of communication among providers and decreases the time available for face-to-face meetings places pragmatic obstacles to achieving this goal.

Death Notification

Many health care providers are understandably anxious about notifying parents/guardians about their child's death. There has been limited research about how best to perform death notification and little professional training is generally provided to health care providers. Often providers "learn" how to perform this critical and sensitive task by direct observation of others who have themselves had limited training and may not be comfortable or particularly skillful. Practically oriented guidance on how to conduct effective death notification and to provide immediate support to survivors is adapted from [1] and shows the steps to conducting effective death notification and providing immediate support.

- Establish contact with parents/guardians as soon as possible after serious clinical deterioration is suspected. Do not delay contact until a time felt to be more convenient (e.g., if the death occurs in the middle of the night, do not wait until the following morning).
- If the family is not present in the hospital, they can be contacted by phone and asked to return to the hospital or someone (e.g., police) can be sent to the home to ask the family to come to the hospital. Notification of the death, though, is best delivered in person and not over the phone.
- If a phone call is used to establish contact, in order to minimize the likelihood that you will be compelled to notify the family of the death over the phone, try to contact the family before the death has been declared (i.e., when the child is showing clinical deterioration or during resuscitation efforts) or have someone else who has not been directly involved in the care call on your behalf (someone not directly involved in the care could make a statement such as: "The health care team told me that your child was having some difficulties breathing, but I don't know any further information. If you came to the hospital now, someone who is taking care of your child will be available to talk with you when you arrive.") If family members demand information on the phone, the caller can state: "Dr. X would prefer to talk with you about this in person when you arrive at the hospital. She is with your daughter now and unable to leave to speak with you."
- Consider inviting additional family members or friends to accompany the parent/guardian to the hospital for notification, especially when a single parent/guardian is involved. Additional family members and friends can provide much needed support and can help notify other relatives and friends. Notify both parents/guardians at the same time whenever feasible.
- Before notifying the family, the physician (or other member of the health care team who will be conducting the notification) should briefly review the basic facts, including the name of the deceased, the relationship to individual(s) that will be notified, the basic circumstances of the clinical deterioration, the

nature of medical care or interventions provided to deal with the worsening clinical status, and the likely cause(s) of the death (if known).

- When the family arrives at the hospital (or site where death notification will be occurring), if possible, have them escorted to a private location. Death notification should be conducted whenever possible in a private setting.

- It is helpful to have the notification be conducted by a physician who was involved in the care, especially if this individual already has a relationship with the family. Inform the patient's primary care provider soon after the death.

- Consider including at least one other professional on the health care team, such as a social worker, chaplain, child life specialist, mental health provider, nurse, etc. One staff person, though, should be in charge of the discussion and the number limited to staff who were directly involved so as not to overwhelm the family.

- Professionals with training and experience in working with children should be involved in the notification process if the patient has siblings or the family will need to inform other children such as cousins, friends, or classmates. It is preferable that the notification of the death be provided to children by family members (such as the parent), as opposed to notification by professionals unknown to the child. Parents may wish, though, for professionals to be present when the children are told, to provide support and to be available to help answer questions. Provide families with written information about how to talk to children about death and how to provide support (such as *After a Loved One Dies: How Children Grieve and How Parents and Other Adults Can Support Them* [2], which can be freely downloaded in English or Spanish (www.nylgriefguide.com) and shared or free print copies ordered).

- Introduce yourself and any other member(s) of the health care team that may be participating by name and title and offer to shake hands.

- Offer seating to the family members; sit close to them and face them so that you can easily maintain eye-to-eye contact.

- Refer to the child who died by name and/or relationship to the survivor (e.g., "John" or "your son"); avoid referring to the person as "the deceased" or "the patient."

- Remember that notification of a death is a process, not an act. Adjust pacing of the discussion to the family's ability to listen to and respond to the information. Do not start by stating that the child is dead—survivors are unlikely to hear any subsequent information.

- Begin the discussion by asking the family what they already have been told or are aware of. Then provide a brief description of the circumstances of the deterioration and the team response. This information helps the family understand the context of the death, which will promote ultimate adjustment. After this brief summary, it is appropriate to give a "warning notice" (e.g., " . . . Your son was having great difficulty breathing, so we gave him some oxygen hoping that it might help. His breathing only became more shallow and less regular. Unfortunately, I have some very difficult news to share with you. Approximately five minutes ago he stopped breathing entirely . . . "), and then proceed fairly quickly to stating that the child died. In many situations, the family will have been present during the time of the clinical deterioration and response and would have been given updates that could serve as a "warning notice" (e.g., "the team has tried giving oxygen to relieve your son's difficulty breathing, but so far unfortunately he is continuing to have a great deal of difficulty breathing").

- Pause after delivering notification of the death to allow the information to be absorbed and to permit the family to begin to express their emotions. Do not try to fill the silence, even though it may seem awkward. Silence is often better than anything you might consider saying. Remain present with the family as they are reacting to the news, or at least make sure that another member of the health care team is able to remain with them.

- Use clear and simple language. Avoid euphemisms (e.g., terminated, expired, passed away, or is no longer with us); state the child died of is dead.

- Don't provide unnecessary graphic details; begin by providing basic information and allow the individual to ask questions for more details.

- If you do not know the answer to a question, say that you do not know. Try to get the answer to the question if possible. Don't give intentionally misleading information or speculate.

- Be conscious of non-verbal communication and cues—both those of the family as well as your own.

- Remain sensitive to cultural differences. Feel free to ask the family how their culture and family deals with a death if you do not know. Be particularly attentive to difficulty the family may have with speaking or understanding English. If there is any doubt that the family is fluent in English, make sure to involve a professional translator. Using family and friends as unofficial translators often leads to inadequate translation in the general medical setting; such reliance on friends and family members as translators for death notification is particularly bur-densome to the friends and family and should be avoided.

- If you are comfortable and think the individual will be as well, consider the use of limited physical contact (e.g., placing a hand on the family member's shoulder or providing a shoulder to cry on). Monitor the individual's body language and, if at all in doubt, ask permission first.
- Anticipate that family members may initially be in shock or denial. Expect additional reactions, such as sadness, anger, guilt, or blame. Acknowledge emotions and allow them to be expressed without judgment.
- Do not ignore or dismiss suicidal or homicidal statements or threats—investigate any such statements (strongly consider the involvement of mental health professionals if there is any concern that the statement may reflect actual intentions) and if concerns persist, take appropriate action.
- Just before and during the notification process, try to assess if the survivors have any physical (e.g., severe heart disease) or psychological (e.g., major depression) risk factors and assess their status once notification has been completed.
- Consider writing down your name and contact information if you are not already well known to the family and invite them to contact you if they think of questions at a later date. Survivors may not be ready to think of or ask questions and may later regret failing to get critical information that may help them understand, and ultimately adjust, to the death.
- Do not try to "cheer up" survivors (e.g., "I know it hurts very much right now, but I know you will feel better within a short period of time"). Instead, allow them their grief. Do not encourage them to be strong or cover up their emotions (e.g., "You need to be strong for your children; you don't want them to see you crying, do you?").
- Feel free to express your own feelings and demonstrate empathy in a sincere and genuine manner, but do not state you know exactly how they feel. Comments such as "I realize this must be extremely difficult for you" or "I can only begin to imagine how painful this must be to hear" can demonstrate empathy; you may wish to avoid such statements as "I know exactly what you are going through" or "You must be angry" (let the individual express their own feelings; don't tell them how to feel) or "I had two children who both died of a car accident at your son's age" (don't compete with the survivor for sympathy). It is fine to provide whatever reassuring information you are able to honestly provide (e.g., "I was with your child throughout this time period

and he seemed to be peaceful and in no pain") but do not use such information as an attempt to cheer them up (e.g., "You should be happy, many children who die from your son's illness die after hours of feeling like they are suffocating. At least your son didn't experience that").

- Feel free to show that you are upset as well. It is fine to cry or become tearful. Parents often feel that their child has been given optimal care when the health care providers show that they care. If you feel, though, that you are likely to be overwhelmed (i.e., sobbing or hysterical), then it is best to identify someone else to do the notification on your behalf.
- After you have provided the information to the family and allowed adequate time for them to process the information, consider asking questions to verify comprehension.
- Offer the family the opportunity to view and spend time with their child's body. A member of the health care team should escort the family to the viewing and remain present, at least initially. (For further information about preparation of the body for viewing, as well as additional recommendations about the death notification process, see [3].)
- Families may not know what they are expected to do next, or how to accomplish the tasks. Offer to help them notify additional family members or close friends. Tell them what needs to be done regarding the disposition of the body, etc. Check to see if they have a means to get home safely (if they have driven to the hospital themselves or were already there at the time, they may not be able to drive back safely) and inquire if they have someone they can be with when they return home.
- Help survivors identify potential sources of support within the community (e.g., member of the clergy, their pediatrician, family members or close friends).
- Take care of yourself. Death notification can be very stressful to health care providers and can lead to a range of reactions, including sadness, anger, guilt, or a sense of responsibility. It is important to offer at least informal support to professionals who provide death notification, especially for professionals who are likely to experience multiple patient deaths, as is the case in pediatric oncology.

The Needs of Siblings and Other Children

Siblings and other children in the extended family (e.g., cousins), as well as friends, are likely to be significantly impacted by the child's death but typically receive little or no support or even explanation [4]. Children's reactions and adjustment to a death depend, in part, on their ability to understand what death means and the implications it has for them personally.

In order to adjust to a death, children need to understand four basic concepts: irreversibility; finality (all life functions cease completely at time of death); inevitability (all living things eventually die); and causality (a realistic understanding of the causes of death) [5, 6]. On average, children learn these concepts between 5 and 7 years of age, but there is wide variability among children based in part on their cognitive abilities, personal experience, and explanations provided [7]. Children who have a terminal illness (see Chapter 18 for a discussion of terminally ill children) tend to have a precocious understanding of the concepts of death [8, 9] and children who have experienced the death of family members or friends, if provided with adequate explanations, may also show an understanding at even younger ages. Even infants and toddlers that are unable to understand death conceptually, can nonetheless sense and respond to emotional distress in caregivers and changes in caregiving that occur when parents/guardians are overwhelmed. They, too, are reacting to their sibling's terminal illness and death. Infant siblings of children with cancer have been shown to experience significant weight loss coinciding with the time of diagnosis, relapse, and death of the sibling with cancer, as well as temporary improvements at the time of remission [10]. Guidance material for parents and other caring adults on how to talk to children about death and how to provide assistance to promote adjustment, such as [2] which can be freely downloaded in English or Spanish (www.nylgriefguide.com) and shared or free print copies ordered, should be offered to families after a death has occurred; books for children and families are also available [11]. Simple misconceptions and literal misinterpretations are not uncommon and may result in long-term fears and anxiety that often can be addressed by clarification, once the misconceptions and misinterpretations are identified. This is one reason it is particularly important to offer children the opportunity to talk about a loss that has occurred. Parents/guardians and other adults who support children are often hesitant to initiate such conversations for fear of upsetting children who are grieving. They need to be reminded that such conversations may allow adults to see children's distress about the death, but the conversations themselves are not the cause of their distress.

Children's reactions to a personal loss are, in many ways, similar to that of adults, even if expressed in a different manner. Just as with adults, they can experience sadness, depression, anxiety, difficulty concentrating or learning, anger, and guilt. Given the common misconception among even school-age children that

cancer is contagious [12], children may have fears that they themselves or others close to them may develop cancer and die; being faced with a personal loss also raises concerns about others dying, even in the absence of such a misconception. Children may become more self-centered; regress or otherwise act less mature; avoid previously enjoyed activities; resist even brief separations from parents/caregivers or other family members (often resulting in school avoidance or clinginess in very young children); engage in risky behaviors (such as tobacco, drug or alcohol use or sexual behavior in older children and teens) or acting out or delinquent behavior; seek inappropriate physical intimacy (such as engaging in premature sexual behavior); or present with physical complaints (such as headaches, stomachaches, or fatigue) and disturbances in sleep or appetite that may be attributed to signs of an underlying physical condition.

Similar to adults, children are likely to wonder what they did, didn't do, or could have or should have done that might have prevented the illness or death. The magical thinking of children and their sense of immanent justice (a belief described by Piaget where good is ultimately rewarded and misdeed, even if just in thought, is punished) results in a nearly universal and profound sense of guilt, even when the reasons appear illogical or irrational to others [13]. Adults often experience similar forms of guilt, but children may have more difficulty understanding (let alone accepting) that their guilt is illogical. It is therefore important to provide outreach to children after a death of a family member has occurred to help them understand the true reason for the death and to provide reassurance that they had no responsibility for the illness or death.

The death of a child from cancer often occurs after a lengthy illness that is physically and emotionally taxing for all family members. During the illness, its treatment, and the immediate period after the death, surviving children are often reluctant to express their worries and concerns and to seek support to have their needs met. As is often seen in children who are terminally ill, they may pretend they either do not understand what is occurring or are having no difficulty with the situation because of a need to protect their parents who are visibly upset or having difficulty coping with the many demands and stresses associated with having a child who is seriously ill or who has died. They may attempt to support their parents at the same time they are most in need of support themselves. Parents who are personally overwhelmed may either need to believe their children are doing well or have little indication from their children to the contrary. Children's adjustment difficulties to a personal loss are therefore often underestimated by parents, guardians, teachers, and others who care for children. They may not present until weeks or months later, often when the parents themselves have begun to return to their regular activities and appear to be coping more effectively. But this does not mean that children do not understand what has happened or are not struggling, as adults are, with what it means. Often it simply indicates that they do not yet feel it is safe to share their concerns with adults and are left to struggle alone. This underscores the need for adults to reach out to children after a death has occurred. At the least, someone should speak to the children without the parent present (for school-age children and adolescents), and/or utilize projective techniques for children who are too young or not yet ready to talk directly, to inquire about what children understand and how they are coping and to offer support. After the death of a sibling or other close family member, this is particularly important. Those working with children with cancer should either personally fulfill this role or ensure that someone else has done so (such as a school counselor or other mental health provider, pediatrician or other pediatric health care provider, member of their faith organization, pediatric bereavement support group, etc.) [14].

Consultation to daycare, schools, afterschool programs, camps, youth groups or other congregate care settings should be offered to provide assistance to teachers, school mental health providers, school administrators, and youth service providers about how to support groups of children after the death of a peer [5, 15]. Guidelines on pragmatic steps to provide notification and support for the death of a member of the school community can be downloaded at the website of the National Center for School Crisis and Bereavement (www.cincinnatichildrens.org/school-crisis) at http://www.cincinnatichildrens.org/svc/alpha/s/school-crisis/guidelines-bereavement.htm. The site also has a PowerPoint slide presentation with presenter notes on supporting grieving students that can be freely downloaded and used for in-service or pre-service training of teachers, other school professionals, and related professionals.

Funeral Attendance

Families should be offered advice at the time of the death (or when appropriate, prior to an anticipated death) about how to support siblings to attend the child's funeral or other commemorative activities. Children, just as adults, can benefit from the opportunity to come together with families and friends at the time of loss to provide and receive support and to honor the individual who has died. While there has not been structured research related to children's attendance at funerals, recommendations can be based on clinical experience.

In general, barring children from participating in funerals and related events may result in resentment and a sense of isolation and engender fantasies about what is so awful that occurs during such events that the children are unable to attend. Instead, it is useful to explain in basic and direct terms what the funeral is and what the children can expect to see or otherwise experience at the event and then invite the children to participate to the extent they wish. Children should not be required or coerced to participate in components of the funeral, such as throwing dirt on the casket or kissing or touching the body of the deceased, or to attend if they feel uncomfortable doing so. It is advisable to assign someone to the children who is familiar with the child and with whom the child feels comfortable, but who is not personally grieving the loss (for example, a babysitter or teacher). This individual can monitor the child's reactions, be readily available to answer the child's questions, and offer to leave or step out when it seems in the best interest of the child. In this way, children can participate to the level they wish; simply standing outside the funeral home and handing out mass cards may serve an important role for the child without being overwhelming. Opportunities for children to play a personally meaningful, but not overwhelming, role in the funeral should also be sought. For example, young children may appreciate the opportunity to help select flowers or pictures of their sibling that can be displayed at the wake or funeral.

Death and Secondary Losses

The death of a child often results in secondary losses that may impact surviving children in the family. Parents may need to work additional hours in order to earn money to replace funds spent during a long illness and treatment or to compensate for missed work during the illness or around the time of death. Or they may still be physically present at home, but may nonetheless be less emotionally available to the surviving children because of their own grief, or due to maladaptive coping techniques (such as increased alcohol or substance use). Life-threatening illness and death of a child may place strains on a marriage, resulting in parental discord that can impact negatively the surviving children. This in turn may cause further financial pressures and require undesired changes in home or school. In addition, parents who are feeling guilt associated with the death of a child or feeling vulnerable to additional losses may alter their parenting of the surviving siblings, which may result in overprotection and/or emotional distancing [16]. It is therefore important to remember that children will not only be responding to the death of their sibling, but will also be responding to all of the secondary losses and stressors that may result from the death of their sibling and the reactions of others within the family. This underscores the importance of making sure that parents have sufficient personal supports so that they can adjust as best as possible to the loss themselves (and can do so without relying heavily on the assistance of older children and adolescents). Support groups for parents who have experienced the death of a child (Compassionate Friends is one such network of self-help groups: www.compassionatefriends.org) and other means of support for parents, especially, but not only, those experiencing complicated mourning, may provide substantial indirect support for the children.

Children who have experienced the death of a sibling also experience other less tangible secondary losses: someone close to them that held unique shared memories; a confidant; someone that knew how to help them with their homework or provide advice on how to interact with peers, etc. It challenges their identity as a brother or sister. It shatters their confidence that the world is fair, just, and safe. The reactions of grieving children themselves may also lead them to have academic difficulties, disruptions in peer relationships (e.g., due to loss of interest in previously enjoyed activities or difficulty in separation from parents), or additional restrictions in social activities (e.g., due to fears and anxieties) that each may result in further stressors or secondary losses. This underscores the needs to ensure that children are connected with support mechanisms that endure beyond the time the pediatric oncology team or hospice program have contact with the family.

A brief discussion with parents around the time of death or the provision of a booklet, no matter how well written, is generally not sufficient to address all of these issues. Bereavement support services for siblings all too often end at the time of the death of the patient, or shortly thereafter. Children will experience ongoing adjustment difficulties that typically last for more than a year. Challenges may be posed by anniversaries (of the child's birth, related to the illness, or the death), disrupted or strained holiday celebrations, or other unanticipated triggers of grief reactions (such as when the sibling hears the favorite song of the child who died or when a lesson on cancer is taught in class). As children develop a more mature understanding of death or a better sense of genetic predisposition, they may begin to worry that they too may develop cancer years later. If it is an older sibling that died, they may become more concerned as they approach the age when their sibling was diagnosed or died. Or they may develop additional concerns or experience a resurgence of their grief when their own children reach those ages. Bereavement is a lifelong process. Access to ongoing support or a source of advice for parents and the surviving children becomes critical to successfully navigate these challenges.

Complicated Mourning

Grief over the death of a family member or close friend is an intense experience and can dominate one's life in the immediate aftermath, whether it is a child or adult who is grieving. But over time, the individual transitions back to a life without the deceased that, although permanently altered, is still meaningful and able—at times—to bring a sense of satisfaction, joy, and accomplishment. Individuals experiencing complicated mourning may fail to adjust over time. They may show extreme reactions, such as extreme and persistent sadness and despair that fails to abate or serious suicidal or homicidal ideations or intentions. They may have difficulty with daily activities that persist weeks or months after the death, demonstrate difficulty in maintaining friendships or other interpersonal relationships, become preoccupied with thoughts of the deceased, or adopt maladaptive responses to the loss such as alcohol or other substance abuse. Therese Rando, PhD [17], identifies characteristics of the death and antecedent and subsequent variables related to the mourner that are common risk factors for complicated grief. Death of a child and, as already noted in the section on anticipatory grieving, death from an overly lengthy illness are two risk factors that are often both present in deaths in pediatric oncology. An additional factor that may be seen in a number of cases in pediatric oncology is death that the mourner perceives as preventable, especially now that most cases of childhood cancer are treatable and curable and family expectations for successful treatment have increased. The remaining risk factor related to the nature of the death is sudden, unexpected death, especially when it is traumatic, violent, mutilating, or random. Often, families experiencing the death of a child from cancer experience three of the four risk factors for complicated mourning that are related to the nature of the death.

Complicated mourning is also more likely to occur when the premorbid relationship with the deceased was markedly angry or ambivalent (which may characterize the death of some adolescent children) or markedly dependent. Prior or concurrent mourner liabilities, especially unaccommodated losses or stressors (such as prior

deaths or pre-existing depression or other mental illnesses) increase the risk of complicated mourning in
response to recent losses. Situations where the mourner
perceives a lack of social support may result in disen-
franchised grief, where there is a perceived invalidation
of the loss, relationship, or the mourner, which also
increases the risk of complicated mourning. This can
occur, for example, if an adolescent peer is not perceived as experiencing a significant loss when a friend
with cancer dies. These risk factors for complicated
mourning should heighten attention to the need for support and ongoing monitoring of adjustment.

The Importance of Self-care

Death of a patient is one of the most stressful personal
and professional experiences faced by pediatric health
care providers. Too often it is assumed that repetitive
exposure alone to patient death diminishes the impact
or even may render someone immune to a response. If
losses are not accommodated and adjustment
achieved, subsequent losses may only be cumulative
and the response heightened. Even among experienced,
competent, and emotionally healthy professionals who
have adequate internal resources and external support
to adjust to prior losses, particular losses can still have
a significant impact. The death of a patient the same
age or similar in some other characteristic as the provider's own child, or one who with whom the provider
has formed a particularly close relationship, for example, may trigger an atypical or more pronounced
reaction—often catching the provider off-guard. Caring for one's patients places caregivers at risk of compassion fatigue. But who would want a caregiver who
actually didn't care about their patients?

Permission and tolerance to discuss and have personal needs met regarding reactions to patient death
are critical [18]. Psychosocial or bereavement rounds
(in contrast to mortality rounds that often look solely
to assign fault and may heighten providers' feelings of
guilt), retreats that address the topic (especially for
trainees or providers early in their careers), and other
formal and informal support services have been utilized to address these needs. But perhaps most importantly, there needs to be a culture within health care
settings that acknowledges the impact and recognizes
the importance of open communication and support.
Individual health care providers, in turn, need to
understand the importance of personal reflection on
the impact of patient death and a commitment to self-
care and to developing mechanisms to communicate
and have met personal needs related to patient death.

References

1. Foltin GL, Schonfeld DJ, Shannon MW (eds.) *Pediatric Terrorism and Disaster Preparedness: A Resource for Pediatricians*. Rockville, MD: Agency for Healthcare Research and Quality, October 2006. http://www.ahrq.gov/research/pedprep/resource.htm.
2. Schonfeld DJ, Quackenbush M. *After a Loved One Dies: How Children Grieve and How Parents and Other Adults Can Support Them*. New York: New York Life Foundation, 2009.
3. Leash RM. *Death Notification: A Practical Guide to the Process*. Hinesburg, VT: Upper Access, 1994.
4. Adams D, Deveau E. When a brother or sister is dying of cancer: the vulnerability of the adolescent sibling. *Death Studies* 1987;**11**:279–295.
5. Schonfeld DJ, Quackenbush M. *The Grieving Student: A Teacher's Guide*. Baltimore, MD: Brookes Publishing, 2010.
6. Schonfeld DJ. Talking with children about death. *Journal of Pediatric Health Care* 1993;**7**:269–274.
7. Speece M, Brent S. Children's understanding of death: a review of three components of a death concept. *Child Development* 1984;**55**:1671–1686.
8. Clunies-Ross C, Landsdown R. Concepts of death, illness, and isolation found in children with leuke-mia. *Child Care Health Development* 1988;**14**:373–386.
9. Spinetta J. The dying child's awareness of death: a review. *Psychology Bulletin* 1974;**81**:256–260.
10. Lansky S, Stephenson L, Weller E, Cairns G, Cairns N. Failure to thrive during infancy in siblings of pediatric cancer patients. *American Journal of Pediatric Hematology/Oncology* 1982;**4**:361–366.
11. Emswiler M, Emswiler J. *Guiding Your Child through Grief*. New York: Bantam Books, 2000.
12. Chin D, Schonfeld D, O'Hare L, *et al.* Elementary school-age children's developmental understanding of the causes of cancer. *Journal of Developmental & Behavioral Pediatrics* 1998;**19**:397–403.
13. Schonfeld D. The child's cognitive understanding of illness. In: Lewis M (ed.) *Child and Adolescent Psychiatry: A Comprehensive Textbook*, 2nd edn. Baltimore, MD: Williams & Wilkins, 1996; pp. 943–947.
14. Lewis M, Schonfeld D. The role of child and adolescent psychiatric consultation and liaison in assisting children and their families in dealing with death. *Child and Adolescent Psychiatric Clinics of North America* 1994;**3**:613–627.
15. Schonfeld D, Lichtenstein R, Kline M, Speese-Linehan D. *How to Respond to and Prepare for a Crisis*, 2nd edn. Alexandria, VA: Association for Supervision and Curriculum Development, 2002.
16. Krell R, Rabkin L. The effects of sibling death on the surviving child: a family perspective. *Family Process* 1979;**18**:471–477.
17. Rando T. *Treatment of Complicated Mourning*. Champaign, IL: Research Press, 1993.
18. Glazer J, Schonfeld DJ. Life-limiting illness, palliative care, and bereavement. In: Martin A, Volkmar F (eds.) *Lewis' Child and Adolescent Psychiatry: A Comprehensive Textbook*, 4th edn. Baltimore, MD: Lippincott Williams and Wilkins, 2007; pp. 971–980.

Part D
Additional Considerations

20

Ethical Considerations in Pediatric Oncology: a Case-Based Psychosocial Overview

Ryan W. Blum, Andrés S. Martin

Introduction: Social and Intellectual Foundations

Bioethics and pediatric oncology have grown into their present forms on the same raw substrate: the increasing power of biomedical science and technology to influence matters of life and death. Wolpe [1] describes the birth of bioethics as the shift in moral power from within the medical profession "toward the moral agency of the patient," a social and epistemic shift which occurred through a series of cultural, legal and professional changes throughout the later twentieth century, largely in response to developments such as ventilation, chemotherapy, organ transplantation, and other medical innovations which affected a person's relationship to their body and to their own life and death as well as that of their loved ones. These changes awarded adult individuals power to help determine their own course through the events of life and death by articulating rights, obligations, and procedural requirements that have been intended to empower individuals in service of the principle of autonomy, a concept variously described as individual liberty, self-determination, or even freedom of choice, and which literally means "self-rule" [2, 3].

But what could it possibly mean for a young child, so dependent on her adult caregivers, and so thoroughly embedded in the family unit, to express the value of autonomy? For children, bioethics must specify their interests through those who care for them, and through their growing, incomplete present abilities to represent themselves. In all cases, the pediatric patient must express their autonomy through others. For children, and in some ethical theories

(such as "care ethics") for any person, autonomy always has its expression in the very relationships, or variations on the relationships, which obviated autonomy in the beginning, and which laid the foundation for its growth. To quote Cassell [4]: "There are no such completely self-determining individuals who are not influenced in the strongest sense by others in their personal and social world . . . Even 'autonomy' and 'freedom of choice' imply relationships." This dialectic–between autonomy and relatedness—is a foundational dynamic of developmental psychology, and it will guide our analysis of the following cases, where decision-making authority, views of a child's best interests, and the very wishes of a child herself all undergo scrutiny.

Informed Consent, Shared Decision-Making, and Parental Authority

In 1947—the same year that Farber discovered that the folate antagonist amiopterin could induce remission in patients with acute leukemia, paving the way for cure rates which continue to rise with each passing decade, currently at around 90% for the most common childhood malignancy, acute lymphocytic leukemia, and 60–70% overall [5]—a three-judge panel convened in Nuremberg to address the terrible crimes perpetrated by members of the German medical and scientific elite on prisoners of Nazi concentration camps, all done under the guise of research and progress. Nuremberg's *doctrine of informed consent* [6], also known as the "classical" doctrine, has served as a template for all

Pediatric Psycho-oncology: Psychosocial Aspects and Clinical Interventions, Second Edition.
Edited by Shulamith Kreitler, Myriam Weyl Ben-Arush and Andrés Martin.
© 2012 John Wiley & Sons, Ltd. Published 2012 by John Wiley & Sons, Ltd.

decisions to accept or decline treatment or to enroll in research:

> The person involved should have *legal capacity* to give consent; should be so situated as to be able to exercise *free power of choice*, without the intervention of any element of force, fraud, deceit, duress, over-reaching or other ulterior form of constraint or coercion; and should have sufficient *knowledge* and *comprehension* of the elements of the subject matter involved as to enable him to make an understanding and enlightened decision.

Today, informed consent is a key protection for patients and research subjects, and it is one of the first major signposts in the long journey patients and their families take in pediatric oncology. Its history, theoretical basis, and practice all show how human values are closely connected to the increasing influence of biomedical technology on our lives, and they reflect the reliance we have come to place on individual autonomy and legalistic practices to ensure the key universal value of *respect for persons*. Furthermore, as we will discuss in depth, informed consent is insufficient because their special vulnerabilities, their incomplete development into decision-makers, and their intimate connection to their family.

Informedness, Honesty

The 2002 Institute of Medicine report, *When Children Die* [7], articulates the three main needs of parents, in the form of requests for information to be used in managing emotions, expectations, and care itself:

(1) "What is happening to me?" "What is happening to my child?"
(2) "What are our choices?" "How can we be good parents?"
(3) "How will you help us?"

The first principle of the International Society of Pediatric Oncology's Psychosocial Issues Working Group's position on informed consent (2003) is one of many professional guidelines which clearly support the first of these priorities, stating that parents have the right to full disclosure of information at the first clinical encounter [8]. Seemingly obvious today, just forty years ago, 90% of American physicians surveyed indicated that they would not tell their adult patients that they had cancer, despite a decades-old legal tradition that affirmed an adult patient's right to accept or decline any treatment. After a series of revolutions affecting moral authority in American medicine, patients grew into a right to honest disclosure of diagnosis and information. In 1977, another survey showed that 97% of the doctors said they would tell a cancer patient of a cancer diagnosis [9].

The Institute of Medicine priorities go beyond supporting informedness by supporting the parents' psychological need to be "good parents" and also by acknowledging their desire to be actively guided by clinicians ("How will you help us?"), a group which remains silent in the classical formulation of informed consent. Beauchamp and Childress [2, p. 80], however, expand the four-element scheme to include two specific elements required to be performed by the clinician, expanding their role into a "guide" and a "safeguard" who must (1) suggest a plan or plans to which the patient or her surrogate must agree, and (2) authorize or approve a subject's final decision to accept or decline a proposed plan. Their version of informed consent [2] has seven required elements:

(1) Legal competence to make decisions
(2) Disclosure of relevant information
(3) Professional recommendation of a plan or possible plans
(4) Understanding the information and proposed plan(s)
(5) Voluntariness of the decision
(6) Consent to accept or decline treatment
(7) A clinician's authorization of the subject's decision.

The clinician taking part in this discussion is expected to play an active role in developing a plan and balancing patient autonomy as a kind of a counselor or guide [9]. This reflects how informed consent should actually be about building trust, sharing authority, and about respecting the rights of an individual in relation to others, as well as the sustenance of their rights in relation to others. In short, at its best, it is a procedure for what is known as *shared decision-making*. Beauchamp and Childress [2] initially criticize the interpretation of informed consent as shared decision-making, arguing that informed consent's protection of the individual patient is a more fundamental function even if this may mean shared decision-making "in ordinary language or law." This reasoning may fall short in pediatric oncology and in pediatrics at large, where respect for individual children is best achieved not through the patient's choice alone.

Case #1: Shared Decision Making and Allison's Heart

The following case illustrates the benefits of detailed parental understanding, as well as the limits on family authority present during at the outset, and indeed during many phases of treatment for most childhood malignancies.

Allison A., the 1-year-old daughter of two research scientists, is brought to the emergency department at night after her mother discovered during an evening bath that her abdomen is full and solid. The next day, a liver biopsy confirms embryonal-type hepatoblastoma, which is considered advanced because of the tumor's size and extent of involvement within the liver itself, where it wraps around a major vessel, making her ineligible for surgery. Her parents are told that she will receive neoadjuvant chemotherapy in hopes of shrinking the tumor for resection or possibly transplantation. In anticipation of starting treatment, Allison's parents—both research chemists working at a local bioengineering firm—spend a sleepless night researching treatments online. They learn that a set of chemotherapy agents commonly used to treat her disease will be tested in a forthcoming national cooperative trial designed to omit the drug doxorubicin, which is notorious for late-onset cardiotoxicity. The next day, they are tearful but composed while meeting with their child's oncologist to discuss and provide consent for her treatment. The oncologist suggests the four-drug regimen because it is what she believes comprises the standard of care. Allison's parents negotiate amicably based on their research, and the oncologist agrees to the three-drug regimen. She begins her treatment that evening.

By becoming meticulously involved in the details of their daughter's initial treatment by researching her cure with the scientific rigor that defines their professional lives, they are able to debate the merits of individual chemotherapy agents with their daughter's oncologist, becoming active participants in decisions to balance chances for cure with risks of rare but serious acute and late side effects which they find particularly concerning. Their staying up all night to learn about her treatments illustrates how, according to Goldstein and colleagues, parents naturally treat their children as an extension of themselves: "Parents normally protect their child's body as if it were their own, and they generally act responsibly in making health care choices for their children" [11]. Importantly, their preferences do not deviate from accepted standards of medical care, which is well established for many diseases at the outset of therapy.

Need all parents be equally well informed? What are the legal and moral requirements for being informed? The American Academy of Pediatrics Bioethics Committee [12] summarizes the requirements for being informed:

[P]atients should have explanations, in understandable language, of the nature of the ailment or condition; the nature of proposed diagnostic steps and/or treatment(s) and the probability of their success; the existence and nature of the risks involved; and the existence, potential benefits, and risks of recommended alternative treatments (including the choice of no treatment).

This basic set of data is fairly standard, but there is some discord over exactly how much a patient legally is entitled to know, and, over and above the law, of what they should be informed [13]. Should the patient be informed of what a provider thinks they ought to know? What the average patient wants to know? These so-called "objective" standards—respectively called the "malpractice" and "material risk" standards—are the two most common legal standards in the US today, depending on state law. Each neglects the needs of individual patients, whose personal values, risk tolerance, and hopes and expectations in treatment and in life, may differ along with their individual information requirements. To satisfy a patient's individual needs is known as a "subjective" standard, which is thought to be the fullest way of dignifying a person, as articulated in one recent judicial opinion quoted by Pope [14]: "[T]o the extent the plaintiff, given an adequate disclosure would have declined the proposed treatment, and a reasonable person in similar circumstances would have consented, a patient's right to self-determination is irrevocably lost" (p. 2).

But relying only on the subjective standard would risk incomplete informedness for patients who are unable to formulate these questions. Indeed, a combination of the two doctrines is preferable: a basic "objective" requirement would provide guidance for patients less educated or empowered, or simply too anxious for their personhood to come to life under stressful circumstances, while the "subjective" one, with some limits based on professional opinion, would help dignify individual persons and their idiosyncratic information needs. We see this standard reflected in the thinking of Allison's parents. They are in touch with the basic information about the trials, including the possibility of cardiac side effects from the anthracycline-class medication doxorubicin, but it is their interest in the late side effects, and the nature of the most recent clinical trials on her disease, which characterizes their thinking here—no surprise, given their status as research scientists. This helps them satisfy their version of what it is to be a good parent—a scientific advocate—and it also recruits the clinician into a supportive, collaborative relationship.

But what if Allison's parents' request fell outside of what the providers felt was medically indicated to her, exposing her to too much risk to satisfy their parents' psychological needs or cultural or religious values? Another way of stating these questions is, who has authority to make decisions for a child, and when should that authority be limited by professional or state authority?

Surrogates, Best Interests, and Shared Decision-Making

With rare exceptions for those who are considered "emancipated" or "mature" [15], minors lack competence to provide informed consent, and therefore require consent to be given by a parent, guardian or other substitute or *surrogate decision-maker*. This dynamic is one major reason why the American Association of Pediatrics' Bioethics Committee [16] declared that "the doctrine of 'informed consent' has only *limited* direct application in pediatrics."

How should surrogates decide? Surrogates are generally held to make decisions based not on what they believe is the right thing to do for themselves, what they wish to do, or what they believe the child should do, but based on what is best for the child. This is known as the *best interest standard*, defined by Buchanan and Brock [17, quoted in 19] as "acting so as to promote maximally the good of the individual." As Kopelman [18] and Diekema [19], for example, point out, the best interest standard has been attacked for a number of reasons, including its lack of specificity concerning diverse cultural values, the vagueness inherent in "knowing" an incapacitated or youthfully incompetent patient's own interests in life, and its various uses as a signpost for treatment and as a threshold for identifying harmful parental choices.

Nevertheless, the best interest standard remains the gold standard for substituted judgment, though critics such as Diekema have proposed splitting its "guidance" and "threshold" functions, and Sulmasy and Snyder [20] propose a more "authentic" substituted interests model, compared with the abstract and possibly deceitful standards of knowing what one would want:

> The key question under best interests is, "What do you think is best for your mother?" Under substituted judgment it is, "What would your mother choose if she could tell us?" The substituted interests model says, "Tell us about your mother." A good surrogate can articulate the patient's authentic values by describing the patient's loves, beliefs, and fundamental moral commitments rather than just specific preferences.

In general, this represents the strong trends in clinical bioethics from a discipline focused on the protection of persons through procedures such as informed consent or advance directives, and towards the value of mediation and psychosocial intervention in mediating disputes.

Best Interests and Relationships in Stem Cell Donation

How exactly are best interests defined? Must they be limited only to medical benefits, or may psychological, emotional or social benefits qualify? One interesting case is that of a minor donating stem cells for transplantation, usually for a sibling with a hematological malignancy. The AAP Bioethics Committee [16] acknowledged that this area has traditionally led to tricky reasoning, largely because a child donor derives no medical benefits from donating his or her stem cells, though he or she incurs non-negligible risk associated with the procedure. If a sibling is donating to his or her brother or sister, the parents are presumed to be acting in the best interests of each child, but their role as surrogates for the donor subject can pose a major conflict of interest favoring the seriously ill child, leading to fears that the donor's wishes may be misrepresented, or that they may have their thoughts or rights ignored altogether in favor of the intervention. Because HLA-matched donors are often difficult to find, the donor may represent the only hope of remission and cure, heightening the emotional and psychological incentives to donate, and potentially contributing to what might be seen as coercion.

Dwyer [21] argued that these interpretations of best interests and surrogate responsibilities are far too strict, and that a minor should be allowed to assume some risk for the benefits accrued in their relationship to a loved one who may survive as a result of their donation. A case history by Lewis [22] details the psychological complexities underlying the gift of a kidney between identical twins; these issues may be less dramatic when considering venipuncture or bone marrow aspiration compared with nephrectomy, but they are still relevant. His analysis shows, largely, that basing the decision on whether or not to allow organ donation on the psychological benefits to the donor, given his or her ways of thinking and understanding the situation, and feelings towards the sibling and parents, is overly simplistic.

Many harbor strong feelings about the use of human biological materials for specific purposes, as illustrated by the profound outrage at the famous case of Marissa Ayala. Marissa was conceived in order to provide stem cells to help cure her older sister, Anissa, who was suffering from chronic myelocytic leukemia. Critics attacked the family for a primary insult to this unborn child, who was conceived to be used for transplantation, as a means to an end. This is the key prohibition in Kantian moral philosophy, and it resonates with the Golden Rule, the I and Thou, and other universal tenets of ethics and behavior. One British politician decried this practice as the "commodification" of children [23].

From follow-up news, it is clear that Marissa Ayala is as loved as any child, though the long-term effects of her unassented gift are unclear. Some have pointed out that it is much better for her to be alive than not, to have a sister to love and hate and learn from than not, to be part of a family that did not experience such a tragic loss, and that the risks were minimized during her procedures (cord blood collection, and then a bone marrow aspiration as a baby.) Savalescu [23] has argued that much of the outcry was the result of underlying attitudes consistent with suspicion of things biological, biomedical, and genetic and not some deep-seated respect for the children into which some of them grow.

Far from routine, this practice marks a certain horizon on which the practice of pediatrics, and medicine at large, is progressing. While Marissa was conceived through natural means with the hope that she would provide a match for her older sister, Spriggs and Savalescu [24] describe how families are proposing to use the reproductive technology of preimplantation genetic diagnosis (PIGD) in order to select for children without certain hereditary diseases, and to select for donors for stem cell transplants, though no oncology cases appear in the public record.

Setting aside the range of arguments is made against these technologies and against the use and commodification of children, there are practical concerns to any sibling donor relationship, which revolve around safeguarding the welfare of the donor. Guidelines such as those of the American Academy of Pediatrics [16] for stem cell donors, which emphasize minimizing risks— though not ensuring absolutely negligible risk—for the donor, will apply widely in these cases. Unnecessary procedures should be avoided, and pain should be minimized and treated appropriately. Children without the ability to speak for themselves may benefit from having a neutral party appointed by the institution, as described by a team from MD Anderson, performing an early pediatric transplant. They chose to appoint a hospital-sponsored surrogate to provide neutral guidance for the donor, since the siblings' parents' conflicts of interest may be amplified by the dire circumstances of the ill child [25].

Another distinct issue which is related to the biological ethics, embodied in the issues of procreative utility and preimplantation genetic diagnosis, is the subject of preserving the fertility materials of children and adolescents undergoing treatments which threaten their fertility. Two recent reviews on this topic outline ways of thinking through these problems [26], and both the AAP and the American Society of Clinical Oncologists recommended in 2008 that all patients of childbearing age whose fertility is threatened by treatments for cancer should be referred to fertility specialists for consultation [27, 28]. This intervention is aimed to ease some of the psychosocial burden of infertility and perceived threats to fertility, which are reported to have a strong effect on self-image and the stability of marriages involving childhood cancer survivors. However, no ethical consensus guidelines exist on the topic, which sparks considerable disagreements about the normative value of the actual technologies, as well as trepidation about the possibility of performing these interventions on younger patients, especially women, whose gametes are formed during fetal development and can be harvested long before any capacities to make decisions emerge. Furthermore, there are significant uncertainties about the long-term health of the patients and, moreover, of these offspring [29].

Case #2: The Limits of Parental Authority

Allison's parents are indeed performing as highly effective surrogate decision-makers, with a detailed subjective knowledge of the risks and benefits of various elements in her treatment. And yet, despite their high level of capacity to perform as surrogates, their only real power at this point in treatment is to debate a relatively small point with regards to a chemotherapy regimen. They would not have the power to decline treatment outright for Allison, nor would they have the right to request medically-nonindicated treatments, no matter what their justification, because doing so would be to put Allison in moral danger, for, according to Goldstein, parents' natural responsibility is sharply limited when and only when children's lives are at stake: "When death is not a likely consequence of exercising a medical choice, there would be no justification for governmental intrusion." This caveat applies widely in pediatric oncology. An oft-quoted judicial maxim supporting this view was articulated by the U.S. Supreme Court in 1944: "Parents may be free to become martyrs themselves. But it does not follow that they are free, in identical circumstances, to make martyrs of their children." These views reflect the fact that children have individual rights separate from parental rights and familial or cultural values, and that respect for these rights may require that parents' choices may be overruled when they critically endanger a child— putting their life at risk and with it, their prospects for developing into a future autonomous individual.

This initial dynamic highlights firstly how high-stakes pediatric oncology is, and how its patients, for all the impressive quoted cure rates for many diseases, are truly walking a fine line between life and death. Parents teeter between primary responsibility for their children and submitting to social and medical norms that will guide their care. Allison's rights, and our respect for her as an individual person, require the representation of her parents, who know her best and hold dear their wishes and plans for her development as a person of immense capability, and it requires the representation of the oncologist who advises and holds in check her parents in case their decisions conflict with Allison's best interests.

Allison's surrogates must not decline an efficacious treatment for any reason, including religious, spiritual, philosophical or moral objections to medical care, because doing so would violate a child's interest in life, and clearly be outside her best interests. This view is supported by positions taken by professional groups such as the American Academy of Pediatrics (1998) as well as by law throughout the United States. Despite this putative consensus, many believe that religious faith outweighs societal norms, which are naturally enforced by the medical team, and by the courts if necessary.

The story of medical neglect based on religious and other non-medical health beliefs repeats itself over and over in stories such as those of Chad Greene and Katie Wernecke [30, 31]. One recent version of this story is that of Daniel Hauser, a 13-year-old Minnesota boy with Hodgkin's lymphoma who began treatment in February 2009 with what his doctors estimated as a 90% chance of cure, but only completed one treatment because, according to the Associated Press [32]:

The Hausers believe that the injection of chemotherapy into Danny Hauser amounts to an assault upon his body, and torture when it occurs over a long period of time . . . They believe that it is against the spiritual law to invade the consciousness of another person without their permission.

The story goes on to point out how this "spiritual law" is not derived from their own religious heritage of Roman Catholicism; it is associated with what they call the "'do no harm' philosophy of the Nemenhah Band," which is a "Missouri-based religious group that believes in natural healing methods practiced by some American Indians" [32].

After a court intervened to force him to receive standard treatment, Daniel and his mother disappeared. The father was reported to say that the two went to Mexico for "alternative" treatment, but they reappeared in California soon thereafter, where Colleen Hauser explained her actions [33]:

"Any mother would do anything to protect their own," says Colleen. She adds that he's on a strict diet with no sugar. He only eats raw fruits and vegetables and eats very little meat. "Daniel is doing really good; he's keeping up whatever he has to do to make sure there's no reoccurrence."

It would be easy to dismiss these beliefs as altogether beside the point, given that Daniel's young life was at stake and the choices being made here were based on specious reasoning without evidence. Though they are marginal health beliefs, the scenario identifies a tension that is, or at least was, present in federal and state law, most notably in an executive order issued by the Nixon administration after the first Child Abuse Prevention and Treatment Act (CAPTA) became law [34]:

In 1974 Congress passed the first Child Abuse Prevention and Treatment Act. Congress debated but rejected the inclusion of religious exemptions to laws requiring parents to provide basic necessities for children, including medical care. However, in formulating the regulations to administer state grants under CAPTA, the Christian Science-influenced Nixon administration required states to have such exemptions in order to qualify for CAPTA grants . . . Faced with loss of federal funds, all 50 states rapidly complied by passing various exemptions in the civil and criminal codes.

Asser and Swan [35] reviewed the prevailing behaviors in the 20 years after these laws came into effect, and found at least 140 deaths resulting from conditions that would have been overwhelmingly likely to have been prevented with available medical care. These incidents have dwindled, many states have reversed their legislation, and the Department of Health and Human services did rescind their order threatening CAPTA defunding, but children continue to be at risk, with very public recent criminal cases now featuring convictions of parents [34].

In general, providers should honor parents' religious, spiritual, and cultural identities as much as possible, unless they conflict with the unalienable right to liberty possessed by their children or others. Among pediatricians, bioethicists, and lawmakers there is broad professional consensus that no parent should ever be allowed to refuse potentially treatment which has a high probability of preserving life of significant function. We live in a society that values life above cultural continuity, but this does not mean that cultural continuity is not an important value. Indeed, children have an inherent right to liberty as well as a future right to self-determination of, among other things, their cultural identity, just as Colleen chose to join the Band when she had been raised, according to the news, as a Roman Catholic.

The second important point about Daniel Hauser is that differences of religious belief can certainly be a sign of cultural difference, but it can also indicate barriers to communication, interpersonal dysfunction, or even mental illness. What were the father's values? How did Daniel relate to the Band's religion, and to his family? Thirteen would likely be old enough for many children to make their opinions known, though they are still deeply dependent on their families. There may be tension among the values of the family or community that could serve as a point of psychosocial intervention, or intervention with the help of colleagues from the chaplaincy.

Case #3: Stress, Research, and Consent

In addition to the lack of direct consent from children and the corresponding need for a surrogate decision-maker whose power is sharply circumscribed by professional authority, there are two other insufficiencies which are critical pieces of decision-making in pediatric oncology: the confounding influence that concurrent consent for treatment and research can have on understanding and decision-making, and the disorienting influence of stress and anxiety, so common in the early stages of diagnosis and treatment for a childhood cancer, which threaten informed, rational, voluntary decision-making.

How can informed consent be properly performed against the backdrop of what is an unimaginably stressful, terrifying experience for children and their families? These potential roadblocks to "valid consent"—not just legally-sufficient informed consent, but consent that involves true respect for and support of a child and family [36]—are potentially overcome, in part, with attention to the underlying cognitive and sociological dynamics that shape decision-making in pediatric oncology.

The dangers, but the usefulness of this limited duty to protect psychological health in the informed consent proceeding, are illustrated by the case of Brian B., a 7-month-old boy who arrived in the hospital with periorbital ecchymoses, anemia, and a palpable abdominal mass, and is subsequently diagnosed with neuroblastoma. During morning rounds the next day, a pediatric psycho-oncology consultation is requested because of the mother's agitation and anxiety the night before during her informed consent discussion with the oncology team, especially around the topic of research enrollment. When we arrive, everyone is calm. His mother reports that she was worried about her child becoming part of "an experiment" but was afraid the team might treat her son and their family differently should they decline to participate. We also learn that she had been visiting her pediatrician a number of times over the past five weeks because her son first "didn't seem right" and subsequently developed more specific symptoms. This young mother of three reports that she had "known for weeks" what the diagnosis would be based on her internet searching. Though her nightmare has come true, now she appears calm and organized and expresses relief at finally being in the hospital where her son can be treated appropriately.

Brian's mother became dysfunctionally, though understandably, anxious after he was brought into the hospital. Her reaction put her at risk for being unable to make the decision, so intense was her ambivalence about joining the study. She described how weeks went by where her son's symptoms progressed undiagnosed, despite seeming to become more specific to what even she could tell was quite serious. Her inability to tolerate the informed consent discussion was the culmination of this process, and it was also the end of uncertainty, at least with respect to Brian's diagnosis; his prognosis would be another matter altogether, for a later time. If her providers had withheld information for her benefit, they may (or may not) have prevented some acute anxiety, but they would have deprived her of the chance to come to terms with the situation, and to develop some degree of psychological relief at the beginning of treatment and hopes for its success.

This quick change from emotion to clarity finds a theoretical explanation reviewed by Volpe in an article on "unexpressed" or emotional needs becoming manifest during the informed consent process. She concludes, following Kahnemann and others, that a patient's initial "impulsive" reaction may be followed by a slower, more analytical way to approach the problem, which may provide more acceptable substance for the process of consent [37]. She recommends that providers "understand that many patients make rapid, intuitive judgments in response to the information they hear, and then return to the information in a more analytic fashion only after they have reacted impulsively." This leads to the following recommendations [37]:

(1) Do not assume that a patient's immediate response to a treatment option or procedure is her or his final answer: revisit the question at a later time. (But be cautious not to be overbearing.)

(2) Allow a patient room to have what might be an overly emotional or vehement response, knowing that the overreaction may be part of the decision-making process and does not always reflect the patient's ultimate answer.

These recommendations largely reflect the major frustration patients report with the consent process: parents want more time spent with a clinician, and more information [38, 39]. Pediatric oncologists, on the other hand, rate "stress" as the main threat to well-performed informed consent [40], presumably attempting to shield parents from more stress by lightening the information load, and either following Volpe's strategy of multiple disclosure points, or else undermining the validity of consent.

Complications in the Relationship between Research and Practice

Overall, Ms. B.'s symptoms recall what Lederberg [41] describes: how ethical dilemmas may sometimes obscure mental health problems, psychiatric consultations may sometimes hide ethical dilemmas, and frequently these two concerns travel together. It is no surprise that Ms. B.'s anxiety "stuck" on an issue that is one of the major threats to proper informed consent in pediatric oncology: the conflicts of interest inherent in what Unguru [42] describes as the "intimate connection between research and practice" in the discipline.

Ms. B is not alone in this respect: Joffe and Simon [43] report the case of "Dan," the father of a young man being diagnosed with ALL, who, like Ms. B., is simply paralyzed when asked to choose whether or not to join a research study, declaring "I don't care," and "You decide!" For patients and family just getting used to the news and environment, these studies may seem like a distraction: Dan is clearly "frustrated and concerned that all this discussion is delaying his son's treatment."

The place of research in clinical care confounds many. Kodish and colleagues [44] discovered that a full 50% of parents "did not understand randomization" despite it being discussed by the vast majority of clinicians. Concepts such as randomization and the "therapeutic misconception"—the mistaken belief that a clinical trial will offer direct medical benefit to the enrollee—have been shown to be consistently confusing to a significant subgroup of adult cancer patients [45, 46], and they prove equally problematic for parents and children to understand.

What could mitigate these difficulties in understanding clinical trials? More time with clinicians, and not the use of forms or even interactive media, is associated with better understanding, according to a review conducted by Flory and Emanuel [47], who laud "direct human contact" and conclude that "informed consent is more than just the action of reading a form and signing it. It is better thought of as a process, ideally a dialogue that takes place over time and largely depends on interactions between human beings." The value of a process of education is captured in one form in the federal requirement for children to provide assent, and adult guardians to provide permission, for enrollment in research [48].

The assent/permission process is best viewed as an ongoing process of joint decision-making whereby any child of greater than seven years of age has the authority to decline to participate in nonbeneficial research, and his or her clinicians are responsible for assessing the child's developmental stage and providing information and guidance that will help his or her participate meaningfully in the decision to participate in research. Joffe *et al.* [49] articulate a clear set of guidelines for this process, including exceptions for incapacity and for studies with clear benefit for the child. A multidisciplinary approach, involving child life specialists to educate the child, social workers and other mental health professionals to counsel the family, and oncologists, nurses, and child mental health professionals to assess and counsel the child, is appropriate to this task, which can be tricky to perform in a way that is truly meaningful [50].

Case #4: Children as Decision-Makers

We have discussed how children's roles in deciding whether or not to join nonbeneficial research studies is protected by federal law and outlined in the process of assent and permission. Children have no similarly protected right to assent for general treatment decisions which is established in federal regulation or law, but there are many arguments for extending the process of assent to include all treatments involving children of a certain age and maturity [51].

How involved should a child be in their care? The case of Abby A., a 12-year-old girl being treated for ALL, shows the virtues and pitfalls of children's involvement in decision-making, and in making premature calculations of risk. Abby is a girl whom the psycho-oncology team had previously seen after providers noted how sad and withdrawn she was, and she was subsequently assigned to a regular therapist and, in the context of familial anxiety and depression, given a trial of an antidepressant. She is now in the hospital for scheduled chemotherapy, seeming down but eager to talk, complaining about how everyone "makes decisions about me without talking to me." She has previously struggled with leg pain and immobility, but is resistant to standing orders for pain medications. Now her pain is much worse. Her oncologist orders her to take an MRI but she refuses, and after a long fight, her mother stops trying to convince her. The next week, her pain is even worse and her doctor simply leaves her no choice. It is discovered that she has a bone infection in her left knee, for which she will need at least six weeks of intravenous antibiotics to cure. "I've had those before, it's no big deal," she tells us.

On the surface, this case seems to show the hazards of eliciting a child's views, since Abby's stated wish not to have the MRI led to the worsening of a serious infection. It also shows the risks potentially hidden in a diagnostic procedure that was initially not expected to be critically important. But her expressed opinion was clearly clouded in anxiety and in isolation and fear—not in her rational sense of her condition and needs. What might have happened if she had been part of the earlier conversations? It might not have decreased her severe anxiety about having an MRI, but maybe these concerns would have emerged before the procedure assumed emergent status. Perhaps she would have felt more involved in her care, and less resistant to the decisions about which she had no say. Clearly, giving her alone the right to choose for herself would be tantamount to abandoning a patient who is immature, worried, and already seriously isolated. But not including her in the proceedings heightens her fear as well. Exactly how involved should a child or adolescent be in in critical decisions about their care? The answer will depend crucially on the child's capacities to understand, reason, and communicate a choice, which will relate to their temperament, emotional and intellectual maturity, their family dynamics, and to their relationships with oncologists, nurses and others. These interrelated tasks—expressing maturity of mind and person, and performing their autonomy within a network of caring others–are captured in the concept of a child's right to provide *assent* to treatment or to being involved in research.

Assent is developed from the concept of consent, which depends crucially on the notion of a person's cognitive abilities known as *capacity*, which is one of the four elements of Nuremberg's classical doctrine of informed consent. How can capacity be assessed? In his review, Appelbaum [52] describes capacity as "the abilities to *communicate* a choice, to *understand* the relevant information, to *appreciate* the medical consequences of the situation, and to *reason* about treatment choices. Gaylin [53] writes that capacity is usefully thought of in the dimensions that limit it, including limits of consciousness, intelligence, rationality, perception, experience, and age. Note that capacity can be determined by any clinician [54], but the equivalent legal concept of *competence* can only be determined by a court. While competence is (almost always) a legally fixed quality of personhood which is acquired at the age of majority, capacity is a dynamic quality that changes as the cognitive abilities of the subject develop, and which depends crucially on the seriousness of the decision being considered. A higher threshold is used for decisions involving significant risk or reward [53].

Appelbaum and Grisso [55]discuss at length how these criteria can be assessed by clinical professionals, focusing on simple subjective assessments in the mental status exam and psychiatric interview, such as asking "What do you believe is wrong with your health now?" to test one's appreciation, and "What makes [a chosen treatment] better than [an alternative option]?" to test a person's reasoning. There are also empirical tools for assessing competence developed by these authors and others [56], but these tools can be limited in scope to assessing only understanding, and they have been infrequently tested in pediatric populations including the medically ill [57, 58].

Clinically, capacity generally grows as a child progresses in his or her development, reflecting a general trend from physical and emotional dependence towards autonomy of mind and body by the time an adolescent transitions into adulthood. These trends are by no means linear, universal, or unalterable, but they do hold generally true. In infancy, a child possesses physical and mental intimacy with her parents. In practice, a young school-aged girl with refractory leukemia might possess capacity to decide in which arm to receive an injection (a changed injection site involving no risks, and small overall benefit) or whether to have intravenous or oral analgesics (small risks, small benefit to changing routes of administration for pain medicine), but she would likely be unable to contemplate the risks and benefits of joining a phase one study or receiving yet another bone marrow transplant for her refractory disease. By late adolescence, it would be unusual, as Gaylin [53] points out, if a patient does not lead or heavily participate in decision-making.

Assent does not strictly require a subject to have capacity. The American Academy of Pediatrics Bioethics Committee [16] presumes that a child's views are important regardless of the incomplete process of their rational and personal development. Instead, it is designed as a developmental process to engage a patient at his or her level of cognitive and emotional development. In the AAP statement, the elements of assent may be summarized as: helping a child form a developmentally-appropriate understanding of their situation and the proposed treatments, making a clinical assessment of their abilities to take this information in, and then actively eliciting their views in a process of shared decision-making with parents and providers [16, pp. 315–316].

Assent has its legal basis only in U.S. federal laws protecting children in human subjects research and not, notably, in any clinical case law or regulation [59, 60]. In research, a child's assent is thought to be binding, largely because involving children in research generally provides them with no real benefit, and thus the risk of their declining involvement is negligible compared with the risks of involving them without their agreement, which may include medical and psychological harms, as well as a growing sense that they are not responsible for themselves. In clinical matters, however, a child's voice may be one among many that aim to state what is in his or her *best interests*. Indeed, one potent argument against eliciting assent from a child such as Abby is that her thoughts may be disregarded if she does not agree with having her MRI, or another critical intervention. Inviting assent to any and all treatment decisions, rather than merely the ones to which they possess capacity to perform may, the critics state, be deceptive [12].

However, we believe that withholding any involvement of a child because of the magnitude of the decision being made would be unfortunate and inhumane. Even if there is no question about whether a child will receive chemotherapy, for example, they may not have a binding right to deliver a decision about their treatment, but they should still be educated in a developmentally-appropriate way about their condition, about the mechanism, risks, benefits, and expected efficacy of chemotherapy, and their input should be elicited because it is their body, because these conversations may reduce resistance and nonadherence later on, and because it will help them grow into more knowledgeable, autonomous persons. If a child strongly disagrees, the process of shared communication with them should not suddenly end, leaving them to feel, as the critics of assent suggest, that they have been misled all along; these disagreements should open further avenues of conversation and work through the disagreements. However, we acknowledge that these "psychosocial" approaches may be limited, in the end, in their effect. That does not mean that they are not crucial ways to engage young patients' deep senses of self and responsibility, helping them express themselves and to grow as persons.

Clearly, there is an important value of protecting a child from information that may be so overwhelming that it is traumatizing. The position of Kunin [61] as well as Simon and Kodish [44] and others includes a careful assessment of what exactly children should be told about their disease, lest they experience psychological harm from the disclosure. For many children, the emotional risks of learning too much will outweigh the benefits of being involved in treatment. Furthermore, these harms may be disproportionately felt by children, whose development depends on security, leading to what some have posited as an obligation to protect them from over-exposure to information, responsibility and its consequences during critical phases of their development.

But there is a group who would probably find relief in being part of conversations with their parents and team, but who are stifled not only by their own fear and immaturity, but by the powerful psychological resistance naturally mounted by any parent to the idea of frankly discussing a child's death with that child herself. In a survey of every family—561 in total—who had lost a child to cancer in Sweden between 1992 and 1997, one-third of parents chose to talk about death with their child, including 16% of parents of dying children under five, 36% between 5 and 9, and nearly half of children over 10. Importantly, none of the parents who chose to talk with children who were thought to suspect that their own death was imminent (55%) regretted this conversation. On the other hand, regrets were shared among only 13% of parents who discussed death with a child who seemed unsuspecting [62].

The powerful resistance experienced by most parents faced with the task of talking with their child, or even with their child's doctors, about that child's possible death, is a major reason why advance care planning does not happen sooner in the course of an illness than has become terminal. Physicians and other clinicians are equally culpable of this tendency, falsely equating advance care planning with giving up. On the contrary, early goal-setting and advance care planning can ease the transition between phases of illness, and it can indicate the inherent dangers in each cancer diagnosis in treatment, without sacrificing any hope to achieve these aims. Interdisciplinary teams are crucial in advance care planning, which should involve representatives from nursing and oncology, as well as child life and child mental health professionals to engage directly with the child herself, preferably not only in tandem with her family but on her own as well. These conversations should take place over time, with general hopes and specific goals unfolding over time. Furthermore, pediatric palliative care teams should be involved early and often in cancer care, helping manage symptoms and contributing to child- and family-centered interdisciplinary care, and preventing the sudden transfer of care to the end of life team, given a child's turn for the worse [63, 64].

Case #6: Grief, Futility, and the Process of Bioethics Mediation

The case of Daniel Hauser describes how parental authority is sharply limited by state authority when a family's ability to protect a child's welfare, in this case because of religious values, places a child at mortal risk. Another way that parental authority has become limited, or at least contested, involves treatments at the end of life, which may, in a professional's best judgment, provide a patient with little or no benefit. Generally, *futility* is the notion that a treatment is unethical because it is medically inappropriate, providing risks without significant possibility of benefit. The idea of futility has a tangled social history [65, 66] with attempts to quantify it empirically largely unsuccessful. Despite the AMA's call for healthcare institutions to adopt policies to determine and adjudicate futility cases [66–69], the status of these policies and institutional ethics committee decisions remains somewhat unresolved [70], though these determinations form the core of many ethics consultation services [71, 72]. These studies and others are discussed within the context of divergent findings in [73].

Overall, this represents an area of resistance by medical professionals to the autonomy of patients to choose each and every intervention. The medical perspective can be summarized as follows: the legal and social victories won by patients and their advocates throughout the twentieth century reward a competent adult the right to accept or decline any proposed treatment, but not to demand any treatment. For example, is it acceptable to perform CPR on a child such as the girl Mercurio [74] describes as "Katherine," an infant suffering from incurable disseminated rhabdomyosarcoma, because her parents request that "everything be done for her"? Her doctors and parents had already agreed to withhold chemotherapy because of the extensive spread of tumor throughout her peritoneum, but their agreement ended when end-of-life care planning had started. As she appeared to be in more and more discomfort despite significant doses of morphine, the neonatology team recommended shifting to comfort care, and withdrawing mechanical ventilation, probably allowing her to die within hours.

Many families facing this terrible situation may decide to allow their child to die in maximum comfort, and to limit the days or weeks she spends suffering on a ventilator, once it is certain that her disease will kill her somehow. Others may equate their agreement to withdraw ventilation or even to limit interventions such as CPR with "giving up." While Burt [75] and others have rightly emphasized mediation between parties in these debates, he is joined by Pope and Waldman [76] in sensing that a small minority of these cases will demand action before resolution is found. See generally also Dubler [77]. Why this may be is illustrated by comparing the case of "Katherine" with another case, that of "T.", a 4-year-old boy with a brain tumor who was unable to finish his previous course of chemotherapy because of complications leading to a stay in intensive care, had a steadily deteriorating neurological examination, and required mechanical ventilation. It was clear to his oncologist, neurosurgeon and intensivist that his tumor was spreading centrally.

Though these determinations have an evolving basis in law, there is largely a consensus that a hospital ethics committee are the ideal body to help resolve these debates, for example, by mediating in disagreements between staff and families, or among staff [78, 79]. Consultations can also help clarify questions, specify which legal and professional norms apply to a given case, and, in some well-circumscribed cases, these groups are also empowered in many institutions to advise doctors on well-circumscribed unilateral decisions about appropriate care, such as supporting doctors to write DNR orders despite a family's objections in the case of a suffering child with a terminal illness, like Katherine.

Some prominent pediatric ethicists disagree with these shifts away from family autonomy [80]. One important reason why the ethics consult for Katherine resulted in a unilateral decision to withhold CPR but that for T. did not, was that Katherine appeared to be suffering, despite considerable attempts at pain management. Were she comfortable enough—even if she required analgesia to the point of sedation for her pain—then the team might have been agreeable to allowing more time for mediation to occur and for her parents' grief to progress.

Conclusion

The foregoing cases represent some of the breadth and depth of ethical issues in pediatric oncology, a specialty that features an uncommon mix of biomedical technology, life and death situations for especially vulnerable patients, and complicated relationships of obligation and dependency through which the individuality of a child finds expression. By looking at these cases from a psychosocial place where normative values, empirical findings, and psychological thinking each occupy a room, we hope to guide clinicians in finding moments of tension and possibilities for intervention, mediation, and relief for the children, families, and providers involved in pediatric oncology.

References

1. Wolpe PR. The triumph of autonomy in American medical ethics: a sociological view. In: DeVries R, Subedi J (eds.) *Bioethics and Society: Sociological Investigations of the Enterprise of Bioethics*. New York: Prentice Hall, 1998; pp. 38–59.
2. Beauchamp TL, Childress JF. *Principles of Biomedical Ethics*, 5th edn. New York: Oxford University Press, 2001.
3. Childress JF. The place of autonomy in bioethics. *Hastings Center Report* 1990;**20**:12–17.

4. Cassell EJ. Unanswered questions: bioethics and human relationships. *Hastings Center Report* 2007;**37**:20–23.
5. Pulte D, Gondos A, Brenner H. Trends in 5- and 10-year survival after diagnosis with childhood hematologic malignancies in the United States, 1990–2004. *Journal of the National Cancer Institute* 2008;**100**:1301–1309.
6. Levine RJ. Directives for human experimentation. In: *Ethics and Regulation of Clinical Research*. New Haven, CT: Yale University Press, 1948/1986; pp. 425–426.
7. Field MJ, Behrman RE (eds.) *When Children Die: Improving Palliative and End-of-Life Care for Children and Their Families*. Washington, DC: National Academies Press, 2003; p. 105.
8. Spinetta JJ, Masera G, Jankovic M, *et al.* Valid informed consent and participative decision-making in children with cancer and their parents: a report of the SIOP working committee on psychosocial issues in pediatric oncology. *Medical and Pediatric Oncology* 2003;**40**:244–246.
9. Schneider C. *The Practice of Autonomy*. Oxford University Press, New York, 1998; p. 5, quoting Higuchi N. The patient's right to know of a cancer diagnosis: a comparison of Japanese paternalism and American self-determination. *Washburn Law Journal* 1992;**31**: 455, 456.
10. Emanuel E, Emanuel L. Four models of the physician–patient relationship. *JAMA* 1992;**261**:2221–2226.
11. Goldstein J, Freud A, Solnit A, Goldstein S. *The Best Interests of the Child: The Least Detrimental Alternative*. New York: The Free Press, 1996; p. 127.
12. Mercurio MR, Adam MB, Forman EN, *et al.* American Academy of Pediatrics Policy Statements on bioethics summaries and commentaries: Part 1. *Pediatrics in Review* 2008;**29**:e1–e8.
13. Katz J. *The Silent World of Doctor and Patient*. New York: The Free Press, 1984.
14. Pope TM. Legal briefing: informed consent. *Journal of Clinical Ethics* 2010;**21**:72–81.
15. Sigman GS, O'Connor C. Exploration for physicians of the mature minor doctrine. *The Journal of Pediatrics* 1991;**4**:520–525.
16. American Academy of Pediatrics Committee on Bioethics. Informed consent, parental permission, and assent in pediatric practice. *Pediatrics* 1995;**95**:314–317.
17. Buchanan AE, Brock DW. *Deciding for Others: The Ethics of Surrogate Decision Making*. New York: Cambridge University Press, 1990.
18. Kopelman LM. The best-interests standard as threshold, ideal, and standard of reasonableness. *Journal of Medicine and Philosophy* 1997;**22**:271–289.
19. Diekema DS(2011). Revising the best interest standard: uses and misuses. *Journal of Clinical Ethics* 1990;**22**:128–133.
20. Sulmasy DP, Snyder L. Substituted interests and best judgments: an integrated model of surrogate decision making. *JAMA* 2010;**304**:1946–1947.
21. Dwyer J, Vig E. Rethinking transplantation between siblings. *Hastings Center Report* 1995;**25**:7–12.
22. Lewis M. Kidney donation by a 7-year-old identical twin child: psychological, legal, and ethical considerations. *Journal of the American Academy of Child and Adolescent Psychiatry* 1974;**13**:221–245.
23. Savulescu J, Boyle RK. Ethics of using preimplantation genetic diagnosis to select a stem cell donor for an existing person *BMJ* 2001;**323**:1240–1243.
24. Spriggs M, Savalescu J. Saviour siblings. *Journal of Medical Ethics* 2002;**28**:289.
25. Burgio GR, Nespoli L, Varrasi G, *et al.* Bone marrow transplantation in children: between therapeutic and medico-legal problems. *Bone Marrow Transplantation* 1989;**4**:34–37.
26. Quinn GP, Murphy D, Knapp C, *et al.* Who decides? Decision making and fertility preservation in teens with cancer: a review of the literature. *Journal of Adolescent Health* 2011;**49**:337–346.
27. Fallat ME, Hutter J. Preservation of fertility in pediatric and adolescent patients with cancer. *Pediatrics* 2008;**121**:1461–1469.
28. American Society of Clinical, Oncology. Recommendations on fertility preservation in cancer patients. *Journal of Clinical Oncology* 2006;**24**:2917–2931.
29. Patrizio P, Butts S, Caplan S. Ovarian tissue preservation and future fertility: emerging technologies and ethical considerations. *Journal of the National Cancer Institute Monographs* 2005;**34**:107–110.
30. Truman JT. Custody of a minor: the Chad Green Case in historical perspective. In: Truman JT, Van Eys J, Pochedly C (eds.) *Human Values in Pediatric Hematology/Oncology*. New York: Praeger, 1986.
31. Associated Press, December 8, 2009. Appeals Court sides with state in cancer girl case. Available at: http://abclocal.go.com/ktrk/story?section=news/state&id=7177562 (Accessed 6 July 2011).
32. Associated Press, May 19, 2009. Judge rules family can't refuse chemo for boy. Available at http://www.msnbc.msn.com/id/30763438/ns/health-childrens_health/t/judge-rules-family-cant-refuse-chemo-boy/ (Accessed 6 July 2011).
33. Wasserman S.March 28, 2010 Daniel Hauser turns 14, is cancer free. Available at http://www.myfoxtwincities.com—Daniel-Hauser-Turns-14,-Is-Cancer-Free-mar-28-2010 (Accessed 5 September 2011).
34. Asser SM. Legalized child abuse: faith healers and child deaths. *Proceedings of the Amazing Meeting* 3, James Randi Educational Foundation, 2005. Online at: http://www.csufresno.edu/physics/rhall/jref/tam3p/05_SA_tam3.pdf.
35. Asser SM, Swan R. Child fatalities from religion-motivated medical neglect. *Pediatrics* 1998;**101**:625–629.
36. Syse A. Valid (as opposed to informed) consent. *Lancet* 2002;**356**:1347–1348.
37. Volpe RL. Patients' expressed and unexpressed needs for information for informed consent. *The Journal of Clinical Ethics* 2010;**21**:45–57.
38. Kodish ED, Pentz RD, Noll RB, *et al.* Informed consent in the children's cancer group. *Cancer* 1998;**82**:2467–2481.
39. Truong TH, Weeks JC, Cook EF, Joffe S. Outcomes of informed consent among parents of children in cancer clinical trials. *Pediatric Blood & Cancer* 2011;**57**:998–1004.
40. Eder ML, Yamokoski AD, Wittmann PW, *et al.* Improving informed consent: suggestions from parents of children with leukemia pediatrics 2007;**119**:e849–e859.
41. Lederberg M. Negotiating the interface of psycho-oncology and ethics. In: Holland JC, *et al.* (eds.) *Psycho-Oncology*, 2nd edn. New York: Oxford University Press, 2010; pp. 625–629.

42. Unguru Y. The successful integration of research and care: how pediatric oncology became the subspecialty in which research defines the standard of care. *Pediatric Blood & Cancer* 2011;**56**:1019–1025.

43. Joffe S, Simon C. Informed consent from the doctor? *Hastings Center Report* 2004;**34**:12–13.

44. Kodish E, Eder M, Noll RB, *et al.* Communication of randomization in childhood leukemia trials. *JAMA* 2004;**291**:470–475.

45. Lidz CW, Appelbaum PS, Grisso T, Renaud M. Therapeutic misconception and the appreciation of risks in clinical trials. *Social Science & Medicine* 2004;**58**:1689–1697.

46. Joffe S, Cook EF, Cleary PD, *et al.* Quality of informed consent in cancer clinical trials: a cross-sectional survey. *Lancet* 2001;**358**:1772–1777.

47. Flory J, Emanuel E. Interventions to improve research participants' understanding in informed consent for research: a systematic review *JAMA* 2004;**292**:1593–1601.

48. Leikin S. Minors' assent or dissent to medical treatment. *Journal of Pediatrics* 1983;**102**:169–176.

49. Joffe S, Fernandez CV, Pentz RD, *et al.* Involving children in decision-making about research participation. *Journal of Pediatrics* 2006;**149**:862–868.

50. Quinn JO, Eder M, Simon C, *et al.* Assent observed: children's involvement in leukemia treatment and research discussions. *Pediatrics* 2002;**109**:806–814.

51. Committee on Bioethics of the American Academy of Pediatrics. Informed consent, parental permission, and assent in pediatric practice. *Pediatrics* 1995;**95**:314–317.

52. Appelbaum PS. Assessment of patients' competence to consent to treatment. *New England Journal of Medicine* 2007;**357**:1834–1840.

53. Gaylin W. The competence of children: no longer all or none. *Hastings Center Report* 1982;**12**:33–38.

54. Jones R, Holden T. A guide to assessing decision-making capacity. *Cleveland Clinical Journal of Medicine* 2004;

55. Appelbaum P, Grisso T. *Assessing Competence to Consent to Treatment: A Guide for Physicians and Other Health Professionals.* New York: Oxford University Press, 1998.

56. Dunn LB, Nowrangi MA, Palmer BW, Jeste DV, Saks ER. Assessing decisional capacity for clinical research or treatment: a review of instruments. *American Journal of Psychiatry* 2006;**163**:1323–1334.

57. Ficke SL, Hart KJ, Deardorff PA. The performance of incarcerated juveniles on the Macarthur competence assessment tool-criminal adjudication (MacCAT-CA) *Journal of American Academy of Psychiatry and Law* 2006;**34**:360–373.

58. Schachter D, Tharmalingam S, Kleinman I. Informed consent and stimulant medication: adolescents' and parents' ability to understand information about benefits and risks of stimulant medication for the treatment of attention-deficit/hyperactivity disorder. *Journal of Child and Adolescent Psychopharmacology* 2011;**21**:139–148.

59. US Department of Health and Human Services. Additional protections for children involved as subjects in research. Federal Registrar; March 8 1993. 45 CFR 46. Available at: http://www.hhs.gov/ohrp/archive/documents/19830308.pdf. (Accessed 6 October 2011).

60. Unguru Y, Sill AM, Kamani N. The experiences of children enrolled in pediatric oncology research: implications for assent. *Pediatrics* 2010;**125**:e876–e883.

61. Kunin H. Ethical issues in pediatric life-threatening illness. *Ethics and Behavior* 1997;**7**:43–57.

62. Kreicbergs T, Valdimarsdóttir U, Onelöv E, *et al.* Talking about death with children who have severe malignant disease. *New England Journal of Medicine* 2004;**351**:1175–1186.

63. Himelstein BP, Hilden JM, Boldt AM, Weissman D. Pediatric palliative care. *New England Journal of Medicine* 2004;**350**:1752–1762.

64. Strong C, Feudtner C, Carter BS, Rushton CH. Goals, values, and conflict resolution. In: Carter BS, Levetown M (eds.) *Palliative Care for Infants, Children, and Adolescents: A Practical Handbook.* Baltimore, MD: Johns Hopkins Press, 2004; pp. 23–43.

65. Luce JM. A history of resolving conflicts over end-of-life care in intensive care units in the United States. *Critical Care Medicine* 2010;**38**:1623–1629.

66. Burns JP, Truog RD. Futility: a concept in evolution. *Chest* 2007;**132**:1987–1993.

67. Plows CW, Tenery RM, Hartford A, *et al.* Medical futility in end-of-life care: report of the Council on Ethical and Judicial Affairs. *JAMA* 1999;**281**:937–941.

68. Bay Area Network of Ethics Committees Nonbeneficial Treatment Working Group. Nonbeneficial or futile medical treatment: conflict resolution guidelines for the San Francisco Bay Area. *Western Journal of Medicine* 1996;**170**:287–290.

69. Halevy A, Brody BA. Multi-institution collaborative policy on medical futility. *JAMA* 1996;**276**:571–574.

70. Pope TM. Medical futility statutes: no safe harbor to unilaterally refuse life-sustaining treatment. *Tennessee Law Review* 2007;**75**:1–81.

71. LaPuma J. An ethics consultation service in a teaching hospital: utilization and evaluation. *Journal of the American Medical Association* 1988;**160**:808–811.

72. Schenkenberg T, Salt Lake City VA's Medical Center's first 150 ethics committee case consultations: what we have learned (so far). *HEC Forum* 1997;**9**:147–158.

73. Bruce CR, Smith ML, Hizlan S, Sharp RR. A systematic review of activities at a high-volume ethics consultation service. *The Journal of Clinical Ethics* 2011;**22**:151–164.

74. Mercurio AR. The role of a pediatric ethics committee in the newborn intensive care unit. *Journal of Perinatology* 2011;**31**:1–9.

75. Burt RA. The medical futility debate: patient choice, physician obligation, and end-of-life care. *Journal of Palliative Medicine* 2002;**5**:249–254.

76. Pope TM, Waldman EA. Mediation at the end of life: getting beyond the limits of the talking cure. *Ohio State Journal on Dispute Resolution* 2007;**23**:143–194.

77. Dubler NN, Liebma CB. *Bioethics Mediation: A Guide to Shaping Shared Solutions.* New York: United Hospital Fund, 2004.

78. AMA Judicial Council. Guidelines for ethics committees in health care institutions. *JAMA* 1985;**253**:2698–2699.

79. American Academy of Pediatrics, Committee on Bioethics. Institutional ethics committees. *Pediatrics* 2001;**107**:205–209.

80. Truog RD. Perspective: is it always wrong to perform futile CPR? *New England Journal of Medicine* 2010;**362**:477–479.

21

When a Parent has Cancer: Supporting Healthy Child Development During Challenging Times

Susan D. Swick, Andrés S. Martin, Paula Rauch

This is a unique chapter in this textbook. In the same way that a child's cancer diagnosis and treatment can have a profound impact on an entire family, a parent's cancer diagnosis and treatment can also pose an unprecedented set of challenges to each of the members of the family. This stress may translate into behavioral, academic or emotional problems in children, conflict within a marriage or even psychological and medical complications in the patient. Although family members may seek out support or treatment once these complications have occurred, it may be possible to prevent them. With practical guidance informed by knowledge of child development and medical illnesses, parents themselves can often manage and minimize the distress their children may feel as a consequence of their parent's illness. Clinicians skilled in providing psychosocial support to pediatric cancer patients may be in a unique position to offer meaningful support and guidance to cancer patients who are also the parents of dependent children.

Parenting At a Challenging Time (PACT)

The PACT (Parenting At a Challenging Time) program was created over ten years ago to address these special parenting concerns with the hope of providing preventive support for children through direct interactions with their parents. Created by the Director of the Child Psychiatry Consultation-Liaison Service at the Massachusetts General Hospital (PR) and staffed by child psychiatrists and child psychologists, parent guidance consultations have been provided to cancer patients and their partners after a referral from their oncologist, nurse, palliative care clinician, or social worker. These clinicians identified their patients as worried about the impact their diagnosis or treatment might have on their children. Most clinicians who provide care to adult patients have limited child development background and knowledge. The PACT program provides adult patients with access to clinicians who have expertise in child development and children's mental health. The clinicians work with parents to help them plan how to support open, honest, child-centered communication at home, preserve their children's routines, protect family time and, when need be, think about end-of-life issues. The goal is to help parents recognize that their knowledge of their children's strengths and personalities and their own established parenting skills apply in this situation as they have before. Practical guidance is offered in ways that might best protect family cohesion and support resiliency in children.

PACT and Pediatric Oncology?

The PACT program currently exists at three hospitals in the U.S., but clearly there are parents of young children facing life-threatening illness throughout the country. These parents are getting their guidance and support from the internet, loved ones, teachers and interested clinicians. Those that they speak with may lack knowledge of child development or experience with serious medical illnesses. We recognize that there may be an untapped resource already available at the medical centers where parents with cancer are getting treatment: clinicians with expertise in child

Pediatric Psycho-oncology: Psychosocial Aspects and Clinical Interventions, Second Edition.
Edited by Shulamith Kreitler, Myriam Weyl Ben-Arush and Andrés Martin.
© 2012 John Wiley & Sons, Ltd. Published 2012 by John Wiley & Sons, Ltd.

development and experience with children and their families coping with serious medical illness, who additionally have fluency with consultative work, working within a medical (rather than mental health or educational) system. Those clinicians who provide psychosocial interventions for families in which a child has cancer possess this unique combination of knowledge and skills. If these clinicians are at hospitals that treat adults as well as children and have interest in providing guidance and support to families facing a parent's serious illness, they could become a treasured resource at their hospital for both these families and the clinicians who currently have little to offer their patients when they ask, "What do I tell my children?"

Background

The National Cancer Institute estimated in 1992 that 24% of adults with cancer were parenting children 18 or younger [1]. Data gathered between 2000 and 2007 suggested that 14% of adult cancer survivors have children 18 years or younger [2]. These data translate to potentially 2.85 million children living with a parent who is a cancer survivor and an additional 562,000 children who are living with a parent who was recently diagnosed with cancer or is in the early phase of treatment. Additionally, it has been estimated that 4–6% of children 18 and younger lose a parent to a terminal illness [3]. Taken together, these data suggest that well over five million children have been affected by parental cancer. When one compares these numbers to the estimated 4.4 million children who are living with ADHD in the United States [4], one can appreciate the enormity of this potential strain on families. Improved and more available diagnostic tests and improved survival rates mean that the number of cancer survivors who are or can become parents will likely increase in the coming decades. There are clearly a large and growing number of families with dependent children in the United States affected by a parent's life-threatening illness and thus there is opportunity for efficient public health interventions here, where focused parent guidance may serve to protect the children from behavioral or emotional complications and reassure parents.

Even though there is limited information about the specific needs and outcomes for these families, there is a growing body of data that suggest that without any support, there may be complications for children coping with a parent's serious illness. Parents consistently underreport their children's level of distress, and children and adolescents self-report significant levels of distress after a parent's diagnosis [5]. Over time, adolescent daughters of mothers with breast cancer appear

to be at particular risk of developing internalizing symptoms (anxiety and depression) [6]. Higher sustained levels of anxiety are reported by children who describe an inability to discuss their parent's illness or decreased time in age-appropriate activities [7]. Complementing these findings is the finding that children who have been given specific, detailed information about their parent's illness report lower levels of anxiety than those children who are not given such specific information [5]. Children whose parents are terminally ill have demonstrated higher rates of depression, anxiety and behavioral changes than their peers [8]. There are limited data on the parents, but what data we have suggest that concern about their children is among the primary concerns of parents diagnosed with cancer, and affects their treatment-related decision-making.

History and Structure of the PACT Program

History

PACT (Parenting At a Challenging Time) is a parent guidance program that was created over ten years ago at the Massachusetts General Hospital Cancer Center (and more recently introduced at the Newton Wellesley Hospital's Cancer Center in Newton, Massachusetts, and at the Smilow Cancer Hospital at Yale-New Haven, in New Haven, Connecticut) in order to address the particular concerns that face parents who are diagnosed with cancer. PACT has provided consultations to parents referred by any member of the multidisciplinary oncology team who noted that a patient was concerned about the impact their diagnosis or treatment might have on their children. A referral may be made at any point in a patient's cancer care, from the time of initial diagnosis through active treatment, remissions and recurrences and even through end-of-life care. PACT clinicians see consultations on an inpatient and outpatient basis and run regular drop-in groups for patients and their spouses. The program is supported by institutional and charitable contributions in order to make the program freely accessible to all referred families, regardless of insurance status.

Parent Guidance Model

PACT uses a parent guidance model of intervention. This is not traditional psychotherapy for families, couples or individual parents or children. It is a supportive intervention that emphasizes identifying and using the parents' existing skills. Parents are recognized as the experts on their own children. They want to be the ones supporting their children through this difficult time, and they are the people best equipped to do so. In the same way that parents may provide the most effective support when their children are cancer patients, they are also going to be the ones their children turn to when they themselves are the patients. Children's questions about a parent's illness are most likely to arise at home and children are going to be most comfortable receiving information and reassurance from their parents, not from an unfamiliar clinician. With guidance and support, parents can effectively manage their children's concerns and can organize the most supportive home environment possible under the circumstances. Most children, while distressed, will not need a psychiatric intervention. For those who do, appropriate referrals can be made by the PACT clinician.

Supportive Approach

The approach of the PACT clinician is supportive: the aim is to identify and then contain parents' strong emotions, rather than to explore them or draw them out. This is often the critical first step towards helping parents realize that they still have the skills to support, comfort, and guide their children through this particular challenge. Although the circumstances may feel extraordinary, their parenting skills remain intact and adequate. This may be similar to the way in which clinicians provide support for parents who are caring for a child with cancer; powerful emotions and anxieties are acknowledged and coping is supported, so that their parenting functions may continue (for all of their children). The PACT clinician learns from the parents about their individual children: their temperaments, developmental maturity, strengths, and vulnerabilities. The clinician will try to learn about prior challenges the family has faced and how they have met them. They discuss what the children have been told about their parent's diagnosis and what they may have observed. The clinician educates the parents about development and their children's likely understanding of and reactions to their diagnosis. Strategies are devised to strengthen communication and emotional support within the family. The clinician helps parents to identify their existing emotional and practical supports and devise strategies to preserve their children's routines and protect family time. The PACT clinician is available to meet with parents as often as is necessary, and will even meet with the children if necessary. But the vast majority of PACT consultations take place over one or two visits. This is typically enough for parents to get practical guidance and informed reassurance. Calmer and more confident, they are able to return to the important task at hand: managing their own treatment while raising their children. If needed, clinicians can provide a referral for ongoing psychiatric treatment or other useful resources within the patient's community.

Two Birds with One Stone: Creating a New PACT Program at Your Institution

We are presented with a prevalent problem: parents of dependent children facing a diagnosis of cancer. Without intervention, a parent's cancer carries a significant risk of distress and disruption for their children. With a fairly straightforward supportive intervention with the parents, both parents' and children's distress may be reduced and family cohesion protected at a critical time. Most patient guidance concerning parenting comes from friends, teachers, pediatricians or the internet. These resources may prove useful, but may lack grounding in child development, children's mental health, or of the particular challenges of cancer. Those hospital-based clinicians who provide guidance to parents of children with cancer could be available to provide this specific service to parents with cancer. Given their specialized expertise in child development, medical illness and its impact on a whole family and mental health interventions, these clinicians are in a unique position to provide this service, either directly or by educating others who are currently caring for cancer patients who are also parents.

It may be simple to present a persuasive argument that a PACT consultation can be an effective means of protecting the mental health of cancer patients and their dependent children, but it is considerably more challenging to find clinicians with the specialized skills necessary to do this work. It can be even more challenging to set up a program that is financially sustainable. It is rare for health insurers to reimburse for a preventive psychiatric intervention for children. In our experience, fundraising around the mission of the program can generate revenue and help support the clinicians' time directly, through charitable contributions. A cancer center or hospital may also decide that PACT is a service that can help set them apart from competing providers, and be willing to underwrite time as they market this aspect of their thoughtful, comprehensive and family-centered patient care. If a hospital is already well staffed by mental health providers, it may be possible to start by adding this type of consultation to the job description of the child psychiatrist, psychologist or social worker who has a special interest in the area. Once it becomes a service that is valued by clinicians and patients, the hospital may be willing to support its continuation and expansion.

It is important to consider the size of a treatment setting in preparing to introduce this program. In small settings, it may be most effective for one provider to focus on individual consultations and educating providers about their availability. In larger settings, it may be effective to begin by offering a drop-in group for parents, with the option of individual consultations, so as to consult to the greatest number of patients. In settings where there are few PACT clinicians, but a large patient population, the clinician should make use of additional resources. It may be most cost-effective to invest in books and use web-based resources as a complement to what a clinician can do individually. Such a clinician should also focus on opportunities to educate other clinicians who are interested in adding these skills to theirs.

After deciding on a funding model and considering how best to use clinical resources, the next challenge is to inform patients and the clinical teams about the service, so that it will connect with those patients who may benefit from it. It may be useful to begin by meeting with the directors of those services caring for these patients (such as surgery, oncology, radiation oncology, palliative care, and social work) and introducing them to the program. If they become committed to the idea of this program, these leaders can facilitate introduction into the appropriate settings within the cancer center. Then it is best to seek out opportunities to introduce this specialized service to those who might refer patients: giving presentations to the chemotherapy nurses, palliative care physicians, oncology fellows or social workers. Any opportunity to speak about this program will improve the likelihood that clinicians will think to ask their patients about their children. That alone is often a helpful experience for families, and it is the first step towards establishing the service as a well-used and respected resource within a medical center. Portable literature, such as pamphlets, bookmarks or postcards, is a common and effective marketing tool. This literature should be geared towards patients, briefly describing the service and its guiding principles or the answers to several common questions, and should provide the number to call and arrange a consultation. Pamphlets can easily be placed in areas where the cancer patients often wait (radiology, chemotherapy infusion suites, etc.) and in a cancer resource room. They can also be left with providers who have heard a presentation, so that they have something to give to patients and remind them of the service.

PACT: Guiding Principles

The idea for the PACT program came from an unmet need within the local community, and the work has always been clinically driven. Over more than ten years of working with parents who are managing a diagnosis and the treatment of cancer, several principles have emerged as being of central importance to the healthy adjustment of children to a parent's illness. These principles guide our work with families and we share them with parents in order to help them organize their efforts with their children.

1. Communication

The first and most important principle that guides our work with parents is that open, honest and child-centered communication within the family is essential to help children manage the anxiety and uncertainty that accompany a parent's diagnosis with cancer. This assertion may seem straightforward, but parents often instinctively want to protect their children by not talking about their illness. This approach may feel protective, but it leaves their children vulnerable to feeling excluded, isolated and worried. Parents may believe they are able to insulate their children from this news, but the home of an ill parent tends to be filled with phone calls and conversations about the illness, treatment options, fears, and talk about prognosis. It is a scenario ripe for overhearing, and the worst way for a child to hear difficult news is to overhear it. They are prone to misunderstandings and will not turn to their parents for further information, clarification or simple support. Children may conclude that a parent's illness is too terrible to be discussed or that they are not valued enough to be included in the discussions. Parents can provide their children with the best protection against uncertainty and anxiety by having open, honest discussions, welcoming questions and providing reassurance.

For communication to be useful, it needs to be honest. This means providing accurate information, using the same language that children might overhear, including the word "cancer." Some parents may feel more comfortable using euphemisms when discussing a serious diagnosis, but these may actually heighten a child's anxiety and cause confusion. Not every detail that has been discussed with physicians must be shared, but it can be helpful to discuss those things that have been or will be observed by the children. For example, helping children anticipate hair loss due to chemotherapy or understand that fatigue is due to the effects of treatment and not the cancer itself, can make those events far less frightening for children. If children have a general sense of what to expect and believe, they will be included in discussions if things change, it is usually very reassuring for them.

The other crucial feature of this communication is that it be child-centered. That is to say that in substance and style, it should be appropriate to the child's developmental age and be focused on their specific concerns. Parents may devise descriptions of cancer, chemotherapy or radiation therapy that will be understandable by their children. Parents should not try to force their children to talk, but should welcome all questions. When their children do ask questions, parents should remain child-centered and not assume they understand the child's underlying concern. Clarifying questions, such as, "What has got you wondering about that?" or "Where did you hear that?" may reveal a different (and sometimes more easily answered) question. Questions also do not require immediate answers. Wondering with their child about the question and reassuring them that, "That's a great question. I don't know. Let me think about it and get back to you," does a wonderful job of keeping the lines of communication open and helping the children to feel reassured, included and supported. Children can be regularly reminded to "never worry alone," and bring any concerns to their parents or other trusted adults.

2. Minimize Disruption

Children are better able to cope and mange anxiety and uncertainty when their routines are preserved. Even under normal circumstances, children depend on predictability and routine for a sense of security: protecting these routines during a parent's serious illness is even more essential to their well-being. Babies, toddlers and preschoolers should have as much consistency as possible: creating a predictable caregiver schedule and a detailed daily itinerary for new caregivers can be very helpful. For slightly older children, school should remain as much of an "oasis of normalcy" as possible, and efforts should be made to assure that children and adolescents can continue with favorite extracurricular activities, hobbies, and socializing. Minimizing disruption is often the result of the well-orchestrated efforts of parents, relatives, friends and neighbors. Helping parents to identify those people who will be most helpful in this regard is essential. Designating a familiar adult, perhaps a classmate's very organized parent, to help keep track of homework assignments, SAT dates or sports practices can help ensure that these things do not get overlooked. Children can be especially distressed by feeling different or unprepared at school when a parent is seriously ill. We recommend that parents have a meeting with the appropriate adults at their children's schools (teachers, principals, guidance counselors) in order to inform them about what is occurring in their family, remind them not to meet their child with long faces, and talk about any special concerns they or the school may have about their children. It can also be helpful for children to choose a "point-person" at school. This is simply the adult they are most comfortable talking to, whom their parents can keep informed about developments in their illness and treatment. This will be the person the child can go to if he or she feels overwhelmed or needs to talk while at school. This is also the person who can gather observations or concerns from other teachers, and in turn share them with the parents, who will appreciate this additional information about how their child is functioning at school during this challenging time.

As with school, designating other adults to help the family minimize disruptions can be a very effective way to support parents and their children during the course of a serious illness. We often suggest that parents consider who of their friends or family would be a good "Minister of Information" or "Captain of Kindnesses." Phone calls from concerned relatives, friends and colleagues can occupy significant amounts of parents' time, usually during the typical family time after school and in the evening. A Minister of Information gets regular updates from the parents and in turn keeps their chosen community informed. Parents then don't have to use their time and energy repeating the same health information to multiple callers. Similarly, a Captain of Kindnesses can keep a list of all the family's needs, from prepared meals to carpool assistance. Then all offers of assistance can simply be referred to this person, to help parents protect their time and ensure that the family gets assistance that they find useful. There are many free online resources (lotsahelping-hands.com is but one) that can facilitate this coordination of efforts so that it is not too big a job, and the Captain may arrange for deliveries to be done in a way that minimizes intrusions during key family times (such as leaving meals in a cooler on the front porch).

3. Protect Family Time

The corollary of minimizing disruptions in a child's and family's routines is to maximize and optimize the meaningful time that a family can spend together. The ill parent often has limited energy and the well parent may have a larger number of parenting responsibilities and increased financial pressures, so making arrangements that protect parents' availability to their children is often necessary. Having a Minister of Information and a Captain of Kindnesses are a few ways to facilitate this. Simply turning the ringer to the telephone off and letting the answering machine handle phone calls during the afterschool hours can help protect the evening mealtime from interruptions, allowing families to catch up on details about school, sports, friends and other topics. Helping parents to consider their important family rituals and routines and choosing those that can be realistically continued can be highly reassuring for children and meaningful for parents.

4. Maximize the Support System

In trying to minimize disruptions and protect family time, a critical strategy is identifying those adults who can be useful resources and making effective use of offers of support from the community of family, friends, colleagues and neighbors that surround a family. Parents benefit from reassurance and direct guidance in utilizing their support systems; used to managing the complicated swirl of activities and responsibilities of parenting, they often expect that they should manage this challenge privately. The simple assertion that now is exactly the time when they should accept offers of help or ask for assistance is often useful. Parents benefit from talking with a clinician about who are (or might become) their reliable supports, within their family or outside of it. Having people who can help with various aspects of the treatment routine (drives to the hospital) or family routine (meals, carpools, school assignments) provides help with flexibility. The parents should also consider how else to take good care of themselves, the healthy parent in particular. Making use of time with friends, an existing therapeutic relationship or simply protecting some time for relaxing activities can greatly enhance the parents' abilities to weather this experience and be as healthy, energetic and available to their children as possible.

In addition to maximizing their own supports, parents should consider their children's support systems. Ensuring consistency in caregivers for infants, toddlers and preschoolers does more than protect their routines, it also ensures emotional consistency. Designating a point person at school for school-age children can be very helpful, as can identifying those adults who might help keep track of homework assignments, projects and activities. Children this age will often "cope by doing" rather than talking, and ensuring that they have caring adults who will facilitate this is protective. Adolescents may need permission to discuss these events and their feelings about them with adults outside of the family. While it is developmentally normal for adolescents to be cultivating relationships with non-related adults, it might feel like a betrayal of their family to discuss this private matter with adults other

than their parents, particularly when their parental relationships have been fraught (which can also be developmentally normal). This is not an intuitive idea for parents, who imagine they do not need to give their teenagers permission to talk to anyone. But this simple strategy is very supportive of healthy adolescent independence and adjustment. Parents can encourage all of their children's healthy relationships with trusted, supportive adults with statements such as, "I'm so happy that you and [the best friend's] mom figured that out together," giving the message that the child's other relationships with adults are appreciated rather than seen as disloyal to the parent.

Supporting the parents' communication with each other is also protective, as parents who work well together with a minimum of marital discord make it easier for a family to adjust to the concerns and inconveniences of an illness. If there is preexisting marital discord or if parents are divorced, it is often more difficult to create a supportive, child-centered approach to the challenge of one parent's illness. If possible, clinicians can meet with parents together to help them plan appropriately to best support their children. Sometimes mutually-respected family members can bridge a parental divide. In special cases, it may become necessary to involve the courts in order to protect the long-term interests of the children, such as when there is an abusive parent or a non-parental adult who has functioned as a parent without the legal designation to do so.

5. Legacy Leaving

All parents facing a serious illness will have thoughts about planning for their children's care in the short-term future. In cases when a parent's illness is terminal, parents will need support to thoughtfully plan for their children's extended future. A PACT clinician can facilitate nuanced planning for a family's emotional adjustment to the loss of a parent. Planning for financial and legal arrangements is essential. The formal details are best done with an attorney, but it can be helpful to consider how this planning can minimize disruption and maximize supports. Moving and changing schools are always disruptive for children and are best avoided in the aftermath of losing a parent. Considering how to provide the surviving parent with supports (having grandparents move closer to the family, for example) can be protective of the surviving family members.

Beyond communicating honestly about their prognosis and what the children may expect in the foreseeable future, parents and children often benefit from considering those things they will want to have said to one another. Parents can be helped to identify those adults who will help their children to lovingly remember the deceased parent. They may want to invite special individuals to be involved in specific aspects of their children's future, such as the mother who designated a female friend who will help a daughter shop for clothes for important events. This is not giving responsibility for their child to any one person, rather it creates a living legacy for a child, who can grow up surrounded by a community of loving adults who are dedicated to their health and happiness. A terminally ill parent may be comfortable anticipating future special events and writing letters for their children. One activity that is often emotionally meaningful and possible even with limited energy is for an ill parent to go through photos with their family, remembering details and dates about the photos that can then be recorded in an album by a spouse or their children. Imagining a future that they will not be a part of is likely to be painful, but parents are also greatly relieved to have the chance to imagine, discuss and plan for this with the support and guidance of an experienced clinician.

PACT: The Practical Approach

Each clinician who does this work develops their own specific and consistent approach for a PACT consultation. This is emotional material. It is organizing for clinicians to have a prepared approach so that they are more fully available to help parents manage their affect. Indeed, parents in turn use this same strategy. Parents who have used the PACT program often comment that it was particularly helpful for them to gather specific phrases to use as they speak and listen to their children about their own cancer diagnosis and treatment. Thus, what follows are some details about our "typical" approach, including specific questions and typical recommendations.

Often when a PACT consultation is requested and scheduled, we will ask for the parents' ages and for the medical diagnosis of the patient and name of the referring clinician. We will ask for the children's ages and whether there is any specific question or concern that the parents have. If possible, the PACT clinician will try to speak with the referring clinician to learn a few more details about the referral, including the patient's treatment plan and prognosis and any special concerns or observations that the clinician may have. We typically recommend that both parents come to the initial consultation, or try to make an inpatient visit when the healthy parent will also be at the hospital. If there are other primary caregivers (a grandparent, a nanny), we may invite that person to participate in the

consultation, as well. We explain that they do not need to bring their children and describe the *parent guidance* nature of our program.

Step 1: Learn about the Parents

After introducing ourselves and the PACT program, we usually begin by asking several introductory questions of the parents. We learn where they live, who lives in the home and what kind of work each parent may do. We often ask about where they are in the process of diagnosis and treatment, so as to be sure we have an accurate appreciation of their understanding. Finding out about *their understanding* of the treatment plan and prognosis is helpful in ensuring that we fully understand the presenting situation. It is helpful to inquire about how the process is going for them, and what they may have found especially difficult. Finally, we will ask about their children's understanding of what is going on currently. As we are speaking with them, we pay attention to their style of communicating with each other, their apparent strengths and vulnerabilities, and their observable level of maturity.

Step 2: Learn about the Children and their Specific Concerns

Once we have learned about what they have told their children (or not told them), we will ask about their children: their ages, temperaments, level of maturity, strengths, and vulnerabilities. We often will ask parents to tell us an anecdote about each child that really captures their personality in order to help us get a detailed picture. We will inquire about how the children get along with each other, about who provides child care for young children or in afterschool hours. We ask who are the other important adults in the lives of their children. We ask about where the children are in school and how they are doing academically and socially. If it has not come up already, we will ask if any of their children has any special medical problems or has been in psychiatric treatment. If they have not volunteered it, we will then ask the parents about how they expect each child will manage their illness. Will they be highly anxious, needing a lot of reassurance? Will they "not get it"? Will they shrug it off and focus on their friends, homework or hobbies? In sketching out a detailed picture of what they expect from each child, parents may discover that they expect their children to cope quite effectively with their illness and treatment. If not, they help the PACT clinician get a nuanced idea of what they are most concerned about, so that we might address their specific apprehensions.

Step 3: Learn About how they have Faced Previous Challenges

The PACT clinician will ask about whether the family has faced any specific challenges in the past, and how they have managed them. Many families, reeling from a cancer diagnosis, will say no, as few problems will seem in the same league as their illness. Still, we inquire. We might clarify this by asking about any other medical problems in a child, parent, grandparent or other close relative. In particular, we will ask if they have faced cancer before, either in a close friend or family member or in the community, where the children might have heard and thought about it. Asking about cancer is especially important, as it may illuminate some of the parents' and children's assumptions about the illness they are facing now.

If they have not faced a medical crisis as a family, we might ask if they have experienced financial difficulties, loss of a job or other related dislocations. Even "normal" problems, such as a child's brief school refusal or troubles with bedtime or a basement flood can be instructive. We may inquire how their family approaches decisions or problems in general: Do they have a family meeting? Do the parents discuss and plan privately? Are their discussions measured or lively? In asking these questions, we are learning about the family's style of coping with stress and also reminding them that they have managed challenging situations before. Although these may seem far removed from the challenge they are currently facing, the skills and principles they brought to (or from) those earlier challenges may be very valuable now.

Step 4: Learn about their Supports

Who is in the parents' support system? Details are very important here. It is informative to find out who was the first person they called when they learned the news of their diagnosis. Who has been the most helpful to them? Is there someone, besides their spouse, who has come to appointments, been calming and reassuring? Is there someone who has already been organizing the response of family members or members of the community? Are there supports they have not used before (through work, their children's school, religious community, etc.)? Of the supports they are using, are there some that present their own challenges (i.e., a supportive grandparent who is also highly anxious or emotional)? It is especially helpful for parents to think about delegating specific aspects of support to different individuals or groups. Who might disseminate information to family members? Who can provide back-up childcare?

Who might be able to drive children to school or soccer practice? Who might coordinate meals from well-wishing neighbors? Who might go to doctor's appointments in case the spouse needs to be at work? Once again, it is valuable for the clinician to have a sense of the family's support network. It is even more valuable for the parents to begin thinking about all of the resources they have available to them, and how best to utilize them during this time.

Step 5: Education about What is Expectable from their Children

Armed with information about the parent's diagnosis and the childrens' ages and temperaments, the PACT clinician can offer their thoughts about what responses the parents might expect from their children to their illness and treatment. We use our knowledge of normal child development and the information we have gathered about these parents' individual children to talk about those normal, healthy responses they can expect and also what red flags the parents might look out for (Table 21.1) We discuss what their individual children are likely to be able to understand and what changes they may be most sensitive to. We emphasize the child's age, temperament and any specific strengths or vulnerabilities we have learned about. This usually leads into a discussion of strategies the parents can use to promote their children's best possible adjustment.

Step 6: Strategies and Scripts

Once we have learned about the medical situation, the parents' style of communication and the children's ages and personalities, we focus on specific strategies to facilitate the family's best possible adjustment to the challenge of a parent's illness. We utilize what we have learned about a particular family, emphasizing our guiding principles. Throughout, the emphasis is on practical suggestions regarding the family's existing supports and identifying and utilizing those parenting skills they already have (Table 21.2). If parents have not been able to tell their children about a diagnosis, we will begin there, trying to better understand their concerns and develop a plan that will address them. Often, simply reassuring parents that children will feel less anxious with information that explains changes they have already noticed prompts these parents to want to speak more honestly with their children. Then we will focus on helping the parents find language that enables them to approach this conversation with greater calm and confidence. If they are speaking honestly with their children, we will consider strategies to

Table 21.1 Typical responses to parent's illness.

Ages	Typical responses to a parent's illness
Infants and toddlers (0–2 years)	• unable to understand or appreciate details of diagnosis, prognosis or treatment planning • sensitive to disruptions in routine or changes in caregivers • behavioral regression (fussiness, difficulty with separations or bedtime)
Preschoolers (3–6 years)	• limited ability to appreciate the details of diagnosis, prognosis and treatment planning • "magical thinking" makes these children vulnerable to misunderstanding and self-blame • even with understanding, may require repeated explanations, given shortened sense of time • disconnection between content and affect (they may be very weepy about small frustrations, and calm or silly when discussing the illness) • themes of illness may become present in their play • sensitive to changes in routines and rules: suspended limits and extra treats can paradoxically worsen behavior
School-age children (7–12 years)	• cognitively able to understand and appreciate most details of a diagnosis, prognosis and treatment planning • understanding will be concrete: may have more difficulty with nuance and uncertainty • lack emotional maturity, so especially prone to anxiety around illness • may seek extensive information to master their anxiety (wanting to visit the hospital, see a surgical scar, etc.) • may become preoccupied with the unfairness of illness • sensitive to the ways an illness may impact their ability to participate and perform in their normal activities (school and hobbies) • cope by doing things, either related to the illness or established activities • may swing between apparent distress and happy engagement in normal activities • may have difficulty articulating strong or difficult feelings
Adolescents (13–18 years)	• fully capable of understanding and appreciating the details of diagnosis, prognosis and treatment planning, including the uncertainty • may turn to friends and other important adults as primary sources of support • may seem very selfish to parents as they fail to pitch in the way parents may expect • may be prone to impulsive risk-taking behavior to manage their distress • prone to guilt and unhappiness as the demands of a parent's illness are at odds with normal developmental tasks • young adults may be less eager to pursue greater independence in this setting

further cultivate a climate of open communication, so none feel forced to speak but all feel included. We will emphasize practical steps that will maximize the parents' and children's support systems, protect children's routines and consider ways for the parents to take good care of themselves. It is impossible to detail all of the questions or scenarios that might arise; this is why it is helpful to have skilled mental health clinicians with special knowledge of child development and the particular strains of medical illness to meet with families and provide individualized guidance. Nonetheless, there are several questions or concerns that come up routinely and deserve special consideration.

Table 21.2 Parenting tips.

Ages	Parenting tips
Infants and toddlers (0–2 years)	• prioritize having consistency in caregivers, at least a predictable schedule of caregivers • create a detailed schedule and instructions re. routines (favorite foods, bedtime routines, etc.) for substitute caregivers to minimize disruptions • maximize opportunities for meaningful time with ill parent, even if it represents a change in routine: make a time for reading together or snuggling when parent feels best, etc.
Preschoolers (3–6 years)	• prioritize consistency in routines, limits, rules and expectations, especially across caregivers • inform other caregivers (preschool teachers, babysitters, etc.) about illness and treatment and child's understanding of it • provide repeated, clear, age-appropriate explanations of what is occurring, especially relating to what the child may be observing • listen for evidence of misunderstandings about the illness or treatment (in discussions, play, etc.) • expect some behavioral regression, manage it with patience and consistent limits
School-age children (7–12 years)	• provide ample opportunities to ask questions and gather information related to illness or treatment • provide opportunities to help at home • prioritize consistency in school and activities (sports, hobbies, etc.) • identify a "point-person" at school to help protect routines while providing emotional support • respect a child's established coping style ("talkers" vs. "do-ers"), but remind them to "never worry alone" • expect distress around unfairness; discussions should acknowledge unfairness and disappointment while providing reassurance and hope • talk about difficult feelings when opportunities arise • watch for signs of intense anxiety
Adolescents (13–18 years)	• provide honest, accurate, timely information and updates about the diagnosis and treatment plans • do not be surprised by concerns that seem selfish ("how will I pay for college?") • give permission for adolescents to speak about the illness with other trusted adults • clearly define any additional expectations of them during this time, limit these if at all possible • identify those adults that might help with important responsibilities and deadlines (SATs, college applications, etc.): "point-person" at school, best friend's parent, etc. • provide opportunities to discuss concerns about practical decisions (money, where to attend college, etc.) that may be affected by the illness • be vigilant for increased risk-taking behavior and do not hesitate to refer for professional evaluation and support • be vigilant for signs that "moodiness" may actually be a mood disorder (deteriorating function at school, withdrawal from friends), and refer for appropriate treatment

PACT: Common Challenges

How Do I Tell My Children?

Whether parents are looking to tell their children about a new diagnosis or about a recurrence or progression of their illness, they often are hoping for guidance on how to speak with their children so as to be both honest and reassuring. Helping parents to prepare for this conversation can be reassuring and organizing, so that they can be calm and clear as well as able to listen to their children. The PACT clinician may start by suggesting that it is best for both parents to be together for this conversation, and that they decide on what they are going to say beforehand (if they are not both present at the consultation). We suggest that it is ideal to tell all of their children at the same time, even if they are of different ages or levels of maturity. This delivers the message that information is being openly shared within the family, and that they are able to face this as a family. It also can create a lot of distress and conflict at a later time if one child learns that another was told first. That said, if it will be difficult to gather the whole family for a meeting, then we would recommend telling the children in sequence. In the time it may take the whole family to gather, there can be a growing worry that something terrible has happened. The goal of the conversation is to lower anxiety, not to increase it. We also often recommend that the discussion take place at home at a time when there isn't pressure to go somewhere soon after. In this way the children are able to retreat to their rooms if they need to be alone, but will still have access to their parents if they want to ask questions or seek comfort.

In considering the specific language parents should use, the PACT clinician emphasizes the importance of not using euphemisms (such as "lump" for cancer). It can be helpful to suggest that any language the children might overhear from adult conversations or phone calls should also be used with their children. Then it is important that parents consider their child's developmental stage and what they will be able to understand. The youngest children can comfortably hear the word cancer as the label for the current challenge. They will then need to know what this illness will mean to their day-to-day routines in the coming days or weeks. School-age children will likely want more detailed information about the nature of the illness and the details of the planned treatments. An effective strategy is to begin by asking about what the children may already know or may have noticed. These observations provide a starting point for the parents' explanation of what the family is facing. The clinician can be helpful in thinking with parents about what their individual children are likely to be able to understand and to

want to know, so that they can be reasonably prepared. Finally, the PACT clinician will help parents to use language that feels like the parents' own, familiar and comfortable, while still age-appropriate and accurate. Prepared with a plan and some specific language, parents can approach a conversation that they may have felt emotional or anxious about with greater calm and confidence. With this preparation, parents can be relaxed, reassuring and more available to their children.

What Happens If I Cry?

Many parents worry that when discussing their diagnosis, treatment or prognosis, they will cry in front of their children, causing more fear or worry. It is valuable to find out if the concerned parent tends to cry easily or not. Parents should acknowledge the fact that they are crying and that they are crying because they wish this weren't happening. It is constructive for children to hear that it is okay to cry when things happen that are sad or worrisome. But they should also acknowledge their hopes and that they are confident that the family will be able to manage this challenge. It is possible to acknowledge sadness while demonstrating that there will still be happiness and hope.

They Aren't Talking About It. Is that Normal?

Creating a climate at home in which communication is open and honest is not the same as requiring children to speak. Once parents have conveyed to their child that they are available and interested in the child's thoughts, it is usually best to let the child initiate discussions. It is also important to respect a child's style of coping and communicating. Some children are talkers and will want to speak with their parents often, whereas others may cope by getting busier with homework or hobbies. What is important is that they are updated with important developments, especially things they are likely to notice, and that they know not to worry alone. It is worthwhile for parents to consider when and where their children are most likely to talk: bedtime, bath time, while cooking dinner or in the car on the way to school. Then at these times, parents can give updates if there is anything to share, and they can "check in" to see if their child has any questions or concerns. Again, there is no right amount of talking, but children should be regularly reminded to never worry alone. Parents might even remind their children of the other adults they can ask questions of, within the family, community or school. If they are addressing their worries only with peers or with Google searches, then they are prone to misinformation and heightened anxiety.

Why Isn't My Adolescent Helping At All?

Parents of adolescents often express frustration that their child seems especially selfish during this challenging time. Parents facing the disruptions of a serious illness would like to be able to lean on their adolescent children for more help with errands, chores, babysitting or driving. It can be constructive to remind parents that while adolescents may be able to appreciate the seriousness of the situation and the ways in which they could be helpful, they are not yet adults. Adolescents are busily working on intimacy, their identity, impulse control and independence. These developmental tasks usually necessitate that adolescents spend more time away from their family while knowing that their family is available to them. Being pulled back into the family by a serious illness can pose a great challenge for them: it is at odds with their pressing needs, but they will feel incredibly guilty if they do not put aside their needs and help. Parents can still make requests for more help, but these should be carefully thought out. In particular, parents should be reminded that responding punitively to their adolescent's "selfishness," will likely make this situation more difficult for their child and may increase the risk of conflict or depression.

Can They Visit In The Hospital?

Parents will often present with practical questions, such as whether their child should visit them in the hospital or be allowed to see where their parent will get chemo. In approaching these questions, it is essential to first consider what the child will likely see in any of these settings. Provided it is logistically feasible and not objectively frightening (seeing a parent who is delirious, for example), it is best to then find out if their child is interested in visiting their parent in a hospital, ICU, hospice, etc. If they are, then it is critical that their parent or other loving adult describes honestly what a visit will be like: the sounds, the things they might see and the way their ill parent may seem (if sedated, or unable to get out of bed). If a child still wants to visit, they should be encouraged and reassured that they are allowed to change their mind at any time. There should be enough adults (for young children) present at the visit, so that if one changes their mind right before or during the visit, they can be accompanied to the gift shop or café while their other parent and siblings can complete their visit. If a child decides that they don't want to visit, they should be provided with reassurance that their parent still knows how much they love them. The child may want to find a different way to feel connected to that parent, with a phone call or a handmade card, for example. If there is something special that they wish to say, then they might write (or dictate) a letter that their other parent can read. The critical factor is that the child has a choice, but no obligation, and that they are provided with the most comfortable way to show their love and feel connected to their ill parent.

What If They Ask If I'm Going To Die?

This is the question that parents are usually the most anxious about having to face from their children. Indeed, it is often a question they have anxiously been asking themselves. It can be useful to start by asking about the parent's sense of their prognosis. In cases where it is early in the process, and the prognosis is likely to be good given what is already known, then we help parents to devise an answer that feels both reassuring and honest. They may be comfortable with a statement such as, "I want to be here for a long time and my doctors have told me that they are confident that they will be able to treat this cancer so that I can be." Parents should be reminded to explore whether their child has another worry underlying this question. A child's underlying concern may be quite easily addressed, and both parents and children will be greatly relieved.

If the situation is one in which a parent's prognosis is considerably worse, it is important to be honest but also reassuring and leaving room for hope. Some parents will say that their illness is serious, acknowledging that the cancer may end their lives. But they acknowledge also that they intend to work with their doctors to have the longest, healthiest life they can. They also might find a way to observe that there are many loving adults surrounding them and that no matter what happens the family will be alright. It can again be useful to find out if their children have specific worries about what might happen if a parent dies. Often these children will be worried about their other parent's health. Although these are difficult conversations, children can benefit greatly from the chance to talk about their sadness and fears. They can get comfort, reassurance and some acknowledgment that while uncertainty is very difficult, it is still possible to be engaged and happy in daily life.

How Do I Tell My Children That I'm Going To Die?

If an illness has become terminal, many parents will wish to protect their children from painful news and will postpone telling them. This strategy is understandable, but there is the risk of children overhearing something or feeling isolated and worried as their parents seem distant and sad. When time with their parent may be limited, it becomes important that children have the opportunity to think about what they may want to say or do with that parent. Often, they may simply want to be with and comforted by their parents.

In considering how to approach this discussion, the challenge is again to find a way for the parents to be honest and yet leave room for appropriate hope, so that the time remaining might have joy and happiness in it.

The PACT clinician will start by determining what the children already know. Is this going to be a shock or has there been a long struggle with a serious illness already? Has uncertainty about the parent's future health been part of the ongoing discussion with the children? We discuss the family's previous losses and religious beliefs to help parents think about their own context for understanding death, anticipating likely questions and possible responses. Helping parents find language they are comfortable with that will also be developmentally appropriate is again practical and organizing. Often parents find language that emphasizes the concrete and faultless nature of what they are facing: "The doctors say that we have done everything we could to fight this illness, but the illness is simply too strong and my body can't fight anymore." They can typically then follow their children's lead, answering their specific questions or simply providing love and comfort. We try to help parents anticipate their children's specific questions, such as time frame, type of death, or custody questions, so they have some chance to think about their responses. The question of "when" often comes up, and we suggest that parents speak in terms of their children's calendar: "the doctors aren't sure, but they think mommy might not be alive by the time you go back to school." It is important to remind children that there is no certainty. The need to offer children some sense of what to expect is weighed against the possibility of having children who are watching the calendar waiting for a dreaded date to arrive.

We also try to help parents think about those things that they especially want their children to hear, know or have from them. What a parent hopes that a child will learn and hold onto must often be said repeatedly, and may need to be entrusted to other adults who will remain available to the children after their parent is gone. The most essential thing that a parent can say to their child if time is limited is that they are deeply loved and why they are loved, those exquisite details that their parent treasures about them. Focusing on the love that exists often helps make meaning and provide comfort during a very sad time in a family's life.

Will My Child Need Therapy?

The great majority of children will neither need nor seek treatment during the course of a parent's illness. Even for those children who lose a parent to an illness, only 20–30% will develop symptoms that will require psychiatric referral within one year of a parent's death, a substantial number, but still a minority. Having the opportunity to meet with a PACT clinician can provide parents with reassurance about their child's well-being while also helping parents to do everything they can to protect their child's well-being. There are some situations, though, in which a psychiatric referral may be helpful or necessary.

High Conflict Families

When there is extensive conflict between the parents or one parent and their in-laws, it can exacerbate the anxieties and disruptions caused by a parent's illness. Should there be a parental loss in a family like this, it may be difficult for the children to grieve with the surviving adults. In this case, it can be protective for a therapist to get involved with the children early, even when the parent is ill, so that they might provide a place for the child to grieve and lovingly remember the deceased parent without the hostility or ambivalence of their family. This is similarly important when there is estrangement between an adolescent and an ill or dying parent. This particular adolescent will benefit from the opportunity to acknowledge the love that is there despite the conflict. If the healthy parent cannot help them do this, then a psychiatric referral can be effective.

Signs of Depression

If a child of an ill or dying parent develops signs of depression and shows impairment in their function in at least two domains (home, academics, friendships), it is a good idea to refer for a psychiatric evaluation. Any child or adolescent who displays dangerous behaviors or expresses suicidal wishes should be referred for a psychiatric evaluation. Adolescents demonstrating increased risky behaviors or substance abuse, or withdrawal from friends and interests may benefit from a psychiatric evaluation. If the healthy (or surviving) parent likewise demonstrates signs and symptoms of depression, especially if these may be affecting their ability to care for their children, they should be offered a referral for a psychiatric evaluation.

Conclusion

A life-threatening illness in a parent will be a difficult, stressful experience for a family with dependent children, but it does not need to be a traumatic one. With guidance from clinicians with knowledge of child development, mental health, parenting and medical illnesses, parents can recognize those skills they already have and plan ways to manage this challenge as a family. Indeed, with this strategic support and guidance, this experience can even be one that helps develop resilience within a family, and in the children in particular. Ideally then, every cancer center would have specially trained clinicians who could provide this guidance to their patients who are also parents. Finding such clinicians and securing funding or reimbursement for this care have been significant barriers to providing this service for patients. This chapter represents recognition that there may be a resource already in place in many hospitals that could begin to provide this service. With a relatively small investment in education, clinicians already providing services to families affected by a child's illness could become available to do consultations to their hospital's cancer centers (or ICUs, Emergency Departments, etc.). Such clinicians could also provide education to others at their institutions (social workers, nurses, palliative care physicians, oncologists) that typically deal only with adults, but are eager to expand their clinical skills to be able to address the parenting concerns of their patients. With a relatively small investment of time, there is potential to make a great difference in the quality of life of many families, even to protect the mental health of many children, children who might otherwise be overlooked.

See Appendix B, Additional Resources, for an introduction to the many resources that are publicly available for families.

References

1. National Cancer Institute. *National Health Interview Survey*. Bethesda, MD: National Cancer Institute, Division of Cancer Control and Population Sciences, Office of Cancer Survivorship, 1992.
2. Weaver KE, Rowland JH, Alfano CM, McNeel TS. Parental cancer and the family. *Cancer*, 2010;**116**:395–4401. doi: 10.1002/cncr.25368.
3. Dowdney L. Childhood bereavement following parental death. *Journal of Child Psychology and Psychiatry* 2004;**41**:819–830.
4. Centers for Disease Control and Prevention. Mental health in the United States: prevalence of diagnosis and medication treatment for attention-deficit/hyperactivity disorder– United States, 2003. *Morbidity and Mortality Weekly Report* 2005;**54**:842–847.
5. Welch AS, Wadsworth ME, Compas BE. Adjustment of children and adolescents to parental cancer. Parents' and children's perspectives. *Cancer* 1996;**77**:1409–1418.
6. Grabiak BR, Bender CM, Puskar KR. The impact of parental cancer on the adolescent: an analysis of the literature. *Psychooncology*. 2007;**16**:127–137.
7. Osborn T. The psychosocial impact of parental cancer on children and adolescents: a systematic review. *Psychooncology*. 2007;**16**:101–126.
8. Siegel K, Mesagno FP, Karus D, *et al.* Psychosocial adjustment of children with a terminally ill parent. *American Academy of Child and Adolescent Psychiatry* 1992;**31**:327–333.

22

Collaborations in Psychosocial Care in Pediatric Oncology: the Middle East as a Case Example

Aziza T. Shad, Maria E. McGee, Matthew G. Biel, Michael Silbermann

Introduction

Pediatric psycho-oncology and pediatric oncology are concurrently evolving subspecialties around the world. In the past, physicians had little option but to focus on thanatology due to the lack of resources in each subspecialty. These focal points are now emerging. However, there exists a significant geographic inequality in the focus of these two interconnected subspecialties between developed (high-income) and developing (middle- and low-income to extreme poverty) countries. In developed countries, these are beginning to focus on the psychosocial, behavioral, physical, spiritual, and existential dimensions of pediatric cancer patients, their parents/caregivers, and their families [1]. At the same time, developing countries often lack the needed financial and clinical resources or have different priorities for the evolution of these subspecialties and other areas of medicine. The advancement of interdisciplinary collaboration and coordination of pediatric oncological care in many developed countries might serve as a possible model for change in developing countries. International collaborations and partnerships between developed and developing countries might help ameliorate significant mental and physical health care disparities in developing countries and contribute fresh cultural insights to developed countries.

Pediatric Cancer in Developed Countries

In developed countries there has been a drastic increase in the survival rates of youth with cancer. There is extensive knowledge about pediatric cancer incidence in many of these countries due to established high-quality population-based registries [2]. In these countries nearly 80% of children and adolescents currently diagnosed with cancer are predicted to be long-term survivors [3]. This is due to progress in medical, radiation, immunological, and surgical oncological interventions, increased interdisciplinary collaboration and coordination of pediatric oncological care, and psychosocial and economic support for affected families [4–8].

With this progress, adverse psychosocial outcomes have often emerged primarily due to the long-term and daily stressors of survival [9]. During and after oncological treatment, youngsters often experience psychological, social, behavioral, and physical challenges [10]. Persistent psychosocial stressors, such as those found in pediatric cancer, are more likely than acute stressors to predispose youth to develop mental disorders [9]. This has somewhat shifted the focus of pediatric oncology in developed countries from a palliative intent to a curative one. It has reoriented pediatric psycho-oncology from concerns related to the impact of impending death to the impact on the quality of life for youth and their families during and after treatment [5, 11].

Pediatric Cancer in Developing Countries

In developing countries, where nearly 80% of the world's children live, pediatric survival rates are significantly inferior to those in developed countries. Despite the fact that pediatric cancers today are highly treatable, it is estimated that only about 25% survive in developing countries because of inadequate medical access, the lack of appropriate medical care, and the lack of the financial resources to develop and

Pediatric Psycho-oncology: Psychosocial Aspects and Clinical Interventions, Second Edition.
Edited by Shulamith Kreitler, Myriam Weyl Ben-Arush and Andrés Martin.
© 2012 John Wiley & Sons, Ltd. Published 2012 by John Wiley & Sons, Ltd.

implement these [3, 12, 13]. Over 60% of the world's pediatric cancer patients have limited or no access to effective oncological treatment [8]. Over 85% of pediatric cancer cases occur in developing countries that use less than 5% of the world's resources. In developing countries, pediatric cancer is generally diagnosed when it is at a relatively advanced stage. Supportive care is inevitably required for successful treatment of pediatric cancer. There have been improved survival rates in pediatric cancer patients receiving treatment protocols in major pediatric cancer treatment centers compared to children who received treatment outside of those centers [14]. In developing countries the challenge is how to bring modern comprehensive pediatric cancer treatment as well as the accompanying need for sub-specialties focused on psychosocial issues.

Industrialized countries generally have the most complete cancer registry data, whereas developing countries often lag far behind. Less is known about pediatric cancer and mortality rates in developing countries; data are lacking in these countries, including those in the Middle East. These countries also suffer from demographic reporting errors often due to complex and elusive factors such as long-standing political strife, military conflict, inaccurate death certificates, misdiagnosis, under-reporting, and the universal challenge of meeting the basic needs of the poor of the Earth for food, water, sanitation, shelter, jobs, and universal medical care [3, 13, 15].

In some parts of developing and developed countries, the absence of an adequate public health infrastructure, high fertility rates, high overall mortality rates in children, poverty, and low childhood cancer cure rates make the question of the availability of relatively sophisticated psychosocial supports for young cancer survivors a conundrum [12]. The profound realities surrounding poverty and extreme poverty make any solution for improvement in mental and physical health care interventions in developing countries even more complex [13].

The Reality of Childhood Poverty in Developing Countries: An Impediment to Psycho-Oncological Care

Extreme poverty serves as a major impediment to appropriate pediatric oncological and psycho- oncological care. External psychosocial needs of impoverished families and their children are likely to be placed on the backburner for needs that require more immediate attention such as food, shelter, education, and standard childhood immunizations. Although extreme poverty can gnaw away at and even devour hope, one of the most vibrant resources in developing countries is the strength of family life and a strong sense of social connectedness. The immediate and extended family plays a strong central role for psychological, social, spiritual, and economic support. In developed countries, the nuclear family predominates, although frequently fractured, and extended family bonds tend to be more tenuous. In developing countries the extended family encompasses a more inclusive and broader definition of "family" than in developed countries. Thus, a family-centered approach to psychosocial and oncological care in developing countries is paramount.

Psychosocial Morbidity and Care for Pediatric Cancer Patients and Their Families

Pediatric cancer is a repetitive and chronic trauma for children/adolescents and their families. It is often a highly stressful, anguish-laden, and burdensome experience somewhat like all psychiatric disorders in youth. It thereby elicits a range of adaptive to maladaptive coping strategies. As a trauma, it impacts on the psychological, social, behavioral, and spiritual domains of youth and their families sometimes with nearly the same vengeance as it bears on their physical health. This places youth and their families at significant risk for a range of short- and long-term psychological, social, behavioral, and spiritual sequelae. Thus, early identification and intervention within the context of family-centered care might diminish or even prevent a lifetime of emotional suffering for these youth and their families [16].

Pediatric psycho-oncology addresses issues related to how youngsters and their families cope with and adapt to the many stressors they might encounter. These could be caused by a range of possibilities such as: (1) the diagnosis of a pediatric cancer as a life-threatening illness; (2) its ensuing life-prolonging treatments (with possible surgical resection, chemotherapy, radiation therapy, or other life-prolonging modalities of care); (3) palliative measures; (4) changes in a youth's level of functioning in multiple domains; (5) reintegration of post-treatment youth back into their schools; (6) family implications of cancer; (7) survivorship/remission; (8) relapses; or (9) the still possible process of dying due to the cancer. Thus, pediatric psycho-oncology essentially addresses the neuropsychiatric sequelae of pediatric cancer along with improving pediatric cancer patients' psychosocial needs of both pediatric oncology patients and their families within a developmental framework [1, 17].

The psychosocial needs of these young patients and their families should be integrated into the pediatric oncological treatment plan, the same as other special-ties involved in pediatric oncological care. This requires encouraging the incorporation of psycho-oncological education into clinical pediatric oncology practice. Pediatric health care providers are in a unique position to identify and help manage psychosocial issues early on. For example, the American Academy of Pediatrics (AAP) has recognized this need in their practice guidelines and has recommended that all pedi-atric oncology patients be treated at major pediatric cancer treatment centers with available psychosocial resources including the availability of child and adoles-cent psychiatrists [18].

A comprehensive interdisciplinary approach to pedi-atric cancer with psychosocial support services from the onset of diagnosis is generally readily available in devel-oped countries and is often unavailable in developing countries, especially in the more marginalized and devalued areas. In developing countries, the availability and accessibility to major pediatric cancer treatment centers, developmentally appropriate mental health care, and other psychosocial resources are at best, limited, and, at worst, non-existent. The most common pathways to care are often rudimentary and include vil-lage health workers, health workers in marginalized urban neighborhoods, traditional healers, nurses, or primary care clinics. Many children and families tend to visit traditional healers prior to visiting a pediatric hospital center [13, 19]. The challenge in such realities is to find ways to support and improve present resources as well as to develop direct access to specialized services in major pediatric cancer treatment centers.

The primary barriers to appropriate psycho-social care in developing countries include: (1) a paucity of resources for child and adolescent mental health treat-ment services; (2) inadequate training and educational programs for mental health care professionals; (3) inadequate mental health training of general practi-tioners and traditional healers, contributing to low rates of detection; (4) a lack of well-organized primary mental health care; (5) a lack of secure funds and gov-ernmental support; (6) a lack of transportation and communication services in rural and urban areas; (7) an irrational fear of the use of opioids in professio-nals and in the public; (8) low awareness of available mental health services; (9) inadequate links between services; (10) a lack of knowledge among urban and rural populations about the causes of and treatments for mental disorders resulting in the underutilization of mental health services; (11) a lack of treatment and referral of mental disorders in traditional and primary care settings; (12) a failure of mental health services to actively identify cases in the community and local hospitals; and (13) a lack of awareness and understand-ing of palliative care needs at public, governmental, and professional levels. In developing countries, the paucity of mental health care resources is compounded by the imbalance of these resources between mental health services in rural settings and those in urban set-tings [13, 19]. The basic reality is how to deal with the question of children with cancer and their psychosocial needs when simultaneously flooded by the reality of malnourished and starving children.

The scarcity of child and adolescent mental health treatment services is a global problem. In developed countries there are problems of geographical mal-distribution of these resources and a great need for them in impoverished community settings. The pres-ence of child and adolescent psychiatrists is a relative rarity outside of developed countries and few are fully trained. For example, in most countries of the African, Eastern Mediterranean, Southeast Asian, and Western Pacific regions, the presence of a child and adolescent psychiatrist is most often in the range of 1 to 4 per mil-lion [20]. This is equally true in most developing coun-tries and needs to be taken into consideration when addressing the psychosocial needs of children and fam-ilies in developing countries.

Pediatric Cancer Pain: A Significant Psychosocial Stressor in Both Developed and Developing Countries

Uncontrolled pediatric cancer pain can have significant repercussions on a youth's quality of life. It is one of the most common symptoms among all cancer patients. Chronic cancer pain is a complex experience and results in significant psychosocial sequelae. Recent studies have concluded that pain appears in 30% of patients in the active stage of treatment, and in two-thirds of patients in advanced stages of cancer [21]. In developed countries, pain might be uncontrolled pri-marily because of physician-related barriers such as misinterpretation of symptoms, lack of identification, or the often extreme difficulty in treating it. In develop-ing countries, pain is often uncontrolled primarily because of restricted access to strong opioids for cancer patients due to excessive cost as well as a sometimes irrational fear of their use [22–24]. Pediatric health care providers need to be educated on the efficacious use of opioids. Global access to opioids is severely lim-ited secondarily to these barriers [25].

Pediatric cancer pain can be misinterpreted as a psychiatric symptom. When perceived as solely psychi-atric, it may be mistreated, undertreated, or even untreated. If any of these occur, it could give rise to various psychiatric symptoms such as anxiety or mood disturbances. Appropriate administration of analgesics can lessen or completely alleviate the "so-called" psychiatric symptoms along with the pain [22–24]. Pediatric health care provider education regarding the presentation of pediatric cancer pain in relation to both a youth's psychiatric symptoms and developmental level can enhance pediatric cancer pain control [22–24].

The Middle East as a Case Example

The Middle East serves as a case example of rampant geographic and socio-economic disparities in the psychosocial and physical needs of pediatric cancer patients and their families. This region is rich in great religions, cultures, philosophy, and science. Yet, it is also a region of great geopolitical furor with people who have endured military conflicts, bitter wars, political strife, torture, economic instability, social upheavals, internal displacement, natural and man-made calamities, and other forms of social injustice such as the devalorization of women. It is also a greatly impoverished region in which many women, men, and children lack access to essential social and medical services. Geographically, it encompasses the developing countries of Western Asia and Northern Africa where Africa, Asia and Europe sometimes intertwine harmoniously and at other times are at war. Opinions vary as to the precise definition of the Middle East. However, there is almost universal agreement that this region is the cradle of our civilization and impacts on religion, science, philosophy, literature, language, art, music, social sciences, archeology, anthropology, history, and medicine. It is the region where the great monotheistic religions had their origin: Judaism, Christianity, and Islam. Despite all of its richness and beauty, presently the resources for pediatric cancer care in the Middle East as a whole are not only inadequate and sparse, but are also directed almost exclusively to pediatric oncological treatment at the expense of not addressing the psychosocial needs of the child and his/her family [26, 27].

The Middle East, like most cultures in the developing world, is allocentric and gives preference to large support networks based on extended family bonds, and perhaps this strong source of support partially buffers Middle Eastern pediatric cancer patients and families against cancer-related stress; along with extended families, strong religious beliefs can effectuate a sense of hope and this in itself can support physical and spiritual healing [28]. Indeed, strong religious beliefs, especially when associated with a loving and embracing God, tend to lower the degree of depression and anxiety in cancer patients and their families [29]. In Middle Eastern communities spirituality can play a prominent role in helping cancer patients and their families cope with the reality of their illness. Physicians should recognize and honor this and integrate it into comprehensive pediatric oncological care.

Presently, the majority of pediatric oncology patients with psychosocial problems are diagnosed and treated by their oncologists rather than by mental health professionals. It is, therefore, important to increase the awareness of pediatric oncologists about the type of developmentally appropriate mental health services needed by patients and how to make them available to patients and their families. Social work professionals in these settings need to proactively develop ways to engage both the pediatric oncologists as well as their families in utilizing these services. The question of how best to integrate psychosocial care into routine cancer care still remains an issue, partly because of the possible stigma associated with cancer in many cultures, the simple lack of awareness of the accompanying psychosocial needs by family members or health workers who have never been able to access such support, or the lack of adequate financial resources to pay for such services [29].

In the Middle East, psychosocial care is increasing, partly due to international collaborative efforts. However, despite this, great disparity still exists in these countries. The treating physician faces many barriers in the management of psychosocial issues. Pediatric psycho-social services in the Middle East are in need of increased development support with child and adolescent psychiatrists and child psychologists, pediatric palliative medicine specialists, facilities, postgraduate education and formal training, opioid legislation and health care policies, negotiation for secure government health insurance with supportive funding provisions, direct access to needed services, and increasing public and professional awareness about the need for pediatric psychosocial services for these patients [19]. An example of a positive step occurred in June 2007, when the Children's Cancer Hospital in Cairo, Egypt, made available to Egyptian children modern pediatric oncology services along with facilities for the first specialized Departments of Social Work and Child and Adolescent Psychiatry. Such a step might serve as a model that other Middle Eastern countries could follow.

International Collaborations and Partnerships: The Middle East Cancer Consortium (MECC)

In developing countries, international collaborations and partnerships have been shown to enhance mental and physical health care. They bring oncological and psycho-oncological expertise and economic and human resources closer to pediatric cancer patients. They provide opportunities for the development of programs and approaches consistent with family-centered care with parent groups, sibling groups, and psychoeducational programs. The overall goals of these efforts are to establish earlier diagnosis, improve a patient's psychosocial and health outcomes, and increase both clinical and basic science research to enhance our understanding of the biological and psychosocial impact of cancer [13].

The Middle East Cancer Consortium (MECC) is a model of international collaboration and partnership for improved oncological care. It was established in May 1996 and is an intergovernmental organization with partnerships between the United States' National Cancer Institute (NCI) and the Ministries of Health of Cyprus, Egypt, Israel, Jordan, the Palestinian Authority, and since June 2004, the Republic of Turkey. MECC's central premise is to put aside any political and religious differences in order to effectively work together with common humanitarian goals [30]. Part of its goals are to help reduce mental health disparities by building mental health care and support services at the community level, to increase the scientific knowledge base, and to reduce the incidence and burden of cancer in the Middle East through the solicitation and support of collaborative research. MECC's overall purposes are to link oncological research and treatment, including its psychosocial dimensions, to share international expertise, to reduce unnecessary duplication of these efforts, and to try to maximize local, regional, and community resources. By doing this, it facilitates trust, participation, and cooperation throughout this tumultuous geopolitical region of the world in the shared campaign against cancer. Since its inception, MECC's major activities have been a Cancer Registry Project (CRP), a Small Grants Program, and a Palliative Care Project (PCP). In 2004, the NCI responded to a request from MECC representatives for support in developing palliative care in the region by initiating a MECC education and training program that specifically addressed these needs [19, 25, 31–33].

The Middle East Cancer Consortium (MECC) and Palliative Care

For the past five years, MECC has been involved in the development of pediatric palliative care programs in the MECC countries, with a special emphasis on

Table 22.1 Pediatric supportive and palliative care provision in MECC.

Pediatric services	Pediatric unit	Pediatric hospital support	Pediatric home care	Total
Cyprus	0	0	0	0
Egypt	0	0	0	0
Israel	1	5	1	7
Jordan	0	1	1	2
Palestinian Authority	0	2	0	2
Turkey	0	0	0	0
Total	1	8	2	11

Source: [19].

psychosocial issues relevant to the region. Following a regional needs assessment of palliative care services, MECC has been able to bring together pediatric oncologists/pediatricians, oncology nurses, social workers, psychologists and spiritual counselors through annual workshops designed to target and address relevant issues related to the delivery of palliative care in the region [28]. Table 22.1 summarizes the small number of or absence of pediatric supportive and palliative care services that were identified in the six participating MECC countries in 2005 [19].

Through the initiative and resources provided by MECC, a Palliative Care Steering Committee has taken the first steps to improve the availability of palliative care knowledge, skills, and services in the Middle East. Although in its infancy, MECC's objective in this project is to improve cancer pain management by changing pain management policy, ensuring analgesic availability, and increasing palliative care education as it relates to physical, psychosocial, emotional and spiritual care for childhood cancer patients and their families [34].

Workshops, almost all held in MECC countries, have been devoted to topics such as: Communication between Care Providers and Families, Stress and Burnout in Care Givers of Cancer Patients, Basics of Pain Management, Alleviation of Fear, Frustration and Sense of Loss through Non-Pharmacological Treatment Modalities, and Cancer Pain, Suffering and Spirituality. The faculty for these workshops are primarily from Israel, the USA, and Europe. All workshops, so far, have been conducted in English and involved didactic presentations, role-playing, and small interactive working groups comprised of members from different MECC countries. Follow-up evaluations from participants and other surveys revealed the following [35]:

(1) Pediatric oncology professionals are not always fully aware of the emotional impact on the family of a child diagnosed with cancer. However, this perception has changed significantly over the past five years.

(2) In most MECC countries, nurses and physicians are the main providers of psychosocial care. The lack of formal training in this area often results in poor communication with families on issues related to pain management and relaying news related to death and dying. Pediatric oncology professionals also experienced significant distress dealing with reactions and emotions of children with cancer and their families.

(3) Nurses generally spend the most time offering to support patients and families. Once a physician has communicated negative diagnostic and/or prognostic information to a patient and family, the nurse often becomes the primary social support. In fact, providing social support is an integral part of nursing care delivery. This makes them more vulnerable to difficult situations arising in clinical practice.

(4) The difference between the role of a social worker and a psychologist in providing psychosocial support is unclear to many health care providers and families. These roles need to be clearly defined.

(5) All pediatric oncology professionals agreed that psychosocial support and intervention is a much needed element in providing comprehensive care to patients and families.

(6) Pediatric oncology professionals seem to recognize that many families have difficulty asking for or availing of psychosocial support, perhaps because there is a stigma attached to it or it is difficult to ask for something that has not yet been experienced. Such support will evolve as health care workers define the place of psychosocial support in pediatric oncological care.

(7) Pain and symptom management play a major role in palliative care. Without the needed knowledge base, caregivers found it stressful to deal with pain and other symptom management.

(8) Pediatric oncology professionals also mentioned staff burnout and emotional stress as key negative outcomes in dealing with dying children and grief-stricken families. This has caused major turn-over in pediatric oncology units.

Pediatric oncology professionals reported that these workshops have fostered a better understanding of the problems they face. This seemed to transcend any religious and cultural differences.

Integrative Pediatric Oncology in the Middle East and the Role of MECC

Integrative pediatric oncology is a holistic approach in which complementary (and unconventional) modalities of care, such as nutrition, nutritional supplementation, energy therapies, aromatherapy, massage therapy, acupuncture, acupressure, music therapy, and mind-body techniques, work side-by-side with conventional modalities of pediatric oncological care, such as surgery, immunotherapy, chemotherapy, and radiation therapy. These approaches are of interest to many pediatric cancer patients and their families. A great number of them seek out and integrate complementary modalities of care while undergoing conventional treatments. They want to and need to explore every available option that might enhance treatment in the hope of boosting their immune system, relieving cancer pain, managing side-effects related to the disease or treatment, and providing psychosocial support for coping with the cancer diagnosis, treatment, and prognosis. Some use unconventional modalities in isolation in hope of a cure. This could subject a pediatric cancer patient to serious risk of harm if it diverts or delays him/her from receiving his/her imminently necessary conventional treatment. Some will desperately pursue a non-evidence-based option that has an infinitesimally small likelihood of positive outcomes because the gift they search for is of immeasurable worth. Most parents/caregivers want to and need to have a sense that they are doing everything possible to help their child be cured, alleviate his/her symptoms, or support him/her during cancer therapy. Integrative approaches provide this for them. In the Middle East, recitations from the Holy Qur'ān along with traditional remedies with herbal medicine are the leading complementary modalities of cancer care [29, 36–39]. Such incantations deserve respect, honor, and study.

In both developed and developing countries, many pediatric cancer centers and pediatric community practices routinely include integrative pediatric cancer care as part of a comprehensive oncological treatment model. This trend is strong in developing countries since these modalities are more readily accessible, have been handed down generation-to-generation, are generally less costly, and are frequently the only available option. However, research is still needed to evaluate the effects of different integrative treatment approaches on pediatric cancer patient outcomes. Not all complementary modalities of care are safe, appropriate, or useful to pediatric cancer patients. Even seemingly helpful complementary modalities of care might not be optimal under some circumstances since they might delay efficacious treatment or cause adverse effects or detrimental interactions with a protocol treatment. Their use among cancer patients varies according to geographical area, gender, disease diagnosis, and cultural beliefs and experiences. Pediatric health care providers need to be aware of these non-conventional modalities along with the evidence regarding their safety and effectiveness and routinely make inquiries of their patients about their possible use particularly for those with ongoing medical problems and those with parents/caregivers who themselves use alternative modalities of care [38].

When developed countries work in international collaborations to share ideas and technology with developing countries, it is imperative that they avoid the endorsement of unacceptable and sometimes deleterious alternative modalities of care. Yet, this should be done within a respectful cultural context and a willingness to study local practices. It is also important to increase the awareness of pediatric health care providers of appropriate and inappropriate alternative modalities of care [38]. The International Society of Pediatric Oncology has recommended that pediatric oncology health care professionals need to possess an awareness of complementary modalities of care that may be physically or psychologically harmful to children and their parents, as well as those that might produce positive therapeutic outcomes. At the same time, health care professionals should avoid any biased reactions that dismiss or discourage the use of non-harmful complementary modalities of care [40].

Indeed, psychosocial supportive practices should gather the fruits of other cultures such as mind–body medicine's interventional strategies. These are being successfully integrated in pediatric oncological patients in developing and developed countries. The concept of mindfulness is an ancient one based on the premise that the mental, emotional, physical, social, and spiritual aspects of a person's life directly influence a person's mental and physical health and well-being. Practicing mindfulness involves a concept of not being distracted by what has already occurred or what might occur. It is essentially an intentional and nonjudgmental state of being present in the here-and-now. The importance of the role of the mind, emotions, and behaviors in health and well-being is fundamental to traditional Chinese, Tibetan, and Ayurveda medicine, as well as other

medical traditions throughout the world. It is a step beyond the conventional industrialized nations' bio-medical model. Regular use of mindfulness practices have been shown to cultivate self-awareness and self-care and, thereby, promote health and well-being through practices such as meditation, relaxation techniques, guided imagery, and repetitive prayer. In pediatric cancer patients it has been specifically used to treat anxiety, mood disturbances, chronic cancer pain, procedural pain, insomnia, nausea, and stress. These have also been utilized to assist patients in practicing healthy coping skills and improving their quality of life. It is important to note that the role of stress in cancer is controversial. There is evidence showing the negative health consequences of sustained stress on health and well-being through profound psychological, behavioral, and physiologic effects. There is also evidence to suggest that chronic stress plays a role in disease progression and that it may contribute to overall mortality. There is no research on its use with children. There are few known risks associated with the use of mind–body techniques. Each time a pediatric patient feels the benefit of a technique they are using; they reinforce a sense of control over their own lives. This counters their feelings of hopelessness, helplessness, and despair [41]. It would be helpful to conduct research in these techniques, especially given the widespread poverty in the world, and attempt to validate which techniques might bring the most positive outcomes.

Conclusion

The primary objective of pediatric psycho-oncology and pediatric oncology in both developed and developing countries is to care for pediatric cancer patients and their families in a collaborative manner, with appropriate attention paid to both their physical and psychosocial needs. This involves the use of an integrative approach. Modern therapeutic strategies, adapted to the developing world's reality, are a primary necessity and can be effectively implemented through international collaborative efforts, including in countries with limited resources or in the throes of political strife.

Through the dynamic leadership and determination of Dr. Michael Silbermann, Executive Director of MECC, who consistently has faced obstacles and barriers to make the Palliative Care initiative a reality, MECC has successfully taken the first steps towards improving the quality of life for children in the Middle East and ameliorating significant mental and physical healthcare disparities in the MECC countries. More research and clinical training are needed to establish culturally sensitive, culturally-appropriate, and family rooted psychosocial support in the care and treatment of the region's youngsters with oncological needs.

References

1. Grassi L, Holland JC, Johansen C, Koch U, Fawzy F. Psychiatric concomitants of cancer, screening procedures, and training of health care professionals in oncology: the paradigms of psycho-oncology in the psychiatry field. In: Christodoulou GN (ed.) *Advances in Psychiatry: Vol. II.* Athens: Beta Publishing Athens, 2005; pp. 59–66.
2. Parkin DM, Whelan SL, Ferlay J, *et al.Cancer Incidence in Five Continents. Vol. VII (IARC Scientific Publications No. 143).* Lyon: International Agency for Research on Cancer, 1997.
3. Kellie SJ, Howard SC. Global child health priorities: what role for paediatric oncologists? *European Journal of Cancer* 2008;**44**:2388–2396.
4. Erickson SJ, Steiner H. Trauma spectrum adaptation: somatic symptoms in long-term pediatric cancer survivors. *Psychosomatics* 2000;**41**:339–346.
5. Last BF, Grootenhuis MA, Eiser C. International comparison of contributions to psychosocial research on survivors of childhood cancer: past and future considerations. *Journal of Pediatric Psychology* 2005;**30**:99–113.
6. *SEER Cancer Statistics Review, 1975–2008.* Bethesda, MD: National Cancer Institute. Available from: http://seer.cancer.gov/csr/1975_2008/, based on November 2010 SEER data submission, posted to the SEER web site, 2011.
7. van de Wetering MD, Schouten-van Meeteren NY. Supportive care for children with cancer. *Seminars in Oncology* 2011;**38**:374–379.
8. Ribeiro RC, Pui CH. Saving the children: improving childhood cancer treatment in developing countries. *New England Journal of Medicine* 2005;**352**:2158–2160.
9. Schrag NM, McKeown RE, Jackson KL, Cuffe SP, Neuberg RW. Stress-related mental disorders in childhood cancer survivors. *Pediatric Blood & Cancer* 2008; **50**:98–103.
10. Kersun LS, Kazak AE. Prescribing practices of selective serotonin reuptake inhibitors (SSRIs) among pediatric oncologists: a single institution experience. *Pediatric Blood & Cancer* 2006;**47**:339–342.
11. Detmar SB, Aaronson NK, Wever LD, *et al.* How are you feeling? Who wants to know? Patients' and oncologists' preferences for discussing health-related quality-of-life issues. *Journal of Clinical Oncology* 2000;**18**:3295–3301.
12. Howard SC, Metzger ML, Wilimas JA, *et al.* Childhood cancer epidemiology in low-income countries. *Cancer* 2008;**112**:461–472.
13. Usmani GN. Pediatric oncology in the third world. *Current Opinion in Pediatrics* 2001;**13**:1–9.
14. Yaris N, Mandiracioglu A, Büyükpamukcu M. Childhood cancer in developing countries. *Pediatric Hematology-Oncology* 2004;**21**:237–253.
15. Freedman LS, Barchana M, Al-Kayed S, *et al.* A comparison of population-based cancer incidence rates in Israel and Jordan. *European Journal of Cancer Prevention* 2003;**12**:359–365.

16. Erickson SJ, Gerstle M, Montague EQ. Repressive adaptive style and self-reported psychological functioning in adolescent cancer survivors. *Child Psychiatry and Human Development* 2008;**39**:247–260.
17. Patenaude AF, Kupst MJ. Psychosocial functioning in pediatric cancer. *Journal of Pediatric Psychology* 2005; **30**:9–27.
18. Corrigan JJ, Feig SA; American Academy of Pediatrics. Guidelines for pediatric cancer centers. *Pediatrics.* 2004;**113**:1833–1835.
19. Bingley A, Clark D. A comparative review of palliative care development in six countries represented by the Middle East Cancer Consortium (MECC). *Journal of Pain & Symptom Managment* 2009;**37**:287–296.
20. World Health Organization, World Psychiatric Association, International Association for Child and Adolescent Psychiatry and Allied Professions. *Atlas: Child and Adolescent Mental Health Resources: Global Concerns, Implications for the Future.* Geneva: World Health Organization, 2005.
21. Sapir R, Cherny NI. *Guide to Pain Management.* Available from: http://mecc.cancer.gov/MECCGuidePainManagement.pdf, 2010.
22. Glare P. Choice of opioids and the WHO Ladder. *Journal of Pediatric Hematology Oncology* 2011;**33**: Suppl 1: S6–S11.
23. Levetown M, American Academy of Pediatrics Committee on Bioethics. Communicating with children and families: from everyday interactions to skill in conveying distressing information. *Pediatrics* 2008;**121**:e1441–e1460.
24. Steif BL, Heiligenstein EL. Psychiatric symptoms of pediatric cancer pain. *Journal of Pain & Symptom Management* 1989;**4**:191–196.
25. Silbermann M. Opioids in Middle Eastern Populations. *Asian Pacific Organization Journal of Cancer Prevention* 2010; MECC Suppl 11 : S1–S5.
26. Daher M. Opioids for cancer pain in the Middle Eastern countries: a physician point of view. *Journal of Pediatric Hematology Oncology* 2011;**33**Suppl 1: S23–S28.
27. UNICEF. *UNICEF Humanitarian Action for Children, 2011: Building Resilience.* Available from: http://www.humansecuritygateway.com/documents/UNICEF_HumanitarianActionforChildren.pdf, 2011.
28. Silbermann M, Hassan EA. Cultural perspectives in cancer care: impact of Islamic traditions and practices in Middle Eastern countries. *Journal of Pediatric Hematology Oncology* 2011;**33**Suppl. 2: S81–S86.
29. Al Sudairy R, Al Omari A, Jarrar M, *et al.* Complementary and alternative medicine use among pediatric oncology patients in a tertiary care center, Riyadh, Saudi Arabia. Paper presented at the "Childhood Cancer and Blood Disorders: Achievements and Challenges Symposium," Post Graduate Center, King Faisal Specialist Hospital and Research Centre (KFSHRC). Riyadh, Saudi Arabia. Oct. 2011.
30. Silbermann M. *The Middle East Cancer Consortium: A Model for a Regional Cooperation Program. Health without Barriers in the Middle East.* Brookdale Institute: Joint Distribution Committee Middle East Program, 2003; pp. 23–30.
31. Silbermann M, *et al.* MECC Workshop on psycho-oncology: The role and involvement of the patient's family. *Journal of Pediatric Hematology Oncology* 2008;**30**:S1–17.

32. Silbermann M, *et al.* Workshop on the stresses and burnout of working with cancer patients, Larnaca, Cyprus, June 22–24 2007, A collection of abstracts. *Journal of Pediatric Hematology Oncology* 2008;**30**:98–115.

33. Silbermann M. Issues in pain management in cancer patients. *Journal of Pediatric Hematology Oncology* 2010; Suppl 32: S419–S439.

34. Moore SY, Pirrello RD, Christianson SK, Ferris FD. Strategic planning by the palliative care steering committee of the Middle East Cancer Consortium. *Journal of Pediatric Hematology Oncology* 2011;**33**Suppl 1: S39–S46.

35. Silbermann M, Khleif A, Tuncer M, *et al.* Can we overcome the effect of conflicts in rendering palliative care? An introduction to the Middle Eastern Cancer Consortium (MECC). *Current Oncology Reports* 2011;**13**:302–307.

36. Ben-Arye E, Ali-Shtayeh MS, Nejmi M, *et al.* Integrative oncology research in the Middle East: weaving traditional and complementary medicine in supportive care. *Support Care Cancer* 2011.

37. Bluebond-Langner M, Belasco JB, Goldman A, Belasco C. Understanding parents' approaches to care and treatment of children with cancer when standard therapy has failed. *Journal of Clinical Oncology* 2007;**25**:2414–2419.

38. Cohen MH, Kemper KJ, Stevens L, Hashimoto D, Gilmour J. Pediatric use of complementary therapies: ethical and policy choices. *Pediatrics* 2005;**116**: 568–575.

39. Kelly KM. Integrative therapies for children with hematological malignancies. *Hematology American Society of Hematology Education Program* 2009: 307–312.

40. Jankovic M, Spinetta JJ, Martins AG, *et al.* Non-conventional therapies in childhood cancer: guidelines for distinguishing non-harmful from harmful therapies: a report of the SIOP Working Committee on Psychosocial Issues in Pediatric Oncology. *Klinische Padiatrie* 2004;**216**: 194–197.

41. Deng GE, Frenkel M, Cohen L, *et al.* Society for Integrative Oncology, *et al.* Evidence-based clinical practice guidelines for integrative oncology: complementary therapies and botanicals. *Journal of Soc Integr Oncology* 2009;**7**:85–120.

Part E
Appendix

Appendix A

Assessment Tools in Pediatric Psycho-oncology

Dafna Munitz-Shenkar, Michal M. Kreitler, Shulamith Kreitler

The preparation of Appendix A, the table of tools in pediatric psycho-oncology, has been inspired by our wish to promote research in pediatric psycho-oncology. There is a general consensus that research is badly needed in this important area. Research depends at least to a certain extent on adequate tools. Appendix A is designed to facilitate access to assessment tools in pediatric psycho-oncology. It presents tools in the following domains: Anxiety and Depression; Behavioral Assessment; Hostility, Aggression and Anger; Health; Fatigue; Quality of Life; Self-Esteem/Self-Concept; Body Image; Hope; Personality; Stress and Post-Traumatic Stress; Cognition; Resilience, Coping and Adjustment; Pain Assessment. Each tool is described briefly, including information about its function, psychometric properties, form of administration, and availability.

The choice of domains and of tools was guided by several criteria. We tried to present tools that are relevant to major domains of research in pediatric psycho-oncology, which have been used in several studies, and have a good psychometric profile.

It is our hope that Appendix A will help to promote research in pediatric psycho-oncology by facilitating the application of the presented tools, by motivating the search for other relevant and useful tools, and by stimulating the development of new tools which are required in a focal domain of study in view of an ever expanding research agenda.

Pediatric Psycho-oncology: Psychosocial Aspects and Clinical Interventions, Second Edition.
Edited by Shulamith Kreitler, Myriam Weyl Ben-Arush and Andrés Martin.
© 2012 John Wiley & Sons, Ltd. Published 2012 by John Wiley & Sons, Ltd.

Table Appendix A Tools in pediatric psycho-oncology.

	Tool	Completed by	Function	Number of Items	Type	Age
Anxiety and Depression	State-Trait Anxiety Inventory for Children (STAIC)	Self-report for children and adolescents.	Screening tool which distinguishes between an anxious personality and anxiety as an emotional state.	20+ 20 items	Three-point scale.	6 to 14 years
	Beck Anxiety Inventory for Youth (BYI-II)	Self-report for children and adolescents.	Screening tool of self concept, anxiety, depression, anger and disruptive behaviour. This tool measures the child's or adolescent's emotional and social impairment in five specific areas.	Five inventories of 20 questions each	Four-point scale	7 to 18 years
	Self-Report for Childhood Anxiety Related Disorders-Revised (SCARED-R)	Self-report for children and adolescents + parents' version.	Sceening tool measures general anxiety, separation anxiety, social phobia, school phobia and physical symptoms of anxiety.	66 items- student version 41 items- parent version	Three-point scale	8 years and older
	Revised Children's Manifest Anxiety Scale (RCMAS-2)–	Self-report for children and adolescents.	Measuring the level and nature of anxiety. Short Form and Audio Administration Option are available.	37 items	Yes/no items	6 to 19 years
	Multidimensional Anxiety Scale for Children (MASC)-+ MASC- 10 short version	Self-report for children and adolescents.	Assessing anxiety symptoms.	39 items +10 items for the short version	Four-point Likert scale	8 to 19 years
	Children's Depression Rating Scale, Revised (CDRS-R)-	Self-report for children and adolescents and a semi-structured interview.	Assessing depression and also taking the first step in the therapeutic process	17 symptoms areas	Seven-point scale	6 to 12 years and 13 to 18 years.
	Weinberg Depression Scale for Children and Adolescents (WDSCA)	Self-report for children and adolescents.	Screening tool can be used as an initial assessment scale and can be repeated to measure response to treatments	56 items	yes/no items	5 to 21 years
	Depression and Anxiety in Youth Scales (DAYS)	Self-report for children and adolescents' + teachers' and parents' versions	Screening tool for depressive and anxiety disorders in children and adolescents.	Parents- 28 items Teachers- 20 items Student self-report- 22 items	Students self-report- 22 items, 4-point Likert scale. Parents scale-28 items true/false scale Teachers scale - 20 items true/false scale.	6 to 19 years
	Children depression inventory (CDI-2) CDI: Teacher (CDI:T) and CDI: Parent (CDI: P)	Self-report for children and adolescents + parents and teachers	Screening tool for depression.	Self-Report scale: 28 items Teacher scale: 12 items Parents scale: 17 items Short version: 12 items	Three-point scale	7 to 17 years

to Complete	Languages[b]	Reliability and Validity	How can you get it?	View Free Online	Authors/Links	Original Reference(s)
20 minutes	English, German, French, Dutch, Spanish, Romanian, Portuguese, Japanese, Turkish, Hebrew, Arabic and Greek	Internal consistency: Cronbach's alphas for the State Anxiety Scale is 0.93, and test-retest correlations range from 0.31 to 0.47, reflecting the transitory nature of state anxiety. Validity for this scale is shown by its correlation with other widely used measures of anxiety in adults.	https://shop.acer.edu.au/acer-shop/UserHelp.page;jsessionid=1E8D54B9BF-F2E0C0BC2CE0C186-BE20D0#quals	No	Charles Spielberger, Ph.D. in collaboration with C.D. Edwards, R. Lushene, J. Montuori, Denna Platzek	[1]
) minutes per ory	English	Internal consistency: Chronbach's Alpha coefficients ranging from 0.86 to 0.96 indicate high internal consistency for all age groups on all scales. Internal consistency for all age groups on all scales. Test-Retest reliability ranged from 0.74 to 0.93 for all age groups and genders on all scales. Validity was found through significant correlations among scales within normative groups and by correlations with other instruments measuring similar characteristics.	http://harcourtassessment.com	No	http://harcourtassess-ment.com	[2]
20 minutes	English, Hebrew	Internal consistency: Cronbach's alpha: 0.94 for the total SCARED-R and ranged from 0.64 to 0.80 for the separate SCARED-R subscales. Validity for this scale is shown by correlation with other used measures of anxiety RCMAS and STAIC.	www.nationwidechil-drens.org/Document/Get/38539	www.beckscales.com birmaherb@msx.upmc.edu		[3]
5 minutes Short composed of the) items less than 5 es	English, Spanish, French	Internal consistency: Cronbach's alphas is 0.92 for Total Anxiety, and test-retest reliability is 0.76 for Total Anxiety. Validity for this scale is shown by correlation with used measures of anxiety; SCARED.		No		[4]
utes + 5 minutes short version	Afrikaans, Dutch, English, French, German, Hebrew, Hungarian, Italian, Icelandic, Lithuanian, Norwegian, Polish, Spanish, Swedish and Turkish.	Test-retest reliability was assessed: at three-week and 3-month times and was found to be satisfactory to excellent. Validity for this scale is shown by correlation with used measures of anxiety and found to be acceptable.	https://www.mhs.com/err.aspx?aspxerrorpath=/ecom/product.aspx			[5, 6]
0 minutes	English, Hebrew	Test-retest reliability was determined by correlation between two time points. Validity for this scale is shown by correlation with used measures of anxiety BDI and found to be acceptable ($r = 0.72$; $P = 0.001$).	It is available for purchase at: http://www.proedaust.com.au/psyc/details.cfm?number=39			[7]
minutes	English	Internal consistency: Cronbach's alphas ranging from 0.89 to 0.93. Validity for this scale is shown by correlation with other measures of Depression; BDI.				[8]
utes	English	Internal consistency: Cronbach's alpha ranging from 0.61 to 0.91. Validity for this scale is shown by correlation with other used measures of anxiety and depression. The average correlation coefficient was reported to be 0.53. and the moderate range of 0.54 to 0.69, was reported.				[9, 10]
15–20 minutes r the short a- 5 minutes	English, Spanish	Evidence of the CDI and Short CDI's strong support for reliability and validity has been established over many years of empirical research. This instrument is mature in the sense	available for purchase at: http://www.pearsonassess-ments.com or https://ecom.mhs.com/(S(0lbca0vhgivv-			[11]

Table Appendix A *(Continued)*

	Tool	Completed by	Function	Number of Items	Type	Age
Behavioral Assessment	Behavior Assessment System for Children, Second Edition (BASC-2)	Self-report for children+ Parent and teacher report + interview for younger children.	Assessing emotional and behavioral status of children and adolescents. Using teachers' and parents' observations of positive or negative behaviors. Teacher Rating Scales (TRS), Parent Rating Scales (PRS), Self-Report of Personality (SRP) and Self-Report of Personality- interview (SRP-I) the Structured. (Developmental History (SDH) form, and the Student Observation System (SOS)).	TRS- 100 to 139 items. PRS- 134 to 160 items. The SRP-Interview (SRP-I).	TRS+PRS; 4-point response format. SRP; 2-point response format (T for True or F for False) and a 4-point response format SRP- 3 separate forms: child (ages 8 to 11), adolescent (ages 12 to 21), and college (ages 18 to 25). SRP1- interview for childre aged 6–7 years; yes/no responses to questions	2 to 21 years
Hostility, aggression and anger	Children's Inventory of Anger (ChIA)	Self-report for children and adolescents.	Assessment of children's anger reactions, expression and effect on personal relationships.	39 items	Four subscale scores: frustration, physical aggression, peer relationships, and authority relations.	8 to 16 years
	Cook–Medley Hostility Scale, children's version (CMHS)	Self-report for children and adolescents.	This instrument has been modified from the adult version to adolescents and children version.	23 items	Four-point Likert scale	10 to 18 years
	Children's Hostility Inventory (CHI)	Parents and teachers report inventory.	Examines aggression and hostility.	38 items	Forced choice	6 to 12 years
	The Eyberg Child Behavior Inventory-revised (ECBI)	Parent rating scale or administered by a professional	Screening Inventory to evaluate parental report of behavioral problems.	36 items	Likert scale	2 to 16 years
	The Anger Expression Scale for Children (AESC)	Self-report for children and adolescents.	Assessing comparisons of anger and anger expression across children with chronic illnesses.	26 items	Four-point Likert scale	7 to 17 years
	Aggression Questionnaire	Self-report for children, adolescents and adults.	Assessing hostility and aggression	34 items	Likert scale	9 through 88
	State-Trait Anger Expression Inventory – 2 (STAXI-2)	Self-report for children and adolescents.	Assessing components of anger and evaluates the role anger might play in certain medical conditions.	57 items	Four-point scales	16 to 19 years
	The Behavioral, Affective and somatic	Nurse report, parent report and patient report.	Assessing acute and short-term outcomes in patients undergoing bone	Nurses and parents- 38 items Child -14 items	Five-point Likert scale	Child form; 4 to 13 years. Nurses and

to Complete	Languages[b]	Reliability and Validity	How can you get it?	View Free Online	Authors/Links	Original Reference(s)
		that there have been a number of fundamental psychometric studies. Further, the CDI has demonstrated consistent correlations with various syndromes, other scales, and replicated predictive relationships. Internal consistency, interrater reliability, and the item-total score correlations were adequate.	fa55gf1dbsjb))/inventory. aspx?gr=edu&prod=c-di&id=pricing&RptGr-pID=cdi			
minutes (TRS RS), 30 minutes +SRP1- 20 es	English, Spanish	Internal consistency: Cronbach's alpha - 0.80 for all forms (TRS, PRS, SRP) in both the general sample and the clinical sample. Internal consistency; ranging from 0.67 to 0.90 and 0.64 to 0.89 for boys and girls, respectively. Validity was established through significant correlations among known reliable and valid scale; Children's Depression Inventory (CDI), Revised Children's Manifest Anxiety Scale (RCMAS), Brief Symptom Inventory (BSI), Beck Depression Inventory-II (BDI-II), and the BASC.	http://ags.pearsonassess-ments.com			[12, 13]
utes	English	Internal consistency: Cronbach's alpha ranging from 0.85 to 0.86. The range of Test-Retest Value: ranging from 0.65 to 0.75. Validity was assessed and found to be acceptable.				[14–17]
utes	English	Internal consistency: Cronbach's alpha ranging from Validity was demonstrated by comparing this tool with other hostility and anger measurements.				[18–20]
0 minutes	English	Internal consistency: Cronbach's alpha - 0.82. Validity was assessed and found to be acceptable.	http://www.yale.edu	No		[21, 22]
minutes	Chinese, English, German, Japanese, Korean, Lebanese, Norwegian, Russian, Spanish and Swedish.	Range of Test-Retest Value: ranging from 0.86 to 0.88; The range of Inter-rater reliability: 0.86 to 0.79; Internal consistency: Cronbach's alpha ranging from 0.88 to 0.95; Validity was assessed and found to be acceptable.	http://www3parinc.com/		The ECBI and accompanying manual and scoring materials may be purchased from PAR Inc.	[23–25]
10 minutes	English	Internal consistency: Cronbach's alpha - 0.83. Validity was assessed by comparing this scale with other used instruments like ChIA, BASC and CHI.	journals.permissions@ox-fordjournals.org			[26]
utes	English	Internal consistency: Cronbach's alpha has a wide range 0.55 to 0.94; Validity was assessed and found to be acceptable				[27–29]
5 minutes to with limited g; 5 minutes to	English	Internal consistency: Cronbach's alpha ranging from 0.73 to 0.95. Validity was demonstrates by comparing this tool with other instruments. The author reports construct-related validity.				[30, 31]
and parents - 15 minutes.	English	Internal consistency of Cronbach's child report: 0.89. Parent ranged from 0.742 to 0.902 and nurses from 0.87.				[32–34]

Table Appendix A (*Continued*)

	Tool	Completed by	Function	Number of Items	Type	Age
Health	Experiences scale (BASES)		marrow transplantation or very intense chemotherapy treatment.			parent forms; 2 to 20 years.
	The Revised Perceived Illness Experience (R-PIE)	Self-report for children and adolescents + parent report.	Mesuring the children's perception of their illness experience and parents' perception.	24 items	Five-point Likert scale	8 to 24 years
	Cognitive orientation of health	Self-report for children and adolescents + Adults' version	Assessing the child's non-conscious motivational tendency to maintain physical health. It is based on the cognitive orientation theory about the manner in which specific beliefs orient behavior and affect physical state	80 items	Statements to which the child is requested to respond by saying if they seem right or not right to him/her.	5 to 18. There is a parallel version for ages 18 and above
	Child Health Questionnaire (CHQ) + Parent form (CHQ-PF50) and parents short version form (CHQPF-28). Child form (CHQCF-87).	Parent report instrument+ children's and adolescents' self-report.	Assessing children's physical, emotional, and social well-being.	Parent form 50 items and short version - 28 items. Child form 87 items.	Likert rating scale	5 to 18 years
	PedsQL Multidimensional Fatigue Scale Acute Version	Self-report for children and parent perceptions of fatigue in pediatric patients.	Measuring fatigue in pediatric patients.	18 items	Likert scale	2 to 18 years.
Fatigue	The Staff Fatigue Scale (SFS)	Staff report on the child's fatigue during the past week.	Staff member's perception of the child's fatigue during the past week.	9 items	Four-point Likert scale	For staff use
	The Parent Fatigue scale (PFS)	Parents' report	Parents' perceptions of fatigue experienced by their child in the past week.	18 items	Five-point Likert scale	For parents' use
	The Child Fatigue Scale (CFS)-	Self-report for children.	Evaluating the child's perception regarding fatigue syndromes during the past week.	14 items, two parts instrument	First part: "yes" or "no" Second part: if the answer is yes for the child, he or she is asked to rate how much the problem bothers him/her on a five-point Likert scale.	7 to 12 years
Quality of Life	The PedsQL 4.0 Generic Core Scale	Self-report for children and adolescents + parent report.	Assessing pediatric quality of life aspects.	23 items	Five-point Likert scale. For ages 5–7 years- a three-point Likert scale.	Ages 5–7, 8–12, 13–18 years and parent forms in regard to children aged 2–4, 5–7, 8–12, 13–18 years
	The PedsQL™ Brain Tumor Module	Self-report for children and adolescents + parent report	Assessing health-related QOL in children undergoing cancer treatments and parents' perceptions of their child's HRQO. Evaluates some cognitive aspects.	24 items	Five-point scale	Parent report for toddlers (ages 2–4), Child self-report includes ages 5–7, 8–12, and 13–18 years.
	PedsQL™ Cancer Module	Self-report for children and adolescents + parent report.	Assessing health related QOL in children undergoing cancer treatments.	27 items	Five-point response scale	Parents' report, and there are child ages 2–4 years, 5–7, 8–12, 13–18 years.

to Complete	Languages[b]	Reliability and Validity	How can you get it?	View Free Online	Authors/Links	Original Reference(s)	
About 15 es.		Parent-nurse correlations showed preliminary evidence of the validity of the measure.					
t 10 minutes	English, Dutch	Internal consistency: Cronbach's alpha- 0.84. Validity was established by comparing this questionnaire with other measures of illness perception..	http://www.holeinthewall-camps.org/Document.Doc?id=99			[35]	
minutes	Hebrew, English, Russian	Internal consistency: Cronbach's alpha >0.90 The questionnaire predicted various physical responses and states of health.	krit@netvision.net.il. The computer program from the author.			[36, 37]	
PF50; 10–15 es CHQPF-28; 5– utes CHQCF- —25 minutes	English, Finnish, French, German, Dutch, Italian, Greek, Honduran, Mexican, Norwegian, Portuguese and Swedish	Internal consistency: Cronbach's alpha - 0.53 to 0.96 Validity was found to be very high.	http://www.healthact.com/survey-chq.php	website www.health-act.com/chq.html		[38]	free online
10 minutes	English, German, French, Dutch, Spanish, Czech, Portuguese, Hungarian, Italian, Norwegian, Polish, Swedish, Hebrew and Croatian.	Internal consistency: Cronbach's alpha - 0.89 child, 0.92 parent report. Validity is shown by comparing this tool with known reliable and valid scales of fatigue.	http://www.pedsql.org			[39, 40]	
nutes or less	English	Internal consistency: Cronbach's alpha- 0.86 Validity for the SFS is shown by correlation with other used measures of fatigue; PFS and CFS.				[41]	
nutes or less	English	Internal consistency: Cronbach's alpha- 0.88. Validity for the PFS is shown by correlation with other used measures of fatigue; SFS and CFS.				[41]	
utes or less	English	Internal consistency: Cronbach's alpha- 0.84. Intensity score range from 0.34 to 0.60. Total correlation ranges from 0.17 to 0.45. Validity for the CFS is shown by correlation with other used measures of fatigue; PFS and SFS.				[41]	
nutes or less	English, Spanish, Dutch, German, French, Hebrew Russian, Italian, Greek, Hungarian, Arabic Portuguese, Turkish and more.	Internal consistency: Cronbach's alpha- child report-ranging 0.72 to 0.88, parent report- ranging 0.87 to 0.93. Validity was demonstrates by comparing healthy children and children with cancer as a group and among children who are on treatment versus off treatment. Validity was also shown by correlation with other used measures of HRQOL.	http://www.pedsql.org			[42]	
nutes	English	Internal consistency: Cronbach's alpha for parent-toddler version and parent-8 to 12 years version $\alpha \geq 0.70$. High correlation was found between this module and PedsQL Generic scale. Validity was established by compeing all the forms of this questionnaire.	http://www.pedsql.org			[43]	
nutes	English, German, Hebrew and Portuguese.	Internal consistency: Cronbach's alpha for all parent report and 13–18 age group; Cronbach's $\alpha \geq 0.70$ and for all other child-report domains ranges from 0.37 to 0.84. Cancer Module Scales (average 0.72 child, 0.87 parent report). Validity was	http://www.pedsql.org			[39]	

Table Appendix A *(Continued)*

Tool	Completed by	Function	Number of Items	Type	Age
The Adolescent Quality of Life Instrument (AQoL)	Self-report for children and adolescents	Assessing quality of life in patients undergoing cancer treatments.	16 items	Likert scale	9 to 20 years
The Miami Pediatric Quality of Life Questionnaire (MPQOLQ)	Parent report questionnaire	Assessing HRQL of pediatric oncology patients undergoing cancer treatments.	56 items	The parents respond twice, first on a five-point Likert scale comparing one's child with other same-aged healthy children and then on a 5-point Likert scale rating the importance of the items.	For parents use
The Royal Marsden Hospital Pediatric Oncology Quality of Life Questionnaire	Parent report instrument	Assessing health-related QOL in children undergoing treatment for cancer and children who have completed treatment. The time period of the questionnaire is one week prior to assessment.	66 items	Four-point Likert scale	Parents' report regarding children ages 3 to 19 years
The Minneapolis-Manchester Quality of Life (MMQL) MMQL-Youth, MMQL-Adolescent and MMQL-Young Adults.	Self-report for children and adolescents + adult form.	Assessing HRQL in childhood-cancer survivors. Three versions. The YF-children between 8 and 12 years. The Adolescent Form and the adult form.	32 items for 8–12 years, 46 items for 13–20 years	Five-point scale. The YF-An interview. The Adolescent Form- self-administered	Three age groups: youth (8–12 years), adolescents (13–20) and young adults (21–45).
The Revised Perceived Illness Experience (R-PIE)	Self-report for children and adolescents + parent report.	Measuring the children's perception of their illness experience and parents' perception.	24 items	Five-point Likert scale	8 to 24 years
The Pediatric Oncology Quality of Life Scale (POQOLS)	Parents' and physicians' reports	Parent report QOL instrument for children attending outpatient clinics or who are hospitalized.	21 items	Seven-point Likert-type scales	5 to 18 years.
CQL - Children's quality of life	Self-report for children and adolescents	Measuring the child's perception of various aspects of their life. Provides a summative score and scores on the following scales: family, school/kindergarten, positive emotions, negative emotions, mastery & independence, cognitive functioning, social functioning, basic needs, stress, body image, self esteem, efficacy, motivation, fun, worries, health.	55 items	Three-point scales, graphically adapted for children	3 to 18 years.
The Child Health Rating Inventories-Hematopoietic Stem Cell Transplantation (CHRIs-HSCT)	Self-report for children and adolescents + parent report.	Measuring health-related QOL specific to children and adolescents undergoing Stem Cell Transplantation.	10 items + 10 items	Five-point Likert scale	5 to 18 years
The Coopersmith Self-Esteem Inventory	Brief self-report questionnaires for children, adolescents and adults.	Measuring level of self-esteem of adolescents.	58 items	8 items which comprise a lie scale. The remaining items are scored on a Like me or Unlike me choice	School form 8 to 15 years. Adult form for 16 years and up
The Tennessee Self-Concept Scale (TSCS)	Self-report for adolescents	Measuring self-concept of adults.	100 items	Five-point Likert scale	13 years and up

Self-esteem/self-concept

to Complete	Languages[b]	Reliability and Validity	How can you get it?	View Free Online	Authors/Links	Original Reference(s)
nutes	English	established by comparing all the forms of this questionnaire. Internal consistency: Cronbach's alpha- ranging from 0.77 to 0.81. The AQoL was found to a reliable, valid and sensitive instrument.				[44, 45]
20 minutes	English	Internal consistency: Cronbach's alpha parents version >0.70, and the internal consistency of the overall scale, Cronbach's alpha ≥0.76. The tool has good validity with regard to diagnostic groups and treatments.	Contact author, F. Daniel Armstrong, Ph.D., Department of Pediatrics (D-820), P.O. Box 016820, Miami, Florida 33101; email: darm-strong@miami.edu			[46]
) minutes	English, Swedish and Dutch	Internal consistency: Cronbach's alpha ranging from 0.80 for 7 of 8 subscales. Validity was established by comparing this instrument with other HRQOL instruments.				[47]
20 minutes	English	Internal consistency: Cronbach's alpha- 0.78, test–retest stability over at least 2 weeks ranged from 0.60 to 0.90. The child form and the parent form have been validated for use in the UK as generic measures of QOL. Construct validity for the child form was assessed and was very high.				[48–50]
10 minutes	English, Dutch	Internal consistency: Cronbach's alpha- 0.84. Validity was established by comparing this questionnaire with other known reliable and valid scales.	http://www.holeinthewall-camps.org/Document.Doc?id=99			[35]
10 minutes	English, Spanish	Internal consistency: Cronbach's alpha ≥0.79 for the total score and two of three domains Good concurrent and discriminant validity as assessed by relations with measures, such as The Child Behavior Checklist.	The measure is available in the central reference			[51]
15 minutes	Hebrew, English, Russian, Arabic	Internal consistency: Cronbach's alpha between 0.85 and 0.92. The reliability was tested by structural equation modeling which yielded a model that showed up consistently in samples of children differing in ethnic-cultural background, religion, gender, age, health, and residential areas.	Available from the author: S. Kreitler krit@-netvision.net.il.			[52]
nutes	English	Internal consistency: Cronbach's alpha >0.70. For age group 5 to 7 years, and 8 to 18 years internal consistency was found to be Cronbach's alpha ≥0.70. Validity within scale was assessed and found to be reasonable.				[53, 54]
ne limit, typically nutes	English, Vietnamese	Internal consistency: Cronbach's alpha ranging from 0.87 to 0.92. Validity results have shown full-scale correlations between Self Perception Profile for Children (SPPC) and the Self Image Profiles (SIP).	http://www.cpp-db.com/			[55]
20 minutes.	English	Internal consistency: Cronbach's alpha ranging from 0.66 to 0.92. The TSCS is considered to have high construct validity and the total self concept score 0.66 (Piers-Harris).				[56, 57]

Table Appendix A (*Continued*)

Tool	Completed by	Function	Number of Items	Type	Age
Self Image Profiles (SIP); SIP-C and SIP-A	Self-report for children and adolescents	Screening instrument that gives a quick assessment of a child's or young person's view of self.	25 items	Six-point Likert scale	7 years to 16 years SIP-C for children aged 7 to 11 years SIP-A for adolescents aged 12 to 16 years.
The Piers-Harris Children's Self-Concept Scale (PHCSCS)	Self-report for children and adolescents.	Measuring of children's self-perceptions in relation to six areas of daily functioning.	60 items	Yes/no items	7 to 18 years
The Multidimensional Self Concept Scale (MSCS)	Self-report instrument for adolescents	Measuring self-perception of children and adolescents.	150 items	Four-point scale	9 to 19 years
The Multidimensional Self Concept Questionnaire for Children	Self-report instrument for children and adolescents	Assessing the child's self image by means of items that refer to different aspects of the self, such as its feelings, thoughts, actions, desires, people and places it likes, etc. Based on the meaning theory of Kreitler and Kreitler.	30 items	Consists of statements about the self and its aspects to which the child is requested to respond by saying if they are important or not so important.	5 to 18 years. There is a parallel version for ages 18 and above.
Rosenberg Self-Esteem Scale (SES)	Self-report for adolescents and adults.	Assessing global self-esteem. The toll consists of statements related to overall feelings of self-worth or self-acceptance.	10 items	Four-point Likert scale+ administered as an interview	High school juniors and seniors
Body Image Self-Perception Profile for Adolescents (SPPA)	Self-report for adolescents	Assessing an adolescent's personal sense of competence.	45 items	Choosing one of two statements and rating whether the statement is "sort of true for me" or "really true for me."	13 years and up
The Self-Perception Profile for Children (SPPC)	Self-report for children.	Assessing social acceptance, athletic competence, physical appearance, behavioral aspects and Global Self-Worth.	36 items	Six-item sub-scale questionnaire.	8 to 12 years
The Multidimensional Body Questionnaire for Children (MDBQ-C)	Self-report for children and adolescents.	Assessing the child's body image by means of items that refer to different aspects of the body, such as its colors, its odors, how it looks, feelings that it evokes, thoughts that it has, its	30 items	The child has to respond to Statements about the body or its part by saying if they seem important or not so important	5 to 18 years. There is a parallel version for ages 18 and above. For 5–7 the items need to be read to the child and

to Complete	Languages[b]	Reliability and Validity	How can you get it?	View Free Online	Authors/Links	Original Reference(s)
: 12 to 25 es. : 9 to 17 minutes	English	Internal consistency: Cronbach's alpha for CIP-C; positive items; 0.69 and negative items 0.79. Validity results have shown full-scale correlations between Self-Perception Profile for Children (SPPC) and Coopersmith Self-Esteem Inventories (CSEI).				[58]
20 minutes.	English	Internal consistency: Cronbach's alpha ranging from 0.88 to 0.93. Concurrent validity results ranged from 0.32 to 0.85. Convergent validity between this scale and The Coopersmith Self-Esteem Inventory - 0.85 and for The Tennessee Self-Concept Scale (TSCS)-0.61.				[59, 60]
30 minutes.	English	Internal consistency: Cronbach's alpha- 0.97 Validity results have shown full-scale correlations between the MSCS and the Coopersmith Self-Esteem Inventory, the Piers-Harris Children's Self-Concept Scale, and the Self Description Questionnaire II ranging from 0.69 to 0.83.				[61]
nutes.	Hebrew, English, Russian	Reliability: Alpha Cronbach >.95; Validity: The questionnaire provided differential scores for children in different states, such as in health and sickness, in intact or divorced families, after success or failure.	For more information and to get the tool: S. Kreitler, krit@netvision. net.il			[62]
nan 5 minutes	English, French, Hebrew and Norwegian	Test-retest correlations are typically in the range of .82 to .88, and Cronbach's alpha for various samples ranging from 0.77 to 0.88. The RSES has been shown to have strong validity for both genders and for different ethnic groups. Convergent validity between this scale and The Coopersmith Self-Esteem Inventory - 0.55.	http://www.bsos.umd. edu/socy/rosenberg.html			[63, 64]
40 minutes	English, Dutch	Internal consistency: Cronbach's alpha ranging from 0.55 to 0.93 for the subscales; Validity results have shown full-scale correlations between Self Perception Profile for Adolescents (SPPA) and Self Perception Profile for Children (SPPC).	Susan Harter, University of Denver, University Park, Denver, CO 80208, Ph: 303 871-2000, shar-ter@du.edu			[65]
nutes	English, Dutch	Internal consistencies: Cronbach's alpha- ranging from 0.78 to 0.84; subscale- ranging 0.71 to 0.86; Validity results have shown full-scale correlations between Self Perception Profile for Children (SPPC) and Self Perception Profile for Adolescents (SPPA).	Susan Harter, University of Denver, University Park, Denver, CO 80208, Ph: 303 871-2000, shar-ter@du.edu			[66]
nutes	Hebrew, English, Russian	Internal consistency: Cronbach's alpha >.95. The questionnaire provided differential scores for children in different physical states, such as with diabetes or in	Get the test in the book or from the author: krit@-netvision.net.il. The computer program from the author.		For more information and to get the tool: S. Kreitler, krit@netvi-sion.net.il	[67, 68]

Table Appendix A *(Continued)*

Tool	Completed by	Function	Number of Items	Type	Age
		function, and activities. It is based on the meaning theory of Kreitler and Kreitler.			his/her responses recorded. Above 7 the child can read and respond by himself/ herself.
Offer Self-Image Questionnaire for Adolescents, Revised (OSIQ-R)	Self-report for adolescents	Assessing variety of aspects of adolescents' self-image.	129 simple statements	Six-point response scale	13 to 19 years
Body-image Instrument (BII)	Self-report for adolescents and young adults with cancer.	Assessing satisfaction with general appearance, body competence, others' reaction to appearance, value of appearance, body parts.	28 items	Five-point Likert scale	12 to 18 years and young adults
Hope Children's Hope Scale (CHS)	Self-report for children and adolescents	Screening tool of hope in children and adolescents.	6 items	Six-point Likert scale	8 to 19 years
Beck Hopelessness Scale (BHS)	Self-administered or verbally administered by a trained administrator.	Measuring negative attitudes about the future. This tool has three major aspects of hopelessness: feelings about the future, loss of motivation, and expectations.	20 items	True or false items	17 to 80 years
Personality Personality Inventory for Youth (PIY)	Self-report for children and adolescents	Assessing emotional and behavorial adjustment, family interaction, and school and academic functioning. The first 80 items of the test can be used as a brief classroom screener to quickly identify students who would show problems if the full inventory were administered.	270 items	Forced choice	9 to 19 years
Child Rorschach Responses - Developmental Trends From Two to Ten Years	Children and adolescents test pictures	A perceptual projective test that provides information about the emotional tendencies of the child, his/ her fears, anger, etc	10 picture cards	The child is shown 10 inkblot cards and is asked to say what he/she perceives in each card	2 to 10 years
Roberts Apperception Test for Children (RATC)	Children	Projective personality measure for adaptive and maladaptive functioning.	16 tests pictures	Pictures	3 to 10 years

to Complete	Languages[b]	Reliability and Validity	How can you get it?	View Free Online	Authors/Links	Original Reference(s)
		chemotherapy, as well as for children suffering from obesity, a broken limb or burned skin. The author reports a good validity to result.				
40 minutes	English, Italian German, Greek, Turkish, Spanish, Croatian, and other languages.	Internal consistency: Cronbach's alpha ranging from 0.83–0.90. The author reports a good validity to result.	For more information regarding this tool, please contact Western Psychological Services (WPS), 12031 Wiltshire Boulevard, Los Angeles, CA 90025-1251. E mail: custsvc@wpspublish.com, or URL: http://www.wpspublish.com.			[69]
utes	English	Internal consistency: Cronbach's alpha ranging from 0.68 to 0.81. Validity is shown by correlation with other used measures; the SF-36 health survey and the pereceived illness experience measure.				[70]
utes	English, Chinese	Internal consistency: Cronbach's alpha ranging from 0.72 to 0.86, with a median alpha of 0.77. The item-remainder coefficients ranging from 0.27 to 0.68, with a median of 0.54 (all ps < .01). The CHS was found to correlate significantly with a modified parent-report version of the Children's Hope Scale across different samples (r > .36 for all samples)	NCTSN Measure Review Database www.NCTSN.org			[71]
) minutes	English, Spanish	Internal consistency: Cronbach's alpha ranging from 0.82 to 0.93. Convergent validity was demonstrated by high correlations with the Hope Scale and the Life Orientation Test (LOT).	http://www.pearsonassessments.com/HAIWEB/Cultures/en-us/Productdetail.htm?Pid=015-8133-609&Mode=summary			[72]
cale, 45 minutes er composed of) items, 15 minute	English	The range of internal consistency: 0.80. valid measure of child and adolescent psychopathology based on the respondent's own perceptions.	http://www.wpspublish.com			[73]
80 minutes	English	The Rorschach's objective scoring system is debatable, hence there is no official data regarding it's reliability and validity.				[74]
80 minutes	English	The standardization sample for this test has been criticized by a number of researchers that have shown that the RATC does not distinguish satisfactorily between clinical and nonclinical populations, but in the Roberts-2 (the second edition of the RATC, published in 2005), new norms, grouped by age and sex, are based on a larger sample of 1,000 children and adolescents, and this test is better representative in terms of gender, ethnicity, and parental education than the original sample. The reliability and validity on both the original and the 2nd edition are doubtful and difficult to determine as in many projective tests.	http://www.wpspublish.com.			[75]

Table Appendix A (*Continued*)

	Tool	Completed by	Function	Number of Items	Type	Age
Stress and Post-Traumatic Stress Disorder	Alexithymia for children	Alexithymia for children and adolescents	Measuring the 3 scales of Alexithymia	20 items	True or false items	5 to 18 years
	Children's Apperception Test – CAT, CAT-S, and CAT-H	Children tests pictures	Measuring aspects of personality. There are three: CAT-A- pictures of animals or humans, CAT-H- pictures of human. CAT-S- pictures of children in common family situations.	31 picture cards	Using of picture cards for orally or writing descriptions. May be used directly in therapy or as a play technique in other settings	3 to 10 years
	The Childhood Cancer Stressors Inventory (CCSI)	Self-report for children and adolescents.	Evaluation of specific stressors experienced by children undergoing cancer treatment.	18 items	True-false items, if true for the child, is asked how much the stressors bother him, on a 4-point scale	School-age child's adjustment to cancer stressors
	The Observation Scale of Behavioral Distress (OSBD).	Observation scale for parents and staff members.	Measuring children's behavioral responses to painful medical procedures.	11 items	Four-point scale	3 to 13 years
	Brief Behavioral Distress Scale (BBDS)	Observation scale for parents and staff members.	Measuring children's cooperation and procedure-related distress undergoing several types of invasive medical procedures.	4 categories	Observational	3 years and up
	The Perceived Stress Scale (PSS)	Self-report for children and adolescents	Measuring the perception of stress. It is a measure of the degree to which situations in one's life are appraised as stressful.	14 items	Five-point scale	12 to 18 years
	Children's PTSD Inventory	An interview for children and adolescents.	Diagnosing Posttraumatic Stress Disorder in children and adolescents.	A structured interview with five subtests	Yes/no items	6 to 18
	Children's Stress Inventory (CSI)	Self-report for children and adolescents.	Assessing stress in children and adolescents	16 items	Interview	9 to 18 years
	Coping Inventory for Stressful Situations (CISS)	Self-report for adolescents and adults.	Measuring three types of coping styles; Task-oriented coping, emotion-oriented coping and avoidance coping	Adult form; 48 items Adolescents form; 21 items	Five-point scale	Adolescent 13 to 18 years and Adult 18 years +.
Cognition	Neurotrax	Self-report for children and adolescents	Assessment of basic cognitive processes available to the child – their nature and strength. The tool is based on the theory of meaning by Kreitler and Kreitler which describes the system of meaning in terms of a set of	11 items	For ages 3–7 the responses need to be written down or recorded; above 10 the child can write by himself	One version for children 3–10, another for 10 to adults

o Complete	Languages[b]	Reliability and Validity	How can you get it?	View Free Online	Authors/Links	Original Reference(s)
0 minutes	English, Hebrew	Cronbach's alpha - 0.85.	For more information and to get the tool: S. Kreitler, krit@netvision. net.il			
5 minutes	English	No statistical information is provided on the technical validity and reliability of the CAT. There is no standardized method of administration as well as the lack of standard norms for interpretation.	http://www.answers.com/ topic/children-s-appercep- tion-test#ixzz1UikCSjmV pictures of human			[76]
20 minutes	English	Internal consistency: Cronbach's alpha ranging from 0.80 to - 0.82. Validity was assessed by comparing the instruments with known reliable and valid scales.				[77, 78]
5 minutes	English	Internal consistency: Cronbach's alpha ranging from 0.68–0.72. Each category yielded an interrater reliability correlation coefficient of ≥ 0.80 over 6 consecutive procedures. Validity was assessed by comparing the instrument with known reliable and valid scales; Children's State Anxiety scores, childen's Pain Thermometer rating of their anticipated pain and their experienced pain. Correlation was found between Parents' distress score and the OSBD.				[79, 80]
5 minutes	English	Kappa coefficients: 0.87 for interfering distress, 0.68 for potentially interfering distress, 0.68 for noninterfering distress, 0.74 for BBDS total distress, and 0.72 for active coping responses. Validity was demonstrated by comparing this tool with the OSBD				[81]
5 minutes	English	Internal consistency: Cronbach's alpha ranging from 0.84 to 0.86. Validity was assessed by comparing the instrument with known reliable and valid scale Life-Event Scores.	mindgarden@msn.com mindgarden@msn.com www.mindgarden.com			[82, 83]
minutes (Test istration time as a function of a history).	English, Spanish and Canadian French	Internal consistency: Cronbach's alpha ranging from 0.80 to 0.83. High levels of perceived correspondence between the Children's PTSD Inventory and the DSM-IV PTSD diagnostic criteria.				[84, 85]
5 minutes	English	Internal consistency: Cronbach's alpha - 0.77	http://www.projectinno- vation.biz/csj_2006.html			[86, 87]
an 10 minutes	English, French, Spanish, Dutch, Icelandic, and Polish.	Internal consistency: Cronbach's alpha ranging from 0.51 to 0.60. Validity was assessed by comparing the instrument with known reliable and valid scales of depression and resilience.	www.mhs.com			[88, 89]
15 minutes	Hebrew, English, Spanish, Greek, French, Arabic, Russian, Czech, Italian, Polish, German	Validity checked by correlations with diverse cognitive acts, including memory, problem solving, giftedness, as well as extroversion, anxiety and other personality and emotional tendencies. Excellent results.	For more information and to get the tool: S. Kreitler, krit@netvision. net.il			[90]

Table Appendix A *(Continued)*

Tool	Completed by	Function	Number of Items	Type	Age
		variables referring to contents, types of relation, forms of relation, referent shifts and forms of expression used in communicating meanings. These variables form patterns underlying various cognitive acts including planning and creativity. A special part of the test may be used for information about personality traits and emotional endencies of the children. The test requires the respondent to communicate the meanings of 11 simple and familiar words, using verbal or any nonverbal means. The communications are analyzed by a computer program which yields for each respondent a profile of the frequencies with which each variable was used.			
Stanford-Binet Intelligence Scales, Fifth Edition (SB5)	An interview for children, adolescents and adults.	Assessing of intelligence and cognitive abilities, visual-motor development. This scale may be used as a screener for neuropsychological impairment.	Four cognitive area scores	Use of template cards with unique figure on each card. The individual is asked to draw each figure	2 to 85+ years
PedsQL™ Cognitive Functioning Scale	Self-report for children and adolescents	Measuring cognitive functioning	6 items	Five-point Likert scale. For ages 5–7 years- a three-point Likert scale.	Ages 5–7, 8–12, 13–18 years and parent forms in regard to children aged 2–4, 5–7, 8–12, 13–18 years
Wechsler Intelligence Scale for Children (WISC)	An interview for children and adolescents	The WISC-IV generates a Full Scale IQ (FSIQ) which represents overall cognitive ability, the four other composite scores are Verbal Comprehension index (VCI), Perceptual Reasoning Index (PRI), Processing Speed Index (PSI) and Working Memory Index (WMI).	There are no items but subsets, as described in the next cell.	Composed of fifteen subtests, including Vocabulary, Similarity, Comprehension, Information, Block Design, Picture Concepts, Letter-Number Sequencing, Matrix Reasoning, Cancellation, Word Reasoning, Digital Span, Letter-Number Sequencing, Arithmetic, Coding and Symbol Search.	6 to 16 years
Wechsler Preschool and Primary Scale of Intelligence, 3rd. ed. (WPPSI-III).	An interview for young children	Verbal IQ is based on Information, Vocabulary, and Word Reasoning.	There are no items but subsets, as described in the next cell.	Composed of 14 subsets, including Block Design, Information, Matrix Reasoning, Vocabulary, Picture Concepts, Symbol Search, Word Reasoning,	2.2 to 7.3 years.

o Complete	Languages[b]	Reliability and Validity	How can you get it?	View Free Online	Authors/Links	Original Reference(s)
minutes	English	Reliability checked for coding by different people and over time (durations of over a year): alpha Cronbach's always above .90 Internal consistency: Cronbach's alpha ranging from 0.90 to 0.92. For the ten subtests, reliabilities range from 0.84 to 0.89. Concurrent and criterion validity data was found.	http://www.minddisorders.com/Py-Z/Stanford-Binet-Intelligence-Scale.html			[91]
utes or less	English	Internal consistency: Cronbach's alpha = 0.88 child report, 0.94 parent report	http://www.pedsql.org			[42]
minutes	Translated or adapted to many languages, and norms have been established for a number of countries, including Spanish, Portuguese (Brazil), Norwegian, Swedish, Finnish, Croatian, French (France and Canada), German (Germany, Austria and Switzerland), English (United States, Canada, United Kingdom, Australia), Welsh, Dutch, Japanese, Chinese (Hong Kong), Korean (South Korea), Greek, Romanian, Slovenian and Italian, Hebrew. Separate norms are established with each translation. (Norway uses the Swedish norms). India uses the Malin's Intelligence Scale for Children (MISIC), an adaptation of WISC.	Standardized and validated in large samples of children, from various sub-sample groups, including gifted children, children with various degrees of mental retardation, children with learning disorders, autistic disorder, ADHD, and more. The test was also corellated with other intelligence tests, such as the WISC-III, WPPS-III, WAIS-III, WASI, CMS, GRS.	http://psychcorp.pearso-nassessments.com			
minutes	Translated and adapted for use with different populations including French (and French Canadian), German, Italian, Swedish,	The reliability coefficients for the WPPSI-III US composite scales range from .89 to .95. The test was validated in large samples of children, including sub-samples such as children with developmental delays, children with	http://psychcorp.pearso-nassessments.com			[92–94]

Table Appendix A (*Continued*)

Tool	Completed by	Function	Number of Items	Type	Age
				Coding, Comprehension, Picture Completion, Similarities, Receptive Vocabulary, Object Assembly, Picture Naming.	
Test of meanings	Self-report for children and adolescents	Performance (fluid) IQ is based on Block Design, Matrix Reasoning, and Picture Concepts. Processing Speed Quotient, or visual-motor, clerical speed and accuracy, includes Coding & Symbol Search. General Language Composite is based on Receptive Vocabulary and Picture Naming Full Scale IQ Assessment of basic cognitive processes available to the child – their nature and strength. The tool is based on the theory of meaning by Kreitler and Kreitler which describes the system of meaning in terms of a set of variables referring to contents, types of relation, forms of relation, referent shifts and forms of expression used in communicating meanings.	11 simple and familiar words, using verbal or any nonverbal means.	The test requires the respondent to communicate the meanings of the words. The communications are analyzed by a computer program which yields for each respondent a profile of the frequencies with which each variable was used.	One version for children 3–10, another for 10 to adults. For ages 3–7 the responses need to be written down or recorded; above 10 the child can write by himself.
Tests for working memory (WMTB-C)	An interview for children and adolescents	Provides an accurate assessment of working memory in children. This tool is based on the Baddeley and Hitch model of working memory, and has been found as useful in identifying children who perform poorly at school, including children with specific learning difficulties such as dyslexia.	Designed to reflect the three component structure of the Working Memory Model proposed by Baddeley and Hitch, Central Executive (CE), Phonological Loop (PL) and Visuo-spatial Sketchpad (VSSP)		5 to 15 years
Cancellation tests	Subjects	Assesses visual search, concentration, visual neglect.	6. Items are pages in which specific items are to be cancelled. There are pages with letters, with digits and with geometric forms, each systematic or nonsystematic.	The subject has one of more digits he has to cross out from a list of numbers. The resulting score consists of the correctly crossed out numbers minus the incorrectly crossed out numbers. Coping figures and drawings.	Since the time a person can hold a pencil and make a line
The Rey-Osterrieth Complex Figure Test (ROCF).	Self-report for children and adolescents. Non-verbal test.	Evaluation of different functions, such as visuospatial abilities, memory,			

o Complete	Languages[b]	Reliability and Validity	How can you get it?	View Free Online	Authors/Links	Original Reference(s)
	Japanese, Canadian, Australian, Hebrew and Dutch	mental retardation, children with language disorders, children with ADHD, and more.				
10 minutes	Hebrew, English, Spanish, Greek, French, Arabic, Russian, Czech, Italian, Polish, German.	Internal Reliability .82–.88. Test retest reliability over periods ranging from 3 days to 3 months .90 (mean of coefficients for different samples) The validity of the test has been broadly tested in studies which confirmed predictions based on the meaning test scores of cognitive acts, such as planning, comprehension of texts and situations, scores in Raven's matrices, memory and creativity.	Get the test in the book or from the author: krit@-netvision.net.il. The computer program from the author.		For more information and to get the tool: S. Kreitler, krit@netvision.net.il	[90, 95]
	Test retest reliability over periods ranging from 3 days to 3 months .90 (mean of coefficients for different samples) English, Hebrew	High reliability was found and correlations between subtest scores indicated high construct validity for the central executive and phonological loop measures. The WMTB-C has been validated against existing well-established tests of achievement, including; British Picture Vocabulary Scale, subtests of the British Ability Scales, Neale Analysis of Reading Ability, Group Arithmetic test and subtests of the Differential Abilities Scales.				[96]
nutes per page	English, Hebrew	Reliability reported to be high (above .85)				[97, 98]
	English	Very good reliability and validity reported.				[99]

Table Appendix A *(Continued)*

	Tool	Completed by	Function	Number of Items	Type	Age
Resilience, Coping and adjustment	The Youth Risk and Resilience Inventory (YRRI)	Self-report for children and adolescents.	attention, planning, and working memory (executive functions). Screening tool to identify adolescents who are at risk of violence and abuse. This tool can measure the adolescent ability to cope with violence or abuse.	54 items	Five-point scale	10 to 19 years
	Motivation for Resilience	Self-report for children and adolescents.	Assessing the child's non-conscious motivational tendency to manifest resilience and overcome crises. It is based on the cognitive orientation theory about the manner in which specific beliefs orient behavior.	40 items	The questionnaire consists of statements to which the child is requested to respond by saying if they seem right or not right to him/her. The statements refer to themes such as getting help from others, relying on others, concealing one's weaknesses. Some of the statements refer to oneself, some to how things should be, some to how things are and some to one's goals and wishes	5 to 18. There is a parallel version for ages 18 and above
	Coping with a Disease (CODI)	Self-report for children and adolescents.	Assessing coping strategies of children and adolescents with chronic health conditions.	50 items organized in the eight scales.	Five-point scale + six open-ended questions	4 to 18 years
	Multidimensional Coping Inventory for Children	Self-report for children and adolescents.	The questionnaire provides information about coping with the disease and treatments, in terms of constructs such as denial, seeking support, seeking information, strengthening oneself, being hopeful, being active or passive.	48 items	One of four kinds: very true, true, not true, not at all true.	4 to 18. Another version, parallel, for adults and those above 18.
	The Pediatric Functional Assessment of Cancer Therapy-Childhood Brain Tumor Survivor (Peds-FACT-Brs)- version 2	Self-report for parents and adolescents.	Assessing emotional social/family well-being and illness experiences, of brain tumor survivor.	37 items	Open questions -Subjects are asked to write their opinions on three statements.	13 to 18 years
	Children's Adjustment to Cancer Index (CACI)	Self-report for children and adolescents	Measuring the child's perception of cancer stressors and adjustment to cancer treatment	30 items	Five-point Likert scale from never to always	7 to 13 years
	Resiliency Scales for Children and Adolescents (RSCA)	Self-report for children and adolescents	Measures children's and adolescents' personal attributes related to resilience	Composed of three scales of 20–24 questions each and ten subscales.	Five-point scale	9 to 18 years

to Complete	Languages[b]	Reliability and Validity	How can you get it?	View Free Online	Authors/Links	Original Reference(s)
20 to 30 minutes	English	Internal consistency: Cronbach's alpha- 0.72 Validity was assessed by comparing the instrument with known reliable and valid scales of depression and resilience.	www.jist.com			[100, 101]
utes	Hebrew, English, Russian	Internal consistency: Cronbach's alpha >.95 The questionnaire predicted the responses of children in difficult situations, some of which dealt with health.	krit@netvision.net.il.		For more information and to get the tool: S. Kreitler, krit@netvision.net.il	[102]
20 to 30 minutes	English, Dutch, German, Greek, and Swedish	Internal consistency: Cronbach's alpha ranging from 0.69 to 0.83. Validity was assessed by comparing the instrument with known reliable and valid scales of coping.				[103]
utes	Hebrew, English, Russian	Internal reliability is .74 (due to the fact that the inventory measures various coping measures, not all of which the child may use); test-retest reliability over 3 months is .95 Validity: Support for the validity of the inventory is based on studies which show high and significant correlations between several specific means of coping as assessed by the inventory and as assessed by other scales, for example, denial.			For more information and for getting the tool: S. Kreitler, krit@netvision.net.il	[102]
20 minutes	English	Internal consistencies Cronbach's alpha- ranging from 0.70 to 0.92. Validity was assessed when correlated with the Revised Children's Manifest Anxiety Scale and Kovacs' Children's Depression Scale and the CHQ-PF-50.	http://www.facit.org			[104]
20 minutes	English	Internal consistency: Cronbach's alpha = 0.91. Validity was assessed by comparing the instruments with known reliable and valid scales.				
utes	English	Internal consistency: Chronbach's alpha ranging from 0.93 to 0.95 Validity correlations of the internal structure for the global scales, found				[105, 106]

Table Appendix A *(Continued)*

	Tool	Completed by	Function	Number of Items	Type	Age
Pain assessment	Pain Experience Questionnaire (PEQ)	Parent report and child self-report.	Assessing the psychosocial impact of chronic pain in children and adolescents. The child PEQ entails the subscales pain severity, pain-related interference, affective distress and perceived social support. The parent version contains the subscales severity of the child's pain, interference and parental affective distress.	3 items	Rating scale	7–18 years
	The OUCHER scale	Self-report for children and adolescents.	Assessing pain in children using two separate vertical scales.	2 scales	Six culturally sensitive faces Faces is scored from 0 to 5. This tool has two scales; numeric scale (i.e., 0–100) for older children and the photographic scale for younger children.	6 years and older
	Faces Pain Scale - Revised	Self-report for children.	Assessing pain in children.	One item	The child selects 1 of 6 sex-neutral faces that reflect their pain which is scored from 0 to 5 or 0 to 10.	4 to 16 years
	The Neonatal Infant Pain Scale (NIPS)	Staff report on neonates' and babies' pain behavior.	Assessing pain in babies. This tool discriminates pain response objectively from other distress reactions that infants manifest.	6 items	Score 0 to 2 points	Neonates and babies
	The Face, Legs, Activity, Cry and Consolability (FLACC)	Staff report on the child's pain behavior.	Assessing pain in babies and children younger than 4 years. The FLACC has been revised specifically for cognitively impaired children ages 4 to 18 years.	5 items	Each behavior is scored from 0 to 2, with the highest possible cumulative score being 10	Up to 7 years
	The Wong-Baker FACES Pain scale	Self-report for children.	Assessing pain in children	One item	Six hand-drawn cartoon-like faces.	4 to 12 years
	Visual Analogue scale (VAS)	Self-report for children and adolescents.	Assessing pain in children. This scale uses either a vertical or horizontal premeasured line (100 mm) to estimate pain	10-point scale	End-points of the 10-centimeter scale were labeled Not Afraid and Very Afraid.	Children 8 years or older
	The Adolescent Pediatric Pain Tool (APPT)	Self-report for children and adolescents.	Measuring pain intensity, pain description and location of pain.	14 items	Graphic rating scale	8–17 years

to Complete	Languages[b]	Reliability and Validity	How can you get it?	View Free Online	Authors/Links	Original Reference(s)
han 5 minutes	English	to be significantly related with each other. Validity was assessed by comparing the instruments with known reliable and valid scales of depression, trait anxiety, and pain.				
han 5 minutes	English	The authors report a reliable instrument with good validity results.	http://www.oucher.org/			[107, 108]
han 5 minutes	English, Arabic, Bulgarian, Chinese, Czech, Dutch, Estonian, French, German, Greek, Hebrew, Hindi, Hungarian, Italian, Japanese, Norwegian, Polish, Portuguese Romanian, Russian, Spanish, Swedish, Thai, Turkish and more	Internal consistency: Chronbach's alpha ranging from 0.83 to 0.90. Validity is supported by a strong positive correlation the visual analogue scale (VAS) ($r = 0.92$, $N = 45$) and the colored analogue scale (CAS) ($r = 0.84$, $N = 45$).	http://www.usask.ca/ childpain/fpsr/			[109, 110]
han 5 minutes	English	Internal consistency: Chronbach's alpha = 0.90 Validation of the Neonatal Infant Pain Scale (NIPS) was shown by positive corelation with hurt rate and oxygen saturation.	http://www.cebp.nl/vault public/filesystem/? ID=1295			[111]
han 5 minutes	English	Internal consistency: Chronbach's alpha- 0.882. Validity is supported by a strong positive correlation with known reliable and valid scales of pain assessment.	http://www2.massgeneral. org/painrelief/pcs pain files/app d flacc.pdf.			[112–115]
han 5 minutes	English + 10 other languages	Reliability was demonstrated $r = 0.791$ (Wong & Baker, 1996); and preference, $2 = 135.81$, $df = 5$, and $p < 0.001$ (Wong & Baker, 1988) for the FACES scale have been demonstrated. Concurrent validity was assessed by the authors. The author reports a good validity results.	http://www1.us.elsevier-health.com/FACES/			[116]
han 5 minutes	English	Construct validity was assessed comparing parent and child, nurse and child, nurse and parent $r = 0.44$, $r = 0.28$, $r = 0.44$, $p < 0.001$, (Abu-Saad, 1990). Validity is supported by a strong positive correlation the Faces Pain Scale- Revised ($r = 0.92$, $N = 45$).	http://www.cebp.nl/vault public/filesystem/? ID=1478.			[117]
han 5 minutes	English	Reliability found to be moderate to high. Validity was assessed by comparing the instruments with known reliable and valid scales of pain assessment.				[118]

References

1. Spielberger CD, Gorsuch RL, Lushene RE. *Manual for the State-Trait Anxiety Inventory*. Palo Alto, CA: Consulting Psychologists Press, 1970.
2. Beck AT. *Cognitive Therapy and the Emotional Disorders*. Madison, WI: International Universities Press, 1976.
3. Muris PM, Merckelbach H, Schmidt H, Mayer B. The revised version of the screen for child anxiety related emotional disorders (SCARED-R): factor structure in normal children. *Personality and Individual Differences* 1999;**26**:99–112.
4. Hagborg WJ. The Revised Children's Manifest Anxiety Scale and social desirability. *Educational and Psychological Measurement* 1991;**51**:423–427.
5. Keller MB, Lavori PW, Wunder J, Beardslee WR, Schwartz CE, Roth J. Chronic course of anxiety disorders in children and adolescents. *Journal of American Academy of Child and Adolescent Psychiatry* 1992;**31**:595–599.
6. March JS, Parker S, Sullivan JD, Stallings KP, Conners CK. The Multidimensional Anxiety Scale for Children (MASC): factor structure, reliability, and validity. *Journal of the American Academy of Child Adolescent Psychiatry* 1997;**36**:554–565.
7. Poznanski EO, Freeman LN, Mokros HB. Children's depression rating scale-revised. *Psychopharmacology Bulletin* 1985;**21**:979–989.
8. Spence SH. A measure of anxiety symptoms among children. *Behavioural Research and Therapy* 1998;**36**:545–566.
9. Brooke SL. Depression and anxiety in youth scale. *Measurement and Evaluation in Counseling and Development* 1995;**28**:162–167.
10. Newcomer PL, Barenbaum EM, Bryant BR. *Depression and Anxiety in Youth Scale*. Austin, TX: PRO-ED, 1994.
11. Kovacs M. *Children's Depression Inventory 2^{TM} (CDI 2): Brief Assessment of Depressive Symptoms in Youth*. London: Pearson Assessment, 2010.
12. Reynolds CR, Kamphaus RW. *Behavior Assessment System for Children: Manual*. Circle Pines, MN: American Guidance Services, 1992.
13. Reynolds CR, Kamphaus RW. *BASC-2: Behavior Assessment System for Children, Second Edition Manual*. Circle Pines, MN: American Guidance Services, 2004.
14. Nelson WM, Finch AJ. Jr. The Children's Inventory of Anger (CIA). Unpublished manuscript, Medical University of South Carolina, Charleston, SC, 1978.
15. Nelson WM, Hart KJ, Finch AJ. Anger in children: a cognitive behavioral view of the assessment-therapy connection. *Journal of Rational-Emotive and Cognitive-Behavior Therapy* 1993;**11**:135–150.
16. Nelson WM, Finch AJ. *Children's Inventory of Anger*. Los Angeles: Western Psychological Service, 2000.
17. Shoemaker OW, Erickson MT, Finch AJ. Jr. Depression and anger in third- and fourth-grade boys: a multimethod assessment approach. *Journal of Clinical Child Psychology* 1986;**15**:290–296.
18. Cook WW, Medley DM. Proposed hostility and pharisaic virtue scales for the MMPI. *Journal of Applied Psychology* 1954;**38**:414–418.
19. Woodall KL, Matthews KA. Changes in and stability of hostile characteristics: results from a 4-year longitudinal study of children. *Journal of Personality and Social Psychology* 1993;**64**:491–499.
20. Liehr P, Meininger JC, Mueller WH, *et al*.Psychometric testing of the adolescent version of the Cook-Medley hostility scale. *Issues in Comprehensive Pediatric Nursing* 2000;**23**:103–116.
21. Kazdin AE, Rodgers A, Colbus D, Siegel T. Children's hostility inventory: measurement of aggression and hostility in psychiatric inpatient children. *Journal of Clinical Child Psychology* 1987;**16**:320–328.
22. Buss AH, Durkee A. An inventory for assessing different kinds of hostility. *Journal of Consulting Psychology* 1957;**21**:343–349.
23. Eyberg SM, Robinson EA. Conduct problem behavior: standardization of a behavioral rating scale with adolescents. *Journal of Clinical Child Psychology* 1983;**12**:347–354.
24. Eyberg S, Pincus D. *Eyberg Child Behavior Inventory & Sutter-Eyberg Student Behavior Inventory: Revised*. Odessa, FL: Psychological Assessment Resources, 1999.
25. Eyberg SM, Ross AW. Assessment of child behavior problems: the validation of a new inventory. *Journal of Clinical Child Psychology* 1978;**8**:113–116.
26. Phipps S, Steele R. Repressive adaptive style in children with chronic illness. *Psychosomatic Medicine* 2002;**64**:34–42.
27. Buss AH, Warren WL. *Aggression Questionnaire: Manual*. Los Angeles: Western Psychological Services, 2000.
28. Archer J, Kilpatrick G, Bramwell R. Comparison of two aggression inventories. *Aggressive Behavior* 1995;**21**:371–380.
29. Buss AH, Perry M. The Aggression Questionnaire. *Journal of Personality and Social Psychology* 1992;**63**:254–459.
30. Spielberger CD. *State-Trait Anger Expression Inventory*. Odessa, FL: Psychological Assessment Resources, 1988.
31. Spielberger CD. *Manual for the State-Trait Anger Expression Inventory*. Odessa, FL: Psychological Assessment Resources, 1988.
32. Phipps S, Hinds PS, Channell S, Bell GL. Measurement of behavioral, affective, and somatic responses to pediatric bone marrow transplantation: development of the BASES scale. *Journal of Pediatric Oncology Nursing*, 1994;**11**:109–117.
33. Phipps S, Dunavant M, Jayawardene D, Srivastiva DK. Assessment of health-related quality of life in acute inpatient settings: use of the BASES instrument in children undergoing bone marrow transplantation. *International Journal of Cancer Supplement* 1999;**12**:8–24.
34. Varni JW, Limbers CA, Bryant WP, Wilson DP. The PedsQL^{TM} Multidimensional Fatigue Scale in pediatric obesity: feasibility, reliability, and validity. *International Journal of Pediatric Obesity* 2010;**5**:34–42.
35. Eiser C, Kopel S, Cool P, Grimer R. The Perceived Illness Experience Scale (PIE): reliability and validity revisited. *Child: Care, Health & Development* 1999;**25**:179–190.
36. Kreitler S, Kreitler H. The psychological profile of the health-oriented individual. *European Journal of Personality* 1991;**5**:35–60.

37. Kreitler S, Kreitler H. Cognitive orientation and physical disease or health. *European Journal of Personality* 1991;**5**:109–129.
38. Landgraf JM, Abetz L, Ware JE. *The CHQ User's Manual*, 1st edn. Boston, MA: The Health Institute, New England Medical Center, 1996.
39. Varni JW, Burwinkle TM, Katz ER, Meeske K, Dickinson, P. The PedsQOL™ in pediatric cancer: reliability and validity of the Pediatric Quality of Life Inventory™ Generic Core Scales, Multidimensional Fatigue Scale, and Cancer Module. *Cancer* 2002;**94**:2090–2106.
40. Varni JW, Burwinkle TM, Szer IS. The PedsQL™ Multidimensional Fatigue Scale in pediatric rheumatology: reliability and validity. *Journal of Rheumatology* 2004;**31**:2494–2500.
41. Hockenberry MJ, Hinds PS, Barrera P, *et al.* Three instruments to assess fatigue in children with cancer: the child, parent and staff perspectives. *Journal of Pain & Symptom Management.* 2003;**25**:319–328.
42. Bastiaansen D, Koot HM, Bongers LL, *et al.* Measuring quality of life in children referred for psychiatric problems: psychometric properties of the PedsQL 4.0 generic core scales. *Quality of Life Research* 2004;**13**:489–495.
43. Palmer SN, Meeske KA, Katz ER, *et al.* The PedsQOL™ brain tumor module: initial reliability and validity. *Pediatric Blood & Cancer* 2007;**49**:287–293.
44. Ward-Smith P, Hamlin J, Bartholomew J, Stegenga K. Quality of life among adolescents with cancer. *Journal of Pediatric Oncology Nursing* 2007;**24**:166–171.
45. Ward-Smith P, McCaskie B, Rhoton S. Adolescent evaluated quality of life: a longitudinal study. *Journal of Pediatric Oncology Nursing* 2007;**24**:329–333.
46. Armstrong FD, Toledano SR, Miloslavich K, *et al.* The Miami Pediatric Quality of Life Questionnaire: Parent Scale. *International Journal of Cancer Supplement* 1999;**12**:11–17.
47. Watson M, Edwards L, von Essen L, *et al.* Development of the Royal Marsden Hospital Paediatric Oncology Quality of Life Questionnaire. *International Journal of Cancer Supplement* 1999;**12**:65–70.
48. Bhatia S, Jenney MEM, Wu E, *et al.* The Minneapolis-Manchester Quality of Life instrument: reliability and validity of the Youth Form. *Journal of Pediatrics* 2004;**145**:36–46.
49. Bhatia S, Jenney MEM, Bogue MK, *et al.* The Minneapolis-Manchester Quality of Life instrument: reliability and validity of the Adolescent Form. *Journal of Clinical Oncology* 2002;**20**:4692–4698.
50. Shankar S, Robison L, Jenney MEM, *et al.* Health-related quality of life in young survivors of childhood cancer using the Minneapolis-Manchester Quality of Life-Youth Form. *Pediatrics* 2005;**115**:435–442.
51. Goodwin DAJ, Boggs SR, Graham-Pole J. Development and validation of the Pediatric Oncology Quality of Life Scale. *Psychological Assessment* 1994;**6**:321–328.
52. Kreitler S, Kreitler MM.The children's quality of life questionnaire: its contents, structure, reliability and validity in different samples of children, in press.
53. Parsons SK, Shih MC, Mayer DK, *et al.* Preliminary psychometric evaluation of the Child Health Ratings Inventory (CHRIs) and Disease-Specific Impairment Inventory-Hematopoietic Stem Cell Transplantation (DSII-HSCT) in parents and children. *Quality of Life Research* 2005;**14**:1613–1625.
54. Parsons SK, Shih M, DuHamel KN, *et al.* Maternal perspectives on children's health-related quality of life during the first year after pediatric hematopoietic stem cell transplant. *Journal of Pediatric Psychology* 2006;**31**:1100–1115.
55. Herz L, Gullone E. The relationship between self-esteem and parenting style: a cross-cultural comparison of Australian and Vietnamese Australian adolescents. *Journal of Cross-Cultural Psychology* 1999;**30**:742–761.
56. Byrne BM. *Measuring Self-Concept across the Life-Span.* Washington, DC: American Counseling Association, 1996.
57. Jamaludin HJ, Ahmad HJ, Rosdi Y, Saifuddin KA. The reliability and validity of Tennessee Self Concept Scale (TSCS) Instrument on residents of drug rehabilitation center. *European Journal of Social Sciences* 2009;**10**:349–363.
58. Butler RJ, Green D. *The Self Image Profiles for Children (SIP-C) and Adolescents (SIP-A). Manual.* London: The Psychological Corporation, 2001.
59. Hawkins SR. The impact of school transition and family cohesion on African American adolescent girls living in resource-poor inner-city communities. Unpublished doctoral dissertation, Howard University, Washington, DC, 1998.
60. Sweitzer E. The relationship between social interest and self-concept in conduct disordered adolescents. Unpublished doctoral dissertation, West Virginia University, WV, 1998.
61. Anstey B. Test review. Evaluation of the Multidimensional Self Concept Scale (MSCS). *Canadian Journal of School Psychology* 1999;**14**:59–65.
62. Kreitler S, Kreitler H. Psychosomatic aspects of the self. In: Honess TM, Yardley KM (eds.) *Self and Identity: Individual Change and Development.* London: Routledge and Kegan Paul, 1987; pp. 338–358.
63. Rosenberg M. *Society and the Adolescent Self-Image.* Princeton, NJ: Princeton University Press, 1965.
64. Robins RW, Hendin HM, Trzeniewski KH. Measuring global self esteem construct validation of a single- item measure and the Rosenberg Self- Esteem Scale. *Personality and Social Psychology Bulletin* 2001;**27**:151–161.
65. Harter S. *Manual for the Self-Perception Profile for Children.* Denver, CO: University of Denver, 1985.
66. Harter S. *Manual for the Self-Perception Profile for Adolescents.* Denver, CO: University of Denver, 1988.
67. Kreitler S, Kreitler H. Body image: the dimension of size. *Genetic, Social and General Psychology Monographs* 1988;**114**:5–32.
68. Kreitler S, Chemerinski H. Body image disturbance in obesity. *International Journal of Eating Disorders* 1990;**9**:409–418.
69. Offer D, Ostrov E, Howard KI. *Offer Self-Image Questionnaire for Adolescents, Revised (OSIQ-R) Manual.* Los Angeles: Western Psychological Services, 1992.
70. Kopel SJ, Eiser C, Cool P, Grimer GF. Brief report: assessment of body image in survivors of childhood cancer. *Society of Pediatric Psychology* 1998;**23**:141–147.
71. Snyder CR, Hoza B, Pelham WE. The development and validation of the Children's Hope Scale. *Journal of Pediatric Psychology* 1997;**22**:399–421.

72. Beck AT, Weissman A. The measurement of pessimism: the Hopelessness Scale. *Journal of Consulting Clinical Psychology* 1974;**47**:861–863.

73. Lacher D, Gruber CP. *Personality Inventory for Youth (PIY) Manual: Technical Guide*. Los Angeles: Western Psychological Services, 1995.

74. Ames LB, Learned J, Metraux, RW, Rodell, JL, Walker RN. *Child Rorschach Responses: Developmental Trends from Two to Ten Years*. Oxford: Brunner/Mazel, 1974.

75. Roberts GE. *Interpretive Handbook for the Roberts Apperception Test for Children*. Los Angeles: Western Psychological Services, 1994.

76. McCoy D. *The Ultimate Guide to Personality Tests*. Inglewood, CA, Champion Press, 2005.

77. Hockenberry-Eaton M, Manteuffel B, Bottomley S. Development of two instruments examining stress and adjustment in children with cancer. *Journal of Pediatric Oncology Nursing* 1997;**14**:178–185.

78. Hockenberry-Eaton M, Kemp V, Dilorio C. Cancer stressors and protective factors: predictors of stress experienced during treatment for childhood cancer. *Research in Nursing and Health* 1994;**17**:351–361.

79. Jay SM, Elliott CH. Behavioral observation scales for measuring children's distress: the effects of increased methodological rigor. *Journal of Consulting and Clinical Psychology* 1984;**52**:1106–1107.

80. Elliott CH, Jay SM, Woody P. An observation scale for measuring children's distress during medical procedures. *Journal of Pediatric Psychology* 1987;**12**:543–555.

81. Slifer KJ, Babbitt RL, Cataldo MD. Simulation and counterconditioning as adjuncts to pharmacotherapy for invasive pediatric procedures. *Developmental and Behavioral Pediatrics* 1995;**16**:133–141.

82. Cohen S, Kamarck T, Mermelstein R. A global measure of stress. *Journal of Health and Social Behavior* 1983;**24**:385–396.

83. Cohen S, Williamson G. Perceived stress in a probability sample of the United States. In: Spacapan S, Oskamp S (eds.) *The Social Psychology of Health*. Newbury Park, CA: Sage, 1988.

84. Saigh PA. The development and validation of the Children's Posttraumatic Stress Disorder Inventory. *International Journal of Special Education* 1989;**4**:75–84.

85. Saigh PA, Yasik AE, Oberfield RA, Green BL, Halamandaris PV, Rubenstein H, *et al.* The Children's PTSD Inventory: development and reliability. *Journal of Traumatic Stress* 2000;**13**:369–380.

86. Bull BA, Drotar D. Coping with cancer in remission: stressors and strategies reported by children and adolescents. *Journal of Pediatric Psychology* 1991;**16**:767–782.

87. Wertlieb D, Weigel C, Feldstein M. Measuring children's coping. *American Journal of Orthopsychiatry* 1987;**57**:548–560.

88. Endler NS, Parker JDA. Multidimensional assessment of coping: a critical evaluation. *Journal of Personality and Social Psychology* 1990;**58**:844–854.

89. McWilliams LA, Cox BJ, Enns MW. Use of the Coping Inventory for Stressful Situations in a clinically depressed sample: factor structure, personality correlates, and prediction of distress. *Journal of Clinical Psychology* 2003;**59**:423–437.

90. Kreitler S, Kreitler H. *The Cognitive Foundations of Personality Traits*. New York: Plenum, 1990.

91. Caruso J. Reliable component analysis of the Stanford-Binet Fourth Edition for 2–6-year olds. *Psychological Assessment* 2001;**13**:827–840.

92. Wechsler D. *The Wechsler Intelligence Scale for Children*, 3rd edition. San Antonio, TX: The Psychological Corporation, 1991.

93. Wechsler D. *The Wechsler Intelligence Scale for Children*, 4th edition. London: Pearson Assessment, 2004.

94. Flanagan DP, Koffman ES. *Essential of WISC IV Assessment*. Chichester: Wiley, 2004.

95. Kreitler H, Kreitler S. Types of curiosity behaviors and their cognitive determinants. *Archives of Psychology*, 1986;**138**:233–251.

96. Gathercole SE, Pickering SJ. Assessment of working memory in six- and seven-year-old children. *Journal of Educational Psychology* 2000;**92**:377–390.

97. Weintraub S, Mesulam MM. Mental state assessment of young and elderly adults in behavioral neurology. In: Mesulam MM (ed.), *Principles of Behavioral Neurology*. Philadelphia: Davis Company, 1985; pp. 71–123.

98. Taylor MA. *The Fundamentals of Clinical Neuropsychiatry*. New York: Oxford University Press, 1999; pp. 357–358.

99. Meyers JE, Meyers KR. *Rey Complex Figure Test and Recognition Trial: Professional Manual*. PAR, Inc.

100. Robinson EA, Eyberg SM, Ross WA. The standardization of an inventory of child conduct problem behaviors. *Journal of Clinical Child Psychology*, 1980; 22–29.

101. Brady RP. *Youth Risk and Resilience Inventory*. St. Paul, MN: JIST Publishing, 2006.

102. Kreitler S. Coping and quality of life in the context of physical diseases. In: Lee AV (ed.), *Coping with Disease*. New York: Nova Biomedical Books, 2005; pp. 81–120.

103. Petersen P, Schmidt S, Bullinger M. Brief report: development and pilot testing of coping questionnaire for children and adolescents with chronic health conditions. *Journal of Pediatric Psychology* 2004;**29**:635–640.

104. Lai JS, Cella D, Tomita T, Bode RK, Newmark M, Goldman S. Developing a health-related quality of life instrument for childhood brain tumor survivors. *Child's Nervous System* 2007;**23**:47–57.

105. Prince-Embury S. The resiliency scales for children and adolescents, psychological symptoms, and clinical status in adolescents. *Canadian Journal of School Psychology* 2008;**23**:41–56.

106. Prince-Embury S. *Resiliency Scale for Adolescents: A Profile of Personal Strengths*. San Antonio, TX: Pearson Education, 2005.

107. Beyer J, Denyes M, Villarruel A. The creation, validation and continuing development of the Oucher: a measure of pain intensity in children. *Journal of Pediatric Nursing* 1992;**7**:335–346.

108. Yeh C. Development and validation of the Asian version of the Oucher: a pain intensity scale for children. *The Journal of Pain* 2005;**6**:526–534.

109. Bieri D, Reeve RA, Champion GD, Addicoat L, Ziegler JB. The Faces Pain Scale for the self-assessment of the severity of pain experienced by children: development, initial validation, and preliminary investigation for ratio scale properties. *Pain* 1990;**41**:139–150.

110. Hicks CL, von Baeyer CL, Spafford P, van Korlaar I, Goodenough B. The Faces Pain Scale: Revised: toward

a common metric in pediatric pain measurement. *Pain* 2001;**93**:173–183.

111. Lawrence J, Alcock D, McGrath P, Kay J, MacMurray SB, Dulberg C. The development of a tool to assess neonatal pain. *Neonatal Network* 1993;**12**:59–66.

112. Merkel SI, Voepel-Lewis T, Shayevitz JR, Malviya S. The FLACC: a behavioral scale for scoring postoperative pain in young children. *Pediatric Nursing* 1997;**23**:293–297.

113. Manworren RC, Hynan LS. Clinical validation of FLACC: preverbal patient pain scale. *Pediatric Nursing* 2003;**29**:140–146.

114. Malviya S, Voepel-Lewis T, Burke C, Merkel S, Tait AR. The revised FLACC observational pain tool: improved reliability and validity for pain assessment in children with cognitive impairment. *Pediatric Anesthesia* 2006;**16**:258–265.

115. Hall JE, Uhrich TD, Barney JA, Arain SR, Ebert TJ. Sedative, amnestic, and analgesic properties of small dose dexmedetomidine infusions. *Anesthesia and Analgesia* 2000;**90**:699–705.

116. Wong D, Baker C. Pain in children: comparison of assessment scales. *Pediatric Nursing* 1988;**14**:9–17.

117. Todd KH, Funk KG, Funk JP, Bonacci PA. Clinical significance of reported changes in pain severity. *Annals of Emergency Medicine* 1996;**27**:485–489.

118. Savedra MC, Tesler MD, Holzemer WL, Ward LA. *Adolescent Pediatric Pain Tool (APPT): Preliminary User's Manual*. San Francisco, CA: University of California, 1989.

Appendix B

Additional Resources

There is an extensive bibliography of articles for professionals listed on the PACT website (see below). Listed here is an introduction to the many resources that are publicly available for families, although the PACT program does not endorse particular books or websites, beyond our own. This list may be a helpful starting point, and we urge families to spend time looking at their hospital's cancer resource room, their local library or their local children's bookstore to find books that will be the best fit for their particular situation and their family.

Books

For Parents

Raising an Emotionally Healthy Child When a Parent Is Sick
P Rauch and AC Muriel. McGraw-Hill; 2006.

When a Parent Has Cancer: A Guide to Caring for Your Children
W Harpham. HarperCollins, 2004.

How to Help Children Through a Parent's Serious Illness
K McCue. St. Martin's Griffin, 1994.

For Children

Butterfly Kisses and Wishes on Wings: When Someone You Love Has Cancer
E McVicker, Self-Published, 2006 (ages 4–10).

Our Mom Has Cancer
A Ackerman and A Ackerman. American Cancer Society, 2001 (ages 7–12).

Promises
E Winthrop. Clarion Books, 2000 (ages 5–8).

Sammy's Mommy Has Cancer
S Kohlenberg. Magination Press, 1993 (ages 3–7).

Websites for Professionals and Families

American Cancer Society (ACS) Provides detailed information on talking to children about a parent's cancer at several different stages, as well as numerous other cancer-related topics. (www.cancer.org).

American Psychosocial Oncology Society (APOS) Provides a free Helpline to connect patients and families with local counseling services, as well as webcasts for professionals on topics such as "LIVESTRONG: A Podcast Series for Young Adults with Cancer" (co-sponsored by the Lance Armstrong Foundation) and "Women Stories Video Series" for breast cancer patients. (www.apos-society.org).

Breast Cancer.org This organization offers medical information about current treatments and research in breast cancer care and survivorship. (www.breast-cancer.org).

CancerCare The mission of this national nonprofit organization is to provide free professional help to people with all cancers through counseling, education, information, and referral and direct financial assistance. They offer online, telephone, and face-to-face support groups to those affected by cancer. (www.cancercare.org).

Cancer.net, from the American Society for Clinical Oncology (ASCO) Offers educational information for patients and families. (www.cancer.net).

Lance Armstrong Foundation (LAF) LAF offers information and services to cancer survivors and the professionals who care for them. (www.livestrong.org).

Pediatric Psycho-oncology: Psychosocial Aspects and Clinical Interventions, Second Edition.
Edited by Shulamith Kreitler, Myriam Weyl Ben-Arush and Andrés Martin.
© 2012 John Wiley & Sons, Ltd. Published 2012 by John Wiley & Sons, Ltd.

Living Beyond Breast Cancer A national education and support organization with the goal of improving quality of life and helping patients take an active role in ongoing recovery or management of the disease. (www.lbbc.org).

National Cancer Institute (NCI) Provides extensive information about cancer, both general and specific and also resources, such as a dictionary of cancer terms and a section on coping with cancer that includes a guide for teens who have a parent with cancer and a section on grief in children. (www.cancer.gov).

Parenting At a Challenging Time (PACT) Program Provides information for parents and professionals, including in-depth discussions of child development, parenting principles, frequently asked questions, practical tips, and referral to additional resources. (www.mghpact.org).

The Truth About Cancer (PBS) Website for the PBS series from 2008 offers links to multiple resources, including an annotated bibliography of cancer-related fiction and non-fiction for children, teens and adults. (http://www.pbs.org/wgbh/takeonestep/cancer/resources-bibliography.html).

The Wellness Community A national, nonprofit organization that provides free online and in-person support and information to people living with cancer and their families. (www.thewellnesscommunity.org).

Young Survival Coalition Through action, advocacy, and awareness, this nonprofit organization seeks to educate the medical, research, breast cancer, and legislative communities and to persuade them to address breast cancer in women 40 and under–and serves as a point of contact for young women living with breast cancer. (www.youngsurvival.org).

Index

Pediatric Psycho-oncology: Psychosocial Aspects and Clinical Interventions, Second Edition.
Edited by Shulamith Kreitler, Myriam Weyl Ben-Arush and Andrés Martin.
© 2012 John Wiley & Sons, Ltd. Published 2012 by John Wiley & Sons, Ltd.